W9-AED-817

PSYCHOTROPIC DRUGS

How to Use This Book

This book is really two books in one. It can be used as a quick clinical reference for specific drugs or for more in-depth information about psychotropic drugs and drug classes.

Part One consists of 17 narrative chapters that provide an overview and basic discussion of the biologic bases of psychopharmacology as well as the uses of psychotropic drugs for specific psychiatric disorders across the lifespan.

Part Two contains a series of brief profiles for more than 100 of the most common psychotropic drugs, listed by generic name in alphabetic order, for quick access in clinical situations. Clinical information and nursing considerations are provided in a consistent format for each drug. Each drug profile provides a reference to the appropriate chapter(s) in Part One should you need further information about the drug.

Three separate indexes are located at the end of the book to speed your access to information. These three indexes are marked with thumb tabs for rapid access and include the:

1. General Index—to help find topics and terms throughout the book.
2. Disorders Index—to locate information about psychotropic drugs used for specific disorders or side effects.
3. Drug Index—to locate entries for all generic and trade names of drugs in the book in alphabetic order, as well as entries for the major psychotropic drug classes.

PSYCHOTROPIC DRUGS

Norman L. Keltner, RN, CRNP, EdD
Associate Professor
School of Nursing
University of Alabama at Birmingham
Birmingham, Alabama

David G. Folks, MD
Professor and Chair
Creighton University Medical Center School of Medicine
University of Nebraska Medical Center College of Medicine
Department of Psychiatry
Omaha, Nebraska

Second Edition
with 40 illustrations

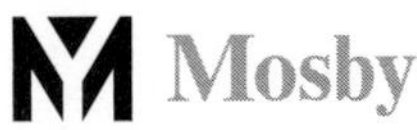

St. Louis Baltimore Boston
Carlsbad Chicago Naples New York Philadelphia Portland
London Madrid Mexico City Singapore Sydney Tokyo Toronto Wiesbaden

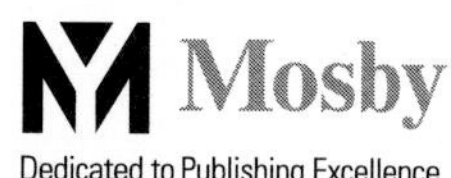

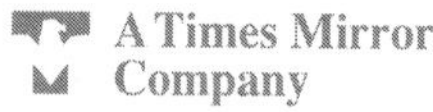

Vice President and Publisher: Nancy L. Coon
Editor: Jeff Burnham
Developmental Editor: Linda Caldwell
Project Manager: Mark Spann
Production Editor: Anne Salmo
Designer: Judi Lang
Manufacturing Manager: Betty Richmond
Cover Design: Centaur Studios

A NOTE TO THE READER:

The author and publisher have made every attempt to check dosages and pharmacologic and nursing content for accuracy. Because the science of pharmacology is continually advancing, our knowledge base continues to expand. Therefore we recommend that the reader always check product information for changes in dosage or administration before administering any medication. This is particularly important with new or rarely used drugs.

SECOND EDITION

Printed in the United States of America
Composition by Clarinda Company
Printing/binding by Western Publishing

Mosby-Year Book, Inc.
11830 Westline Industrial Drive
St. Louis, Missouri 63146

Library of Congress Cataloging in Publication Data

Keltner, Norman L.
Psychotropic drugs / Norman L. Keltner. David G. Folks — 2nd ed.
p. cm.
Includes bibliographical references and indexes.
ISBN 0-8151-4968-9
1. Mental illness—Chemotherapy. 2. Psychotropic drugs.
3. Psychopharmacology. I. Folks, David G. II. Title.
[DNLM: 1. Psychotropic Drugs—pharmacology.
2. Psychopharmacology. 3. Mental Disorders—drug therapy. QV 77.2
K29p 1996]
RC483.K45 1996
616.89′18—dc20
DNLM/DLC
for Library of Congress

96-1047
CIP

97 98 99 00 01 / 9 8 7 6 5 4 3 2 1

Contributors

LELAND N. ALLEN III, MD
Carraway Methodist Medical Center
Birmingham, Alabama

F. CLEVELAND KINNEY, PhD, MD
Associate Professor of Psychiatry and Behavioral Neurobiology
School of Medicine
University of Alabama at Birmingham
Birmingham, Alabama

LAWRENCE SCAHILL, MSN, MPH
Associate Research Scientist
Assistant Clinical Professor of Nursing
Child Study Center
Yale University
New Haven, Connecticut

RICHARD A. SUGERMAN, PhD
Professor of Anatomy
College of Osteopathic Medicine of the Pacific
Pomona, California

Reviewers

ANDREA C. BOSTROM, PhD, RN
Associate Professor
Kirkhof School of Nursing
Grand Valley State University
Allendale, Michigan

BARBARA J. LIMANDRI, RN, CS, DNSc
Advanced Practice Psychiatric-Mental Health Nurse
Associate Professor
School of Nursing
Oregon Health Sciences University
Portland, Oregon

Preface

We wrote the first edition of *Psychotropic Drugs* in response to what we believed was a growing need for accurate, concise, and up-to-date psychopharmacologic information for clinicians and students of the health professions. Responses to our efforts have been favorable on all sides. The fact that we have written a second edition indicates sufficient sales of the book by our publisher. More importantly, personal contacts have underscored our hopes that the book would meet people's needs. Without fail, individuals we have met at conferences and in hospitals and letters we have received have reinforced our initial thinking.

The second edition has retained the format of the first, but the contents have been updated. For instance, at the first writing SSRIs were still relatively new on the market. Today SSRIs are first-line drugs used to treat depression, anxiety, and obsessive-compulsive disorder, and the second edition reflects this broader usage. Likewise, antipsychotic drug treatment is evolving with the advent of serotonin/dopamine antagonists such as risperidone. Still, for all classes of psychotropic drugs, the traditional agents are given full treatment and continue to serve as a springboard for understanding the new. In other words, we attempt to present new information while anchoring it within the context of classic discussions developed over the years.

The book is divided into two parts, each uniquely contributing to an overall comprehensive discussion of chemical interventions in psychiatric care.

Part One, "Clinical Psychopharmacology," provides a narrative presentation in 17 chapters that will enable both the recent graduate and the experienced clinician to better integrate the wide-ranging nature of psychopharmacology into practice. Part One is further divided into four units, each organized around a significant conceptual theme.

Unit I introduces the reader to psychotropic drugs and provides a brief historical perspective of these agents. In addition, chapters that review neuroanatomy and neurotransmitter mechanisms are so presented as to immerse those a bit "rusty" and challenge those who are more conversant with brain biology.

Unit II, "Drugs Used in the Treatment of Mental Disorders," focuses on the major categories of drugs used in psychiatric care. Each chapter begins with an introductory review establishing the need for the drug, followed by a discussion of pharmacokinetics, administration and dosage, side effects, and clinical implications. Clinical implications include therapeutic versus toxic serum levels, use in pregnancy, interventions for side effects, drug interactions, and patient education considerations.

Unit III, "Drug Issues Related to Psychopharmacology," reviews electroconvulsive therapy, drugs of abuse, central nervous system stimulants, and drugs used to treat extrapyramidal side effects of psychotropic drugs.

Unit IV, "Developmental Issues Related to Psychotropic Drugs," includes chapters on the psychopharmacologic treatment of children, adolescents, and elderly persons.

Part Two, "Psychotropic Drug Profiles," features quick, handy profiles for more than 100 psychotropic drugs. Each drug is profiled according to several selected categories such as classification, indications, contraindications, pharmacokinetics, and interactions. The combination of this feature with the extensive narrative explanation in Part One is unique among books on this topic.

This book can be used both as a textbook and as a reference tool. The reader can use the drug profiles when information is required quickly and then, by noting the referent chapter listed at the beginning of each profile, can follow up with more concentrated study as time permits. The book is designed to meet the needs of both the on-duty clinician and the student of psychopharmacology.

Acknowledgments

The second edition of *Psychotropic Drugs* could not have materialized without the help and dedicated efforts of our contributors. Again, Drs. Richard Sugerman and F. Cleveland Kinney have added their expert understanding of neuroanatomy and neurophysiology to the beginning chapters of this book. Dr. Leland Allen, with his clinical base in internal and emergency medicine, provides invaluable insights into the chapter on drugs of abuse. Finally, Larry Scahill, with his strong research and clinical background in child and adolescent psychiatry, completely reworked those chapters to yield a concise yet complete accounting of child and adolescent psychopharmacologic issues. We remain appreciative of the talents of our contributors and thank them for sharing their knowledge through our book.

NLK and DGF

Although many people help an author capture in words his or her understanding of the world, I will just say a collective thank you and move on to a note of dedication. This book is dedicated to the memory of my best friend, Cledy (Tim) Wallace. Tim died in 1995 at age 49. Tim and I had been boyhood friends and although I left "home" 15 years ago, not a week went by that we did not talk on the phone. Additionally, our families spent a week together each summer at a family conference in California. Tim and I thought alike and had the same oddball sense of humor. We shared a long history, dating back to our growing up days in Manteca, California. He was my strongest encourager and took great pride in my accomplishments. More than anything else, relationships make life meaningful. Tim Wallace will be forever missed.

NLK

Contents

CLINICAL PSYCHO-PHARMACOLOGY

PART ONE

UNIT I

Introduction to Psychotropic Drug Use

CHAPTER 1

Psychiatric Care and Contemporary Treatment

"A large gathering of madmen inspires an undefinable thoughtful tenderness when one realizes that their present state derives only from a vivid sensitivity and from psychologic qualities that we value highly."

Philippe Pinel, Dec. 11, 1794 (quoted in Weiner, 1992)

The modern era of psychiatric care, including the discovery and use of psychotropic drugs, can be traced from events occurring near the end of the eighteenth century. The work of several individuals, including Philippe Pinel (1745-1826) in France, William Tuke (1732-1822) in England, and Dorothea Dix (1802-1887) in the United States, is particularly noteworthy because their efforts laid the foundation for compassionate and scientific treatment of people with mental illness. This era of treatment is referred to as the period of enlightenment and is considered the first of four significant benchmarks in the historical development of psychiatric care. Before this time people with mental illness were frequently abused or neglected, or both.

Rosenblatt (1984) writes of the assistance, banishment, and confinement (the ABCs) of the pre-enlightenment era. Assistance included efforts to help families cope with the problems of living with a mentally disordered family member. Banishment, or driving individuals with mental illness away from the "healthy," was a more common approach to mental illness and led to wandering bands of "lunatics," who frightened the public and stole or begged from them for survival. Just as often, however, these wandering bands were victimized by "sane" society. Confinement was the most calculated approach of the pre-enlightenment era. People with mental illness were often chained indiscriminately, the old to the young, men to women, the insane to the criminal or pauper, and by some accounts the living to the dead. Confinement and the natural progression of this practice led to distorted and uninformed views of mental illness; for example, people with mental illness were thought to be immune from normal biologic stressors such as cold, heat, and hunger (Foucault, 1973). Whether such thinking was representative of the times or merely a rationalization for withholding resources is not documented. Nonetheless, people with mental illness suffered greatly. They were deprived of basic biologic needs, that is, shelter, clothing, and food, while their basic emotional needs were also being unmet. Confined mental patients, for example, were placed on display for the paying public and forced to oblige their keepers in many vile and inhumane ways. This widespread abuse and neglect of individuals with mental illness ultimately stimulated a reaction among those who were enlightened—Pinel, Tuke, and Dix—that led to the first of the four significant benchmarks in psychiatric care.

BENCHMARKS IN PSYCHIATRIC CARE: THE ROAD FROM CONFINEMENT TO COMMUNITY

Benchmarks in psychiatric care are significant time periods during which converging forces led to a unique view of mental illness (Figure 1-1). The four benchmarks are the period of enlightenment, the period of scientific study, the period of psychotropic drugs, and the period of community mental health care. Each period represents a definite change in public perception of mental health or psychiatric problems; these changes in perception have led to new strategies and interventions to treat mental illness. A thorough investigation of these benchmarks is beyond the scope of this book. However, a brief description of the relationship between important events and the advent and use of psychotropic drugs is provided.

Period of Enlightenment (Caring)

"One cannot ignore a striking analogy in nature's ways when one compares the attacks of intermittent insanity with the violent symptoms of an acute illness. It would in either case be a mistake to measure the gravity of the danger by the extent of trouble and derangement of the vital functions. In both cases a serious condition may forecast recovery, provided one practices prudent management."

Philippe Pinel, Dec. 11, 1794 (quoted in Weiner).

The period of enlightenment is so named because reformers Pinel, Tuke, Dix, and others rejected the common reasoning of the day and substituted a humane approach to the care of people with mental illness. Affected individuals were no longer considered animal-like but instead were to be treated as fellow humans deserving of adequate shelter, clothing, and food, which would be provided in a dignified manner. Pinel became superintendent of the French institutions Bicêtre for men and later, Salpêtriére for women. Dismayed by the living conditions at these institutions, he unchained the shackled, clothed the naked, fed the hungry, and disposed of whips and other instruments of cruel treatment. Pinel showed great understanding of his charges. His address to the Society for Natural History in Paris on December 11, 1794, readily demonstrates his vast insights into mental illness (Weiner, 1992). Tuke, on the other hand, developed a private institution to care for the psychiatric needs of his English Quaker brethren. He established the York Retreat in 1796, a facility in which moral treatment was instituted and maintained to help mentally ill people. Dix, an American reformer, visited the York Retreat and, on returning to the United States, launched an effective campaign to change the treatment of people with mental illness. She played a direct role in the opening of 32 public mental hospitals.

The period of enlightenment was significant because the first evolutionary step toward a humane and scientific way of thinking was accepted, paving the way for the

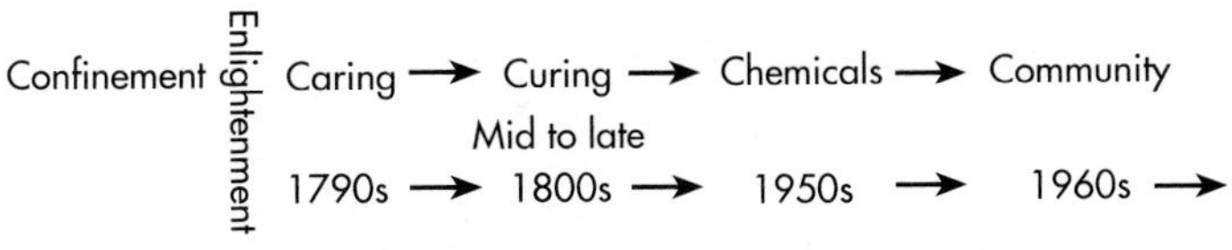

Figure 1-1 Evolution of psychiatric care (The 5 Cs).

discovery of contemporary treatments, including psychotropic drugs. People with mental illness were now included in the human family, no longer to be chained and beaten but to be accorded dignity and access to humane treatment. This period also set the stage for the period of scientific study.

Period of Scientific Study (Curing)

The second benchmark in the evolution of psychiatric care was the period of scientific study. The period of enlightenment represented a change in the way people perceived mentally ill individuals. During the period of scientific study, clinicians such as Kraepelin (1856-1926), Freud (1856-1939), and Bleuler (1857-1939) made significant contributions to the body of knowledge about mental illness. These individuals not only were concerned with providing a humane atmosphere but also wanted to study mental illnesses and develop treatment strategies. The thrust of this period therefore was moving beyond caring to curing. Kraepelin, a gifted and thorough neurologist, carefully studied the course of serious mental illness. *Kraepelin, it could be said, laid the groundwork for those who study mental illness from a biologic perspective.* Freud, through years of observation and treatment, developed an approach to working with patients—the psychoanalytic approach—that is still used and, more importantly, is the foundation for many other psychodynamic and psychotherapeutic approaches. Bleuler and others provided unique contributions to our understanding of mental illness, including description of symptoms, course, etiology, prognosis, and treatment. *Freud, Bleuler, and others laid the groundwork for those who study mental illness from a psychologic perspective.*

The significance of the period of scientific study was the concerted effort to identify causes and cures for emotional disturbances. The predominant approach that evolved from the work of Freud and his followers was a therapy based on dialogue with patients, such as psychoanalysis, individual therapy, and group therapy, that is still being used, studied, and refined today. The predominant approach that evolved from the work of Kraepelin and other neurologists was somatic, including the development of drug therapy, electroconvulsive therapy, and other nonpsychodynamic interventions.

Period of Psychotropic Drugs (Chemicals)

The milieu of theory development and scientific advances superimposed on a humane regard for people with mental illness further led to the discovery of psychotropic drugs (Box 1-1). In 1949 John Cade, an Australian physician, discovered lithium was effective in treating bipolar illness. In the early 1950s chlorpromazine (Thorazine) was developed and found effective in treating patients with schizophrenia and other psychoses. In the late 1950s Ayd (1957; 1991) and Kuhn (1958) published the first articles on antidepressant therapy. Hence within one decade three major classes of psychotropic drugs—antimanic, antipsychotic, and antidepressant—were discovered. These compounds significantly advanced the treatment of people with bipolar illness, psychosis, and depression, respectively.

The significance of this period of psychotropic drugs was noted particularly as patients began to take these drugs consistently; the demand for observation, food and shelter, and ongoing treatment by a professional staff decreased. For example, in 1955, shortly after the introduction of chlorpromazine, state hospitals reached a peak census of 558,922 patients, but by 1992 that population had dropped to 103,000 (Lamb, 1992), representing a drop of 80% (Appleby et al, 1993). Many mental health professionals believe the single most significant factor affecting this

Box 1-1 Significant Points in the Evolution of Psychotropic Drugs

1930s Benzodiazepines are first synthesized by Sternbach.
1948 Rapport, Green, and Page isolate "serotonin" from beef serum.
1949 John Cade, an Australian psychiatrist, reports on the efficacy of lithium in mania.
1949 The U.S. Food and Drug Administration bans lithium because of deaths in patients with cardiac disease.
1951 Chlorpromazine is developed as a nonsedating antihistamine. Laborit and others report diminished surgical anxiety in conscious patients.
1952 Delay and Deniker, two psychiatrists working with Laborit, administer chlorpromazine to a manic patient with successful results.
1952 Iproniazid, a derivative of the anti-tuberculosis agent isoniazid, is identified as a monoamine oxidase inhibitor (MAOI).
1953 Bein isolates reserpine from rauwolfia. Reserpine, effective in treating psychosis, causes severe depression related to depletion of norepinephrine.
1954 Lehman publishes the first American article on chlorpromazine in the *Archives of Neurology and Psychiatry.*
1955 Researchers alter the molecular structure of chlorpromazine, developing new antipsychotic agents, e.g. haloperidol and fluphenazine.
1957 The first papers appear on MAOIs as antidepressants.
1957 Haloperidol (Haldol) is developed.
1958 Kuhn publishes the first article on tricyclic antidepressants in the *American Journal of Psychiatry.*
1960 Harris presents the first paper on the effectiveness of benzodiazepines in *The Journal of the American Medical Association.*
1970 The ban on lithium is lifted in the United States.
1980s A new class of antidepressants is developed, the selective serotonin reuptake inhibitors (SSRIs).
1980s The antiepileptic drugs carbamazepine and valproate are reported to have mood-stabilizing properties.
1990s Clozapine (Clozaril) and risperidone (Risperdal), the first truly new antipsychotic agents in 40 years, are released in the United States.
1990s Tacrine (Cognex), a drug used to treat patients with Alzheimer's disease, is made available. Studies indicate that about 20% to 30% of cases improve.

From Ayd FJ: The early history of modern psychopharmacology, *Neuropsychopharmacology* 5(2):71, 1991; Kuhn R: The treatment of depressive states with G 22355 (impramine hydrochloride), *Am J Psychiatry,* 115(5):459, 1958; Rifkin A: Extrapyramidal side effects: a historical perspective, *J Clin Psychiatry,* 48(9):3, 1987.

decrease was the introduction of psychotropic drugs. The concept of least restrictive alternative treatment milieu was a by-product of this period, and the fourth benchmark—the period of community mental health care—evolved.

Period of Community Mental Health Care (Community)

If the first three periods represent the *evolution* of psychiatric care, the period of community mental health care represents a *revolution*. A multitude of converging factors resulted in public demand for reforms in the mental health care system: films and books depicted an isolated, leaderless, and often cruel state hospital system that was perhaps contributing to the cause and perpetuation of mental illness; the promise of "talking" patients back to health was losing appeal as the public began to demand and expect faster results; and new emphasis on patient rights began to significantly affect the infrastructure of the public hospital, which previously had been immune to outside interference and criticism. However, the most influential factor contributing to the closing of many state hospital beds was the development of psychotropic drugs. As previously mentioned, patients were helped tremendously by these drugs insofar as patients were more amenable to psychodynamic treatment and other less restrictive formats. Behaviors that necessitated inpatient care and locked units, that is, agitation, withdrawal, delusions, hallucinations, suicidal ideations, and the like, were significantly relieved by the introduction or institution of psychotropic drugs. These agents enabled patients to respond more appropriately; to cooperate; and to comply with physicians, nurses, psychologists, and social workers. Because dialogue with professionals occurred only a few times per week and the aforementioned "problem" behaviors were better controlled, the economically attractive alternative of outpatient care was now possible.

Although the concept of community mental health care provides a five-pronged approach to treatment modalities and levels of care, the outpatient dimension has been the most widely used. The development and success of psychotropic drugs were largely responsible for the advent of this fourth benchmark in psychiatric care. Today many affected individuals, who only 40 years earlier would have been committed to a state hospital for treatment, are able to lead productive lives in or near their own homes because of the efficacy of psychotropic drugs and community-based care.

The significance of the period of community mental health care has not yet been fully revealed. Neither the promise of psychotropic drugs nor the dream of community mental health care has been realized. The consequences of depopulating state hospitals, often referred to as *deinstitutionalization*, and the subsequent rise in mental illness among an ever-growing homeless population, the overuse of emergency psychiatric services, and the flight of professionals from the community mental health arena remind us that much work remains to accomplish the objectives of the community approach. Because the promise of psychopharmacology is not yet realized, researchers continue to develop new drugs. This ongoing research and development of drugs remain critical elements in the care of individuals with mental illness or psychiatric disturbances.

Remarks

The foregoing discussion is meant to serve as a historical foundation for the remainder of this book and to describe, albeit briefly, social and scientific factors associated with the development and use of psychotropic drugs today. The four benchmarks in psychiatric care have been chosen to illustrate the steady movement by the psychiatric community to develop humane (benchmark 1), scientific (benchmark 2) treatment (benchmark 3) in an optimal therapeutic environment (benchmark 4). Those who have discovered and developed psychotropic drugs owe a conceptual debt to Pinel and Tuke for changing the world's view of people with mental illness and to Freud and the early scientists who studied mental illness and were determined to find a cure. The community mental health movement has demonstrated to the psychiatric community and to the lay public that drug therapy alone is insufficient for many psychiatrically disordered individuals. Continuing research is needed to identify more effective treatment approaches and to refine existing therapeutic interventions and techniques, including the research and development of new psychotropic agents.

REFERENCES

Appleby L, et al: Length of stay and recidivism in schizophrenia: a study of public psychiatric hospital patients, *Am J Psychiatry* 150:72, 1993.

Ayd FJ Jr: A preliminary report on marsilid, *Am J Psychiatry* 114:459, 1957.

Ayd FJ Jr: The early history of modern psychopharmacology, *Neuropsychopharmacology* 5(2):71, 1991.

Foucault M: *Madness and civilization,* New York, 1973, Vintage.

Kuhn R: The treatment of depressive states with G 22355 (imipramine hydrochloride), *Am J Psychiatry* 115:459, 1958.

Lamb HR: Is it time for a moratorium on deinstitutionalization? *Hosp Community Psychiatry* 43(7):669, 1992.

Rifkin A: Extrapyramidal side effects: a historical perspective, *J Clin Psychiatry* 48(9):3, 1987.

Rosenblatt A: Concepts of the asylum in the care of the mentally ill, *Hosp Community Psychiatry* 35:685, 1984.

Weiner DB: Philippe Pinel's "Memoir on Madness" of December 11, 1794: a fundamental text of modern psychiatry, *Am J Psychiatry* 149(6):725, 1992.

CHAPTER 2

Neuroanatomy

RICHARD A. SUGERMAN
F. CLEVELAND KINNEY

The nervous system is artificially divided into the central nervous system (CNS) and the peripheral nervous system (PNS). A careful review of Figure 2-1 will improve the reader's understanding of this chapter. The CNS (Figure 2-2) is composed of the brain, which fills the cranial vault, and the spinal cord, which lies within the vertebral canal. The CNS is frequently presented as if the brain and spinal cord were separate entities; however, they are logically viewed as one functional unit. Motor information is transmitted from the cerebrum down the spinal cord and ultimately to the body musculature; sensory information from the body and muscles ascends the spinal cord to higher levels. Integration of information takes place throughout the CNS.

CENTRAL NERVOUS SYSTEM

The CNS may be divided into three sections based on embryologic development: the prosencephalon, the mesencephalon, and the rhombencephalon. The prosencephalon, or forebrain, is further separated into the telencephalon (cerebrum) and the diencephalon (thalamic nuclei).

Telencephalon (Cerebrum)

The telencephalon (cerebrum) consists of two hemispheres that constitute the bulk of the nervous system; these cerebral hemispheres are composed of the cerebral cortex, certain limbic structures, the corpus striatum, and a multitude of nervous system pathways. The cerebral cortex (Figure 2-3) is divided into four lobes, the frontal, temporal, parietal, and occipital lobes. The insular cortex (Island of Reil) is buried deep within the frontal, parietal, and temporal lobes and lies at the depth of the lateral fissure. The cingulate gyrus is associated through its length with the frontal, parietal, and temporal lobes. The corpus striatum (Figure 2-4) is made up of the caudate nucleus and the lentiform nucleus (putamen and globus pallidus). It is involved in motor functions and is described later in this chapter. The pathways formed by axons from neurons in the cerebral cortex transmit information throughout the CNS. Some of these pathways form the corpus callosum (Figures 2-3 and 2-4), which interconnects the two cerebral hemispheres, internal capsules (Figure 2-4), and the corona radiata, through which pass motor and sensory information, as well as many other pathways interconnecting the four cerebral lobes.

Diencephalon (Thalamic Nuclei)

The diencephalon (thalamic nuclei) (Figure 2-5) is made up of (1) the epithalamus, which is composed of several small nuclei and the pineal gland, (2) the dorsal

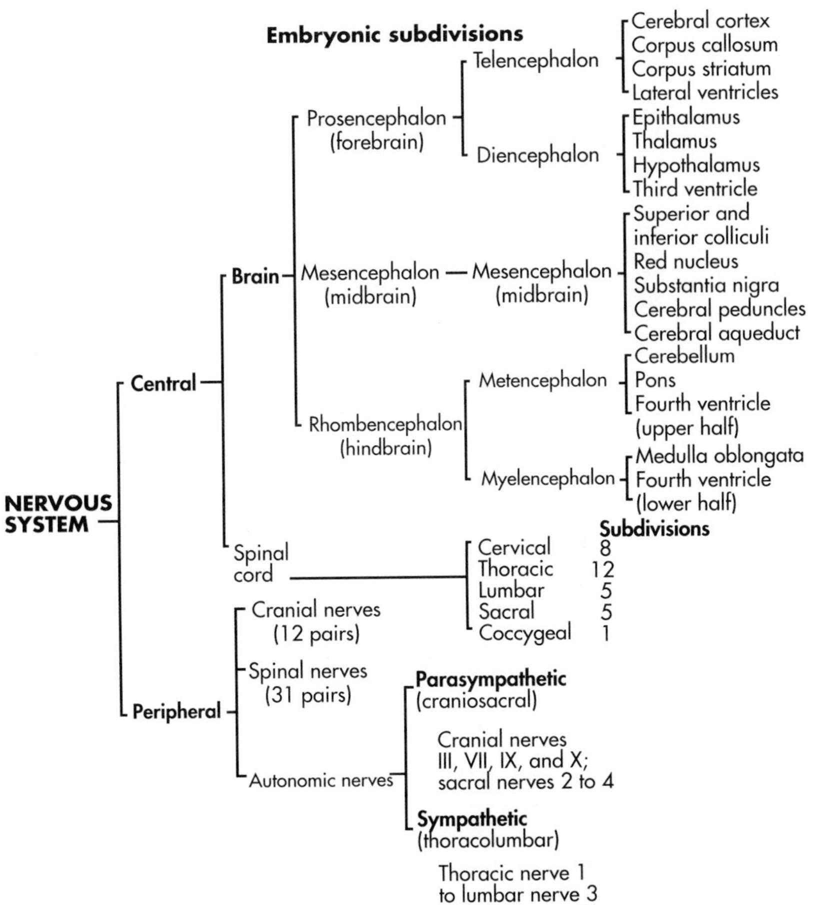

Figure 2-1 Major divisions of the nervous system.

thalamus, which is the major sensory relay nuclear area to and from the cerebral cortex, (3) the hypothalamus, which maintains homeostasis, and (4) the ventral thalamus, which functions primarily with the basal ganglia. The hypothalamus (Barr and Kiernan, 1988) is a tiny structure inferior to the dorsal thalamus, which is a major sympathetic-parasympathetic visceral integration center. It functions in part as a chemoreceptor by "sampling" cerebrospinal fluid and blood. The hypothalamus controls and influences functions such as body temperature regulation, food and water intake, gastrointestinal activity, respirations, and cardiovascular and endocrine functions. The hypothalamus has two modes of affecting the pituitary gland. The first mode is by the production of releasing or inhibiting factors that pass into the pituitary portal system, that is, capillary beds in the hypothalamus and pituitary gland, which are interconnected by a portal vessel. These factors are thus transmitted to the anterior pituitary, where they cause the release or inhibition, or both, of anterior pituitary hormones into the blood. The second mode is by the direct projection of hypothalamic neurons on the posterior pituitary, in which the

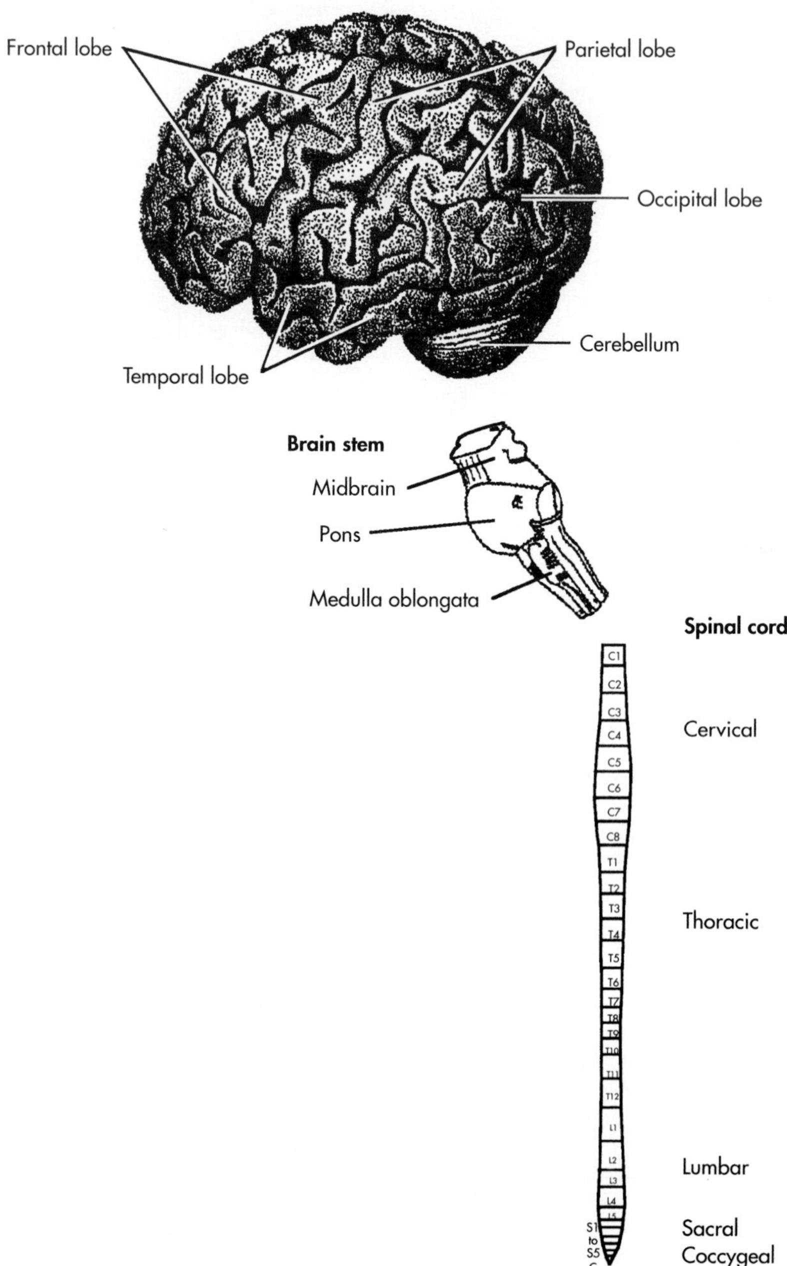

Figure 2-2 Expanded view of the central nervous system showing the major components. (From Berne RM, Levy MN: *Physiology,* ed 2, St. Louis, 1988, Mosby.)

Frontal lobe
Cingulate gyrus
Parietal lobe
Cerebral aqueduct
Parieto-occipital sulcus
Occipital lobe
Calcarine sulcus
Cerebellar hemisphere
Vermis of cerebellum
Fourth ventricle
Corpus callosum
G
R
S
Interventricular foramen
Temporal lobe
Diencephalon (forming wall of third ventricle)
Midbrain
Medulla
Pons
Brain stem

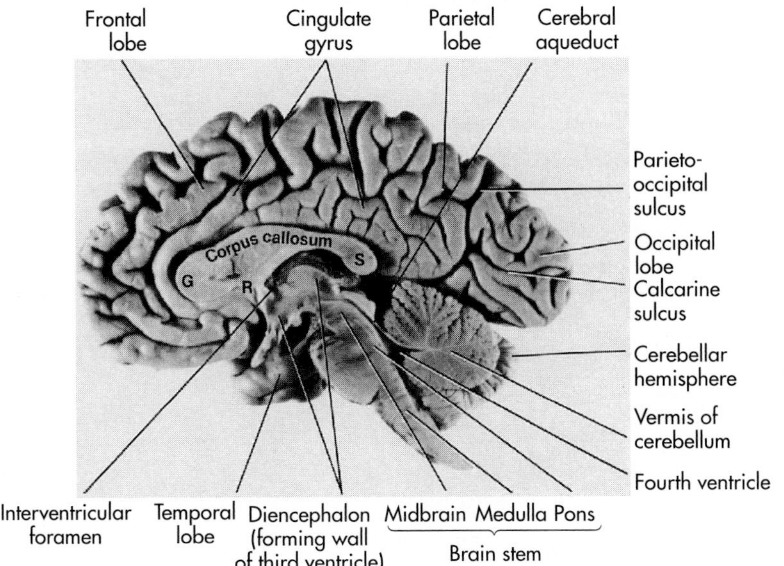

Figure 2-3 Major regions of the cerebrum, cerebellum, and brain stem as seen in the saggital plane. *R, G,* and *S* indicate the rostrum, genu, and splenium, respectively, of the corpus callosum. (From Nolte J: *The human brain,* ed 3, St Louis, 1993, Mosby.)

Genu of corpus callosum
Head of caudate nucleus
Lateral ventricle (anterior horn)
Internal capsule (anterior limb)
Septum pellucidum
External capsule
Extreme capsule
Ventral tier nuclei
Claustrum
Putamen
Dorsomedial nucleus
Globus pallidus
Pulvinar
Tail of caudate nucleus

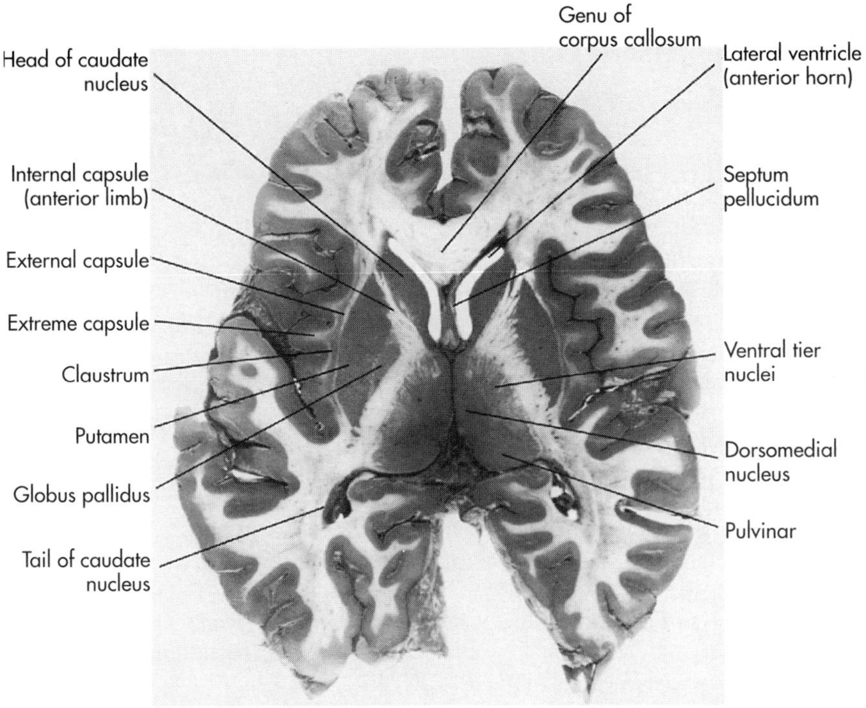

Figure 2-4 Basal ganglia and surrounding structures as seen in an approximately horizontal section. (From Nolte J: *The human brain,* ed 3, St Louis, 1993, Mosby.)

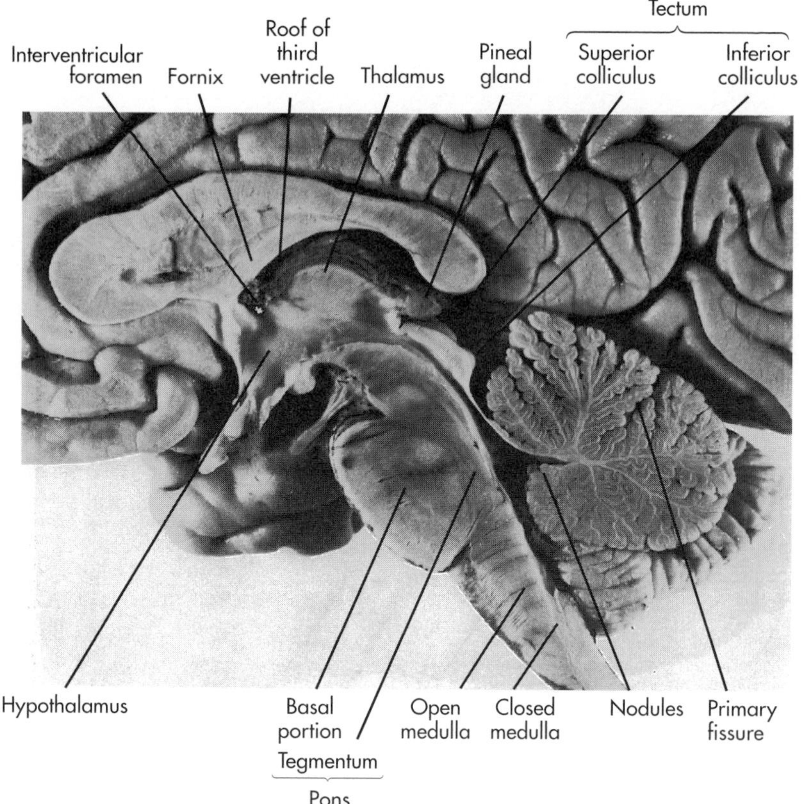

Figure 2-5 Major features of the diencephalon, brain stem, and cerebellum as seen in the sagittal plane. (From Nolte J: *The human brain,* ed 3, St Louis, 1993, Mosby.)

neurons release their hormones directly into the pituitary blood supply (portal system).

Brain Stem, Cerebellum, Reticular Formation, and Spinal Cord

The brain stem, cerebellum, reticular formation, and spinal cord reside beneath the forebrain. The brain stem is a collective term for the midbrain, pons, and medulla oblongata. The cerebellum is an expansive area attached to the posterior surface of the pons and resembles its Latin name, "little brain." The most caudal portion of the CNS is the spinal cord.

Brain stem. The midbrain (Figure 2-6) is the caudal (inferior) continuation of the CNS below the forebrain. It is about 1.5 cm long and is significantly narrower than the forebrain. The midbrain consists of the tectum, the tegmentum, the cerebral peduncles, and the associated substantia nigra. The red nuclei and substantia nigra are large structures in the midbrain that can be seen by the naked eye on examination. The red nuclei may be seen on freshly cut brains as large, vaguely reddish, round circles; the substantia nigra, as its name implies, is black. The black col-

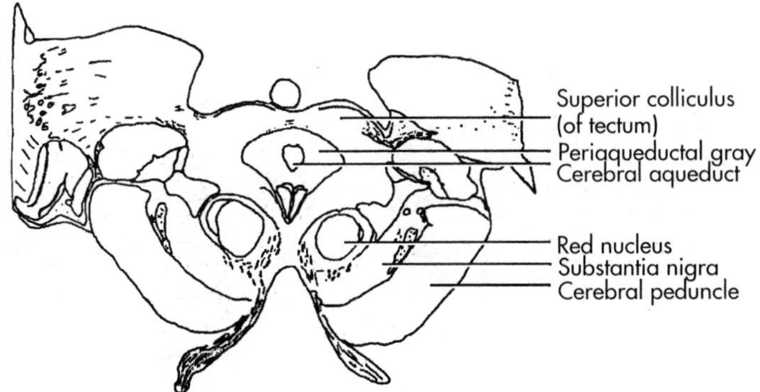

Figure 2-6 Cross section through superior colliculus of the midbrain.

oration is caused by melanin pigment found in neurons within the substantia nigra. These nuclei are covered further in the discussion of the motor systems. The basis pedunculi (cerebral peduncles) are basically a continuation of axons from motor neurons that project from the cerebral cortex through the corona radiata and internal capsule. The pedunculi form prominent bulges on the anterior (ventral) surface of the midbrain.

The hindbrain is composed of the pons, medulla oblongata, and cerebellum. The pons is an expansive area approximately 2.5 cm long that lies between the midbrain and the medulla oblongata. Some of the fibers in the basis pedunculi continue into the pons near the ventral surface of the brain stem, where many of them synapse in pontine nuclei. The pontine nuclei, in turn, project their axons to the cerebellum.

The medulla oblongata is about 3 cm long and narrows until it is continuous with the cervical spinal cord at the level of the foramen magnum. The motor fibers from the cerebral cortex continue on the anterior surface of the medulla oblongata. These fibers are known collectively as the pyramids because they form two pyramidal bulges. The decussation of the pyramids, that is, the crossing of the motor pathways contralaterally (to the opposite side), takes place at the lower level of the medulla oblongata. The pons and the medulla oblongata contain the central nuclei associated with the last 8 of the 12 cranial nerves and also contain autonomic control centers.

Cerebellum. The cerebellum consists of two hemispheres separated by a central portion called the *vermis*. The cerebellar hemispheres and most of the vermis simultaneously receive (through complex ascending pathways from the spinal cord) sensory input from muscles and joints. They also receive motor signals from the cerebral cortex that indicate how the muscle is being directed. The various areas of the cerebellum then communicate with the cerebral cortex to coordinate the final motor activity. These cerebellar areas function to coordinate muscle synergy and activity, but they do *not* initiate movements. The cerebellum also functions to maintain equilibrium. The central processing of balance information occurs in a small part of both the vermis and each cerebellar hemisphere.

Reticular Formation. The reticular formation resides within the brain stem. It comprises a discontinuous series of large nuclei located within the mesencephalon that extends interiorly through the pons and the medulla oblongata, as well as many

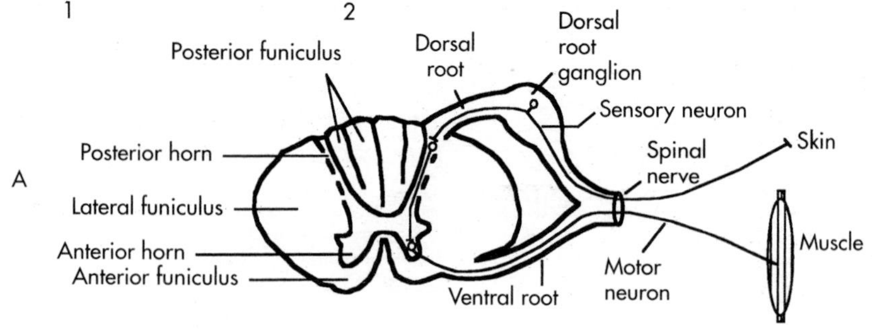

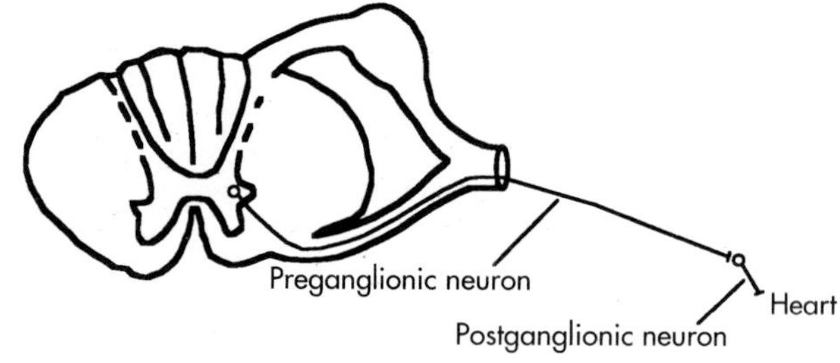

Figure 2-7 **A,** Cross section through a sacral segment of spinal cord. *1,* Basic subdivisions of horns and funiculi columns. *2,* Somatic components of a spinal nerve. **B,** Cross section through a sacral segment of spinal cord. Parasympathetic (visceral) motor components.

multisynaptic ascending and descending neural pathways. The reticular formation may be conceived of as a primitive brain buried deep within the brain stem. Input from most sensory pathways passes into the reticular formation, where it is integrated and then projected to the thalamus or the hypothalamus, or both. There are also descending reticulospinal tracts to the spinal cord. The reticular formation is a polysynaptic integration area that affects motor, sensory, and visceral functions. The functional relationship between cell bodies that arise from the reticular formation and are involved in norepinephrine, serotonin, acetylcholine, and dopamine synthesis is fundamental to understanding the anatomy of behavior. These systems and projection fields are further discussed in Chapter 3, Neuropharmacology and Psychotropic Drugs.

Spinal Cord. The spinal cord is approximately 42 to 45 cm in length and 1 cm in diameter. In the normal adult the spinal cord ends between lumbar vertebrae L1 and L2. Internally the spinal cord (Figure 2-7, *A*) is divided into gray and white matter, cell bodies, and cell processes. The gray matter is shaped like an H and fills the central portion of the cord. The posterior (dorsal) part of the H, or posterior (dorsal) horn, is concerned with sensory information, and the anterior (ventral)

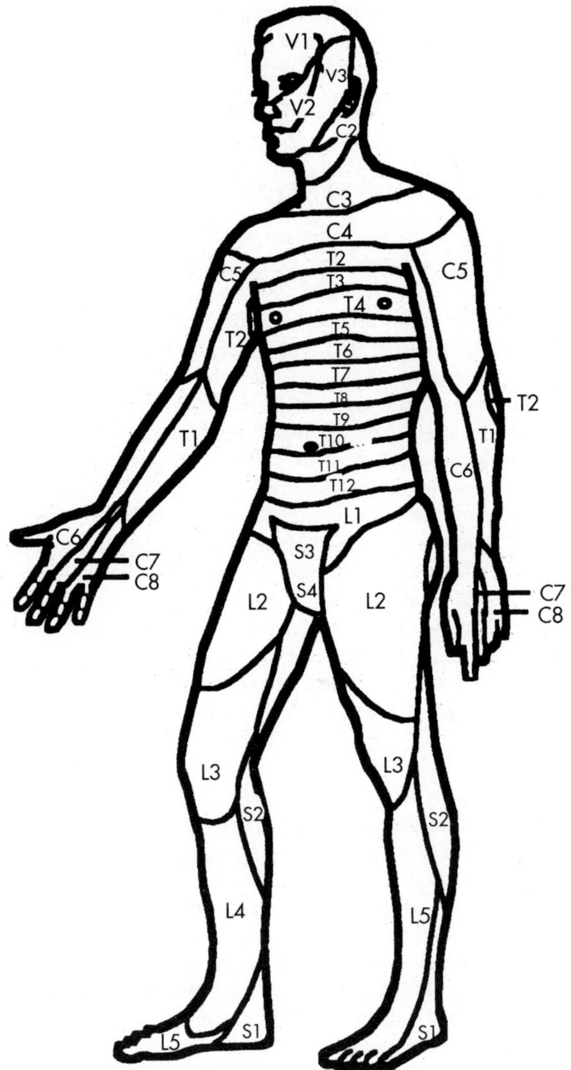

Figure 2-8 Dermatomes. Cutaneous distribution of spinal nerves. (Courtesy Richard Sugerman.)

part of the H, or anterior (ventral) horn, is related to somatic (skeletal muscle) and visceral motor actions. The white matter is divided into posterior, lateral, and anterior areas (funiculi). In general the posterior area contains ascending sensory pathways; the lateral and anterior areas transmit both ascending sensory and descending motor pathways. According to all theories on pain pathways, pain information ascends in both the anterior and lateral areas.

The spinal cord is organized in segments. There are 8 cervical, 12 thoracic, 5 lumbar, and 5 sacral segments and 1 coccygeal segment. This arrangement is reflected in the dermatomes of the body (Figure 2-8). For example, sensory nerves from the fourth and twelfth thoracic vertebrae (T4 and T12) subserve a narrow band of skin at the level of the nipples and the umbilicus, respectively. A transection of the spinal cord at the fourth cervical vertebra (C4) results in *quadriplegia,* a total loss of motor and sensory functions from the level of the superior surface of the shoulders and below.

PERIPHERAL NERVOUS SYSTEM

The peripheral nervous system is composed of 31 pairs of spinal nerves and 12 pairs of cranial nerves. The peripheral nervous system can be divided into a motor nervous system and an autonomic nervous system. The spinal nerve is considered to be a prototype for the entire peripheral nervous system. The spinal nerve (Figure 2-7, *A*) contains motor and sensory neurons. The motor axons originate from neurons in the ventral horn, pass through the ventral root into the spinal nerve, and terminate in skeletal (somatic) muscle, cardiac muscle, smooth (visceral) muscle, or glands. The spinal cord receives sensory information from exteroceptors, proprioceptors, and interoceptors. This information travels from sensory organs through the spinal nerve and dorsal root before synapsing in the dorsal horn of the cord. The exteroceptors transmit sensations of pain, touch, and temperature; the proprioceptors are responsible for joint, muscle, and tendon perceptions. These sensory modalities are consciously perceived. All these receptors are transducers, that is, they change sensory modalities into action potentials, which are generated by the receptive neurons. The cranial nerves may be considered practically as modified spinal nerves. Some cranial nerves are primarily motor, others are mainly sensory, and still others are a mixture of somatic and visceral, motor and sensory.

Autonomic Nervous System

The autonomic nervous system (Figure 2-9) receives interoceptor input and transmits visceral motor output. The autonomic nervous system is further divided into the parasympathetic (craniosacral) and the sympathetic (thoracolumbar) nervous systems. The parasympathetic nervous system is divided into cranial and sacral portions. The cranial part has neuronal components within the oculomotor, facial, glossopharyngeal, and vagus nerves, whereas the sacral part is composed of neuronal elements located in the second through fourth sacral nerves. The sympathetic nervous system is associated with the spinal nerves in a continuous column from the first thoracic nerve to the third lumbar nerve. Although sympathetic neurons originate within the thoracic portion and part of the lumbar portion of the spinal cord, they innervate effector organs throughout the body. The anatomy of the visceral motor portion of the autonomic nerves differs from that of the somatic motor nerves. Each somatic motor neuron projects its axon out of the spinal cord and innervates a skeletal muscle. Each neuron has its cell body in the anterior (ventral) horn of the spinal cord. The visceral nerve is made up of two neurons that are referred to as the *preganglionic* and *postganglionic* neurons (Figure 2-7, *B*). The preganglionic neurons of the autonomic nervous system have their cell bodies in the gray matter of the spinal cord and brain stem but are located for the most part slightly dorsal to somatic neurons. In the spinal cord the myelinated axon of the preganglionic neuron joins with the axons of the somatic motor neurons in the ventral root but soon leaves the spinal nerve to enter the sympathetic chain ganglia. The axon of the preganglionic neuron synapses on the dendrites or cell body of the postganglionic neuron. The cell bodies of the postganglionic neurons are organized into either ganglia or plexuses. When many neuronal cell bodies are in a connective tissue capsule outside

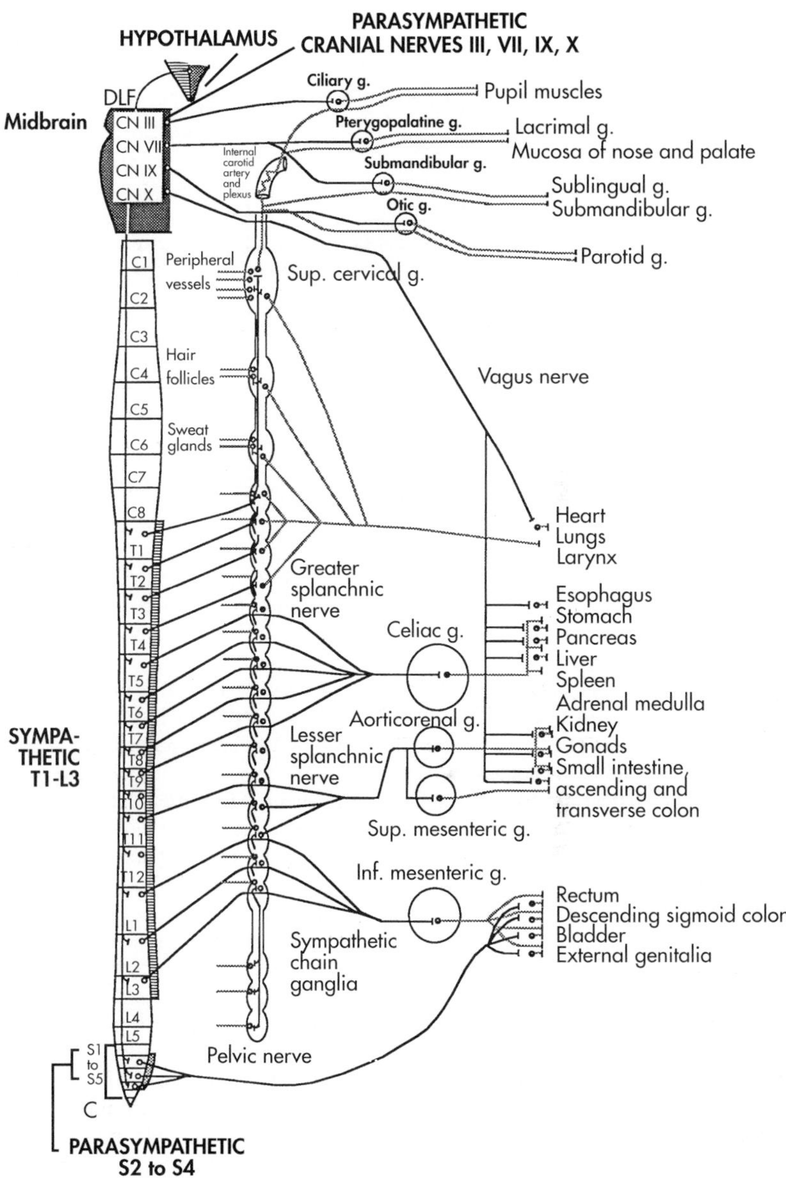

Figure 2-9 Diagram of the entire autonomic nervous system. Sympathetic portions of the central nervous system are shown as horizontally lined areas; the parasympathetic portions are shown as stippled areas. Preganglionic neurons are represented as solid lines, and postganglionic neurons are represented as dashed lines. The dorsal longitudinal fasciculus *(DLF)* interconnects the hypothalamus.

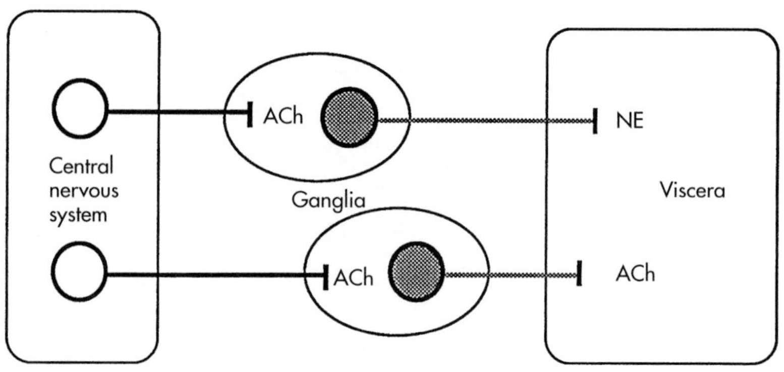

Figure 2-10 Major differences between the sympathetic and parasympathetic systems. The axons of preganglionic sympathetic neurons end in ganglia near the spinal cord, whereas those of preganglionic parasympathetic neurons travel a longer distance and reach ganglia near the innervated organ. The preganglionic neurons of both systems use acetylcholine (ACh) as their neurotransmitter, but at the synapses of postganglionic neurons the parasympathetic system uses ACh, and the sympathetic system uses norepinephrine (NE). (From Nolte J: *The human brain,* ed 3, St Louis, 1993, Mosby.)

the CNS, they are called a *ganglion.* If the cell bodies are spread out, as in the wall of the gut, they are called a *plexus.* The sympathetic chain ganglia, the largest of the autonomic structures, run parallel to the vertebral column and extend from the base of the skull to the end of the coccyx.

Preganglionic neurons use acetylcholine as their neurotransmitter (Figure 2-10). The postganglionic neurons send their lightly myelinated axons to their effector organs, smooth muscle, cardiac muscle, or glands. In general the parasympathetic postganglionic neurons use acetylcholine, and the sympathetic postganglionic neurons use norepinephrine as their neurotransmitters.

SUPRASPINAL MOTOR PATHWAYS

The term *supraspinal motor pathways* refers to pathways concerned with motor activity that involve cortical and subcortical (including brain stem nuclei) structures. The motor aspects of peripheral nerves and spinal reflexes are not discussed in this section. The three major motor systems traditionally include the corticospinal tracts (pyramidal system), corticobulbar pathways, and the basal ganglia system (extrapyramidal system). These systems function as an integrative whole in accomplishing motor activity.

The corticospinal tract originates primarily in the precentral gyrus, the most caudal gyrus of the frontal lobe, with contributions from adjacent cortical areas. The motor strip located within the precentral gyrus is often called the *primary motor cortex* and has an inverted body pattern in the form of a homunculus *(little man)* (Figure 2-11). The foot and leg muscles are represented on the medial surface of the precentral gyrus, and in order, descending over the lateral surface of the gyrus, are the buttock, thorax, arm, hand, and facial muscles. This somatotopic organization is

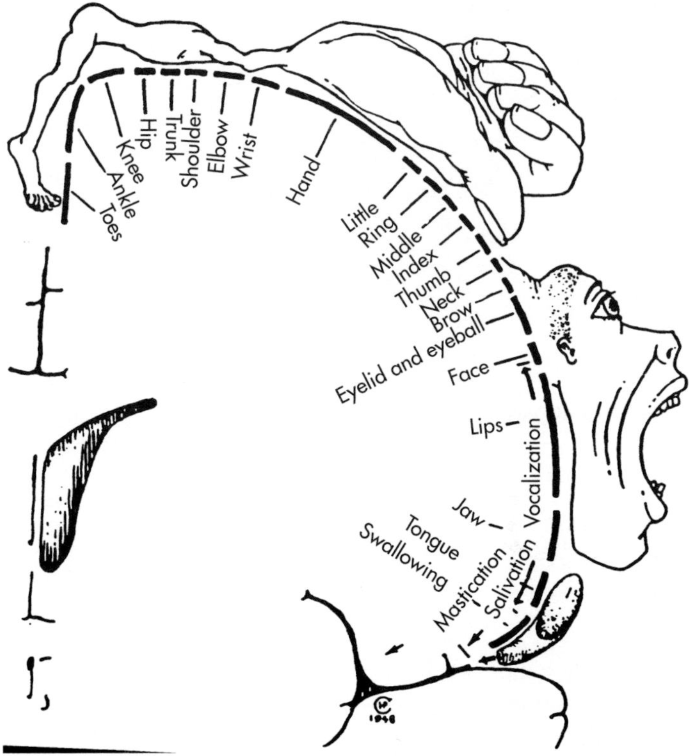

Figure 2-11 Homunculus of the precentral gyrus. This is a frontal section depicting the relative amount of cortex subserved in controlling the motor functions of various body areas. (From Penfield W, Rasmussen T: *The cerebral cortex of man,* New York, 1950, Macmillan.)

maintained throughout the CNS. Motor and sensory information are both organized throughout the nervous system in specific patterns.

The cortical neurons (Figure 2-12) project from the precentral gyri ipsilaterally (same side) through the corona radiata, the internal capsule, and the middle three fifths of the cerebral peduncles (basis pedunculi), thence they are interspersed within the basal pons and ultimately form the pyramids at medulla oblongata levels. In the inferior medulla oblongata about 70% of the pyramidal fibers decussate (cross) contralaterally, forming the lateral corticospinal tract, which ultimately synapses either directly or indirectly on alpha motor neurons in the spinal cord. Therefore the right cerebral cortex gives rise to the left lateral corticospinal tract and vice versa. This pathway controls voluntary, precise motor movements.

The corticobulbar pathways synapse on brain stem motor nuclei associated with the cranial nerves. The pathways have their origin in the precentral gyrus or immediately adjacent areas and descend through the corona radiata, the genu of the internal capsule, the cerebral peduncles, the basal pons, and the medulla oblongata. The vestibular nuclei and their associated ascending and descending connections help coordinate conjugate eye movements, balance, and primarily extensor muscle groups of the body. The descending pathway from the vestibular nuclei (located in the caudal pons and medulla) is called the *lateral vestibulospinal tract* and descends

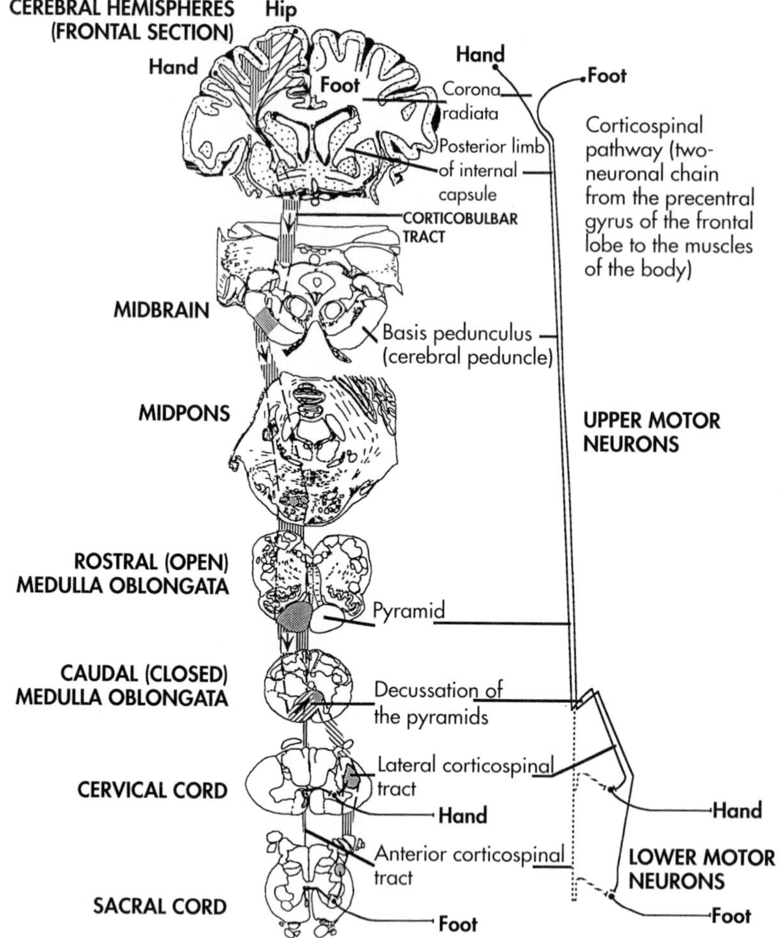

Figure 2-12 Distribution of the corticospinal tract (long pathway) and corticobulbar tract (short pathway). *Left,* Actual representation; *right,* schematic.

ipsilaterally in the brain stem and spinal cord, synapsing ipsilaterally on extensor motor neurons. This pathway helps us to stand erect and to maintain balance.

Basal Ganglia

The basal ganglia give rise to the extrapyramidal system; these projections do not pass through the pyramidal tracts. The extrapyramidal system is composed of a group of nuclei deep within the telencephalon and their projection pathways, which interrelate motor activities of the cerebral cortex, cerebellum, and brain stem. The descending output of this system originates largely from the globus pallidus, with synapses in course on the red nucleus and adjacent nuclei. The descending pathways terminate on motor (ventral horn) neurons within the spinal cord.

Generally the corticospinal tract *controls* precise, voluntary movements, and the basal ganglia, in conjunction with the cerebellum, *stabilize* motor movements.

Lesions of the basal ganglia result in abnormal motor movements such as those seen in Parkinson's disease.

The basal ganglia may be defined in many ways. A strict anatomic definition of the basal ganglia is outlined as follows:

I. Corpus striatum
   A. Caudate nucleus
   B. Lentiform nucleus
      1. Putamen
      2. Globus pallidus
II. Claustrum
III. Amygdala

It could be argued that the claustrum and amygdala are not truly dimensions of the basal ganglia. Structures that are interconnected with the basal ganglia are (1) the red nucleus, (2) the thalamus, (3) the cerebral cortex, and (4) the reticular formation.

A simplified illustration of many of the interrelationships of the nuclei and tracts of the basal ganglia is presented in Figure 2-13. The pathways, shown in the form of neurons projecting to anatomic areas, give only general basal ganglia relationships and do not fully represent all pathways.

A lateral view of the left cerebral hemisphere, including the precentral and postcentral gyri, is represented in Figure 2-13, *A*. Neurons located in the frontal and parietal lobes and neurons close to the precentral and postcentral gyri project their axons to the striatum, that is, the caudate nucleus and the putamen. These axons traverse the corona radiata and the internal capsule. These projections from the cortex are transmitting motor information to the striatum. The caudate nucleus in part (Figure 2-13, *B*) integrates this information and projects it to the putamen.

The neurons of the putamen distribute their axons within the putamen to the globus pallidus, which is subdivided into internal and external sections, and to the substantia nigra (Figure 2-13, *C*) through the striatonigral pathway. Most neurons within the putamen secrete gamma-aminobutyric acid (GABA) as their primary neurotransmitter and are referred to as GABA (gabanergic) neurons. Gamma-aminobutyric acid is an inhibitory neurotransmitter. The putamen also receives projections from dopamine-secreting neurons located within the substantia nigra via the nigrostriatal tract.

The globus pallidus sends a significant number of gabanergic axons to the subthalamic nucleus, the substantia nigra, the red nucleus, and the nuclei of the dorsal thalamus (DeLong, 1989).

The subthalamic nucleus projects glutaminergic neurons (excitatory neurons) to the globus pallidus and to the putamen (not illustrated). The pallidal neurons, whose axons pass to the red nucleus (Figure 2-13, *C*), stimulate two pathways (the rubrospinal and reticulospinal tracts), which are the primary pathways by which the basal ganglia ultimately influence the brain stem and spinal cord.

The rubrospinal tract (*rubro,* red) originates in the red nucleus and descends into the cervical spinal cord contralaterally, where it terminates on ventral horn cells.

Information from the basal ganglia passes to the dorsal thalamus and then, by way of thalamocortical fibers, through the internal capsule and corona radiata, to terminate on the premotor cortex, immediately anterior to the precentral gyrus. Although not illustrated in Figure 2-13, the motor cortex incorporates and uses this information when discharging through the corticospinal tract.

There are three major feedback loops within the basal ganglia. The one already discussed involves a circuit of synapses from the frontoparietal cortex to the striatum; impulses then pass from the putamen to the globus pallidum, from the globus pallidum to the dorsal thalamus, and from the dorsal thalamus to the cortex. The second loop is from the globus pallidus to the subthalamic nucleus and then to the globus pallidus, and the third loop is from the putamen to the substantia nigra and then back to the putamen. The third circuit is of great interest to clinicians. The striatonigral pathway has already been mentioned as a gabanergic pathway passing from the putamen to the substantia nigra. These neurons synapse on dopaminergic neurons in the substantia nigra, which in turn sends axons to the putamen via the nigrostriatal pathway. The dopaminergic neurons are believed to synapse on acetylcholine (ACh) neurons intrinsic within the putamen. These ACh neurons then excite the previously mentioned putamen gabanergic neurons. The interaction of dopamine, ACh, and GABA and their relative concentrations are important in the control of movement disorders (Afifi and Bergman, 1986). Clinical neuropharmacologists and clinicians who treat problems within this system use drug therapy, brain implants, and psychosurgery.

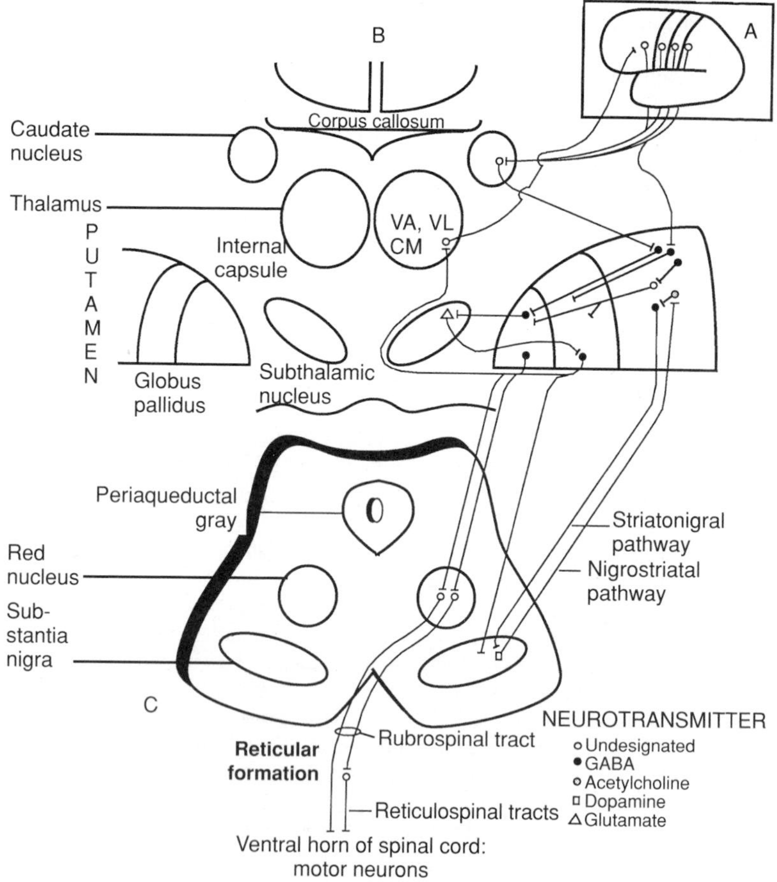

Figure 2-13 Basal ganglia system and its interconnections, including identified neurotransmitters. **A,** Left view of cerebral hemisphere. **B,** Coronal section of brain through corpus striatum. **C,** Midbrain. *VA,* Ventral anterior; *VL,* ventrolateral; and *CM,* centromedian thalamic nuclei.

LIMBIC LOBE

The limbic lobe (Figure 2-14) is the portion of the telencephalon that forms a border, or limbus, between the telencephalon and diencephalon. The limbic lobe frequently has been referred to as the rhinencephalon, or "nose-brain," because it is intimately involved with the perception and transmission of olfactory impulses. The so-called limbic lobe is not a separate anatomic division within the CNS but comprises structures that are found in the frontal lobe and pass through the parietal lobe, as well as structures found within the temporal lobe. The limbic lobe is concerned with the use of visceral functions for survival mechanisms and with the development of preferential visceral functions that are involved in eating and sexual activity. Structures most commonly included in the limbic lobe are (1) the olfactory nerves, (2) the olfactory bulbs and olfactory tracts, or striae, (3) the cingulate gyrus, (4) the amygdala, (5) the parahippocampal gyrus, (6) its underlying hippocampal formation, (7) the major projection bundle from the hippocampus, the fimbria-fornix, and (8) the preoptic area. To understand the limbic lobe one must have some appreciation of its connections. Mitral cells in the olfactory bulbs that are receiving olfactory impulses from the nasal mucosa transmit these impulses along the olfactory striae. The medial olfactory tract or stria terminates largely in the parolfactory area of Broca. The impulses are relayed from the parolfactory area of Broca (the septum) to the hypothalamus by way of the medial forebrain bundle. It is well known and documented that the hypothalamus and the discharges from it are concerned with visceral responses to olfactory stimuli. Thus olfactory impulses, which ultimately reach the hypothalamus, influence the major discharge of two pathways from the hypothalamus, the dorsal longitudinal fasciculus and the hypothalamotegmentoreticular pathways. Both of these pathways descend through the brain stem to terminate on cranial nerve parasympathetic and motor nuclei concerned with visceral impulses such as feeding. Hence there is a multisynaptic pathway by

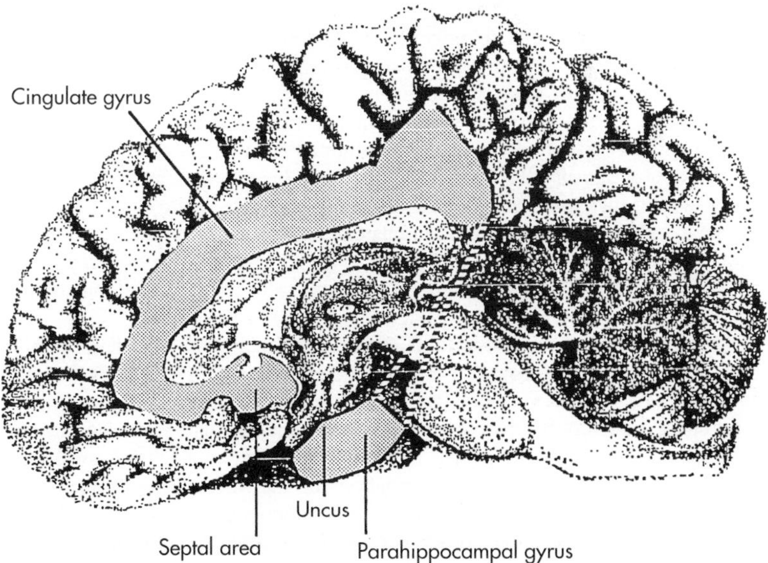

Figure 2-14 Limbic lobe as seen from a medial midsagittal view of the brain. (From Nolte J: *The human brain,* ed 3, St Louis, 1993, Mosby.)

which olfactory impulses may pass from the primary receptive areas within the telencephalon into the brain stem so that we might salivate in response to olfaction. Olfaction related to higher cortical functions is largely accomplished through the connections of the lateral olfactory tract. Olfactory impulses are transmitted along the lateral olfactory tract to terminate principally in the corticomedial amygdaloid nucleus and in the prepyriform cortex. From the corticomedial amygdaloid nucleus there are interconnections with the basolateral amygdaloid nucleus. From the basal lateral amygdaloid nucleus these impulses are transmitted into the temporal lobe to the parahippocampal gyrus. The parahippocampal gyrus, in turn, projects these impulses to the underlying hippocampal formation, which, through the cornu ammonis, gives rise to the fimbria-fornix. The fimbria-fornix projects mainly to the mammillary bodies of the hypothalamus. The major projections from the mammillary bodies are through the mammillothalamic tract (bundle of Vicq d'Azyr), which terminates in the anterior nucleus of the dorsal thalamus; however, the mammillary bodies are also interconnected with other hypothalamic nuclei and thus may influence the discharge of the descending pathways previously mentioned. It must be remembered that the temporal lobe contains primary auditory cortex and auditory association cortex. The temporal lobe also receives long association bundles from both the occipital and parietal lobes. Thus the temporal lobe is stimulated by connections from many widely varying cortical areas. These impulses are transmitted to the hippocampal gyrus and to the hippocampal formation and take part in the stimulation of the fimbria-fornix.

Not only is the amygdala connected with the parahippocampal gyrus but also there are direct projections from the amygdala into the hypothalamus by way of the ventral amygdalohypothalamic tract. Thus olfactory impulses that reach the amygdala may not only ultimately stimulate the various structures within the medial temporal lobe but also may influence the discharge of the hypothalamus through this pathway. It is often thought, and has been stated, that the amygdala is concerned with visceral impulses related to pleasurable and discriminatory activities. Bilateral lesions of the amygdala result in what is known as a *Klüver-Bucy* syndrome. The pure state is usually not seen in humans and was described originally in experimental studies performed on monkeys. Bilateral destruction of the medial temporal lobes, including the amygdala, results in an animal that is frequently placid. These animals have a tendency to examine everything in their environment by using their oral cavities. They also may lose sexual discrimination, and their eating preferences are altered. Occasionally these animals, rather than being placid, are extremely aggressive and hostile; this behavior has sometimes been referred to as "sham" rage. Trauma in human beings may result in bilateral damage to the temporal lobes, and in such cases a combination of these symptoms is often seen. Herpes encephalitis, which has a predilection for the temporal lobes, may also result in a combination of these various symptoms.

One cannot discuss the connections of the medial temporal lobes and the hippocampus without considering those structures included in what has become known as *Papez's circuit.* This circuit includes a number of important interconnections among the temporal lobe, the hypothalamus, the cingulate gyrus, and its underlying long association bundle, the cingulum. Impulses, as stated previously, are transmitted from the hippocampal formation through the fimbria-fornix to the mammillary bodies. From the mammillary bodies impulses are projected to the anterior nucleus of the dorsal thalamus by way of the mammillothalamic tract. The anterior nucleus of the dorsal thalamus relays these impulses by way of anterior thalamic radiations, which pass through the anterior limb of the internal capsule to the cingulate gyrus. The cingulate gyrus gives rise to the cingulum, which then transmits impulses that pass along its length through the isthmus and ultimately into the temporal lobe, where it terminates in relation to the hippocampal gyrus. As stated previously, there are interconnections between the parahippocampal gyrus and the hippocampal formation. Because impulses may be transmitted along both directions through this circuit, it may be said to be a "two-way street." It is now known that bilateral lesions of Papez's circuit, particularly those involving the fornix, result in profound loss of recent memory. It is well documented that the removal of tumors from the third ventricle, which interrupts the fornix bilaterally, results in a patient who is no longer able to lay down new or recent memory. Bilateral lesions of the hippocampal formation also have been noted to have this profound result. Patients with these kinds of injuries may have intact long-term memory, but their ability to make new memories is frequently severely impaired. Thus it is thought that the integrity of Papez's circuit is vital for the ability to learn.

REFERENCES

Afifi AK, Bergman RA: *Basic neuroscience: a structural and functional approach,* ed 2, Baltimore, 1986, Urban & Schwarzenberg.

Barr ML, Kiernan JA: *The human nervous system: an anatomical viewpoint,* Philadelphia, 1988, JB Lippincott.

DeLong MR: Symposium. Basal ganglia: structure and function, *Soc Neuroscience* 15(1):952, 1989 (abstract).

ADDITIONAL READINGS

Berne RM, Levy MN: *Physiology,* ed 3, St Louis, 1993, Mosby.

Crill WE: The milieu of the central nervous system. In HD Patton et al, editors: *Textbook of physiology,* vol 1, Philadelphia, 1989, WB Saunders.

Doane BK, Livingston KF, editors: *The limbic system: functional organization and clinical disorders,* New York, 1983, Raven.

Franck JAE et al: The limbic system. In HD Patton et al, editors: *Textbook of physiology,* vol 1, Philadelphia, 1989, WB Saunders.

Isaacson RL: *The limbic system,* New York, 1982, Plenum.

Lindsley DF, Holmes JE: *Basic human neurophysiology,* New York, 1984, Elsevier.

Narabayashi H: Stereotaxic vim thalamotomy for treatment of tremor, *Eur Neurol* 29:29, 1989.

Neuwelt EA, editor: *Implications of the blood-brain barrier and its manipulation,* vol 2, *Clinical aspects,* New York, 1989, Plenum.

Nolte J: *The human brain: an introduction to its fundamental anatomy,* ed 3, St Louis, 1993, Mosby.

Papez JW: A proposed mechanism of emotion, *Arch Neurol Psychiatry* 38:725, 1937.

Rowland LP: Blood-brain barrier, cerebrospinal fluid, brain edema, and hydrocephalus. In Kandel ER, Schwartz JH: *Principles of neural science,* New York, 1985, Elsevier.

Squire LR: Mechanisms of memory, *Science* 232:1612, 1986.

CHAPTER 3

Neuropharmacology and Psychotropic Drugs

RICHARD A. SUGERMAN

Neuropharmacology has been a subject of study since the discovery that smoking or ingesting substances could lead to profound effects on consciousness, sensorium, and mood. Purification of plant alkaloids, for example, morphine, cocaine, and reserpine, affect the nervous system significantly. Moreover, psychotropic drugs have been produced synthetically for decades, following the serendipitous discovery of lithium salts in 1949. These efforts have resulted in a significant number of drugs being used for psychiatric effects. In fact, 20% of all prescriptions written are for psychotropic drugs. Antihistamines, sympathomimetics, and various other over-the-counter agents are also used to affect the nervous system.

Eighty percent of the U.S. population uses psychoactive drugs for nonmedicinal purposes (Hyman and Nestler 1993). Alcohol and tobacco mostly account for recreational drug use. However, 20% of the population abuses illegal substances such as cocaine, opiates, stimulants, hallucinogenics, or marijuana. These psychotropic drugs significantly affect society and the lives of many individuals and their families.

Neuropharmacology involves the blood-brain barrier, which is unique to the CNS. A homeostatic balance is essential to brain function. Thus the blood-brain barrier controls fluctuations of ions and other substances, for example, K^{+}, Ca^{++}, and metabolites. Transporters facilitate transfer of substances such as glucose and amino acids. Lipophilic compounds also cross the blood-brain barrier quite readily. This process is used in drug delivery to the nervous system. Overall, the complexity of the brain, as described in Chapter 2, Neuroanatomy, makes treating neuropsychiatric disorders challenging. The basic processes, as such, will be described in this chapter.

Neurons are the basic subunit of the nervous system. They transmit information by sending action potentials, or waves of electrical depolarization, down their processes and on to other neurons. Most action potentials travel from one neuron to another by sending a chemical called a *neurotransmitter* across a minute space (or synapse), which separates these cells, to evoke the next action potential. It is in or around this synapse that many drugs act on the nervous system.

SYNAPTIC TRANSMISSION

Figure 3-1 depicts two neurons. The first neuron is the presynaptic neuron, and its axon is going to a dendrite of the second neuron, or postsynaptic neuron. The presynaptic membrane often has on its surface synaptic boutons, button- or bulb-shaped projections on the end of the axon, that are directly opposite the postsynaptic membrane. Synaptic boutons are about 1 m in diameter and contain synaptic vesicles carrying neurotransmitters. An action potential arriving at a synaptic bouton

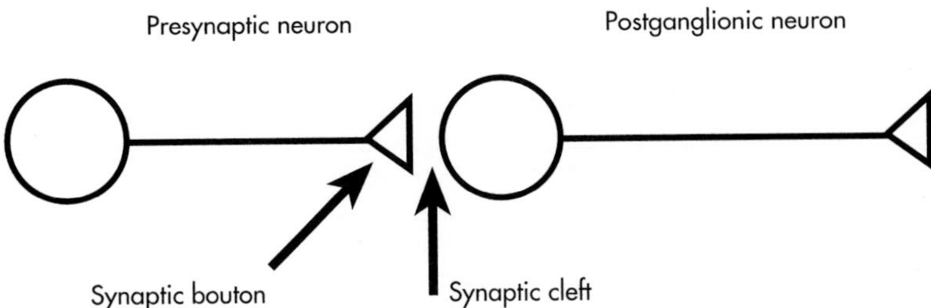

Figure 3-1 Two-neuron chain showing the presynaptic and postsynaptic neurons interconnected by a synapse. The synapse is composed of a synaptic bouton *(triangle)*, which is on the presynaptic membrane, the synaptic cleft, and the postsynaptic membrane, which in this instance is the dendrite or cell body *(circle)* of the postsynaptic neuron.

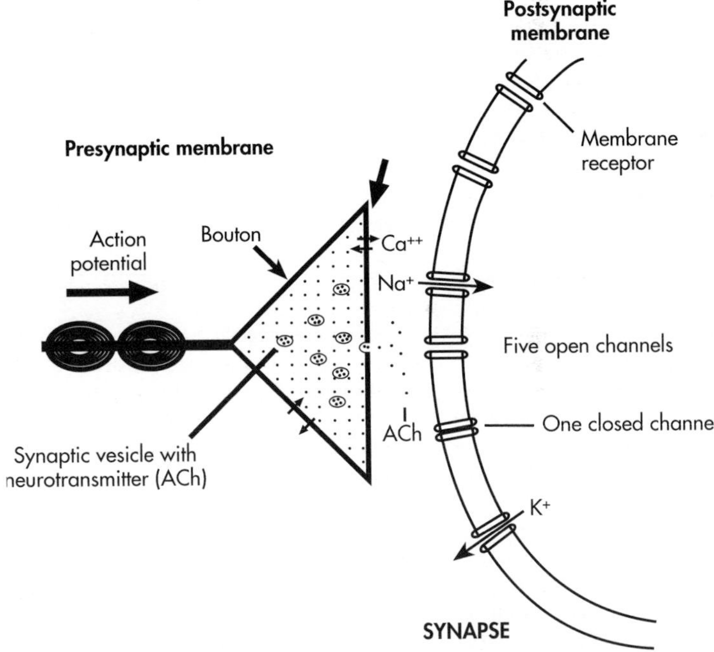

Figure 3-2 An action potential opens calcium ion channels and allows Ca^{++} to enter the presynaptic membrane (bouton). The Ca^{++} triggers the vesicles to fuse with the membrane and release the neurotransmitter acetylcholine (ACh) into the synaptic cleft. Two molecules of ACh then bind with an ACh receptor on the postsynaptic membrane of the target cell, which allows sodium (Na^{+}) influx and potassium (K^{+}) efflux through opened channels in the target cell membrane. The channels are normally closed, except when activated by the ACh-receptor complex.

(Figure 3-2) causes a change in the membrane potential of the bouton by opening calcium channels and allowing extracellular calcium (Ca^{++}) to enter the bouton. The increased intracellular calcium in the bouton triggers the vesicles to fuse with the bouton's cellular membrane and release the transmitter into the synaptic cleft, a 20-nm space between the cells. The neurotransmitter then diffuses across the synaptic cleft to the postsynaptic membrane of the next neuron, where it binds only to specific receptors. For example, the neurotransmitter acetylcholine (ACh) binds only with the ACh receptors on the postsynaptic membrane of the next neuron. This binding allows sodium ions into and potassium ions out of opened channels. If enough ACh diffuses to the postsynaptic membrane (receptors), an action potential can be generated by the postsynaptic neuron. Most neurotransmitters, after binding to the receptors, are quickly and actively "reuptaken" by the presynaptic boutons or surrounding glial cells. ACh is an exception to this general principle. It is broken down in the synaptic space by the enzyme acetylcholinesterase. The rapid degradation of ACh allows only a short burst of activity at the postsynaptic membrane.

Types of Synapses

At one time neuroscientists were aware of only a few types of synapses. The classic axon synapsed on the dendrites, somas (cell body), and axons—the axodendritic, axosomatic, and axoaxonic synapses, respectively. With the advent of the electron microscope scientists found somatosomatic and dendrodendritic synapses. In addition, electron micrography has allowed scientists to find reciprocal synapses between two neurons, for example, dendrodendritic (Shepard, 1983). These reciprocal synapses probably form minuscule local positive or negative feedback loops. Furthermore, many neurons receive input from more than 1000 other neurons. Thus the true complexity of the neuronal milieu begins to be appreciated.

MEMBRANE RECEPTORS

Receptors are cell membrane proteins that react to specific neurotransmitters. These proteins are depicted as hollow tubes that extend their openings between the extracellular and intracellular spaces. These openings are referred to as *pores* or *channels*. When a neurotransmitter binds with its specific receptor, a conformational change takes place that opens or closes the channel to the flow of specific ions, for example, sodium, potassium, and chloride. The ACh receptor molecule is a glycoprotein with a molecular weight of 268,000 and five separate polypeptides that extend into the extracellular space (Hille, 1989). The exposed polypeptides help in providing the specificity for the receptors. Classically, pharmacologists working with ACh have operationally defined ACh receptors as either nicotinic or muscarinic, depending on whether the alkaloid nicotine or muscarine has an excitatory (agonistic) effect at the synapse. For example, ACh receptors that are stimulated by nicotine are *nicotinic*, and ACh receptors that are stimulated by muscarine are *muscarinic*. Acetylcholine receptors at the neuromuscular junction of skeletal muscle and in sympathetic ganglia are nicotinic, whereas ACh receptors found on effector organs such as glands, smooth muscle, and cardiac muscle are muscarinic. Therefore ACh has more than one type of receptor. In addition, the excitatory effects of ACh at the receptors can be blocked selectively by different agents or antagonists. For example, nicotinic receptors on skeletal muscle are selectively blocked by curare, whereas muscarinic receptors are blocked by atropine. Thus the presence of specific agonists and antagonists for the membrane receptors has enabled scientists to classify receptors for ACh and other neurotransmitters into more than one type. Scientists now know that there are many different types of receptors that are specific for individual neurotransmitters.

Mechanisms of Receptor Action

When a neurotransmitter binds with a receptor, ion channels are opened or closed, allowing specific ions to start or stop moving across the postsynaptic membrane and evoking local changes in the membrane potential. In neuron excitation, when a sufficient amount of neurotransmitter binds with a threshold-level number of receptors, an action potential takes place and travels along the entire length of the neuron. When the neurotransmitter-receptor complex results in direct change of the membrane potential, it is referred to as *first messenger transmission.* First messenger transmission requires only a few milliseconds to initiate its changes to the cell membrane. First messenger transmission also can initiate a series of intracellular reactions by triggering *secondary messenger transmission,* which causes not only delayed ion channel opening or closing but also the regulation of many cell functions. These secondary messengers are cell membrane proteins that relay the "message" from the neurotransmitter-receptor complex to a chain of chemical reactions in the neuroplasm of the cell (Patton, 1989). Thus hormones and neurotransmitters can activate intracellular mechanisms to initiate cell division, protein synthesis, and the like. First messenger transmission can be viewed as evoking rapid, *direct* membrane changes and secondary messenger transmission as a slower, *indirect* process with broad applications.

NEUROTRANSMISSION

Neuron Excitation and Inhibition

Neuron excitation of the postsynaptic membrane is caused by the stimulation of the receptor by the neurotransmitter. This stimulation causes an influx of sodium ions into the neuron, resulting in depolarization of the postsynaptic membrane. Inhibition is caused by an efflux of potassium ions or an influx of chloride ions, or both, that causes a hyperpolarization of the postsynaptic membrane. Neurotransmitters are sometimes classified as excitatory or inhibitory, *but the mechanism of action actually depends on the postsynaptic receptor.* Acetylcholine can be either excitatory or inhibitory, depending on the receptor that it activates.

Defining Neurotransmitters

The following specific criteria are used to define a chemical as a neurotransmitter:

1. The chemical must be found in the presynaptic boutons and must be released when the neuron is stimulated.
2. The chemical must somehow be inactivated after it is released. Two mechanisms of inactivation have been found. The most common is reuptake of the chemical by the presynaptic membrane, and the second is the degradation of the chemical by an extracellular enzyme.
3. If the chemical is applied exogenously at the postsynaptic membrane, the effect will be the same as when the presynaptic neuron is stimulated. The quantity of chemical applied must be in a reasonable concentration.
4. The chemical applied to the synapse must be affected in a manner similar to that of the normally occurring chemical.

ACTION AND SYNTHESIS OF NEUROTRANSMITTERS

Neurotransmitters have been divided into four major groups or systems: *cholinergics, monoamines, neuropeptides,* and *amino acids* (Table 3-1). In this section neurotransmitters are classified by major group or system, and their sites of action, their modes of synthesis, and their mechanisms of action are discussed. Neurotransmitters occur

Table 3-1 Classification of Neurotransmitters and Pathways

Neurotransmitter	Chemical transmitter	Location found	Major pathways
Cholinergic systems	ACh	Myoneural junctions, postganglionic neurons, autonomic ganglia, parasympathetic postganglionic neurons	Basal nucleus of Meynert to cerebral cortex, septal area (rostral to hypothalamus) to hippocampus
Monoamine systems	Catecholamines		
	Dopamine		Nigrostriatal
	Norepinephrine	Locus ceruleus	Locus ceruleus (in pons) to thalamus, cerebral cortex, cerebellum, and spinal cord; lateral midbrain to hypothalamus and basal forebrain
	Epinephrine		Central tegmental tract
	Serotonin	Raphe nuclei	Central brain stem nuclei up to forebrain and down to spinal cord
Neuropeptides	Enkephalins	Spinal cord, hypothalamus, midbrain, and the like	
	Endorphins	Spinal cord, hypothalamus, midbrain, and the like	
	Substance P	Spinal cord, hypothalamus, and many other places	
	Somatostatin, VIP, CCK, ACTH, neurotensin, angiotensin II, and others		
Amino acids	GABA	Most neurons, indicating ubiquitous distribution	
	Glycine	Spinal cord, brain stem, and many other CNS areas	
	Glutamate	Widely distributed in the CNS	
	Asparate	Hippocampus, dorsal root ganglion	

ACh, Acetylcholine; *ACTH,* adrenocorticotropic hormone; *CCK,* cholecystokinin; *CNS,* central nervous system; *GABA,* gamma-aminobutyric acid; *VIP,* vasoactive intestinal polypeptide.

in neurons and tracts in too many locations to discuss in detail; therefore only significant anatomic locations are mentioned.

Cholinergic System

The neurotransmitter in the cholinergic system is ACh (Mathews and Van Holde, 1990; Taylor and Brown, 1989). Acetylcholine is found in the peripheral nervous system (PNS) at the myoneural junction of skeletal muscle, in autonomic ganglia and at parasympathetic postganglionic-effector synapses, and in the central nervous system (CNS) within the spinal cord, basal ganglia, and cerebral cortex. Several pathways in the brain have been identified as ACh tracts. The basal nucleus of Meynert projects fibers to the cerebral cortex and has been implicated as a site of lesion in Alzheimer's disease. The septal area, an area rostral to the hypothalamus, sends ACh fibers to the hippocampus. Acetylcholine is synthesized by the union of acetylcoenzyme A (acetyl-CoA) and choline in the axonal boutons and stored in synaptic vesicles (Figure 3-3, *A*).

As stated earlier, ACh is released from the presynaptic membrane, crosses the synaptic cleft, and attaches to its receptor. Acetylcholinesterase in the synaptic cleft breaks down the ACh into its component molecules (Figure 3-3, *B*). Much of the choline in the bouton is obtained by reuptake from the synaptic cleft and is used subsequently for ACh synthesis. It was also stated earlier that ACh has two major categories of membrane receptors, nicotinic and muscarinic. Both nicotinic and muscarinic receptors can be further divided into subtypes, which are beyond the scope of this review. The nicotinic receptors are found at the postsynaptic membrane at the myoneural junction and, rarely, in the CNS. The muscarinic receptors are located on parasympathetic effector organs and in the CNS. Nicotinic receptors appear to be excitatory in function and use first messenger transmission. The muscarinic receptors trigger secondary messenger transmission and can affect the postsynaptic membrane in a number of ways, including membrane hyperpolarization.

Monoamine Systems

Neurotransmitters containing one amine group are called *monoamines* (Mathews and Van Holde, 1990; Weiner and Molinoff, 1989). These include the catecholamines (dopamine, norepinephrine, and epinephrine), serotonin, and histamine. The term *adrenergic* refers to neurons activated by catecholamines, which are adrenalin-like substances also derived from the adrenal gland. The catecholamines are common neurotransmitters that are widely dispersed in the CNS and PNS. Dopamine neurons project from the substantia nigra to the putamen via the nigrostriatal pathway, a major pathway affected in Parkinson's disease. Additional dopamine sites are located in the caudate nucleus, amygdala, and temporal lobe. High concentrations of dopamine appear to be involved in schizophrenia. Norephinephrine cells in the locus ceruleus (in the pons) send their processes to the thalamus, cerebral cortex, cerebellum, and spinal cord. Norepinephrine is also the neurotransmitter of the sympathetic postganglionic neurons. Epinephrine (adrenalin) is found in neurons that run from the red nucleus to the medulla oblongata in the central tegmental tract. Serotonin is found in central midbrain nuclei and in neuronal processes up to the forebrain and down to the spinal cord. The catecholamines are all derived from tyrosine (Figure 3-4).

Tyrosine is found in the neurons, where it is converted to levodopa (L-dopa) and then to dopamine. Dopamine is then taken up into storage vesicles and converted to

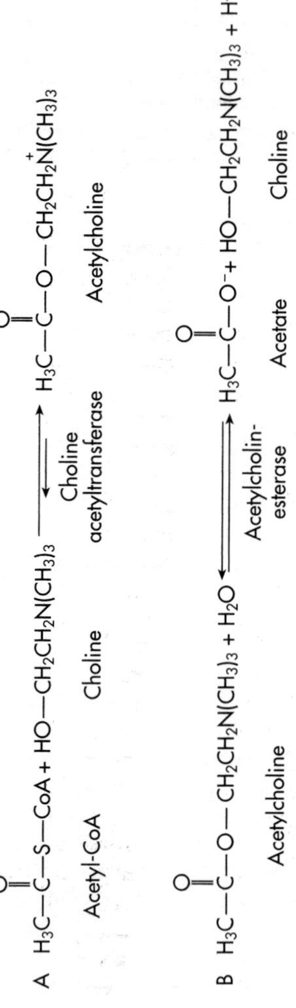

Figure 3-3 **A,** Synthesis of acetylcholine and **(B)** its subsequent breakdown, facilitated by acetylcholinesterase.

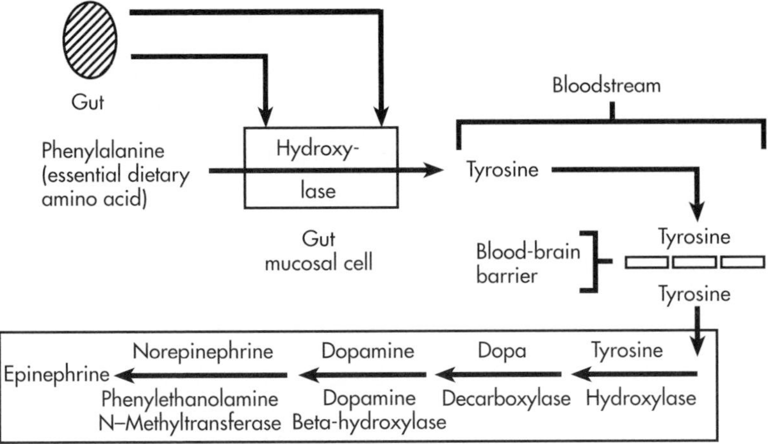

Figure 3-4 Normal synthesis of the catecholamines.

norepinephrine within these vesicles. There are several classes of catecholamine receptors (five dopaminergic receptors and four adrenergic receptors), and these receptors appear to influence ion channels by secondary messenger mechanisms. Many of these receptors affect the postsynaptic neurons by stimulating adenylate cyclase to convert adenosine triphosphate (ATP) to cyclic adenosine monophosphate (AMP). Cyclic AMP is an important secondary messenger.

Serotonin (5-hydroxytryptamine) is derived from tryptophan within the CNS. Serotonin receptors have been described as activating secondary messenger transmission. Serotonin is involved in the spinal pain pathway, in facilitating motor activity, and possibly in modulating human behavior. Both norepinephrine and serotonin have been implicated in depression.

Histamine is found in low quantities in the brain. Its precursor is histidine, which is the chemical that crosses the blood-brain barrier. Histamine neurons are located primarily in the hypothalamus, and their processes extend to many CNS areas. The receptors for histamine initiate secondary messenger transmission. Histamine is believed to be involved in body functions such as the regulation of biorhythms and thermoregulation and in neuroendocrine functions.

The monoamines can be excitatory or inhibitory transmitters, depending on the action mediated by their receptors. These receptors primarily give rise to secondary messenger transmission that can be slow-acting initially but have an extended duration of action. Therefore, for a full understanding of the action of neurotransmitters, one needs to understand the action of the specific receptors.

Neuropeptides

Neuropeptides are proteins that act as neurotransmitters or hormones. These are highly diverse proteins that have a common ability to excite or inhibit the activity of cell membranes. This discussion is limited to the neuropeptides that act as neurotransmitters in the CNS. Some of these proteins are released from their neurons in a manner similar to that of other transmitters. However, these neurotransmitters may enter either synaptic clefts or the bloodstream (pituitary hormones). Receptors on the postsynaptic membrane initiate secondary messenger transmission. Neuropeptides have been found to be released in conjunction with other neurotransmitters. For example, ACh and vasoactive intestinal polypeptide (VIP) have been shown to be released from cortical neurons at the same boutons (Detwiller and Crill, 1989). Therefore the principle that one neuron releases one neurotransmitter (Dale's principle) does not reflect current information. Theoretically, then, one might expect to find multiple transmitters from the same neuron working synergistically or antagonistically on the postsynaptic receptors. Hence the quantity and distribution of the receptors are important in forming neural circuits.

The synthesis of neuropeptides is hypothesized to be performed in one of two ways: by messenger ribonucleic acid (mRNA) or by enzymatic action. Large neuropeptides are proteins that originate from the interaction of mRNA with polyribosomes on the endoplasmic reticulum in the cell body. Because these proteins will be involved in secretory processes, they are transported to the Golgi apparatus as prohormones, where they are packed in membranes and shipped by axonal transport to the cell processes for storage, degradation to the active molecule, and release (Holaday, 1985; Schwartz, 1985). Small neuropeptides can be synthesized by means of enzymatic action through glycolysis, the citric acid cycle, and related mechanisms.

Opioids. In 1975 Hughes et al discovered that the brain contained its own opioid system and that the system appeared to be involved with pain and pleasure. The receptors of this system are stimulated by endogenous, opioid-like chemicals and morphine and can be blocked by naloxone, a narcotic antagonist. The chemicals are called *endorphins* and are defined as endogenous molecules of the body that have an opioid-like action. The term *endorphin* encompasses a large group of diverse neuropeptides. In this section beta-endorphin and a smaller group of endorphins called *enkephalins* are discussed. These chemicals are widely distributed throughout the CNS.

Beta-endorphin, which contains 31 amino acids, is an excellent representative of the endorphin group. It has been found to be 48 times as potent as morphine. Beta-endorphin has been localized to the hypothalamus, with projecting processes to the midbrain and other CNS locations. It is synthesized from the prohormone proopiomelanocortin, which is broken down in vesicles into adrenocorticotropin, or adrenocorticotropic hormone (ACTH), beta-lipotropin, and a number of other active neuropeptides. Beta-lipotropin is further processed into beta-endorphin and another peptide. Under stress, beta-endorphin and ACTH are released simultaneously into the blood, which helps demonstrate the common prohormone origins (Kelly, 1985).

Enkephalins are specific endorphins. They are all pentapeptides. Enkephalins are widely distributed throughout the CNS in primarily small neurons that are locally active. The prohormones for enkephalins are proenkephalin and prodynorphin. The synthesis is similar to that of endorphin formation in that a number of neuropeptides are formed when the cell dismantles the prohormones. The enkephalins have been implicated in physiologic areas such as pain perception, taste and olfaction, arousal, emotional behavior, vision and hearing, neurohormone secretion, motor coordination, and water balance (Dorsa, 1989; Holaday, 1985; Kutchai, 1993; Simon and Miller, 1989).

Substance P. Substance P was discovered in 1931 from the precipitate of horse brain. It is composed of a chain of 11 amino acids. The activity of substance P was shown at that time to be similar to that of ACh, but it was not blocked, as ACh is, by atropine. Substance P is found in great quantities in the ventral horn of the spinal cord and is widely distributed throughout the CNS. In the spinal cord it appears to be the neurotransmitter of the small-diameter, peripheral pain neurons (Dorsa, 1989).

Somatostatin. Somatostatin is produced inside the brain and in D cells of the pancreas. It is composed of a chain of 14 amino acids. One fourth of the brain somatostatin has been localized to the hypothalamus, and it is also found in the small-diameter, peripheral pain neurons with substance P. Somatostatin is both a hormone and a neurotransmitter. Somatostatin affects the postsynaptic membrane by hyperpolarizing (inhibiting) the membrane (Dorsa, 1989; Erulkar, 1989).

Other Neuropeptides

Vasoactive intestinal polypeptide
Cholecystokinin
Adrenocorticotropic hormone
Neurotensin
Angiotensin II

Amino Acid Transmitters

The amino acid transmitters are a special group of amino acids that are normally found in cells. They are formed, like many other amino acids, as products during the normal cellular processes of glycolysis and the citric acid cycle (Figure 3-5) (Mathews and Van Holde, 1990). These chemicals include gamma-aminobutyric acid (GABA), glycine, glutamate, and aspartate. GABA and glycine are well-known inhibitory transmitters; glutamate and aspartate are excitatory transmitters. These amino acid transmitters are widely distributed throughout the nervous system.

GABA receptors have been localized on all neurons that have been investigated (Detwiller and Crill, 1989), which indicates a ubiquitous distribution in the nervous system. GABA receptors are designated *A* and *B* (Gottlieb, 1988). Type A receptors function by first messenger transmission, whereas type B receptors use the indirect secondary messenger transmissions. Both receptors, when activated, result in an influx of chloride ions into the neuron, which causes hyperpolarization of the membrane potential, that is, inhibition. Glial cells, which form a dense network around neurons, have an affinity for GABA, and by removing it from the synaptic cleft, they prevent GABA buildup (Gottlieb, 1988; Crill, 1989). GABA is synthesized by the decarboxylation of glutamate (Figure 3-5) via alpha-ketoglutaric acid from the citric acid cycle.

Glycine has been localized in the cerebellum, brain stem, and spinal cord. Both glycine and GABA have been isolated from the two types of Renshaw cell, from interneurons, and in the spinal cord. The receptor for glycine uses the fast-acting first messenger transmission. The storage mechanism within the neuron for both glycine and GABA has not yet been determined. The mechanism for inhibition is the same as that described for GABA. Glycine is synthesized directly from serine, which is derived from glycolysis (Figure 3-5) (Detwiller and Crill, 1989; McGeer and McGeer, 1989). Glutamate has been found in the cortex, hippocampus, cerebellum, and spinal cord. Two receptor types have been classified, N-methyl-D-aspartate (NMDA) and non-NMDA. Both receptors evoke first messenger transmission to cause depolarization of the membrane potential, that is, excitation. When glutamate loses an ammonium ion, glutamine is formed. Glutamine is readily diffusible into the blood and the cerebrospinal fluid. Therefore measuring the glutamine level in

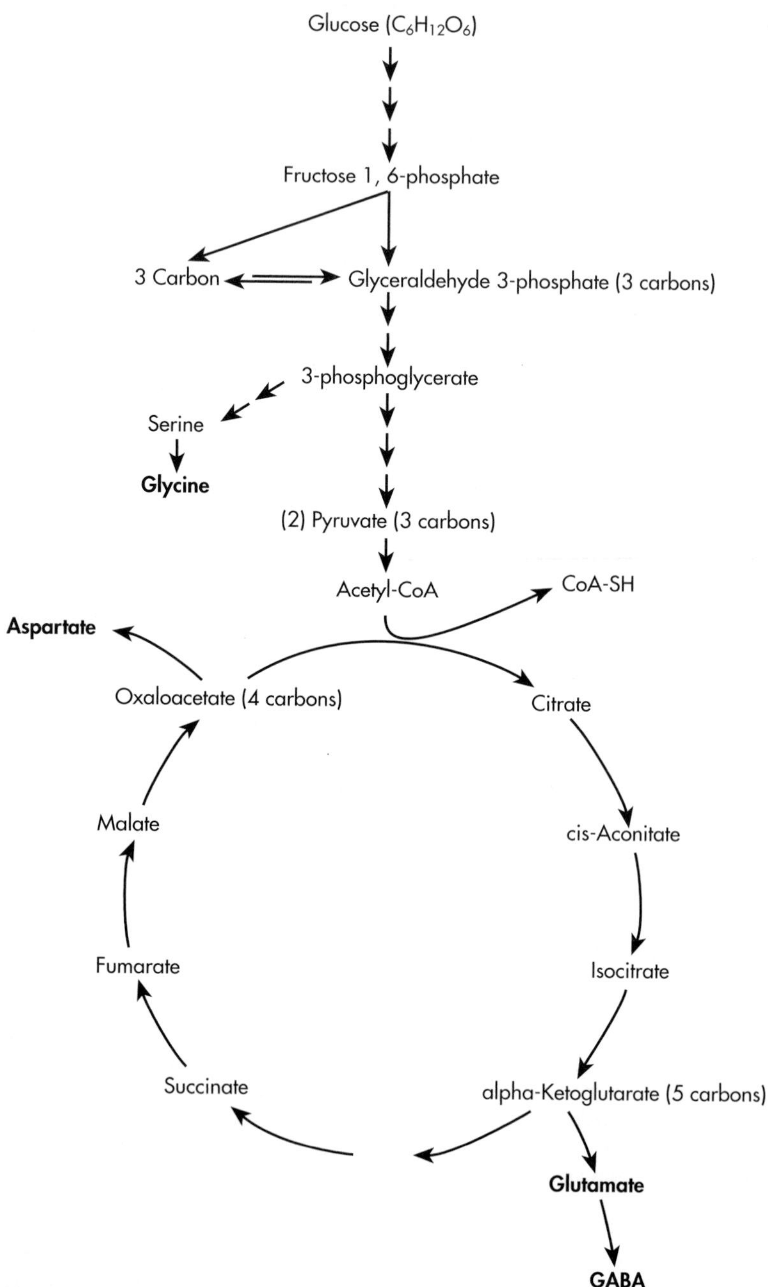

Figure 3-5 Reactions of glycolysis and the citric acid cycle and synthesis of glycine, aspartate, glutamate, and gamma-aminobutyric acid.

the cerebrospinal fluid provides an indicator of the ammonia concentration in the brain. High ammonia concentrations in the brain can lead to coma (McGeer and McGeer, 1989).

Aspartate is found in the hippocampus and the dorsal root ganglion. Its activity is similar to that of glutamate. Asparate is synthesized (Figure 3-5) directly from oxaloacetic acid, again a primary chemical in the citric acid cycle. It is difficult to distinguish between glutamate and asparate by means of current technology.

NEUROTRANSMITTERS AND NEUROCHEMISTRY OF BEHAVIOR

It is important to recognize that all neurotransmitters and pathways have multiple functions. Only a few are discussed in this review. Further, more than one neurotransmitter may be released at any synapse. When this occurs the synergistic effect or a differential effect may take place. Finally, receptors act to select which transmitter will activate or inhibit the neuron. The following section discusses some of these neurotransmitters with respect to the neurochemistry of behavior. Additionally, the functional neuroanatomic pathways rising from the reticular formation (see Chapter 2, Neuroanatomy) are known to be involved in the integration, modulation, and regulation of several neurotransmitter systems, for example, acetylcholine, norepinephrine, serotonin, and dopamine. Our basic understanding of these systems is useful when considering the actions and effect of pharmacologic agents. Moreover, current neurophysiologic studies, postmortem studies, and molecular genetics studies are seeking to further clarify the role of these systems in the behavioral neurobiology of pharmacologic agents.

In this chapter neurochemical systems have already been characterized with respect to their neurochemical transmission and communication between presynaptic and postsynaptic receptors. Additionally, the potential for transmission at the postsynaptic receptor site through ion channels and the influence of second messenger systems have been discussed. Also, projections arising from the reticular formation, including the locus ceruleus, dopaminergic tracts such as the arcuate nucleus, and serotonergic tracts, including raphe nuclei, have been presented in Table 3-1 and are important in understanding the proposed effects of psychotropic drugs.

The neurochemistry of many behaviors and mechanisms of several classes of psychotropic agents may best be understood through an appreciation of the interaction among the neuroanatomic structures and the interplay of the neurochemical systems, especially in the case of certain pharmacologic compounds that have been discovered or developed along these conceptual frameworks. For example, the initial observations further leading to the neurochemical explanations of many behaviors were stimulated in the 1950s by Labrec, a French anesthesiologist, who was trying to invent a cocktail to relieve anxiety and stress associated with surgical procedures. In Labrec's work with a chemist to invent a new antihistamine, chlorpromazine was identified as the active ingredient of his cocktail. The cocktail was then given to schizophrenic and psychotic patients in a French asylum and shown not only to calm the patients but also to reduce the other symptoms, that is, hallucinosis, paranoia, and agitation, in these patients. This experiment resulted in the dramatic changes discussed in Chapter 1, Psychiatric Care and Contemporary Treatment, and many historical advances; in addition, it led to the neurochemical studies of chlorpromazine and other chemicals, which were believed to be possibly useful in clinical practice.

Chlorpromazine, from the phenothiazine class, or family, was found to be similar in structure to dopamine, especially in its ring structure and tailed nitrogen. The molecule was found to fit, or interact, with the dopamine receptor and to act as a dopamine antagonist, preventing transmission of dopamine impulses believed responsible for schizophrenic and other psychotic symptoms. It was observed that a concentration of approximately 600 mg per day was necessary for the desired clinical effect, probably because of its relatively low affinity for the dopamine receptors. Other drugs in the phenothiazine family found later included triflupromazine, trifluoperazine, fluphenazine, and others that were much more potent, had a higher affinity for the receptor, and were much more likely to be clinically effective at lower doses. Two potent nonphenothiazine drugs were haloperidol and thiothixene. These agents are discussed fully in Chapter 4, Schizophrenia and Other Psychoses.

Further study of the phenothiazine family of agents resulted in additional delineation of the dopaminergic tracts. The mesolimbic and mesocortical tracts were identified as the main ones responsible for schizophrenic behavior. The nigrostriatal tract was involved in symptoms that were identified with Parkinson's disease. Thus when chlorpromazine is administered to a patient, it interacts with dopamine receptors in the terminal portion of the striatum and can result in extrapyramidal symptoms that mimic Parkinson's disease. These symptoms are referred to as *pseudoparkinsonian* symptoms and include dyskinetic movement, dystonia, and other frank parkinsonian symptoms. The development of tardive dyskinesia, which is discussed in detail in Chapter 4, Schizophrenia and Other Psychoses, as well as other undesired effects, results from the "upregulating" of dopamine receptors, particularly D_2 receptors.

As with the discovery of antipsychotic agents, the antidepressant drugs were discovered serendipitously. After the success of treating patients with tuberculosis using isonicotinic acid was established, pharmaceutical companies began seeking to create similar compounds. This research resulted in the development of iproniazid, which underwent clinical trials. The moods of tuberculous patients who had been taking this drug for 3 to 4 months improved significantly, although the tuberculosis did not. Iproniazid, which acts as a monoamine oxidase (MAO) enzyme inhibitor, had many effects on neurotransmitters, including the potentiation of norepinephrine and serotonin, neurotransmitters thought to play a key role in depression. Because it took 3 to 4 months to see these effects, these drugs did not have significant abuse potential and this class of drug (MAO inhibitors) was later developed as a conventional antidepressant (see Chapter 5, Mood Disorders). Another pharmaceutical company attempted to develop alternative forms of chlorpromazine and developed a compound called mipradine. When they tested this drug, they found that it was also successful for treating depression. This compound was the predecessor to the tricyclic antidepressants and was later noted to block the reuptake of various biogenic amines.

The discovery of the MAO inhibitors and tricyclic antidepressants resulted in further consideration of depression as an illness in which both mood and behavior were affected and induced by neurochemical changes. The biogenic amine theory of depression resulted from this thinking. Subsequent hypotheses included the serotonin hypothesis, which was developed after it was found that the concentrations of specific serotonin metabolites (5-hydroxyindoleacetic acid [5-HIAA]) in the cerebral spinal fluid of depressed patients was biomodally distributed. This simply means that one group had normal levels of 5-HIAA, and the other had low 5-HIAA levels. This finding indicated that low serotonin synthesis and turnover were occurring in one subgroup of depressed patients. Because the vast majority of serotonin is produced in the central nervous system by the raphe nuclei that supply the limbic system and frontal cortical system, this distribution made serotonin a likely suspect in the cause of depressive illness. Tricyclic antidepressants prevented the reuptake of this neurochemical from the synapse by the presynaptic terminal, which in turn increased the relative amount of serotonin in the synapse and corrected the relative deficiency. The initial result was a greater-than-normal response because of the supersensitivity of the serotonin receptor site. In short, these receptor sites were hungry for serotonin and these pharmacologic agents, the MAO inhibitors and the tricyclic antidepressants, enabled those receptors to have an increased supply.

Subsequently the norepinephrine hypothesis of depression was developed. The major nuclei of the norepinephrine production are found within the locus ceruleus. This structure, the virtual command-and-control center of norepinephrine, sends projections to the limbic system and cortex in a manner similar to that of serotonin. Norepinephrine was also deemed to be important in certain depressive syndromes, particularly when a decrement of norepinephrine production was occurring. It was proposed that certain agents, in particular, tricyclic antidepressants, acted with norepinephrine as they did with serotonin. That is, they blocked the reuptake of norepinephrine at the presynaptic terminal and supersensitized the postsynaptic membrane. Thus a greater synaptic supply of norepinephrine was available.

The action of the tricyclic antidepressants showed a lag time of approximately 2 to 5 weeks before any effects of treatment were seen. Furthermore, the amount of neurotransmitter in the synapse increased *immediately* because of the block of the reuptake by the presynaptic terminal. However, the changes in the sensitivity of the postsynaptic receptors occurred *over time.* This seems to be the critical step in how this class of agents has its clinical effect. Additionally, effects at differential receptor sites are now thought to be critical to the clinical efficacy of these and other antidepressant compounds, including novel agents such as bupropion and newer agents such as the selective serotonin reuptake inhibitors.

Many other agents that affect neurotransmitter systems outlined in this chapter are discussed in chapters specific to disorders. For example, generalized anxiety disorder that occurs in patients with persistent, severe, and disabling anxiety involves the GABA–benzodiazepine chloride system. Psychostimulants such as amphetamines and methylphenidate (Ritalin) may cause brief periods of euphoria but are more commonly used to treat attention deficit hyperactivity disorder. These drugs increase the amount of synaptic dopamine, suggesting that this disorder may be caused by too little dopamine. It has also been noted that when psychostimulants are given to schizophrenic patients, their condition worsens significantly.

Other connections between neurotransmitter systems and identified psychiatric disorders include the role of ACh and other cholinergic systems in memory processes. The degeneration of cholinergic neurons of the basal nucleus of Meynert into the hippocampus is one of the many features found in Alzheimer's disease. Endorphins and enkephalins are known to be important in pain perception. Cholecystokinin and neurotensin may also be important in schizophrenia. Somatostatin may be found to be deficient in Alzheimer's disease. These neurochemical systems, as they are being explored, have certainly furthered our understanding of the biology of behavior, including the cause and course of many significant neuropsychiatric syndromes.

A final discussion of neurochemistry and the neurotransmitter systems as they relate to psychotropic agents might include current genetic and postmortem studies. For example, it is known that there is a significant increase in D_2 receptors in the CNS in schizophrenics, and in patients with Alzheimer's disease, plaques and tangles may disrupt neurotransmitter systems. The core symptoms of both schizophrenia and Alzheimer's disease, as well as a host of psychiatric complications, are thought to be caused by these neurochemical deviations from normal.

The introduction of computerized tomography, magnetic resonance imaging, and other imaging techniques, including single photon emission computerized tomography and positron emission spectroscopy, may also be useful in examining structural and functional defects in individuals who have major psychiatric syndromes. These technologies have also been useful, through the use of radioisotopes, in the study of the influence of pharmacologic agents on certain receptor sites and structures. These technologies allow us to view the inside of the brain, including the ventricular system, receptor sites, and brain tissues. Positron emission spectroscopy scanning with the use of radioisotopes, which are taken up readily into the cells, may also enable the evaluation and assessment of metabolic disturbances and the relative value of pharmacologic agents in correcting these defects. For example, obsessive-compulsive disorder is known to be characterized by the hypermetabolism of the striatum and frontal cortex. Drugs such as clomipramine (Anafranil) and fluvoxamine (Luvox) are known to correct this functional defect.

Molecular genetics, through which certain disorders based on specific chromosomal defects can be identified, may be useful in developing certain genetic pharmacologic and chemical agents that can correct these defects. The identification of disease genes, in combination with molecular tools, may result in the development of more effective treatments for mental illness. Also, the availability of genotype studies will allow identification of individuals at risk for neuropsychiatric disorders. Identification of disease genes and/or proteins with potential roles in psychiatric disorders could enable delineation of (1) regulation by specific psychotropic drugs, (2) anatomic specificity, that is, expression or drug regulation in specific brain regions implicated for a psychiatric disorder, and (3) differential expression or regulation in genotypic annuals serving as a model for psychiatric disorders. These techniques may allow the discovery and development of novel drugs and targeted actions. Cloning of genes, regulation of genes and transgenic models, that is, linkage studies, may result in psychotropic drugs that prevent the expression of psychiatric disorders (Friedmann, 1989). This could certainly open up further development of chemical treatments for psychiatric disorders. Identifying the gene, cloning it, getting the DNA to express its protein product, and figuring out how the protein affects behavior may ultimately correct abnormal function. This is indeed an interesting time in the neurochemistry of behavior and is largely accountable for the National Institutes of Health deeming the 1990s "the decade of the brain."

REFERENCES

Crill WE: The milieu of the central nervous system. In Patton HD et al, editors: *Textbook of physiology,* vol 1, Philadelphia, 1989, WB Saunders.

Detwiller PB, Crill WE: Synaptic transmission. In Patton HD et al, editors: *Textbook of physiology,* vol 1, Philadelphia, 1989, WB Saunders.

Dorsa DM: Neuropeptides as neurotransmitters. In Patton HD et al, editors: *Textbook of physiology,* vol 2, Philadelphia, 1989, WB Saunders.

Erulkar SD: Chemically mediated synaptic transmission: an overview. In Siegel GJ et al, editors: *Basic neurochemistry,* New York, 1989, Raven.

Friedmann T: Progress toward human gene therapy, *Science* 244:1275-1281, 1989.

Gottlieb DI: GABAergic neurons, *Scientific American* 258:82, 1988.

Hille B: Neuromuscular transmission. In Patton HD et al, editors: *Textbook of physiology,* vol 1, Philadelphia, 1989, WB Saunders.

Holaday JW: *Endogenous opioids and their receptors: current concepts,* Kalamazoo, Mich, 1985, Upjohn.

Hughes H et al: Identification of two related pentapeptides from the brain with potent opiate agonist activity, *Nature* 258:577, 1975.

Hyman, SE, Nestler EJ: *The molecular foundations of psychiatry,* Washington D.C., 1993, American Psychiatric Press, Inc.

Kelly DD: Central representation of pain and analgesia. In Kandel ER, Schwartz JH, editors: *Principles of neural science,* New York, 1985, Elsevier.

Kutchai HC: Cellular physiology. In Berne RM, Levy MN, editors: *Physiology,* ed 3, St Louis, 1993, Mosby.

Mathews CK, Van Holde KE: *Biochemistry,* Redwood City, Calif, 1990, Benjamin-Cummings.

McGeer PL, McGeer EG: Amino acid neurotransmitters. In Siegel GJ et al, editors: *Basic neurochemistry,* New York, 1989, Raven.

Patton HD: The autonomic nervous system. In Patton HD et al, editors: *Textbook of physiology,* vol 1, Philadelphia, 1989, WB Saunders.

Schwartz JH: Chemical messengers: small molecules and peptides. In Kandel ER, Schwartz JH, editors: *Principles of neural science,* New York, 1985, Elsevier.

Shepard GM: *Neurobiology,* New York, 1983, Oxford University.

Simon EJ, Miller JB: Opioid peptides and opioid receptors. In Siegel GJ et al, editors: *Basic neurochemistry,* New York, 1989, Raven.

Taylor P, Brown JH: Acetylcholine. In Siegel GJ et al, editors: *Basic neurochemistry,* New York, 1989, Raven.

Weiner N, Molinoff PB: Catecholamines. In Siegel GJ et al, editors: *Basic neurochemistry,* New York, 1989, Raven.

UNIT II

Drugs Used in the Treatment of Mental Disorders

CHAPTER 4

Schizophrenia and Other Psychoses

"At home I was living a nightmare. I was totally afraid to move in bed. I seldom felt more terrified at any time in my life than I did that time. The slightest movement seemed to arouse the anger of the voices. I lived in shock 2 or 3 weeks, was unable to get some peace, and often came in late for work in the morning. I thought that someone in the office had bugged me, and the bugs, or voices, bothered me during work. Ultimately I was fired. . ."

Suzanne Jeffery, 1993.

HISTORICAL CONSIDERATIONS

Schizophrenia is the diagnostic category defined by the *Diagnostic and Statistical Manual of Mental Disorders, Fourth Edition (DSM-IV)* criteria (American Psychiatric Association, 1994) that describes a psychiatric disorder characterized by social withdrawal and disturbances in thought, motor behavior, and interpersonal functioning. The *DSM-IV* criteria are depicted in Box 4-1. Individuals with schizophrenia may appear dull and colorless, dependent and apathetic, emotionally isolative, or agitated and threatening; these and other characteristic symptoms determine which subtype is assigned, that is, paranoid, catatonic, disorganized, undifferentiated, or residual (Box 4-2). The cost in human suffering is incalculable. It is known that about 1% of the population meets conventional criteria for schizophrenia (Regier et al, 1993; Rice, Kelman, and Miller, 1992). Economic costs are estimated in the tens of billions of dollars each year.

Morel was the first to assign a name to the psychiatric symptoms described in the preceding paragraph . In 1856, while treating an adolescent boy, he used the phrase *démence précoce* (precocious senility) to describe the group of observed symptoms. Over the next several years Kahlbaum, Hecker, and Kraepelin contributed the diagnostic terms *catatonia, hebephrenia,* and *paranoia,* respectively. Kraepelin, the best scientist of the group, engaged in a rigorous study of a variety of disorders now recognized as schizophrenia. He noted the symptomatic commonalities among catatonia, hebephrenia, and paranoia, and in 1896 grouped them under the label *dementia praecox.* Kraepelin (1919) believed schizophrenia resulted from neuropathologic disturbance and attempted to distinguish florid symptoms from those characterized by persistent losses or deficits. Kraepelin envisioned a progressive deteriorating course for patients suffering from the latter. These individuals, he recognized, experienced a disabling trajectory of impairment and had little hope of recovery (Andreasen et al, 1990). Kraepelin described the fundamental deficit in schizophrenia as "annihilation of the will" (Lewine, 1990).

The term *schizophrenia* was not developed until the 1900s when Bleuler used it in his book subtitled *The Group of Schizophrenias.* Bleuler (1950) argued against the use of the term *dementia praecox.* Because schizophrenia does not always follow a course of deterioration, *dementia* is an inappropriate term, and because schizophrenia does not always begin in early life, *praecox* is inappropriate as well. Bleuler's contribution

Box 4-1 DSM-IV Criteria for Schizophrenia

A. Characteristic symptoms (at least two of the following):
   Delusions
   Hallucinations
   Disorganized speech
   Grossly disorganized or catatonic behavior
   Negative symptoms
B. Social/occupational dysfunction: work, interpersonal, and self-care functioning is below the level achieved prior to onset
C. Duration: continuous signs of the disturbance for at least 6 months
D. Schizoaffective and mood disorders are not present and are not responsible for the signs and symptoms
E. Not caused by substance abuse or a general medical disorder

Modified from the American Psychiatric Association: *Diagnostic and statistical manual of mental disorders,* ed 4, Washington, DC, 1994, The Association.

broadened Kraepelin's concept by focusing on symptoms rather than strictly clinical outcomes. Kraepelin's paradigm of schizophrenia did not incorporate recovery. For example, on finding an individual who had "recovered," Kraepelin believed the individual had never actually experienced schizophrenia. Because of Bleuler's wider grouping, pessimism eased, and some clinicians began to record improvements in their patients. Bleuler, largely influenced by Freud and other psychodynamic theorists, explored psychologic explanations for schizophrenia, yet he never abandoned the biologic theories of Kraepelin.

In recent years a resurgence of interest in biologic research has resulted in renewed respect for Kraepelin's work. In fact, even the dated term *dementia praecox* is experiencing renewed support. Kopelowicz and Bidder (1992) suggest that it is the best diagnostic term to describe about 10% of the schizophrenic population who do experience a decidedly deteriorative course. In contrast, the introduction of the *Diagnostic and Statistical Manual of Mental Disorders, Third Edition (DSM-III)* in 1980 resulted in the view that Bleuler's contributions, albeit significant, had softened the diagnostic criteria and obscured the deteriorating course of the illness. This "softening" possibly led to overdiagnosis, particularly in blacks and lower socioeconomic groups (American Psychiatric Association, 1980; Jones and Gray, 1986).

DSM-IV TERMINOLOGY AND CRITERIA

Science attempts to classify, categorize, and subordinate. Beginning with Morel in 1856 and continuing until today, psychiatric scientists have attempted to divide schizophrenia into homogeneous subtypes (Kendler, Gruenberg, and Tsuany, 1988). Early categorizing efforts yielded the subtypes catatonic, hebephrenic, paranoid, and *simple* schizophrenia. Paranoid and catatonic subtypes are still reflected in the current official diagnostic classification system given in Box 4-2.

The most clinically useful subtyping approach, in our view, is derived from Kraepelin's work. As noted above, Kraepelin differentiated between florid symptoms (positive symptoms) and those characterized by loss/deficit (negative symptoms). Biologically oriented diagnosticians such as Strauss, Carpenter, and Bartko (1974),

Box 4-2 DSM-IV Criteria for Schizophrenia Subtypes

Paranoid:
A. Preoccupation with one or more delusions or frequent auditory hallucinations
B. None of the following is prominent: disorganized speech, disorganized behavior, flat or inappropriate affect, catatonic behavior

Disorganized:
A. All of the following are prominnent: disorganized speech, disorganized behavior, flat or inappropriate affect
B. Does not meet criteria of catatonic type

Catatonic:
At least two of the following are present:
A. Motoric immobility, waxy flexibility, or stupor
B. Excessive motor activity (purposeless)
C. Extreme negativism or mutism
D. Peculiar movements, stereotypy of movements, prominent mannerisms, or prominent grimacing
E. Echolalia or echopraxia

Undifferentiated:
Characteristic symptoms are present, but criteria for paranoid, catatonic, or disorganized subtypes are not met.

Residual:
A. Characteristic symptoms (criterion A) are no longer present; criteria are unmet for paranoid, catatonic, or disorganized subtypes
B. There is continuing evidence of disturbance, such as the presence of negative symptoms or criterion A symptoms, in an attenuated form (e.g., odd beliefs, unusual perceptual experiences)

Modified from the American Psychiatric Association: *Diagnostic and statistical manual of mental disorders,* ed 4, Washington, DC, 1994, The Association.

Andreasen and Olsen (1982), Andreasen et al (1990), Crow (1980), and others have developed two subtypes, positive and negative schizophrenia. This dichotomy is based on well-designed research. Positive, or type 1, schizophrenia presents a different constellation of symptoms than does negative, or type 2, schizophrenia. Type 1 is positive in the sense that symptoms are an embellishment of normal cognition and perception: the symptoms are "additional." Positive symptoms are believed to be caused by a subcortical dopaminergic process (too much dopamine) affecting limbic areas. Type 2 is labeled negative because symptoms are essentially an absence of what should be, that is, lack of affect, lack of energy, and so forth. Type 2 is thought to be nondopaminergic or perhaps even hypodopaminergic in frontal cortical areas (Ereshefsky and Lacombe, 1993) and to be caused by cortical structural changes. Cortical changes such as cerebral atrophy and increased ventricular vol-

Box 4-3 Symptoms and Pathoanatomy of Positive and Negative Schizophrenia

Type I
Positive symptoms
- Hallucinations
- Delusions
- Abnormal thought form
- Bizarre behavior
- Develops over a short time

Pathoanatomy
- Hyperdopaminergic process
- No structural changes

Type II
Negative symptoms
- Alogia (poverty of speech)
- Affective flattening
- Anhedonia (lack of pleasure)
- Attentional impairment
- Avolition (poor motivation)
- Asocial behavior
- Anergia (lack of energy)

Pathoanatomy
- Nondopaminergic process
- Structural changes:
  - Increased ventricular brain ratios (VBRs)
  - Decreased cerebral blood flow (CBF)

ume are similar to those changes found in Alzheimer's disease. Neurobiologic changes reported in the literature include decreased cerebral blood flow, a hypometabolic state (particularly in the dorsolateral prefrontal cortex), increased ventricular-brain ratios, a 5% reduction in brain weight, a slight decrease in brain length, and neuronal loss in cortical areas (Roberts, Leigh, and Weinberger, 1993). Basic differences between type 1 and type 2 are listed in Box 4-3.

According to biologic theory, antipsychotic drugs (drugs that effectively block dopamine receptors) are likely to be more beneficial for individuals with positive schizophrenia (a hyperdopaminergic process). Because negative schizophrenia is more related to a structural defect and not as specifically related to disturbances in dopamine function, the use of dopamine-blocking drugs or traditional antipsychotics is relatively less effective and their continuous administration more controversial (Johnson, 1990). Accordingly, the more flagrant the psychotic symptoms characteristic of positive schizophrenia, the greater the likelihood of a positive response to an antipsychotic drug.

ANTIPSYCHOTIC DRUGS

Antipsychotic drugs are used to treat the symptoms of psychosis and various other manifestations of mental illness. These drugs are particularly important in the prevention of relapse, but rates of compliance are low. Table 4-1 presents a comparative description of these drugs. Chronic mental illness, specifically, schizophrenia accompanied by symptoms of florid psychosis, and acute agitation in mania or in other psychotic or motor-disturbed patients are the major targets of these compounds (Harris, 1981; Overall et al, 1989). Other uses are acknowledged and discussed briefly in this chapter.

Table 4-1 Antipsychotic Drugs

Antipsychotic agent	Approximate equivalent oral dose (mg)*	Adult daily dosage range (mg)	Sedation	Extrapyramidal symptoms	Anticholinergic effects	Orthostatic hypotension	Concentration (ng/mL)
Phenothiazines							
Aliphatic phenothiazines							
Chlorpromazine (Thorazine)	100	30-800	+++	++	++	+++	30-500
Promazine (Sparine)	200	40-1200	++	++	+++	++	
Triflupromazine (Vesprin)	25	60-150	+++	++	+++	++	
Piperidine phenothiazines							
Mesoridazine (Serentil)	50	30-400	+++	+	+++	++	
Thioridazine (Mellaril)	100	150-800	+++	+	+++	+++	
Piperazine phenothiazines							
Fluphenazine (Prolixin, Permitil)	2	0.5-40	+	+++	+	+	0.13-2.8
Perphenazine (Trilafon)	10	12-64	+	+++	+	+	0.8-1.2
Trifluoperazine (Stelazine)	5	5-80	+	+++	+	+	
Butyrophenone							
Haloperidol (Haldol)	2	1-15	+	+++	+	+	5-20

Thioxanthenes							
Chlorprothixene (Taractan)	100	75-600	+++	++	++	++	
Thiothixene (Navane)	4	8-30	+	+++	+	+	2-57
Dibenzoxazepine							
Loxapine (Loxitane)	10	20-250	++	+++	+	++	
Dihydroindolone							
Molindone (Moban)	10	50-225	+	+++	+	+	
Dibenzodiazepine							
Clozapine (Clozaril)	50	300-900	+++	+	+++	+++	>350†
Benzisoxazole							
Risperidone (Risperdal)	N/A	4-16	+	0/+	+	+	
Diphenylbutylpiperidine							
Pimozide (Orap)	0.3-0.5	1-10	++	+++	++	+	

*Many clinicians believe that for most schizophrenic patients the effective dosage should be at or above 400 mg/day of chlorpromazine or its equivalent. (From Beresford TP, Hall RCW: *Psychiatr Med* 8[4]:1, 1990.)

†Perry JP et al found that 64% of treatment-resistant schizophrenic patients improved. (From Perry JP et al: *Am J Psychiatry* 148[2]:236, 1991.)

Incidence of side effects: +++ = high; ++ = moderate; + = low; 0/+ = very low.

History

In 1950 French scientists synthesized chlorpromazine (Thorazine) from another phenothiazine, promethazine (Phenergan), while attempting to develop an antihistamine (Ayd, 1991). This new medication caused mild antihistaminic effects but was highly sedating. Labroit, a physician, used the drug to calm anxious surgery patients. He observed, ". . . a slight tendency to sleep and above all a disinterest for what goes on around him" (Ayd, 1991). Not long after, two other French physicians, Delay and Deniker, administered chlorpromazine to 38 patients. The discovery of antipsychotic drugs is attributed to these men.

Chlorpromazine was introduced in public hospitals in about 1954. Before the use of antipsychotic drugs in these facilities, hundreds of thousands of patients with severe psychiatric disturbances were hospitalized under sometimes poor conditions. Social isolation, physical restraint, and occasional treatment with aggressive measures, for example, psychosurgery or lobotomy, were employed. These treatments rarely restored the patient to a state that enabled productive social or occupational functioning, and affected individuals often were unable to interact reasonably with others.

Although some of the hopes and expectations for antipsychotic drugs have not been realized, these drugs have had a dramatic impact on psychiatric care and therapeutic outlook. Their use in the psychiatric community has resulted in earlier and more effective treatments; many of the ineffective or restrictive treatments have been abandoned, and the number of long-term hospitalizations has declined from more than 558,000 patients in 1955, before the widespread use of antipsychotic drugs, to 103,000 in 1992 (Lamb, 1994). In short, patients who previously would have been hospitalized are now living and functioning well socially and occupationally, largely because of the efficacy of antipsychotic drug treatment. However, the large homeless population (estimated at 600,000 on any given night) includes many previously hospitalized, mentally ill persons (Federal Task Force on Homelessness and Severe Mental Illness, 1992). This reality indicates that psychopharmacologic treatment alone is not enough and is ideally combined with other social, behavioral, and psychotherapeutic approaches.

The drugs discussed in this chapter are generally called antipsychotic agents, but they also have been referred to as *major tranquilizers, ataractics* (that is, drugs that produce calmness or serenity), or *neuroleptics*, because they can also produce neurologic symptoms (Keltner, 1993). Further, these drugs cause a certain apathy toward the environment and a diminution of emotion and affect (Olin, 1995).

Three Classification Systems: Molecular, Potency, Typicality

Antipsychotic drugs can be generally classified in three ways. The first and most accurate system is based on chemical and structural class. These drugs have diverse chemical properties and are considered equieffective, that is, they all effectively reduce various psychiatric symptoms. Drug differences are mainly attributed to a drug's potential for sedation and other side effects. For instance, because of chemical class differences, the type, intensity, and frequency of side effects vary among individual antipsychotic drugs. Also, when a drug is "not working," a switch to a drug of a different class is appropriate to take advantage of these molecular differences. There are eight distinct chemical classes for antipsychotic drugs.

A second means of classifying antipsychotic drugs is based on potency. This system is admittedly less "scientific" than subgrouping by means of chemical class but has gathered support because of its clinical utility. Essentially, some drugs are required in much higher doses to achieve clinical results similar to those of other drugs. For example, about 100 mg of chlorpromazine is required to achieve the same clinical effect as 2 mg of haloperidol (Haldol). Drugs that are one to four times as potent as chlorpromazine are designated as *low potency,* and those 20 or more times as potent, *as high potency* (Gomez and Gomez, 1990). Accordingly, chlorpromazine is referred to as a low-potency antipsychotic drug and haloperidol as a high-potency one.

In clinical practice it appears that low-potency antipsychotic drugs produce more frequent and intense anticholinergic side effects and are more likely to produce orthostatic symptoms; in contrast, high-potency antipsychotic drugs are more likely to produce more frequent and intense extrapyramidal side effects (EPSEs). Admittedly, this classification system is less inclusive and leaves a few drugs in a "medium potency" group from which this generalization cannot be made. Interestingly, anticholinergic agents are used to treat EPSEs, and antipsychotic drugs with more potent anticholinergic effects are known to produce fewer EPSEs. In other words, low-potency agents seem to have a "built-in" treatment for extrapyramidal side effects.

The third approach to classifying antipsychotics contrasts traditional or typical antipsychotics with newer or atypical antipsychotics. Typical antipsychotic agents include all of those drugs developed from the advent of chlorpromazine until about 1990—the year clozapine (Clozaril) was released. Two atypical antipsychotics, clozapine and risperidone (Risperdal) are now available. Typical antipsychotic drugs block dopamine D-2 receptors in the limbic system and striatum, thus accounting for both their antipsychotic and extrapyramidal effects (Matsubara et al, 1993). Atypical antipsychotic drugs have been defined as those with low capacity to cause EPSEs (Borison et al, 1992) or sedation (Kerwin, 1994) and that antagonize serotonin 5HT-2 receptors (Ereshefsky and Lacombe, 1993; Roth, Ciaranello, and Meltzer, 1992). Although this definition continues to evolve, the latter property (5HT-2 antagonism) appears to have the most support. Because serotonin can inhibit dopamine release, drugs that block serotonin have the potential to therapeutically liberate dopamine.

Neurochemical Theory of Schizophrenia

Although various theories of schizophrenia exist and are vigorously debated, the neurochemical theory affords the best explanation for the effectiveness of antipsychotic agents (Thompson, 1990). This view is referred to as the *dopamine theory.* Yaryura-Tobias, Diamond, and Merlis (1970) observed that L-dopa worsened the symptoms of schizophrenia. Coupling this observation with the fact that the dopamine antagonist chlorpromazine was an effective antipsychotic, Matthysse (1977) conceptualized the so-called dopamine theory of schizophrenia. This theory states that schizophrenia and psychotic symptoms, for example, hallucinations and delusions, are caused by increased levels of dopamine in the brain. The atypical antipsychotics, through their more novel mechanism of action, have prompted researchers to rethink this traditional view of schizophrenia as a purely hyperdopaminergic disorder (Remington, 1993). More recent studies indicate a role for another neurochemical, serotonin, and hence a role for antiserotonergic drugs such as clozapine and risperidone. The notion of a serotonergic process was first discussed by Woolley and Shaw in 1954 but was overshadowed by the more conceptually pleasing dopamine theory until recent years.

The addition of a serotonergic understanding clarifies the clinical and neurochemical question: Why do traditional antipsychotic drugs help patients with positive symptoms, for example, hallucinations and delusions more than patients with negative symptoms, for example, flat affect and apathy? Essentially, positive schizo-

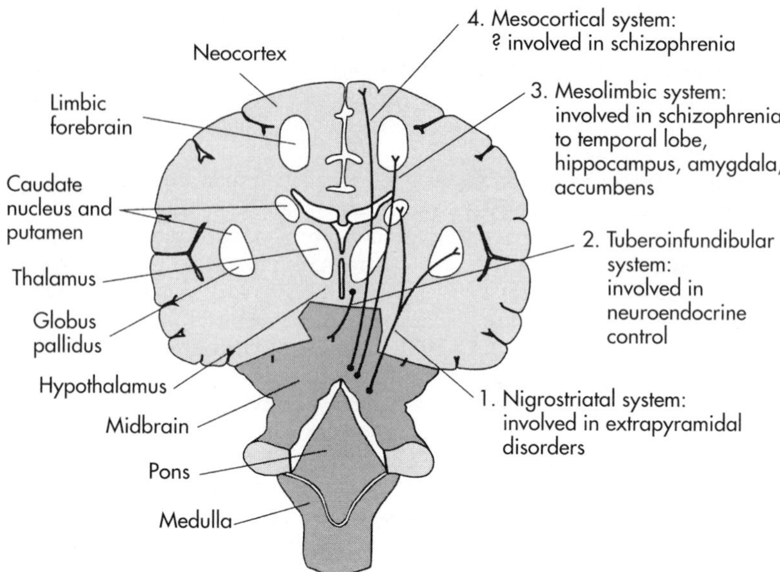

Figure 4-1 Four dopaminergic tracts important for understanding the actions of antipsychotic drugs. **1,** Nigrostriatal system: when antipsychotic drugs antagonize this system, a pseudoparkinsonism or extrapyramidal effect occurs. **2,** Tuberoinfundibular system: when antipsychotic drugs antagonize this system, the dopamine inhibition of the hypothalamic hormone prolactin is lifted and can lead to gynecomastia and galactorrhea. **3,** Mesolimbic system: when antipsychotic drugs antagonize this system, a decrease in the symptoms of schizophrenia occurs (primarily positive symptoms). This is the effect that makes these drugs antipsychotic. **4,** Mesocortical system: when antipsychotic drugs antagonize this system, it is thought the disorder can be worsened in some patients. Risperidone is thought to antagonize serotonin in the cortex which, in turn, liberates dopamine there. That is, it is suspected that a mesocortical hypodopaminergic state may contribute to negative symptoms. Much remains to be understood about the role, if any, of the mesocortical dopaminergic tract in schizophrenia. (From Roberts GW, Leigh PN, Weinberger DR: *Neuropsychiatric disorders,* London, 1993, Wolfe Publishing.)

phrenia may be a hyperdopaminergic disorder of the limbic region of the brain, and negative schizophenia may be a hypodopaminergic disorder of the frontal cortex. Hence drugs that block dopamine in limbic areas (D-2 receptors primarily) will modify positive symptoms, and drugs that block serotonin 5HT-2 in cortical areas will liberate dopamine. Typical antipsychotics antagonize dopamine receptors limbically, and atypical antipsychotics antagonize serotonin 5HT-2 receptors in the cortex. Figure 4-1 briefly describes the dopamine antagonizing effects of antipsychotic agents on four major dopaminergic tracts.

Pharmacologic Effects (Therapeutic Effects)

Chlorpromazine and the other antipsychotic drugs are used primarily to treat psychiatric disorders, specifically, schizophrenia and other mental illness associated with psychotic or motor disturbances. Well-designed clinical research has produced impressive evidence for their effectiveness. Not all patients respond, but many who do have the potential to live their lives unencumbered by the oppressive symptoms of psychosis. Psychosis is a phenomenon of brain activity. Therefore a drug that affects psychosis acts primarily in the central nervous system (CNS). Tolerance to an antipsychotic effect is uncommon. Peripheral nervous system (PNS) effects are discussed in the section on side effects (undesired effects). Chlorpromazine, a phenothiazine and the prototype antipsychotic agent, is discussed extensively, and a more condensed discussion of the other drugs is included.

Central nervous system effects. Central nervous system effects include sedation, emotional quieting, and psychomotor slowing; thus at one time these drugs were generally referred to as major tranquilizers. This emotional quieting enables the patient to take advantage of other forms of therapeutic intervention, for example, the therapeutic relationship and the therapeutic milieu.

Other CNS effects include a sedating quality that decreases insomnia and sleep disturbances frequently observed in persons with psychoses. Whether the sedating effect itself or being freed from disturbing thoughts, or a combination of the two, enhances sleep is not precisely known. Not all antipsychotic drugs are equally sedating. High-potency drugs are less sedating than are the low-potency drugs. For example, haloperidol and fluphenazine (Prolixin) are not generally sedating yet are quite effective. Thus the effectiveness of antipsychotic agents results from more than just their tranquilizing qualities.

Psychiatric Symptoms Modified by Antipsychotic Drugs

Antipsychotic drugs are prescribed because other people note a patient's behavior to be disturbed (objective symptoms) or because the individual is experiencing psychotic symptoms (subjective symptoms) and seeks relief. As previously discussed, traditional antipsychotic drugs are effective in treating the positive symptoms of schizophrenia (given in Box 4-3). Positive symptoms include hallucinations, delusions, and to some extent acute motor and thought disturbances. Negative symptoms are less responsive to traditional antipsychotic drug therapy but have proven susceptible to the newer atypical antipsychotics. Negative symptoms include those that develop insidiously such as flat or restricted affect, verbal paucity or laconic speech, and a lack of drive or volitional, goal-directed activity. Unfortunately, neuroleptics can cause apathy, so differentiating a drug effect from negative symptoms can be difficult at times. Improvement in objective and subjective symptoms or in positive and negative signs of schizophrenia is the yardstick by which progress is gauged. Psychotic symptoms associated with other disorders, for example, mania, depression, organic mental syndromes, or disorders of cognitive impairment, may also respond well to antipsychotic drugs.

Perceptual disturbances. As a general rule the more bizarre the behavior associated with psychosis, the more likely that an antipsychotic drug will be found beneficial. Hallucinations and illusions usually diminish or remit with the use of these drugs. Even when symptoms are not fully eradicated, antipsychotic drugs may enable the individual to understand that hallucinations and illusions are, indeed, not real or can be tolerated without influencing behavior.

Thought disturbances. The use of antipsychotic drugs may also improve reasoning and decrease ambivalence and delusions or suspiciousness. Because disturbed reasoning, ambivalence, and delusional thinking may produce frustration and behavioral consequences, an antipsychotic agent can free the patient from these symptoms while improving the ability to communicate and cooperate with others.

Motor disturbances. Individuals with schizophrenia and other psychotic disorders are frequently found to be hyperactive or agitated because of internal turmoil and, perhaps, because of the disturbed neurobiology. Antipsychotic drugs may slow or normalize psychomotor activity. Low-potency drugs such as chlorpromazine are inherently sedating, and this effect may be particularly useful for agitated and combative persons.

Altered consciousness. Mental confusion found among psychotic and schizophrenic patients is possibly caused by the anxiety and disturbed processing of thought associated with psychosis. Some mental health professionals believe these symptoms are among the most disabling. Antipsychotic drugs may be effective in decreasing disturbances of thought and in clearing mental confusion.

Interpersonal disturbances. Schizophrenic patients often have a history of asocial behavior and social withdrawal and may have few if any close personal relationships. Inconsistent relationships with family members are common as well. Individuals with schizophrenia may invest little energy in their appearance and may be oblivious to their behavior. When combined with introspective, self-focused speech and the resultant ineffective communication patterns, isolation is reinforced. Antipsychotic drugs, together with other forms of therapy, may enable patients to become less self-focused and to divert their attention from themselves to others. The socially damaging introspectiveness may simply be caused by the considerable energy expended to maintain some degree of equilibrium in the face of psychologic turmoil. This pattern may parallel the regression and lack of attention given to appearance or behavior when an individual is ill. For the psychotically disturbed individual, antipsychotic drugs often can reduce the inner turmoil, freeing psychic energy for more effective interpersonal relationships and for establishing and maintaining a therapeutic relationship.

Affective disturbance. Affective symptoms alone are not treated with antipsychotic drugs, but flat affect, inappropriate affect, or lability of affect seen in schizophrenia may respond to antipsychotic drug therapy.

Other Uses and Effects

The site of neuronal control of nausea and vomiting is the chemoreceptor trigger zone, which is well supplied by dopaminergic receptors. When these receptors are stimulated with dopamine, nausea and vomiting occur. Because antipsychotic drugs block dopamine, most phenothiazines are effective antiemetics. Prochlorperazine (Compazine) is prescribed primarily for its antiemetic qualities. Chlorpromazine also is used to prevent nausea and vomiting during surgery, for intractable hiccups, and as adjunctive therapy for tetanus. Antipsychotic drugs also block PNS muscarinic acetylcholine receptors and alpha-adrenergic receptors, which are responsible for some of the side effects discussed later.

Pharmacokinetics

Absorption after oral intake of antipsychotics is variable. Peak plasma levels are usually seen within 2 to 4 hours (Olin, 1995). A tranqulizing effect from chlorpromazine occurs within 60 minutes of administering an oral dose and within 10 minutes of giving an intramuscular dose. However, the actual antipsychotic effect may not be realized for several weeks or months. Antipsychotics are highly lipophilic and accumulate in fatty tissue, from which they are released slowly. They also accumulate in regions of high blood supply such as the brain and lungs (Olin, 1995). Traces of metabolites are found in the urine months after therapy has stopped, which may explain why patients who abruptly stop their medication continue to experience an antipsychotic effect for a time. This slow release from fatty stores may also account for noncompliance, because the patient who stops taking this medication does not experience an immediate return of symptoms.

Antipsychotics are highly bound to plasma proteins (91% to 99%) so the proportion that crosses the blood-brain barrier may be negligible, that is, only a fraction of the drug ingested accounts for its effect. Interestingly, antipsychotics may have an increased effect in older individuals who have decreased protein-binding capabilities.

Antipsychotics are metabolized in the liver and have a half-life of 10 to 30 hours or more. Impaired hepatic function extends their half-life and therefore their effect.

Although many individual antipsychotic drugs are available, no one drug is more effective than another. Some patients, however, show a differential and individual response: one patient may respond best to chlorpromazine and another to haloperidol. Therefore the choice of antipsychotic drug is usually based on the physician's preference and experience, for example, the likelihood, based on the patient's previous response to a certain drug, that another drug will be helpful, and an educated guess about the potential for a particular agent to produce unwanted side effects. Because the nurse has prolonged contact with inpatients and periodic contact with outpatients, few psychiatric professionals have a better opportunity to assess both desired and undesired responses that affect the selection of the best drug for a particular patient. Additionally, because nearly half of all orders for antipsychotic medications are written as needed, the nurse may have added reason to evaluate the response to these drugs (Blair, 1990).

Most antipsychotic drugs are available in oral and parenteral forms. Oral administration is the favored route for a variety of reasons, not the least of which is patient preference. Tablets, however, have consistently created a problem because they may be "cheeked." Cheeking occurs when an individual places the tablet to one side of the mouth and pretends to swallow it. Moreover, an estimated 46% of patients, both inpatients and outpatients, take less of their medications than prescribed (Blair, 1990). Noncompliance is perhaps the single most important cause of symptom exacerbation, relapse, and rehospitalization. As shown in Box 4-4, psychiatric patients may not comply with their medical regimen for several reasons, including the stigma of illness or the sick role, paranoid fears of poisoning, or unpleasant reactions or side effects. Many inpatient units use liquid forms of antipsychotic and other psychotropic drugs to reduce noncompliant tendencies. However, liquids or concentrates may have an unpleasant taste and should be diluted. Two other issues related to cheeking and noncompliance are decompensation and hoarding.

For severely disturbed patients, chlorpromazine 25 mg 3 times a day is a usual starting dosage and is typically increased every 1 or 2 days by 20 to 50 mg, up to a daily dose of 400 mg. The daily dose may range from 30 to 800 mg.

Parenteral and depot forms. Another form of administration is the parenteral route (Table 4-2). Parenteral drugs are usually employed to treat acutely dis-

Box 4-4 Issues in Antipsychotic Therapy

Relapse

There is a consensus that about one third of all schizophrenic patients will relapse over a 2-year period, even when taking prescribed levels of antipsychotic drugs. Johnson* suggests that antipsychotic medication be continued for at least 12 months after remission. Among all schizophrenic patients relapse rates are expected to be as high as 50% in the first year and 20% in the second year after hospitalization.†

Noncompliance

Van Puttent,‡ in a much quoted paper, stated that 24% to 63% of outpatients and 15% to 33% of inpatients do not take the prescribed amounts of antipsychotic drugs. In general, extrapyramidal side effects and, specifically, akathisia were the primary cause of noncompliant behavior. Interestingly, in a study by Lund and Frank,† the authors found that psychiatric nurses believe noncompliance to be an educational issue, whereas the patients themselves give many reasons for noncompliant behavior.

*Johnson DAW: *Drugs* 39(4):481, 1990.
†Lund VE, Frank DI: *J Psychosoc Nurs* 29(7):6, 1991.
‡Van Putten T: *Arch Gen Psychiatry* 31:67, 1974.

Table 4-2 Parenteral Antipsychotic Drug Use

Drug	Parenteral administration (intramuscular)
For acute agitation*	
Chlorpromazine (Thorazine)	Initially 25 mg, repeated in 1 hour as needed; switch to oral dose as soon as possible
Haloperidol (Haldol)	Initially 2 to 5 mg, repeated every 1 to 8 hours as needed
For long-term maintenance or noncompliant behavior	
Fluphenazine decanoate (Prolixin decanoate)†	Initially 12.5 to 25 mg, maintenance dosage based on response; repeated every 2 to 4 weeks
Haloperidol decanoate (Haldol decanoate)†	Initially 10 to 15 times the oral dose of haloperidol (but should not exceed 100 mg); usually maintenance dosage of 50 to 200 mg every 4 weeks

*See Chapter 9, Acute Psychoses and the Violent Patient, for a complete review.
†Long-acting antipsychotics.

turbed patients or those who represent significant compliance risks. Both haloperidol and fluphenazine are available in long-acting or depot-injectable forms that require injection as seldom as once per month. Recent studies indicate a specific role for depot injections as prophylaxis for bipolar disorder (Littlejohn, Leslie, and Cookson, 1994; White, Cheung, and Silverstone, 1993). These depot compounds

Box 4-5 Patient Responses Suggesting a Possible Drug Change

1. Is the patient able and willing to comply with the original drug therapy as ordered? The potential therapeutic value cannot be established if the patient is noncompliant.
2. Has the drug currently being prescribed been given a fair trial with respect to dosage and time interval? Daily therapy at an effective dose for 3 to 6 weeks (or more) may be needed before a drug's effectiveness can be ascertained. The emphasis on short hospital stays may make evaluation of a response more difficult.
3. If a change of medication is indicated, is the new agent from a different chemical class (or subclass of the phenothiazines) so that the patient benefits from any inherent differences between classes? Drugs within a class or subclass act similarly and may offer no therapeutic advantage; for example, fluphenazine and trifluoperazine are both high-potency piperazine phenothiazines.

are particularly beneficial in community outpatient clinics and have several advantages and disadvantages (Barnes and Curson, 1994).

Advantages of depot compounds are:

1. Overcoming noncompliance
2. Reduction of bioavailability and metabolism of oral antipsychotic drugs
3. Achievement of stable plasma levels

Disadvantages of depot injections include:

1. Inability to withdraw drugs rapidly should problems develop
2. Lengthy process to adjust dosage

Antipsychotics available in parenteral form include the following:

Chlorpromazine (Thorazine)
Chlorprothixene (Taractan)
Fluphenazine (Prolixin)—depot form available
Haloperidol (Haldol)—depot form available
Loxapine (Loxitane)
Mesoridazine (Serentil)
Perphenazine (Trilafon)
Promazine (Sparine)
Thiothixene (Navane)
Trifluoperazine (Stelazine)
Triflupromazine (Vesprin)
Prochloperazine (Compazine)

When a patient is not responding to an antipsychotic drug, reassessment is necessary. Three principles guide assessment of the patient's response and raise the possibility of a change of drug. These principles are listed in Box 4-5.

Side Effects

The antipsychotic drugs produce numerous side effects because of PNS and CNS actions (given in Box 4-6). Side effects caused by PNS autonomic blocking, that is,

Box 4-6 Side Effects of Antipsychotic Drugs and Appropriate Clinical Interventions

Peripheral nervous system effects

Constipation

Encourage high dietary fiber and increased water intake; give laxatives as ordered.

Dry mouth

Advise patient to take sips of water frequently; provide sugarless hard candies, sugarless gum, and mouth rinses.

Nasal congestion

Give over-the-counter nasal decongestant if approved by physician.

Blurred vision

Advise patient to avoid potentially dangerous tasks. Reassure patient that normal vision typically returns in a few weeks, when tolerance to this side effect develops. Pilocarpine eyedrops can be used on a short-term basis.

Mydriasis

Advise patient to report eye pain immediately.

Photophobia

Advise patient to wear sunglasses outdoors.

Hypotension or orthostatic hypotension

Ask patient to get out of bed or chair slowly. He or she should sit on the side of the bed for 1 full minute while dangling feet, then slowly rise. If hypotension is a problem, measure blood pressure before each dose is given. Observe to see whether a change to another antipsychotic agent is indicated.

Tachycardia

Tachycardia is usually a reflex response to hypotension. When intervention for hypotension (previously described) is effective, reflex tachycardia usually decreases. With *clozapine,* hold the dose if pulse rate is greater than 140 pulsations per minute.*

Urinary retention

Encourage frequent voiding and voiding whenever the urge is present. Catheterize for residual fluids. Ask patient to monitor urine output and report output to nurse. Older men with benign prostatic hypertrophy are particularly susceptible to urinary retention.

Urinary hesitation

Provide privacy, run water in the sink, or run warm water over the perineum.

Sedation

Help patient get up early and get the day started.

Weight gain

Help patient order an appropriate diet; diet pills should not be taken.

Agranulocytosis

A high incidence of agranulocytosis (1% to 2%) is associated with *clozapine.* White blood cell count (WBC) should be performed weekly. When baseline WBC is less than 3500 cells/mm^3, treatment should not be initiated. After treatment begins, a WBC of less than 3000 cells/mm^3 and a granulocyte count of less than 1500 cells/mm^3 indicate treatment interruption to monitor for infection. If no signs of infection are present, treatment can resume. If WBC is less than 2000 cells/mm^3 and granulocyte count is less

Box 4-6 Side Effects of Antipsychotic Drugs and Appropriate Clinical Interventions—cont'd

than 1000 cells/mm^3, stop therapy and do not rechallenge the patient. If infection develops, antibiotics should be prescribed.

Central nervous system effects

Akathisia

Be patient and reassure patient who is "jittery" that you understand the need to move and that appropriate drug interventions can help differentiate akathisia and agitation. Since akathisia is the chief cause of noncompliance with antipsychotic regimens, switching to a different class of antipsychotic drug may be necessary to achieve compliance.

Dystonias

If a severe reaction such as oculogyric crisis or torticollis occurs, give antiparkinson drug (e.g., benztropine mesylate [Cogentin]) or antihistamine (e.g., diphenhydramine [Benadryl]) immediately, as needed, and offer reassurance. Intramuscular route will be needed if a severe reaction occurs.

Drug-induced parkinsonism

Assess for the three major parkinsonism symptoms—tremors, rigidity, and bradykinesia—and report to physician. Antiparkinson drugs will probably be indicated.

Tardive dyskinesia

Assess for signs by using the Abnormal Inventory Movement Scale (AIMS). Drug holidays may help prevent tardive dyskinesia. Because antipsychotic drugs may mask tardive dyskinesia, their use should be reviewed. Anticholinergic agents will worsen tardive dyskinesia, so question their indiscriminate prophylactic use. However, young men taking large doses of high-potency antipsychotic drugs (e.g., haloperiodol) are one group in which prophylactic use of antiparkinson drugs may be more prudent than not using them.†

Neuroleptic malignant syndrome

Be alert for this potentially fatal side effect. *Routinely* take temperatures and encourage adequate water intake among all patients on a regimen of antipsychotic drugs and *routinely* assess for rigidity, tremor, and the like.

Seizures

Seizures occur in approximately 1% of patients receiving antipsychotic drug treatment. *Clozapine* causes an even higher rate, up to 5% of patients taking 600 to 900 mg/day. For dosages of clozapine greater than 600 mg/day a normal EEG should be performed. If a seizure occurs, it may be necessary to discontinue clozapine. See Chapter 7, Seizure Disorders, for appropriate antiepileptic therapy.†Jaretz, Flowers, Millsap: *Perspect Psychiatr Care* 28:19,1992.

*Jaretz, Flowers, Millsap: *Perspect Psychiatr Care* 28:19, 1992.

†American Psychiatric Association Task Force on Tardive Dyskinesia: *Am J Psychiatry* 137:1163, 1980.

Table 4-3 Anticholingeric Effect on Cranial Nerves with Parasympathetic Functions

Cranial nerve	Parasympathetic function	Anticholingeric effect
III	Constricts pupils	Mydriasis (dilates pupils)—blurred vision
	Alters shape of lens	Impairs accommodation
VII	Salivation	Dry mouth
	Lacrimation	Decreased tearing
	Nasal mucous secretion	Dry nasal passage
IX	Salivation	Dry mouth
	Nasal mucous secretion	Dry nasal passage
X	Slows heart rate	Tachycardia
	Promotes peristalsis	Slows peristalsis—constipation
	Constricts bronchi	Dilates bronchi

anticholinergic and antiadrenergic, actions are more likely to be caused by low-potency forms such as chlorpromazine (Richelson, 1984). Extrapyramidal symptoms in the CNS are more likely to be caused by high-potency drugs such as haloperidol.

Peripheral nervous system effects. Anticholinergic PNS effects are related to the blockade of parasympathetic functions of several cranial (Table 4-3) and other parasympathetic nerves. Dry mouth (cranial nerves [CN] VII and IX), blurred vision (CN III), photophobia (CN III), and decreased lacrimation (CN VII) are common and often can be managed with nondrug interventions. Mydriasis (CN III) can increase intraocular pressure, which can aggravate glaucoma. Other relatively common anticholinergic effects are constipation and urinary hesitance. Patients with a history of glaucoma or prostatic hypertrophy are not ordinarily placed on regimens of these drugs. Tachycardia (CN X) is another PNS effect, and patients with cardiovascular disease should be carefully evaluated before these drugs are prescribed. Sudden death related to arrhythmias and decreased cardiac output has been reported with antipsychotic drugs. Thioridazine (Mellaril) has been implicated in more cases of sudden death than has any other antipsychotic drug (Mehtonen et al, 1991).

Hypotension is the major antiadrenergic effect of antipsychotic drugs. Hypotension often occurs when the individual stands or changes position suddenly (orthostatic hypotension). Orthostatic symptoms occur most often in elderly persons (Gomez and Gomez, 1990). Thus precautions against falls must be instituted. Additionally, hypotension may cause a reflex tachycardia in a tachycardia-prone heart (because of CN X blockade) that can, in turn, cause general cardiovascular inefficiency. Thus low-potency antipsychotic drugs are usually not prescribed for individuals with severe hypotension, heart failure, or a history of arrhythmias.

Central nervous system extrapyramidal side effects. EPSEs develop in up to 75% of patients receiving antipsychotic medications (Blair, 1990), and up to 50% of readmissions are related to these side effects (Blair and Dauner, 1993a). Abnormal involuntary movement disorders develop because of a drug-induced imbalance between two major neurotransmitters, dopamine and acetylcholine (ACh). As

Box 4-7 Guidelines for Minimizing EPSEs

1. Antipsychotic drugs are used for approved indications, that is, they are not used, for example, to treat anxiety.
2. The dose for certain patients is limited. Elderly persons, for instance, are especially susceptible to hypotension and tardive dyskinesia and should be prescribed antipsychotics in dosages 25% to 50% of that recommended for younger adults.*
3. As with all drugs, but especially because of a dose-EPSE relationship, the lowest effective dose of an antipsychotic drug is given. Because these drugs are metabolized primarily in the liver, persons with reduced liver function as a result of old age or liver disease should be given lower doses than normal.
4. Drug holidays, brief periods when the patient is taken off a regimen of drugs, can decrease side effects without jeopardizing the therapeutic value of the drug.
5. After 1 year of continuous antipsychotic drug therapy the patient is gradually weaned from the drug. This taper allows the treatment team or clinician to evaluate the current need for the drug and also permits detection of an emerging tardive dyskinesia.

*Gregory C, McKenna P: Pharmacological management of schizophrenia in older patients, *Drugs and Aging* 5(4):254, 1994.

dopamine D-2 receptors are antagonized or occupied at levels between 60% and 75%, an optimal clinical effect occurs. As occupancy levels approach 90% of D-2 receptors, EPSEs develop (Sedvall, 1995; Seeman and Van Tol, 1994) because the balance between dopamine and ACh is markedly altered. This imbalance seems to be caused more readily by high-potency antipsychotic drugs, for example, haloperidol. EPSEs may be characterized as akathisia, dystonias, dyskinesias, akinesias, and drug-induced parkinsonism. Neuroleptic malignant syndrome and tardive dyskinesia (TD), a late-appearing dyskinesia, also may result from dopamine depletion and are the most serious side effects and (in the case of TD) the least treatable. Guidelines for minimizing EPSEs are listed in Box 4-7.

Akathisia. "Akathisia is an EPSE that results from antipsychotic medication and is by far the most dramatic; akathisia may also be the most dangerous . . .," according to Dauner and Blair (1990). Akathisia, literally "the inability to sit" (Blair and Dauner, 1992), is an unpleasant subjective and objective response to antipsychotic drugs. It is the most common EPSE (about 50% of all EPSEs) and probably accounts for more noncompliant behavior than do the other side effects. Some clinicians believe that a majority of patients receiving antipsychotic drugs have akathisia.

Akathisia was first described in 1911, long before antipsychotic drugs were available, suggesting that other variables may contribute to its occurrence.

Subjectively the patient often feels jittery or uneasy. He or she may report a lot of "nervous energy." *Objectively* the patient is restless and cannot sit still, even during group activities, and assaultive behavior can result. Planasky and Johnston (1971) found that 79% of suicidal schizophrenic patients had akathisia. Restlessness and verbal reflections of subjective anguish can be misinterpreted as a worsening of the psychotic process. Agitated patients frequently come to the emergency department because of a psychiatric illness. Because akathisia can present as agitation, the ER nurse should not mistake the two because of treatment differences (Foley, 1993). *If additional antipsychotic medication is given, (that is, a dose "as needed," because of this misinterpretation, the patient will suffer much more.* Akathisia may respond to anticholinergic drugs (see Chapter 14, Drugs Used to Treat Extrapyramidal Side Effects) such as trihexyphenidyl (Artane) or benztropine (Cogentin) but can also be resistant to this intervention. Benzodiazepines, for example, lorazepam, may also be useful. However, Keepers and Casey (1986) pointed out that other approaches, including waiting for tolerance to develop and decreasing the dosage of the antipsychotic agent, may be the best way to treat akathisia.

Dystonias. Dystonic reactions may cause rigidity in muscles that control posture, gait, or ocular movement. Remington et al (1990), in a small prospective study ($N = 41$), found that 67% of schizophrenic patients taking parenteral haloperidol became dystonic. In oculogyric crisis, a type of dystonic reaction, the eyes roll back, causing a frightening experience. Torticollis, another dystonic reaction, is a contracted state of the cervical muscles, producing torsion on the neck. A laryngeal-pharyngeal dystonia, which is associated with gagging, cyanosis, respiratory distress, and asphyxia (particularly in young men), is life threatening. Up to 46% of patients who do not receive prophylactic anticholinergic drugs develop dystonic reactions (Tesar, 1993). All these conditions respond to intramuscular anticholinergic drugs or may respond to intramuscular or intravenous diphenhydramine (see Chapter 14, Drugs Used to Treat Extrapyramidal Side Effects).

Akinesia. Akinesia refers to an absence of movement and a diminished mental state. More often a state of bradykinesia, or a slowing of movement, exists. Akinesia is experienced by about 33% of patients taking antipsychotic drugs (Van Putten and Marder, 1987). Movement is difficult to initiate and difficult to maintain. The patient lacks spontaneity in movement and speech. Paradoxically these same symptoms (for different reasons) are common in schizophrenia, the focus of treatment. Historically health care professionals have occasionally mistaken bizarre postures caused by EPSEs for exacerbation of schizophrenic symptoms. The dilemma is real. If a manifestation of schizophrenia is occurring, more medication may be indicated; if the condition is an EPSE, more medication will worsen the symptoms.

Drug-induced parkinsonism. Antipsychotic drug therapy can produce the constellation of symptoms peculiar to parkinsonism: tremors, rigidity, and bradykinesia. Antipsychotic drugs can intensify existing "naturally occurring" parkinsonism, and therefore these drugs are avoided if at all possible for persons with this condition.

Dyskinesias and tardive dyskinesia. *Dyskinesia* refers to abnormal, involuntary skeletal muscle movements, which usually produce a jerky motion. Treatment with any antipsychotic drug involves the risk of tardive dyskinesia, which is a serious side effect. The term *tardive* means "late-appearing." Typically TD appears after months or years of drug usage; however, TD can appear sooner. Although EPSEs, much like parkinsonism, are caused by a dopamine deficiency, TD theoretically is caused by hypersensitivity to dopamine (and, possibly, cholinergic deficit). In a sense TD is the pharmacologic opposite of the EPSEs (Lieberman et al, 1988). Therefore, although anticholinergic antiparkinsonism drugs, for example, trihexyphenidyl and benztropine, are beneficial for the other EPSEs, they may exacerbate TD. Tardive dyskinesia is thought to affect about 15% to 25% of the patients who receive antipsychotic drug treatment; however, current research (Yassa et al, 1990) suggests even higher levels (34%) of this illness.

Tardive dyskinesia usually affects the muscles of the mouth and face and can also occur in the trunk and extremities. Signs of tardive dyskinesia include lip smacking, grinding of the teeth, rolling or protrusion of the tongue, tics, and diaphragmatic movements, which may impair breathing. These involuntary movements are generally coordinated, fluctuate in severity, and disappear during sleep. Patients with TD are three times as likely to have an impaired gag reflex. Tardive dyskinesia is most often severe in young men and most common in women over age 70 (Appleton, 1988).

Because TD is considered irreversible (except in the early stages, when it is more appropriately termed *withdrawal dyskinesia*), a physician should be notified and the patient or family, or both, be educated when TD is suspected. The Abnormal Involuntary Movement Scale (AIMS) provides a mechanism for assessing TD. The dopamine agonist bromocriptine (Parlodel) has been used to treat this side effect, as has clonazepam (Klonopin) and vitamin E (which apparently works by neutralizing free radicals). However, no highly effective treatment approach has yet been established so prevention and early recognition remain the most important tools for clinicians. Nonpsychotropic drugs such as metoclopramide (Reglan) have also been inplicated in TD.

Neuroleptic malignant syndrome. A final side effect or adverse event worthy of discussion is neuroleptic malignant syndrome (NMS), an underdiagnosed adverse response to antipsychotic drugs (Keltner and McIntyre, 1985). NMS may occur in as many as 1% (some research estimates run as high as 2.4%) of patients receiving antipyschotic drugs; of this number from 14% to 30% may die (Hooper, Herren, and Goldwasser, 1989). Blair and Dauner (1993b), after a review of relevant studies, indicate these percentages translate into 1000 to 4000 NMS-related deaths per year in the United States. NMS is most often associated with high-potency antipsychotic drugs, especially when prescribed with a large loading dose. Deng, Chen, and Phillips (1990), in a large prospective study (9700 inpatients), found fluphenazine decanoate (Prolixin decanoate), when used without an antiparkinson agent, to be a major risk factor. However, NMS is not related to toxic drug levels and may occur after only a few doses. Onset can occur within minutes or take months after drug initiation. NMS is essentially caused by decreased dopamine transmission, and treatment seems to be to give dopamine agonists.

Neuroleptic malignant syndrome shares some symptoms with the EPSEs. Hyperthermia, muscular rigidity, tremors, impaired ventilation, muteness, altered consciousness, and autonomic hyperactivity are observed. Perhaps the cardinal symptom is elevated body temperature. Temperatures as high as 42.2° C (108° F) have been reported, although those between 101° F and 103° F are more likely. Historically risk factors associated with NMS have been young adulthood, male sex, nonschizophrenic illness, and high-potency drugs. Because many patients do not associate these symptoms with their antipsychotic medication, emergency room and primary care providers may be contacted first. These health care professionals should always rule out NMS in their patients taking antipsychotics who develop high temperatures. Pharmacologic treatment has included bromocriptine, dantrolene (Dantrium), and amantadine (Symmetrel) (see Chapter 14, Drugs Used to Treat Extrapyramidal Side Effects).

Other side effects. Other side effects that may occur in association with antipsychotic drugs include hyperglycemia, jaundice, blood dyscrasias, susceptibility to hyperthermia, blue-gray skin rash, sun-sensitive skin (sunburn), nasal congestion, wheezing, galactorrhea (seepage from breast), gynecomastia (enlarged breast in either sex), impaired ejaculation, and amenorrhea. A CNS effect that is not an extrapyramidal symptom is memory loss. Because the cholinergic system is implicated in memory and learning, anticholinergic antiparkinsonism drugs and low-potency antipsychotic drugs could play a role in this cognitive symptom. The atypical antipsychotic, clozapine, causes agranulocytosis in 1% of the persons who take it (Barrett, Ormiston, and Molyneux, 1990). Agranulocytosis, a potentially fatal disorder, is discussed more thoroughly later in the chapter.

Prophylactic treatment of EPSEs. Prophylactic use of anticholinergic agents has been debated because these drugs have their own set of side effects and a potential for abuse. Nonetheless, Tesar (1993) finds prophylactic administration particularly effective in preventing dystonic reactions. In his study only 13% of patients receiving prophylactic anticholinergic drugs experienced dystonias compared with 46% not taking anticholinergics. Because 90% of dystonic reactions occur within the first 5 days of treatment, anticholinergics can be discontinued fairly soon for most patients. Typical anticholinergics used for EPSEs are trihexyphenidyl 2 to 5 mg or benztropine 2 mg by mouth or intramuscularly for patients beginning high-potency antipsychotic treatment.

Implications

Individual profiles for each antipsychotic can be found in Part Two of this book.

Therapeutic versus toxic levels. Overdoses of antipsychotic drugs are seldom fatal but are even less likely with high-potency agents. Symptoms of overdose include severe CNS depression (somnolence to coma), hypotension, and EPSEs. Restlessness or agitation, convulsions (antipsychotic drugs lower the seizure threshold), hyperthermia, increased anticholinergic symptoms, and arrhythmias also indicate an overdose. Treatment is mostly supportive, with gastric lavage to empty the stomach, amphetamine for severe CNS depression (although a risk of seizure is incurred), and antiparkinson drugs for severe EPSEs. Norepinephrine can be used for severe hypotension. *Epinephrine aggravates hypotension.*

Use in pregnancy. Although the risks to the fetus are statistically low, exposure to antipsychotic drugs during the first trimester should still be avoided. During the remainder of the pregnancy, the lowest possible dose is desirable. If possible, antipsychotic drugs should be discontinued to reduce the risk of transient neonatal toxicity (Cohen, 1989).

Side effects. Peripheral nervous system anticholinergic and antiadrenergic effects of antipsychotic drugs are troublesome but are not always as serious or as disturbing to the patient as the CNS EPSEs. Nurses are often the first psychiatric professionals to observe side effects. Box 4-6 lists several specific interventions the nurse can provide to ameliorate the side effect or prevent serious consequences.

Interactions. Antipsychotic drugs compromise and are compromised by many other drugs (Watsky and Salzman, 1991). Because these drug-drug interactions can be serious, it is important, first, to know potential offending agents and, second, to advise the family and patient accordingly. Agents such as alcohol, antihistamines, antianxiety drugs, antidepressants, barbiturates, meperidine, and morphine have additive effects that can cause profound CNS depression. The clinician should check prescriptions for the possible inadvertent combination of these and the an-

Box 4-8 Adverse Interactions of Antipsychotics with Other Drugs

Amoxapine, fluoxetine
Increase EPSEs

Amphetamines
Decrease antipsychotic effect

Anticholinergic antiparkinson drugs
Increase anticholinergic effect; delay onset of the effects of oral doses of antipsychotics; possess potential to increase risk of hyperthermia

Barbiturates, nonbarbiturate hypnotics
All cause respiratory depression and increase sedation; all decrease antipsychotic serum levels; hypotension

Benzodiazepines
Increase sedation; respiratory depression with lorazepam and loxapine

Beta-adrenergic blocking agents (propranolol)
Effect of either or both drugs increased

Cimetidine
Chlorpromazine absorption decreased; increased sedation with chlorpromazine

Diazoxide
Can cause severe hyperglycemia

Dopaminergic antiparkinson drugs (e.g., bromocriptine)
Antagonize the antipsychotic effect

Guanethidine
Control of hypertension is decreased

Insulin, oral hypoglycemics
Control of diabetes is weakened

L-dopa
Decreased antiparkinson effect of L-dopa; may exacerbate psychosis

Lithium
Decreases antipsychotic effect; may cause neurotoxicity when combined with haloperidol; lithium toxicity may be masked by antiemetic effect of antipsychotic drugs; increases EPSEs

Continued

Box 4-8 Adverse Interactions of Antipsychotics with Other Drugs—cont'd

Narcotics
Hypotension with chlorpromazine and meperidine; increased sedation; hypotension augmented; respiratory depression augmented

Phenytoin
May increase phenytoin toxicity; decreased antipsychotic blood serum levels

Trazodone
Additive hypotension with phenothiazines

Tricyclics
Possible ventricular arrhythmias with thioridazine; possible increased blood serum levels of both; hypotension; sedation; anticholinergic effect; increased risk of seizures.

tipsychotic drugs and should advise the patient to avoid both alcohol and certain over-the-counter medications, for example, cold medications and sleep aids.

Because antacids decrease absorption of antipsychotic drugs, administer these agents 1 to 2 hours after an oral antipsychotic drug has been given.

Be aware of other drugs that interact adversely with the antipsychotic drugs. Box 4-8 lists these other drugs.

Patient education. Patient education is important when caring for people who are taking antipsychotic drugs. Use discretion in selecting the content of education sessions, because patients may become anxious about potential side effects. Focus on symptoms that can be seen or felt. Some patient education issues have been discussed throughout this chapter. Recommendations not previously mentioned include the following:

- Avoid hot tubs, hot showers, and hot tub baths, because hypotension may occur and may cause falls.
- Avoid abrupt drug withdrawal, thereby reducing the risk of EPSEs.
- Use sunscreen to prevent sunburn.
- Adhere to the drug regimen as prescribed. Noncompliance is the primary cause of symptom exacerbation.
- Pay attention to and communicate symptoms of sore throat, malaise, fever, or bleeding. Such signs and symptoms may indicate the emergence of a blood dyscrasia.
- Adopt appropriate dress in hot weather and increase fluid intake to avoid heat stroke.

Chemical Class and Structure of Specific Drugs

With the possible exceptions of clozapine and risperidone, true therapeutic differences among antipsychotic agents have not been substantiated. Any differences among individual drugs are those of sedation and side effects (Johnson, 1990) as aforementioned in Table 4-1.

Phenothiazines. The phenothiazines are divided into three subclasses: aliphatics, piperidines, and piperazines.

Aliphatics: chlorpromazine, promazine, and triflupromazine. The aliphatics are more sedative and more likely than other phenothiazines to produce orthostatic hypotension. Chlorpromazine has been described previously in detail. The other two drugs, *promazine* (Sparine) and *triflupromazine* (Vesprin), are seldom ordered.

Piperidines: thioridazine and mesoridazine. Thioridazine is almost as old as chlorpromazine and historically has been the largest-selling antipsychotic in the United States (Wysowski and Baum, 1989). It is frequently ordered, and many patients respond to it or tolerate it. Thioridazine is sometimes prescribed for the short-term treatment of depression accompanied by anxiety in adult patients and for agitation, anxiety, depressed mood, tension, sleep disturbances, fears, and other symptoms in geriatric patients. In children with severe behavioral problems marked by combativeness, thioridazine has been therapeutic. As a group piperidines have a lower risk of EPSEs, but important concerns about eye toxicity exist. For example, in prescribing thioridazine, the maximum daily dose is 800 mg. At higher doses there is a risk of pigmentary retinopathy, which decreases visual acuity, impairs night vision, and is characterized by pigment deposits on the fundus. Mesoridazine is not prescribed as often as thioridazine but has the advantage of being available as an injectable and is more easily metabolized. Mesoridazine is sometimes preferred in alcohol abusers or other persons with liver disease. Elderly persons are highly sensitive to mesoridazine-induced hypotension.

Piperazines: fluphenazine, trifluoperazine, and perphenazine. Piperazines are moderately sedative; they seldom cause orthostatic hypotension but do cause significant levels of EPSEs. The two most often prescribed piperazines are fluphenazine and trifluoperazine. Fluphenazine, a high-potency antipsychotic, is available in a long-acting or depot form. Fluphenazine decanoate, the long-acting form, is beneficial for patients who do not comply with a daily oral medication regimen. An injection can be given every 2 to 4 weeks. Fluphenazine hydrochloride has a "regular" duration and is available in tablet, concentrate, and "regular-acting" parenteral forms. Restrictions for diluting the concentrate are given in Table 4-4.

Trifluoperazine is prescribed relatively often. It is available in tablets and concentrate and for parenteral use and is indicated for excessive anxiety, tension, agitation, and psychotic manifestations.

Perphenazine is often used with antidepressants for patients who are both psychotic and depressed. It can be given separately or is available in a fixed-dose combination with amitriptyline (Elavil). The fixed-dose combination of perphenazine and amitriptyline is Triavil. This combination drug is seldom prescribed.

Butyrophenone: haloperidol. Haloperidol is in the butyrophenone chemical class of antipsychotic drugs. It is a high-potency drug (2 mg of haloperidol is equivalent to 100 mg of chlorpromazine) and tends to cause EPSEs but has fewer anticholinergic side effects than do the low-potency agents. Haloperidol is a frequently prescribed antipsychotic and is used extensively in older adults (because of fewer anticholinergic and hypotensive effects) and in pediatric psychiatry. Haloperidol is also used for Gilles de la Tourette's syndrome, which is characterized by facial grimaces; tics; purposeless movements of the upper body, shoulder, and arms; copro-

Table 4-4 Liquids Compatible with Liquid Antipsychotic Agents

Medication	Compatible liquid	Incompatible liquid
Haloperidol	Water, apple juice, orange juice, tomato juice, cola sodas	Coffee, tea, saline, lithium citrate
Loxapine	Orange juice, pineapple juice, grapefruit juice, Tang, Kool-Aid (lemon, raspberry), cola, 7-Up, coffee (preferably with cream and sugar)	No data
Thioridazine	Acidic juices (orange, grapefruit), acidified tap water	Water, milk, coffee, tea, nonacidic juices (apple, grape, pineapple, prune), cola, orange drink, lithium citrate
Molindone	Orange juice, apple juice	No data
Thiothixene	Water, milk, prune juice, apricot juice, tomato juice, pineapple juice, cranberry juice, grapefruit juice, orange juice	Cola sodas, apple juice
Fluphenazine	Water, orange juice, pineapple juice, prune juice, tomato juice, grapefruit juice, apricot juice, decaffeinated noncola soda, V-8 juice	Coffee, tea, cola, apple juice
Mesoridazine	Water, orange juice, grape juice, cranberry juice, grapefruit juice	No data
Trifluoperazine	Water, milk, coffee, tea, grapefruit juice, orange juice, pineapple juice, prune juice, tomato juice, soda, orange syrup, simple syrup	Lithium citrate
Chlorprothixene	Water, milk, coffee, fruit juices, carbonated beverages	No data
Chlorpromazine	Water, milk, orange juice (made from frozen concentrate), apricot juice, grapefruit juice, prune juice, tomato juice, V-8 juice, lemon-lime soda	Coffee, tea, apple juice, cola, root beer, diet ginger ale, lithium citrate
Perphenazine	Water, saline, homogenized milk, orange juice, grapefruit juice, pineapple juice, apricot juice, prune juice, tomato juice, 7-Up, carbonated orange drink, V-8 juice	Coffee, tea, cola, apple juice

Modified from Geller JL, Gaulin BD, Barreira PD: A practitioner's guide to use of psychotropic medication in liquid form, *Hosp Community Psychiatry* 43(10):969, 1992.

lalia (frequent extreme profanity); and echolalia (repetition of words spoken to patient).

Whereas dosages of up to 100 mg per day of haloperidol have been given for psychosis, Rifkin et al (1991) found that smaller dosages of more than 10 mg per day had no additional benefit. This phenomenon is related to what is known as a therapeutic window. Bernardo et al (1993) found serum levels below or above the range 4 to 22 ng/mL are not as beneficial. In other words, both undermedicating and overmedicating decrease the therapeutic value of haloperidol.

Haloperidol decanoate is a long-acting depot form and can be given every 2 to 4 weeks (or with longer intervals). This preparation is particularly beneficial for patients with compliance difficulties.

Thioxanthenes: chlorprothixene and thiothixene. Chlorprothixene and thiothixene have different potencies. Chlorprothixene is similar to chlorpromazine or the aliphatic phenothiazines in potency. Thiothixene is 20 times as potent as chlorpromazine, or more like the piperazine phenothiazines. Thiothixene is prescribed relatively often. Thiothixene exhibits weak anticholinergic properties but relatively powerful EPSEs.

Dibenzoxazepine: loxapine. Loxapine is available in capsule, concentrate, and parenteral forms. The concentrate is unpleasant and should be diluted with orange or grapefruit juice shortly before administration. Specific EPSEs have been reported in approximately 20% of patients, particularly during the first few days of treatment. Specific EPSEs include akathisia and symptoms of parkinsonism—tremors, rigidity, sialorrhea, and masked facies. As with other agents, reduction of the loxapine and administration of an antiparkinson drug usually control these manifestations.

Dihydroindolone: molindone. Molindone (Moban) is about 10 times as potent as chlorpromazine and is used exclusively to treat psychosis. Some studies indicate that molindone may be the ideal antipsychotic agent because it has fewer overall side effects than the other antipsychotic drugs (Richelson, 1984). Available only for oral administration, molindone has several unique properties; for example, it provokes heavy menstruation in previously amenorrheal women and contains calcium ions that can interfere with the absorption of tetracycline antibiotics or phenytoin (Dilantin).

Atypical Antipsychotics or Serotonin/ Dopamine Antagonists (SDAs)

Since 1952 when chlorpromazine was introduced, psychiatric researchers have continually sought to develop a better drug. Meltzer (1993) defines better as "more effective with fewer side effects." However, in the United States, since 1975 only two new antipsychotics have been approved by the FDA for retail sale: clozapine in 1990 and risperidone in 1994 (Keltner and Folks, 1991; Kane, 1994). During the 40 years between the introduction of chlorpromazine (1950s) and clozapine (1990s), the "molecule manipulators," to borrow a catchy phrase from Ayd (1991), developed a multitude of "traditional" antipsychotics. (Chapter 1, Psychiatric Care and Contemporary Treatment, outlines these historical developments briefly.)

A commonality among traditional antipsychotics is their ability to antagonize dopamine D-2 receptors (Matsubara et al, 1993). Before long researchers realized that blocking D-2 receptors alone could not effectively alter symptoms of schizophrenia (Keltner, 1995). This conclusion was based on several observations:

1. Dopamine blockade occurs rapidly, but chemical improvement occurs slowly (weeks to months) (Hollister, 1994).
2. A substantial number of schizophrenic patients do not improve (10% to 20%) or relapse within 1 year (20% to 30%) (Perry et al, 1991).
3. Patients who do improve often suffer serious side effects (Hollister, 1994).
4. Up to 30% of patients with chronic or persistent mental illness and exhibiting negative symptoms show little improvement with traditional antipsychotic drugs (Remington, 1993).

These observations fueled the search for a better antipsychotic.

Dibenzodiazepine: clozapine. Although it was first introduced in 1960, clozapine was not marketed in the United States for three decades (Safferman et al, 1991) because of its potentially fatal side effect, agranulocytosis. Clozapine is a dibenzodiazepine derivative and has pharmacologic features unique among antipsychotic drugs. Whereas traditional antipsychotic drugs block dopamine D-2 receptors, clozapine produces a weaker blockade of D-2 receptors but has a more significant blockade of dopamine D-1 and D-4 receptors and of serotonin 5HT-2 receptors (Kane, 1993). It has a low affinity (about 20% receptor occupancy) for dopamine D-2 receptors (Kerwin, 1994). This low affinity probably explains the relative lack of EPSEs associated with clozapine.

Clozapine's primary importance is that patients resistant to other antipsychotics have responded to it (Meltzer, 1989). Approximately 10% to 20% of schizophrenic patients are not responsive to traditional antipsychotics, and another 20% to 30% who are initially responsive to antipsychotics other than clozapine relapse within 1 year. Some studies suggest that as many as 64% of treatment-resistant schizophrenic patients show a favorable response to clozapine (Perry et al, 1991). Lawson (1992) credits clozapine with pushing forward the acceptance of a biologic approach to treatment.

Some estimates suggest there are 200,000 suitable candidates for clozapine (Salzman, 1990). Although clozapine has been used for some time in Europe and China to treat schizophrenia, it was not approved in the United States until 1990, largely because of the seriousness of the side effect agranulocytosis. Agranulocytosis is a sudden and severe drop in the number of white blood cells that can lead to death, which is usually caused by overwhelming infection. The period of maximum risk is 4 to 18 weeks (Safferman et al, 1991). A study in 1986 revealed that agranulocytosis develops in about 1% to 2% of patients who take clozapine and that of these, 35% die. Since clozapine's approval in 1990, 416 cases of agranulocytosis have been reported, and 13 deaths have occurred as of July 1995 (Sandoz, Inc., oral communication, July 10, 1995).

Clinical implications. Until the advent of clozapine, all antipsychotic drugs were considered equally effective. Some drugs helped some people more than other drugs, but one could not say, for instance, that haloperidol was superior to chlorpromazine. Clozapine is the first drug for which an improved rate of response is suggested. However, because of the high risk of bone marrow suppression or bone marrow failure and death, certain precautions must be observed by the clinician and patient. Although clinicians agree that clozapine treatment succeeds where treatment with other neuroleptics fails, its efficacy for purely negative symptoms is unknown (Safferman et al, 1991).

Frequent monitoring of white blood cells and platelets. When white blood cells and platelets are monitored frequently, impending bone marrow failure can be detected early, thus greatly reducing the risk associated with infection.

Prominent side effects. Sedation, hypersalivation, dizziness, tachycardia, hypotension, and constipation are the most frequent side effects of clozapine treatment. Hypersalivation (sialorrhea) affects up to 30% of patients taking clozapine and can be extremely bothersome and embarrassing (Jaretz, Flowers, and Millsap, 1992). Just as important are the side effects that do not occur. A report issued in 1992 by the American Psychiatric Association could not trace one case of tardive dyskinesia to clozapine. In fact, some evidence exists that suggests clozapine actually has a therapeutic effect on existing tardive dyskinesia (Littrell and Magill, 1993). Additionally, clozapine reduces the seizure threshold. Up to 5% of patients taking between 600 and 900 mg per day experience seizures.

Weekly distribution. Clozapine should be distributed to the patient once a week to ensure that monitoring standards are followed.

Clinical criteria. Pelonero and Elliot (1990) have outlined the following guidelines for the selection of patients who could benefit from clozapine:

1. Treatment-resistant schizophrenia or severe, persistent tardive dyskinesia, or both are present.
2. No medical contraindication, such as blood dyscrasia, epilepsy, or hepatic or renal disease, is present.
3. The patient has the ability to give informed consent.
4. The patient is able to comply with the treatment regimen and monitoring protocols.

When clozapine was first given FDA approval in 1990, a rigid manufacturer monitoring system was required. This system, referred to as the Clozaril Patient Management System, was cumbersome and costly. The mandate to provide this system drove up the cost of Clozaril to about $9000 a year (Griffith, 1990), preventing some public agencies from using this medication (Bergmann, 1990). Noting this concern, political and other forces succeeded in streamlining the monitoring system to cut costs in half.

In May 1991 physicians and pharmacists were allowed to monitor clozapine patients according to locally developed systems. These systems must include a requirement for a weekly white blood cell count. In addition, they must require that no more than 1 week's supply of clozapine be given to each patient and that patients being taken off a regimen of clozapine be monitored for a minimum of 4 weeks.

Benzisoxazole: risperidone. The newest antipsychotic, approved in 1994, is risperidone (Risperdal). Risperidone, like traditional antipsychotic drugs and unlike clozapine, blocks D-2 receptors, albeit somewhat weakly. However, risperidone blocks 5HT-2 potently (Ereshefsky and Lacombe, 1993). It is theorized that blocking 5HT-2 in cortical regions of the brain frees dopamine in that area, thus improving negative symptoms of schizophrenia. It simultaneously blocks D-2 receptors in the limbic tract, thus reducing positive symptoms. The therapeutic advantage of risperidone is critically important to some patients—risperidone ameliorates positive symptoms (hallucinations, delusions, bizzare behavior, and thought disorders) like traditional antipsychotics and is also effective in diminishing negative symptoms associated with cortical dopamine deficiencies (alogia, flattened affect, avolition, and anergia) (Awouters et al, 1990; Borison et al, 1992; Brown et al, 1993). This efficacy in treating negative symptoms is attributed to risperidone's antiserotonergic properties (Bleich et al, 1988; Chouinaird and Arnott, 1993; Claus et al, 1992; Mok and Yatham, 1994).

Side effects. Risperidone has an affinity for alpha-1 adrenergic receptors, causing orthostatic hypotension. It is thought that alpha-1 blockade may play a role in risperidone's antipsychotic effect as well (Sleight, Koek, and Bigg, 1993). This mechanism for producing an antipsychotic effect is not fully understood. Risperidone has little affinity for histamine H-1 (hence little sedation) and adrenergic alpha-2 receptors. Risperidone does not bind to cholinergic muscarinic receptors so anticholinergic effects are not a problem (Land and Salzman, 1994). Risperidone does not appear to cause agranulocytosis, significant EPSEs, tardive dyskinesia, or neuroleptic malignant syndrome (Borison et al, 1992). Although the overall safety of risperidone is not known, Brown (1993) reported the case of a 29-year-old man who ingested 100 to 240 mg of the drug in a failed suicide attempt. Brown did, however, note ECG and electrolyte changes in this individual.

Side effects, including insomnia, agitation, headache, anxiety, and rhinitis, appear routinely among recipients of risperidone. Less commonly reported side effects include sedation, dizziness, constipation, nausea, and tachycardia.

Pharmacokinetics. Risperidone is rapidly absorbed from the gastrointestinal tract; it reaches plasma levels in about 1 hour (Keltner, 1995). The half-life of risperidone and its active metabolite (9-hydroxyrisperidone) is 24 hours. The metabolite is equally as potent as the parent compound (Land and Salzman, 1994).

Efficacy. A number of large-scale studies have found risperidone to be an effective antispychotic for both positive and negative symptoms (Addington et al, 1993; Claus et al, 1992; Marder and Meibach, 1994).

Box 4-9 Potential New Antipsychotic Drugs

Multireceptor blocking drugs (atypical)
Sertindole
Amperozide
Zotepine

Selective D-2/D-3 antagonists
Remoxipride
Raclopride
Amisulpiride
Savoxepine

Partial D-2 agonists (autoreceptor agonists)
Roxindol

Serotonergic agents
Ritanserin

5HT-3 antagonists
Ondansetron

Glutamate/sigma receptor agonists
Milacemide
Rimcazole

From Hollister LE: New psychotherapeutic drugs, *Clin Psychopharmacol* 14(1):50-63, 1994.

Box 4-10 Dopamine Receptors

Dopamine receptors are the target when treating schizophrenia and parkinsonism. Dopamine antagonists (i.e., antipsychotic drugs) block dopamine receptors and are useful in treating schizophrenia. Dopaminergic drugs stimulate dopamine receptors and are useful in treating parkinsonism. L-dopa, a dopamine precursor, and bromocriptine, a dopamine agonist, are examples of dopaminergic agents.

There are five dopamine receptor subtypes and a number of variants of some of these. Dopamine receptors can be broadly divided into D-1 like receptors and D-2 like receptors. D-1 like receptors are D-1 and D-5. D-2 like receptors are D-2, D-3, and D-4. Most antipsychotics block D-2 receptors, but clozapine has a greater affinity for D-4 receptors. In schizophrenia, the D-2 and D-3 receptor density is increased by 10%, and the D-4 receptor density is increased 600%. Consequently, drugs, such as clozapine, that block D-4 receptors may have the greatest potential in the treatment of schizophrenia.

Following is a listing of dopamine receptor subtypes and their variants:

D-1 like:

D-1
D-5
D-5 pseudo-1
D-5 pseudo-2

D-2 like:

D-2L
D-2S
D-2 Ala96
D-2 Ser310
D-2 Cys311
D-3
D-3 Gly9
D-3 nf
D-3 TM4 d
D-3 TM3 d
D-4.0
D-4.1
D-4.2
D-4.3
D-4.4
D-4.5
D-4.6
D-4.7
D-4.8
D-4.9
D-4.10
D-4 d

Modified from Seeman P, Van Tol HHM: Dopamine receptor pharmacology, *Trends Pharmacol Sci* 15(7):264-270, 1994.

Administration. Marder and Meibach (1994) determined that the most beneficial dosage of risperidone for adults was 6 mg per day. The manufacturer recommends a twice daily dosing schedule of 1 mg on Day One, 2 mg on Day Two, and 3 mg on Day Three and beyond. Elderly patients may need a reduced amount of risperidone (Mannens et al, 1993). Significant EPSEs can occur at higher than recommended dosages.

Drugs in the Evaluation Phase

Holister (1994) identifies the new agents that are being clinically tested for possible use as antipsychotics. These drugs are listed in Box 4-9.

REMARKS

The dopamine hypothesis of schizophrenia states that the illness is caused by excessive levels of dopamine in the brain. Box 4-10 describes the complexity of the dopamine neurotransmitter system. Antipsychotic drugs block dopamine receptors, which accounts for the ability of these drugs to effectively combat the excessive level of dopamine. Antipsychotic drugs are most accurately classified according to chemical structure; however, a classification system based on potency seems to offer clinical utility. A third system contrasts traditional D-2 receptor blockers and atypical serotonin/dopamine antagonists. Antipsychotics sedate, quiet emotions, and slow psychomotor agitation while alleviating major symptoms of schizophrenia and psychoses, that is, alterations in perception, thought, consciousness, affect, and the like.

Antipsychotic drugs produce three major side effects: anticholinergic side effects, extrapyramidal side effects, and to a lesser extent, hypotension. For the most part anticholinergic side effects are annoying, whereas EPSEs and severe hypotension with orthostasis are often serious. Low-potency antipsychotics, such as chlorpromazine, tend to produce anticholinergic side effects and hypotension, whereas high-potency antipsychotics, such as haloperidol, produce EPSEs.

Overdoses of antipsychotics, especially the high-potency agents, are seldom fatal, but drug interactions with other CNS depressants such as alcohol can be serious. All health care professionals with direct responsibilities for patient care should be alert for signs and symptoms of EPSEs, including tardive dyskinesia and neuroleptic malignant syndrome.

The newer atypical antipsychotics, clozapine and risperidone have antiserotonergic properties that putatively liberate dopamine in cortical regions. Negative symptoms are susceptible to these new agents and when added to this low potential for EPSEs, tardive dyskinesia, and in the case of risperidone, few anticholinergic effects, these agents are becoming increasingly popular among clinicians.

REFERENCES

Addington DE et al: Reduction of hospital days in chronic schizophrenia patients treated with risperidone: a retrospective study, *Clin Therapeutics* 15:917, 1993.

American Psychiatric Association: *Diagnostic and statistical manual of mental disorders,* ed 3, Washington, DC, 1980, The Association.

American Psychiatric Association: *Diagnostic and statistical manual of mental disorders, ed 4,* Washington, DC, 1994, The Association.

Andreasen NC, Olsen S: Negative vs. positive schizophrenia, *Arch Gen Psychiatry* 39:789, 1982.

Andreasen NC et al: Positive and negative symptoms in schizophrenia: a critical reappraisal, *Arch Gen Psychiatry* 47:615, 1990.

Appleton WS: *Practical and clinical psychopharmacology,* Baltimore, 1988, Williams & Wilkins.

Awouters F et al: Functional interaction between serotonin-S-2 and dopamine-D-2 neurotransmission as revealed by selective antagonism of hyper-reactivity to tryptamine and apomorphine, *J Pharm Exper Ther* 254(3):945, 1990.

Ayd FJ: The early history of modern psychopharmacology, *Neuropsychopharmacology* 5(2):71, 1991.

Barnes TR, Curson DA: Long-term depot antipsychotics: a risk-benefit assessment, *Drug Safety* 10(6):464, 1994.

Barrett N, Ormiston S, Molyneux V: Clozapine: a new drug for schizophrenia, *J Psychosoc Nurs Ment Health Serv* 28:24, 1990.

Bergmann GT: Clozapine: will states ration care? *State Health Reports* 57:1, 1990.

Bernardo M et al: Monitoring plasma level of haloperidol in schizophrenia, *Hosp Community Psychiatry* 44(2):115, 1993.

Blair DT: Risk management for extrapyramidal symptoms, *Quality Review Bulletin, J Quality Assurance* 17:116, 1990.

Blair DT, Dauner A: Dangerous consequences: neuroleptic-induced tardive akathisia, *J Psychosoc Nurs Ment Health Serv* 30(3):41, 1992.

Blair DT, Dauner A: Nonneuroleptic etiologies of extrapyramidal symptoms, *Clin Nurs Spec* 7(4):225, 1993a.

Blair DT, Dauner A: Neuroleptic malignant syndrome: liability in nursing practice, *J Psychosoc Nurs Ment Health Serv* 31(2):5, 1993b.

Bleich A et al: The role of serotonin in schizophrenia, *Schizophr Bull* 14:257, 1988.

Bleuler E: *Dementia praecox or the group of schizophrenias.* Translated by Zinkin J, New York, 1950, International Universities Press.

Borison RL et al: Risperidone: clinical safety and efficacy in schizophrenia, *Psychopharmacol Bull* 28(2):213, 1992.

Brown K et al: Overdose of risperidone, *Ann Emergency Med* 22(12):140, 1993.

Chouinard G, Arnott W: Clinical review of risperidone, *Can J Psychiatry* 38(3):S89, 1993.

Claus A et al: Risperidone versus haloperidol in the treatment of chronic schizophrenic inpatients: a multicenter double-blind comparative study, *Acta Psychiatr Scand* 85(4):295, 1992.

Cohen LS: Psychopharmacology: psychotropic drug use in pregnancy, *Hosp Community Psychiatry* 40:566, 1989.

Crow TJ: Molecular pathology of schizophrenia: more than one disease, *Br Med J* 280:66, 1980.

Dauner A, Blair DT: Akathisia: when treatment creates a problem, *J Psychosoc Nurs Ment Health Serv* 28(10):13, 1990.

Deng MA, Chen GQ, Phillips MR: Neuroleptic malignant syndrome in 12 of 9,792 Chinese inpatients exposed to neuroleptics: a prospective study, *Am J Psychiatry* 147:1149, 1990.

Ereshefsky L, Lacombe S: Pharmacological profile of risperidone, *Can J Psychiatry* 38(3):S80, 1993.

Federal Task Force on Homelessness and Severe Mental Illness: Outcasts on Main Street, Washington, 1992, Interagency Council on the Homeless.

Foley JJ: Considerations in the use of benzodiazepines and antipsychotics in the emergency department, *J Emer Nurs* 19(5):448, 1993.

Geller JL, Gaulin BD, Barreira PD: A practitioner's guide to use of psychotropic medication in liquid form, *Hosp Community Psychiatry* 43(10):969, 1992.

Gomez GE, Gomez EA: The special concerns of neuroleptic use in the elderly, *J Psychosoc Nurs Ment Health Serv* 28:7, 1990.

Griffith EEH: Clozapine: problems for the public sector, *Hosp Community Psychiatry* 41:837, 1990.

Harris E: Antipsychotic medication, *Am J Nurs* 81:1316, 1981.

Hollister LE: New antipsychotic drugs, *J Clin Psychopharmacol* 14(1):50, 1994.

Hooper JF, Herren CK, Goldwasser H: Neuroleptic malignant syndrome, *J Psychosoc Nurs Ment Health Serv* 27:13, 1989.

Jaretz N, Flowers E, Millsap L: Clozapine: nursing care considerations, *Perspect Psychiatr Care* 28:19, 1992.

Jeffrey S: Clozapine: how it changed my life, *J Psychosoc Nurs Ment Health Serv* 31(4):44, 1993.

Johnson DAW: Pharmacological treatment of patients with schizophrenia: past and present problems and potential future therapy, *Drugs* 39(4):481, 1990.

Jones BE, Gray BA: Problems in diagnosing schizophrenia and affective disorders among blacks, *Hosp Community Psychiatry* 37:61, 1986.

Kane J: Newer antipsychotic drugs: a review of their pharmacology and therapeutic potential, *Drugs* 46(4):585, 1993.

Kane J: Risperidone, *Am J Psychiatry* 151(6):802, 1994.

Keepers GA, Casey DE: Clinical management of acute neuroleptic-induced extrapyramidal symptoms. In Masserman JH, editor: *Current psychiatric therapies,* New York, 1986, Grune & Stratton.

Keltner NL, McIntyre CW: Neuroleptic malignant syndrome, *J Neurosurg Nurs* 17:362, 1985.

Keltner NL, Folks DG: Clozapine: miracle or mirage? *Perspect Psychiatric Care* 27(3):35, 1991.

Keltner NL: Antipsychotic drugs. In Shlafer M, Marieb E, editors: *The nurse, pharmacology, and drug therapy,* Menlo Park, Calif, 1993, Addison-Wesley.

Keltner NL: Risperidone: the search for a better antipsychotic, *Perspect Psychiatric Care* 31(1):30, 1995.

Kendler KS, Gruenberg AM, Tsuany MT: A family study of the subtypes of schizophrenia, *Am J Psychiatry* 145:57, 1988.

Kerwin RW: The new atypical antipsychotics, *Br J Psychiatry* 164:141, 1994.

Kopelowicz A, Bidder TG: Dementia praecox: inescapable fate or psychiatric oversight? *Hosp Community Psychiatry* 43(9):940, 1992.

Kraepelin E: *Dementia praecox and paraphrenia, with historical introduction (1919).* Translated by Barclay RM, New York, 1971, RE Krieger.

Lamb HR: Deinstitutionalization at the crossroads, *Hosp Community Psychiatry* 45:1434, 1994.

Land W, Salzman C: Risperidone: a novel antipsychotic medication, *Hosp Community Psychiatry* 45(5):434, 1994.

Lawson WB: Drugs versus other therapies, *Hosp Community Psychiatry* 43(1):84, 1992.

Lewine RRJ: A discriminate validity study of negative symptoms with a special focus on depression and antipsychotic medication, *Am J Psychiatry* 147:1463, 1990.

Lieberman J et al: Pharmacologic characterization of tardive dyskinesia, *J Clin Psychopharmacol* 8(4):254, 1988.

Littlejohn R, Leslie F, Cookson J: Depot antipsychotics in the prophylaxsis of bipolar affective disorder, *Br J Psychiatry* 165(6):827, 1994.

Littrell K, Magill AM: The effect of clozapine on pre-existing tardive dyskinesia, *J Psychosoc Nurs Ment Health Serv* 31(9):14, 1993.

Lund VE, Frank DI: Helping the medicine go down, *J Psychosoc Nurs Ment Health Serv* 29(7):6, 1991.

Mannens G et al: Absorption, metabolism, and excretion of risperidone in humans, *Drug Metab Dispos* 21(6):1134, 1993.

Marder SR, Meibach RC: Risperidone in the treatment of schizophrenia, *Am J Psychiatry* 151(6):825, 1994.

Matsubara S et al: Dopamine D-1, D-2, and serotonin-2 receptor occupation by typical and atypical antipsychotic drugs in vivo, *J Pharm Exper Ther* 265(2):498, 1993.

Matthysse SW: The role of dopamine in schizophrenia. In Usdin E, Hamburg DA, Barchas J, editors: *Neuroregulators and Psychiatric Disorders,* New York, 1977, Oxford University Press.

Mehtonen et al: A survey of sudden death associated with the use of antipsychotic or antidepressant drugs: 49 cases in Finland, *Acta Psychiatr Scand* 84:58, 1991.

Meltzer HY: Duration of a clozapine trial in neuroleptic-resistant schizophrenia, *Arch Gen Psychiatry* 46:672, 1989.

Meltzer HY: New drugs for the treatment of schizophrenia, *Psychiatr Clin North Am* 16(2):365, 1993.

Mok H, Yatham LN: Response to clozapine as a predictor of risperidone response in schizophrenia (letter), *Am J Psychiatry* 151(9):1393, 1994.

Olin BR: *Drugs facts and comparisons,* ed 49, St. Louis, 1995, Wolters Kluwer.

Overall JE et al: Justifying neuroleptic drug treatment, *Hosp Community Psychiatry* 40:749, 1989.

Pelonero AL, Elliot RL: Ethical and clinical considerations in selecting patients who will receive clozapine, *Hosp Community Psychiatry* 41:878, 1990.

Perry PJ et al: Clozapine and norclozapine plasma concentrations and clinical response of treatment refractory schizophrenic patients, *Am J Psychiatry* 148(2):231, 1991.

Planasky K, Johnston R: The occurrence and characteristics of suicidal preoccupation and acts in schizophrenia, *Acta Psychiatr Scand* 47:473, 1971.

Regier DA et al: The de facto U.S. mental and addictive disorders service system: epidemiologic catchment area prospective 1-year prevalence rates of disorders and services, *Arch Gen Psychiatry* 50:85, 1993.

Remington GJ: Clinical considerations in the use of risperidone, *Can J Psychiatry* 38(3):S96, 1993.

Remington GJ et al: Prevalence of neuroleptic-induced dystonia in mania and schizophrenia, *Am J Psychiatry* 147:1231, 1990.

Rice DP, Kelman S, Miller LS: The economic burden of mental illness, *Hosp Community Psychiatry* 43(12):1227, 1992.

Richelson E: Neuroleptic affinities for human brain receptors and their use in predicting adverse effects, *J Clin Psychiatry* 45:331, 1984.

Rifkin A et al: Dosage of haloperidol for schizophrenia, *Arch Gen Psychiatry* 48:166, 1991.

Roberts GW, Leigh PN, Weinberger DR: *Neuropsychiatric disorders,* London, 1993, Mosby.

Roth BL, Ciaranello RD, Meltzer HY: Binding of typical and atypical antipsychotic agents to transiently expressed 5-HT1C receptors, *J Pharm Exper Ther* 260(3):1361, 1992.

Safferman A et al: Update on the clinical efficacy and side effects of clozapine, *Schizophr Bull* 17(2):247, 1991.

Salzman C: Notes from a state mental health director's meeting on clozapine, *Hosp Community Psychiatry* 41:838, 1990.

Sandoz, Inc.: *Oral communication,* July 10, 1995.

Sedvall G: PET studies on the neuroreceptor effects of antipsychotic drugs, *Current Approaches to Psychosis* 4:1-3, 1995.

Seeman P, Van Tol HH: Dopamine receptor pharmacology, *Trends Pharmacol 57 Sci*15(7):264, 1994.

Sleight AJ, Koek W, Bigg DC: Binding of antipsychotic drugs at alpha 1A- and alpha 1B-adrenoceptors: risperidone is selective for the alpha 1B-adrenoceptors, *Eur J Pharmacol* 238(2-3):407, 1993.

Strauss J, Carpenter WT, Bartko J: The diagnosis and understanding of schiophrenia, Part III: speculation on the processes that underlie schizophrenic symptoms and signs, *Schizophr Bull* 1:61, 1974.

Tesar GE: The agitated patient, Part II: pharmacologic treatment, *Hosp Community Psychiatry* 44(7):627, 1993.

Thompson LW: The dopamine hypothesis of schizophrenia, *Perspect Psychiatric Care* 26(3):18, 1990.

Van Putten T, Marder SR: Behavioral toxicity of antipsychotic drugs, *J Clin Psychopharmacol* 7:243, 1987.

Watsky EJ, Salzman C: Psychotropic drug interactions, *Hosp Community Psychiatry* 42(3):247, 1991.

White E, Cheung P, Silverstone T: Depot antipsychotics in bipolar affective disorder, *Int Clin Psychopharmacol* 8(2):119, 1993.

Woolley D, Shaw E: A biochemical and pharmacological suggestion about certain mental disorders, *Proc Natl Acad Sci USA* 40:228, 1954.

Wysowski DK, Baum C: Antipsychotic drug use in the United States: 1976-1985, *Arch Gen Psychiatry* 46(10):929, 1989.

Yassa R et al: Factors in the development of severe forms of tardive dyskinesia, *Am J Psychiatry* 147:1156, 1990.

Yaryura-Tobias YA, Diamond BI, Merlis S: The actions of L-dopa on schizophrenic patients (a preliminary report), *Curr Ther Res* 12:528, 1970.

CHAPTER 5

Mood Disorders

HISTORICAL CONSIDERATIONS

Mood or affective disturbances reflect the normal human condition and manifest as a symptom, a syndrome, or a specific diagnostic disorder. *Descriptions of depression* have been noted since ancient times. The term *melancholia* is attributed to Hippocrates, who thought the malady resulted from the influence of black bile and phlegm on the brain, which darkened the spirit. *Descriptions of bipolar disorder* can be traced to early in the second century, when Aretaeus of Cappadocia recognized the association between melancholia and mania. It was not until the end of the 1800s that another major contribution to our understanding of mood disorders was developed. In 1896 Kraepelin separated the functional psychoses into two groups, dementia praecox and manic-depressive psychosis. Subsequently patients with chronic depression were included (Winokur, 1972). Freud in 1917 published *Mourning and Melancholia,* which described his theories of depression (Freud, 1957). He noted that depression and grief had in common the process of mourning, that is, the response to the loss of a love object. He further observed that although grief was a healthy response, it differed from melancholia in that the latter involved intense expression of ambivalent, hostile feelings formerly associated with the object.

The controversy concerning endogenous (biologic) versus reactive depressions (reactions to life events) undoubtedly arose as a result of the differing viewpoints of Kraepelinians and Freudians. A large part of the existing literature assumes that the two basic forms of depression do indeed exist. However, clinical observations in the past two decades indicate that primary mood disorders are more appropriately divided into bipolar and unipolar forms. Other mood or affective spectrum disorders have been identified and subclassified as minor forms of mood disturbances (Goodwin and Guze, 1984).

SCOPE OF THE PROBLEM

Estimates of the prevalence of mood disturbances depend on the sample of the population studied and on the definition of the illness. Lifetime incidences as high as 18% for major depression have been reported. The Epidemiological Catchment Area (ECA) studies, sponsored by the National Institutes of Mental Health, found much lower lifetime incidences of 6.7%, 3.7%, and 5.7% for New Haven, Conn.; Baltimore; and St. Louis, respectively (Myers et al, 1985). The prevalence of bipolar disorder has been investigated primarily through treatment cases because it occurs less frequently. The ECA studies revealed a 6-month incidence ranging from 0.4% to 0.8% for men and from 0.4% to 0.9% for women.

Women are at greater risk than men for major depression, and the patient age at onset is usually the late twenties. No differences are found among races in its distribution. Differences among social classes and familial differences have been shown; depression is most common in lower socioeconomic groups and is most likely to emerge in individuals with a positive family history of depression. Negative events are often identified as precipitators or as having occurred before the onset of a depressive disorder.

The occurrence of bipolar disorder is equal between men and women and among races; the patient age at onset is typically the early twenties. This disorder is most common in higher socioeconomic groups and in religious communities, for example, Old Order Amish. Family history is particularly important insofar as genetic contributors are present, and often a positive family history is found among affected individuals. The relative effect of life events on the onset of an episode is currently unknown.

Primary mood disorders are the psychiatric problem for which patients are most frequently admitted to hospitals and to many psychiatric clinics. The National Institute on Mental Health estimates that 17.5 million individuals in the United States suffer from major depression or bipolar mood disorder at a cost to society of $30 billion. Mood disturbance is also a common reason for psychiatric consultation; secondary depression or mania is frequently found among elderly and medically ill individuals or among substance abusers who are referred for consultation.

DIAGNOSTIC CONSIDERATIONS

Diagnostic criteria for major depression and mania (bipolar disorder) are presented in Boxes 5-1 and 5-2.

Minor forms of depression include dysthymic disorder and adjustment disorder. Mania subtypes include hypomania, mixed, and rapid cycling. These syndromes and subtypes of depression and mania are frequently treated with pharmacotherapy. Residual categories or subsyndromal mood disturbance may also be a focus of treatment. It is recognized that a mood disturbance may be related to psychologic problems, may be a component of another major psychiatric disorder, or may be associ-

Box 5-1 Diagnostic Criteria for Major Depression

1. Five of the following are present:
   - Depressed mood*
   - Lack of pleasure or loss of interest*
   - Appetite disturbance or weight loss/gain
   - Sleep disturbance
   - Motor agitation or retardation
   - Fatigue or loss of energy
   - Guilt or worthlessness
   - Concentration difficulties or indecisiveness
   - Suicidal ideation or thoughts of death
2. Distress or impairment in social, occupational, or other areas of functioning
3. Symptoms not caused by substances or general medical conditions, or normal grief and bereavement

*Must have one of these symptoms to qualify.
Modified from American Psychiatric Association: *Diagnostic and Statistical Manual of Mental Disorders,* ed 4, Washington DC, 1994, The Association.

Box 5-2 Diagnostic Criteria for Bipolar Disorder: Mania

1. Euphoric, expansive, or irritable mood associated with social or occupational impairment
2. Three or more of the following are present:
   - Grandiosity
   - Decreased need for sleep
   - Pressured or hyperverbal speech
   - Flight of ideas or racing thoughts
   - Distractibility
   - Motor agitation or increased activity
   - Excessive involvement in activities
3. Not caused by a primary psychotic disorder, substances, or a general medical condition

Modified from American Psychiatric Association: *Diagnostic and Statistical Manual of Mental Disorders,* ed 4, Washington, DC, 1994, The Association.

ated with a seasonal pattern (American Psychiatric Association, 1994). Some individuals with depression may meet conventional criteria for melancholia, the most severe form of depression. Melancholia is characterized by agitation, somatic or nihilistic delusions, loss of pleasure in all or almost all activities, excessive anhedonia, increased depression in the morning, early morning awakening, and excessive or inappropriate guilt.

Major Depression

The chief complaint of patients with major depressive disorder is usually psychologic, that is, mood disturbances or feelings of worthlessness, or despair or ideas of self-harm. However, a significant portion of depressed individuals also complain of somatic disturbances combined with dysphoric mood. They may also describe themselves as having irritability, fearfulness, worry, or discouragement. Patients who somatize have a tendency to minimize feelings of dysphoria and focus on insomnia and anorexia, the so-called vegetative disturbances (Ford, 1983; Stone and Folks, 1992). Agitation may be so overwhelming in some depressed individuals that other symptoms of mood disturbance go unnoticed. In contrast, some patients may have prominent motor retardation to the point that they become mute or even catatonic. Psychotic symptoms, for example, suspiciousness and perceptual disturbances, may complicate a depressive episode. Delusions or hallucinations, or both, may or may not be congruent with the mood disturbance per se. Depressed patients may or may not be able to identify precipitating events that have contributed to the illness. In fact, some of the "precipitators" actually may have occurred *after* the onset of depressive symptoms. For instance, a failed marriage may be either the cause of or the result of depression.

A variety of biologic correlates are known concomitants of depression, such as reduction in slow-wave sleep, shortened rapid eye movement (REM) latency, and increased REM density. Neuroendocrine disturbances, for example, alterations in the response to dexamethasone or thyrotropin releasing factor, may also be present, but a discussion of these parameters is beyond the scope of this book.

Bipolar Disorder

The cardinal features of mania are euphoria, hyperactivity, and disturbances of thinking and speech, that is, flight of ideas and pressured speech (Box 5-2). Many bipolar patients are primarily irritable. Manic patients may have mixtures of manic and depressive symptoms, that is, mixed subtype. Psychotic symptoms, especially persecutory and grandiose delusions, hallucinations, or ideas of reference, also complicate mania.

Suicide and Other Risks

There is a clear association between mood disturbance and suicide; in fact, 50% to 70% of people who commit suicide are found retrospectively to have had symptoms characteristic of depression. Of those who are depressed it is suggested that approximately 15% eventually die by suicide (Guze and Robins, 1970). Disregarding suicide, patients with primary mood disturbance still show an increased mortality when compared by age and sex with members of the general population (Kerr, Schapira, and Roth, 1969). Alcoholism and poor judgment are other risks of primary affective disorders, especially among manic patients. The postpartum period is significant also, especially in women with bipolar disorder, who are likely to have episodes of depression or mania during the postpartum period.

Diagnostic Dilemmas

Depressed patients may show impairment in concentration and short-term but not long-term memory (Sternberg and Jarvik, 1976). Sometimes the memory impairment associated with depression mimics dementia. This condition is referred to as *pseudodementia* (Table 5-1). Distinguishing between primary mood disturbance and grief can be difficult (Table 5-2). Differential diagnosis includes anxiety disorders,

Table 5-1 Comparison of Dementia and Depression

Feature	Dementia	Depression
Onset	Insidious, indeterminate	Rapid, abrupt
Symptom duration	Longer	Shorter
Mood	Variable	Depressed
Cognitive deficits	Consistent	Inconsistent
Mental status assessment	Wrong answer	Refuses to attempt answer
Neurologic deficit	Aphasia, apraxia, agnosia	None

Table 5-2 Comparison of Grief and Depression

Grief	Depression
Guilt/self-reproach	Guilt/self-reproach
Somatic symptoms	Somatic symptoms
Duration of 6 months or less	Greater than 6 months' duration
Remains functional	Becomes debilitated
Usually not suicidal	Possibly suicidal

hypochondriasis or other somatoform disorders, and other major psychiatric syndromes such as schizophrenia, dementia, and delirium. Syndromes in which a mood disturbance is secondarily induced as a side effect of drugs or substances as a complication of general medical problems are also prominent and must be considered in the differential diagnosis. Personality disorder, especially borderline, histrionic, narcissistic, or antisocial, must be considered. In many cases depression will coexist with a general medical condition or substance use disorder or a personality disorder. Pharmacotherapy and other forms of treatment are indicated for these cases similar to those without comorbidity.

TREATMENT CONSIDERATIONS

Depression

The management of depression ideally combines an indicated drug treatment together with other interventions. Insight-oriented psychotherapy, for example, may involve examinations of motives and feelings; cognitive psychotherapy may focus on defects in the individual's perception of self, the environment, or future outlook. Other forms of psychotherapy, including interpersonal, behavioral, group, and marital therapy, may contribute significantly to positive patient outcome. Studies have repeatedly shown that psychotherapy is more efficacious than nontreatment and that the combination of psychotherapy and antidepressant medication is more efficacious than either drug treatment alone or no treatment. Some patients do not wish to receive drug treatment, and many patients cannot tolerate the side effects of antidepressant medication. Still others may not wish to enter into any form of psychotherapy and should not be denied treatment with antidepressant medication.

No definitive data suggest that patients will recover as a result of one type of treatment rather than another or that an individual with a particular subtype of depression will benefit from drugs or psychotherapy, or a combination of the two. However, the best approach to the management of major depressive illness is often drug treatment or electroconvulsive therapy (ECT), or both. Choosing the most suitable antidepressant medication for a particular patient remains more of an art than a science. It is not yet clear how antidepressant medication shortens depressive episodes, and ECT may be the most effective treatment available for depression, especially major depression as discussed in Chapter 11, Drugs Used for Electroconvulsive Therapy. Generally ECT is no more dangerous than treatment with drugs.

Bipolar Disorder

Mania may be effectively treated with antipsychotics, mood stabilizers or alternative agents, or ECT. Of these methods ECT is probably the least effective. Lithium or valproate are the drugs of choice, but antipsychotic or anxiolytic agents may be particularly useful in active or agitated manic patients. The usefulness of lithium or valproate or other alternative agents such as carbamazepine (Tegretol) may be limited to the treatment of acute mania. However, growing evidence suggests that these drugs may reduce morbidity, that is, they may prevent depression as well as mania (Keltner and Folks, 1991).

Other Mood Disorders

The use of drugs to treat other mood disturbances depends largely on the "target" symptoms that are present. The identification of target symptoms and a rationale for treatment are considered carefully before therapy is instituted. Patients with dysthymic disorder, adjustment disorder with depressed mood, cyclothymia, or other subsyndromal mood disturbances may benefit greatly from drug treatment. Substantial data to support this conventional wisdom does not exist but remains the subject of further studies.

ANTIDEPRESSANTS

Historical Considerations

The introduction of pharmacologic agents with antidepressant action in the 1950s revolutionized our thinking about the causes, pathogenic mechanisms, and management of depressive illness. As a consequence, many patients with depressive illness were able to function normally and lead productive lives. Electroconvulsive therapy, developed in the 1930s, remains an effective and safe modality for treatment of depressions that fail to respond to pharmacotherapy and is discussed in Chapter 11, Drugs Used for Electroconvulsive Therapy.

Before the 1950s and after the initial development of ECT, amphetamines to treat psychomotor retardation and barbiturates to treat agitation were used in patients with depression. Although amphetamines and barbiturates are still used in the initial treatment of depression in medically ill, abulic, or demented patients, there is little reason to use these drugs in most cases. Moreover, the use of amphetamines with severe depression is not indicated and may actually worsen any associated agitation or psychosis, or both (see Chapter 13, Drugs Used to Stimulate the Central Nervous System).

The antidepressant actions of the monoamine oxidase inhibitors (MAOIs) were discovered serendipitously in the 1950s; these drugs were the first to have a true mood-elevating effect. Clinical pharmacologists also began to observe and correlate changes in brain chemistry with changes in mood and behavior. This, in turn, led to theories about the mechanisms of action of these drugs and the biologic contributors to psychiatric illness (Goodman and Charney, 1985). Subsequently in the 1960s the tricyclic antidepressant compounds (TCAs) were introduced to treat depression. The TCAs first developed were actually an outgrowth of attempts to find more effective antipsychotic drugs that were chemically related to the phenothiazines. The tricyclics remain as a viable pharmacologic treatment of depressive illness, although newer agents have been developed and introduced. Depending on molecular configuration, some of these newer agents are more correctly identified as bicyclic or tetracyclic. To reduce repetition, an encompassing classification, "heterocyclic," has been developed to embrace bicyclic, tricyclic, and tetracyclic antidepressants. Although these categories are not identical, it is common for all to be referred to as *tricyclic antidepressants,* or TCAs, in the literature. Figure 5-1 shows the chemical structures of many currently available antidepressants. Tables 5-3 and 5-4 show the dosage range, reuptake inhibition, half-life, and the relative effects resulting from cholinergic, histaminergic, alpha-adrenergic, and dopaminergic blockade (discussed in the section on side effects).

All of the antidepressant agents depicted in Tables 5-3 and 5-4 are effective in alleviating the symptoms of depressive illness. Melancholia, including sadness and hopelessness, as well as vegetative, somatic, and motor symptoms, is responsive to drug treatment. The ability to re-engage in social, occupational, and relationship functioning and to recapture quality of life are among the many benefits that may be derived from antidepressant therapy. Patients generally experience an improvement in energy level, a decrease in fatigue and psychomotor symptoms, and the disappearance of suicidal thoughts.

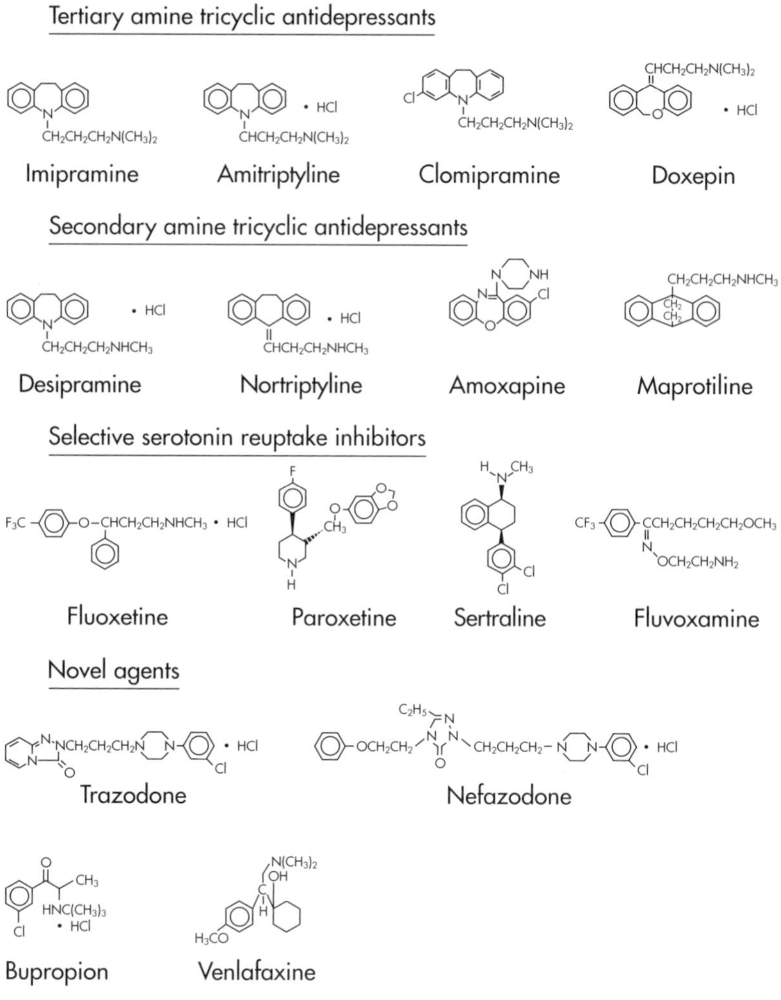

Tertiary amine tricyclic antidepressants

Imipramine Amitriptyline Clomipramine Doxepin

Secondary amine tricyclic antidepressants

Desipramine Nortriptyline Amoxapine Maprotiline

Selective serotonin reuptake inhibitors

Fluoxetine Paroxetine Sertraline Fluvoxamine

Novel agents

Trazodone Nefazodone

Bupropion Venlafaxine

Figure 5-1 Chemical structures of heterocyclic antidepressants.

Neurochemical Theory of Effectiveness

Although a number of theories concerning the cause of depression have been promulgated, the efficacy of antidepressants is best understood from a neurochemical and neurobiologic perspective. The biogenic amine theory of depression essentially implies that an imbalance or a relative deficiency exists of certain neurotransmitters or biogenic amines, for example, serotonin and norepinephrine. Specifically, deficiencies of these substances result in a neurochemical imbalance. Perhaps alterations exist in the functioning of the receptor site or the secondary messenger systems that modulate the activity of the receptor site postsynaptically, hence the term *neuromodulator.*

Table 5-3 Antidepressant Dosage, Neurotransmitter Effect, and Half-life of Selected Agents

Drug	Adult starting daily dosage/range(mg)	Neurotransmitter effect† Serotonin	Norepinephrine	Half-life (hours)
Heterocyclics				
Amitriptyline	25 tid/75-300	3	1	31-46
Amoxapine	50 bid/100-300	1	3	8-30
Clomipramine	25 hs/75-200	4	1	19-37
Desipramine	25 tid/75-300	1	5	12-24
Doxepin	25 tid/75-300	2	1	8-24
Imipramine	25 tid/75-300	3	2	11-25
Maprotiline	25 tid/75-300	1	2	21-25
Nortriptyline	25 bid/50-200	2	3	18-44
Protriptyline	10 bid/40-60	2	5	67-89
Trazodone	50 tid/150-450	2	0	4-9
Trimipramine	25 tid/75-300	1	1	7-30
SSRIs				
Fluoxetine	20/10-60	4	0	48-216‡
Fluvoxamine*	50-100/100-300	4	0	15-19
Paroxetine	20-30/20-60	5	1	21
Sertraline	50/25-200	4	0	26-98‡
Novel agents				
Bupropion	75 bid/150-450	0	0/1	8-15
Nefazodone	50 bid/100-600	3	0	2-4
Venlafaxine	37.5 bid/150-450	3	2	5-11‡

* Although an antidepressant, fluvoxamine's approved indication in the United States is for obsessive compulsive disorder.
†Relative intensity of effect on scale of zero to five based upon Richelson, 1994.
‡With active metabolite.

Psychopharmacologic treatment is based on the restoration of normal levels of neurotransmitter systems:

1. by blocking neurotransmitter uptake in the nerve ending
2. by inhibiting neurotransmitter breakdown and
3. by reducing stimulation at the site of the receptor.

Reduction of the beta-adrenergic receptor stimulation occurs through norepinephrine pathways or by normalizing/regulating receptor function and neurotransmission. Whether the amine-potentiating actions of antidepressants are either necessary or sufficient to account for the clinical actions of antidepressants remains uncertain. Thus considerable risk is taken when simply developing new antidepressants by screening for a chemical compound's ability to inhibit the uptake of norepinephrine or serotonin or to otherwise alter neurochemical transmission. Nonetheless, this type of circular reasoning is tempting in view of the apparent association of these drugs' effects and the clinical response (Baldesserini, 1985).

Four new-generation agents, fluoxetine (Prozac), sertraline (Zoloft), paroxetine (Paxil), and fluvoxamine (Luvox) are classified as selective serotonin reuptake inhibitors (SSRIs) and show great promise for patients with depression. Clomipramine (Anafranil), a TCA, possesses selective beneficial effects in the treatment of obses-

Table 5-4 Comparison of Drugs that Inhibit Serotonin Reuptake

	Half-life (mean)	Half-life (metabolic)	Activity of metabolite	Cytochrome inhibition	Impairment of drug metabolism	Reuptake inhibition (K_i)*		
						Serotonin	Norepinephrine	DA
Fluoxetine (Prozac)	2-3 days	7-9 days	Equal to F	+ + + +	+ + + +	25	500	4200
Fluvoxamine (Luvox)	15 hr	Inactive	0	+	+ + +	6.2	1100	>10,000
Paroxetine (Paxil)	21 hr	Inactive	0	+ + + + +	+ + +	1.1	350	2000
Sertraline (Zoloft)	26 hr	2-4 days	Minimal	+	+	7.3	1400	230
Venlafaxine (Effexor)	5 hr	11 hr	Equal to V	±	±	21	64	280
Clomipramine (Anafranil)	32 hr	69 hr	CM/serotonin DCM/NE	±	+	7.4	96	91

Antidepressant					
Heterocyclics	**Cholinergic**	**Histaminergic**	**+1 adrenergic**	**+2 adrenergic**	**Dopaminergic**
protriptyline	+3	+2	+3	+1	+1
trimipramine	+2	+4	+2	+/0	+1
SSRIs					
fluvoxamine	0	0	+/0	+/0	+1
paroxetine	+/0	0	0	0	+1
Novel agents					
nefazodone	0	0	0	0	0
venlafaxine	+1	+/0	+2	+/0	+1

* The smaller the K_i value, the greater the inhibition of the neurotransmitter reuptake (i.e., fluvoxamine is a more potent inhibitor of serotonin reuptake than is fluoxetine).
DCM=desmethylclomipramine
NE=norepinephrine

sive-compulsive disorder by blocking the reuptake of both norepinephrine and serotonin. A newer agent, venlafaxine (Effexor), also significantly inhibits both serotonin and norepinephrine reuptake. Furthermore, some effective antidepressants neither primarily block the uptake of monoamines nor inhibit monoamine oxidase but probably exert subtle influences on neuronal processes; nefazodone (Serzone) and bupropion (Wellbutrin) are good examples of these drugs. Thus it would seem that antidepressants with similar actions on neurotransmitters may be selectively beneficial for dissimilar disorders and that antidepressants with dissimilar actions on neurotransmitters may be selectively beneficial for similar disorders. These differences raise doubts about the biogenic amine theories of depression.

Although the influence of monoamines is the most studied neurochemical aspect of mood disorders, other important receptor interactions are also useful in predicting clinical side effects and potential toxic effects (Table 5-4). These effects account for nontherapeutic actions of antidepressants. Variable effects in blocking the reuptake of norepinephrine and serotonin, and other effects, undoubtedly account for some of the variability in side-effect profiles as well as the therapeutic effects.

TRICYCLIC, HETEROCYCLIC, AND SECOND-GENERATION ANTIDEPRESSANTS

Pharmacokinetics

The tricyclic, heterocyclic, and newer second-generation antidepressant agents are well absorbed from the gastrointestinal tract and are usually given orally. Imipramine and amitriptyline are available in parenteral forms. Antidepressant compounds are metabolized in the liver, and some metabolites have active antidepressant effects and are marketed as such. For example, desipramine is a metabolite of imipramine; nortriptyline is a metabolite of amitriptyline.

Peak plasma concentrations of antidepressants are generally reached in 3 to 4 hours. Tricyclic, heterocyclic, and other antidepressant compounds are water soluble and are highly bound to plasma proteins. Their effects are caused by a small fraction of free drug; thus even a small increase in free drug is potentially significant.

Individuals with diminished liver function, decreased plasma proteins, and decreased total body water are at special risk for elevated serum levels. Antidepressant compounds are also relatively lipophilic but are avidly bound to tissue and plasma proteins, making it virtually impossible to remove the heterocyclic agents by hemodialysis, thereby adding to the danger of acute overdoses.

The ratio of parent tricyclic compound to the active secondary amine products varies markedly among patients by as much as fiftyfold (Baldesserini, 1985). After a fixed dose of antidepressant drug is administered, the plasma levels of active agents may vary by tenfold to twentyfold among individuals. Assays of antidepressant compounds may not be reliable, but such measurements do help to confirm patient compliance with medication regimens and may be useful in evaluating unexpected or untoward clinical outcomes.

Tolerance to many of the side effects of heterocyclic and other antidepressant compounds, for example, sedation and the autonomic effects, is usual. Occasional symptoms suggestive of physical dependence have been reported, especially after a discontinuation of the drug, and a withdrawal syndrome consisting of malaise, chills, coryza, and muscle ache has been described. Therefore gradual withdrawal is considered a reasonable and standard practice. These compounds are eliminated in a manner similar to that of antipsychotic compounds.

The individual and structural characteristics and pharmacologic properties of the antidepressant medications are shown in Figure 5-1 and Tables 5-3 and 5-4. A discussion of the side effects or undesirable effects may begin with comparing tricyclic antidepressants with newer drugs and the MAOIs.

Side Effects

Patients for whom TCAs are prescribed have both peripheral and central nervous system side effects (Box 5-3).

Peripheral nervous system effects. Peripheral nervous system (PNS) side effects include anticholinergic effects on the peripheral autonomic nervous system, which often affect patient tolerance and may also affect compliance; these side effects include dry mouth and visual disturbances, including blurred vision, tearing, and photosensitivity resulting from mydriasis. These symptoms are more annoying than dangerous; however, the narrow mydriatic action of the tricyclics can precipitate an acute attack of glaucoma. Moreover, TCAs should not be prescribed for individuals with narrow-angle glaucoma. Other anticholinergic side effects include slowing of the gastrointestinal tract, which can lead to constipation, and slowing of bladder function, which can bring about hesitancy or urinary retention. Elderly individuals are most susceptible to these side effects (see Chapter 17, Psychopharmacology for Elderly Persons).

Anticholinergic effects on the cardiovascular system are common enough to warrant some consideration. Tachycardia, reflex tachycardia, and arrhythmias can lead to myocardial infarction or heart block or both. Essentially the potential reduction in cardiac conduction time is of greater concern than is the potential for inducing arrhythmias except in patients who have a pre-existing arrhythmia or bundle branch block. The tricyclic antidepressants possess a quinidine-like effect and may actually prove to be beneficial for patients with arrhythmia. In any event, patients with a history of cardiac problems should be carefully evaluated and closely monitored when receiving treatment with a tricyclic antidepressant. The secondary amine TCA, nortriptyline, has gained some favor in the treatment of persons with cardiac conditions because of its ability to be monitored by means of serum level determinations and because of its relatively favorable profile with respect to the potential for causing orthostasis and other hemodynamic instabilities. Newer agents are much less likely to result in cardiovascular side effects.

Central nervous system effects. A number of effects on the central nervous system (CNS) have been reported with the TCAs. Sedation is common but sometimes represents a "fringe therapeutic benefit," because insomnia frequently accompanies depression. Less pleasant CNS effects include confusion, disorientation, delusions, agitation, hallucinations, and lowering of the seizure threshold. These neuropsychiatric side effects are probably caused by CNS anticholinergic effects and may be found in as many as 5% to 15% of patients (Meador-Woodruff, 1990). These CNS effects are more likely to occur when serum TCA levels are elevated. Other potential CNS effects include anxiety, insomnia, nightmare, ataxia, and tremors. Some patients report nightmares so terrifying that they avoid sleep even though they are sleep deprived.

Implications

Therapeutic versus toxic levels. Tricyclic antidepressants do not produce euphoria and are nonaddictive, so their potential for abuse is minimal. However,

Box 5-3 Side Effects and Nursing Interventions for Tricyclic Antidepressants

Peripheral nervous system effects

Dry mouth

Advise frequent sips of water, hard candies, sugarless gum.

Mydriasis

Advise wearing of sunglasses outdoors.

Diminished lacrimation

Suggest artificial tears.

Blurred vision

Caution about driving and potential for falls. The patient should remove objects in the house that might be tripped over (e.g., throw rugs and small tables).

Eye pain

Advise patient to report eye pain immediately, since it may indicate an acute glaucoma attack. All elderly persons should be screened for glaucoma before treatment with TCAs is initiated.

Urinary hesitancy or retention

Monitor fluid intake. Patient should be told to avoid putting off urinating. Running water or pouring water over the perineum can stimulate urination. Catheterization may be needed.

Constipation

Monitor fluid and food intake. Urge patient to heed the urge to defecate. A high-fiber diet and large amounts of water (2500 to 3000 ml per day) are helpful.

Anhidrosis

Decreased sweating can lead to increased body temperature. Adequate fluid intake, appropriate clothing, and sensible exercise should be stressed.

Cardiovascular effects

Tricyclic antidepressants are contraindicated during the recovery phase of myocardial infarction.

Orthostatic hypotension

Advise patient to assume sitting position on side of bed, to wait and dangle feet for 1 full minute, then to rise slowly. Patients should not stand in one position too long and should avoid hot showers and tub baths. Elderly patients may require assistance at these times.

Central nervous system effects

Sedation

Caution patient about driving.

Delirium or mania

Discontinue the drug and call the physician.

Suicidal patients

Observe patients closely, since TCAs may increase energy for suicide.

Table 5-5 Tricyclic Antidepressant Blood Levels

Drug	Range (ng/mL)	Relationship
Imipramine and desipramine (combined levels)	150-250	Linear
Desipramine	150-250 100-155	Linear; plateau above 250 ng/mL; ?therapeutic window
Amitriptyline and nortriptyline (combined levels)	100-250 130-220	Linear; ?therapeutic window
Nortriptyline	50-140	Curvilinear; therapeutic window
Protriptyline	80-240	Linear; ?therapeutic window
Doxepin and desmethyldoxepin	120-250	Linear; ?therapeutic window
Maprotiline	150-250	Linear

Clinical application of TCA blood level monitoring (1) is not necessary in routine treatment with imipramine and amitriptyline, for which a linear relationship exists; (2) is useful in elderly patients who achieve higher levels with standard doses; (3) is useful in nonresponders who may not be taking medication properly; and (4) is necessary in titrating dosage of tricyclic drugs such as nortriptyline, for which a curvillinear therapeutic window exists. There are inadequate data to reliably correlate plasma drug concentration with therapeutic response for amoxapine, trimipramine, and trazodone.

overdose of these agents is a real issue. TCA overdose accounts for 25% to 50% of all hospital admissions for psychotropic overdose (Harsch and Holt, 1988). The difference is slight between a therapeutic dose and a health-impairing or lethal dose. As little as 10 to 30 times the daily dose can be fatal. TCA serum levels should be monitored, and because many clinicians do not attempt to memorize all acceptable therapeutic plasma values, the information in Table 5-5 should be kept available. Toxic blood levels may result in sedation, ataxia, agitation, stupor, coma, respiratory depression, and convulsions. Exaggeration of side effects previously mentioned can also occur. Cardiovascular reactions can occur suddenly and cause acute heart failure. On the other hand, cardiovascular reactions can be delayed, that is, they can occur after recovery from overdose. For these reasons all TCA overdoses should be considered serious, and the patient should be admitted to a hospital for monitoring. However, some studies suggest that imipramine also has antiarrhythmic properties. Imipramine's arrhythmic and antiarrhythmic properties underscore the need for more knowledge about TCAs.

TCAs have a paradoxic effect. Although they are effective antidepressants, they also can energize suicidal patients. Apparently, as TCAs begin to exert their antidepressant effect, patients who otherwise might be too depressed to act on suicidal thoughts slowly begin to accrue the energy to act in self-destructive ways. Because of the potential lethality of TCAs, it is common for outpatients to be restricted to a 7-day supply when suicide is a risk. Inpatients should be watched for hoarding. Interventions for TCA overdose are given in Box 5-4.

Use in pregnancy. Depressive symptoms such as loss of appetite can interfere with fetal development by preventing adequate fetal weight gain. During pregnancy, TCAs with low anticholinergic effects, such as nortriptyline and desipramine, are preferred to those with high anticholinergic effects. The TCAs must be tapered off before delivery to avoid transient perinatal toxicity (Cohen, 1989).

Box 5-4 Interventions for TCA Overdose

Monitor blood pressure, heart rate and rhythm, and respirations.
Maintain patent airway.
Monitor cardiovascular system with electrocardiogram.
Induce vomiting or gastric lavage with activated charcoal to prevent further drug absorption (for up to 24 hours).
Sodium bicarbonate (hypertonic, 1 M) IV has been used effectively to treat cardiac arrhythmias and hypotension. If cardiac arrhythmias do not respond, lidocaine or phenytoin may be used. If hypotension does not respond, fluid expansion and vasopressors (e.g., dopamine) may be required.

Modified from Keltner NL. In Shlafer M, Marieb E, editors: *The nurse, pharmacology, and drug therapy,* Redwood City, Calif, 1989, Addison-Wesley.

Side effects. TCAs, as noted previously, can cause many CNS and PNS side effects. Although some are simply annoying, others are significant—even dangerous—and warrant clinical attention. A common CNS effect is sedation. Sedation can be beneficial for depressed patients who have insomnia, and a drug such as amitriptyline (Elavil) can be ordered, to take advantage of its sedating properties. In other situations, such as when a patient must continue to work, sedation can present an array of problems, from dozing off at work to impairment of driving. Protriptyline (Vivactil) can be ordered for patients who experience unacceptable sedation. This one side effect underscores the need for individual consideration when prescribing TCAs. Box 5-3 lists interventions.

Interactions. Several serious drug interactions occur with TCAs. These interactions can be categorized as CNS depression, cardiovascular and hypertensive interactions, and additive anticholinergic effects.

Central nervous system depression. When taken with drugs such as the antipsychotics, benzodiazepines, sedatives, antiepileptics, alcohol, and some antihypertensives (for example, beta-blockers, clonidine, and reserpine), TCAs can increase CNS depression.

Cardiovascular and hypertensive effects. Cardiovascular arrhythmias or hypertension can occur when sympathomimetic drugs that increase norepinephrine levels in the synaptic cleft are given with TCAs. Interactants to avoid include norepinephrine, dopamine, ephedrine, and phenylpropanolamine, which is a major component of over-the-counter weight-loss stimulants. Monoamine oxidase inhibitors, another class of antidepressants, must also be avoided for similar reasons. The MAOI-TCA combination, although perhaps not as lethal as once thought, can cause a severe reaction, including high fever, seizures, and a fatal hypertensive crisis. Because MAOIs are not typically prescribed unless TCAs fail, care should be taken when switching the TCA-resistant patient to MAOIs. A minimum of 14 days should occur between the time TCAs are discontinued and MAOIs are given. TCAs block the release of several antihypertensives from presynaptic cells, thus contributing to the failure of antihypertensives to control hypertension.

Additive anticholinergic effects. An "atropine-poisoning" effect can occur when TCAs are mixed with other anticholinergic drugs. Especially troublesome drugs include antipsychotic drugs, atropine, scopolamine, anticholinergic-antiparkinson drugs, and antihistamines. Elderly persons are at special risk for this interaction, and all the central and peripheral anticholinergic effects mentioned in the side effects section can be intensified.

Patient education. Besides the teaching related to side effects, the following areas of education are worth discussing with the patient and his or her family:

A "lag period" of 2 to 4 weeks occurs before full therapeutic effects are experienced.

Certain interactants must be avoided, including over-the-counter products (see the section on interactions).

Abrupt discontinuation of TCAs can cause nausea, headache, and malaise.

Eye pain must be reported immediately.

SPECIFIC TRICYCLIC ANTIDEPRESSANTS

Tertiary amines. Tricyclic antidepressants are usually divided into tertiary and secondary amine TCAs (based on their structure). *Imipramine* (Tofranil) is the oldest of the TCAs. Imipramine has relatively high anticholinergic and sedative effects. However, none of the newer antidepressant agents has proved to be more effective. Imipramine pamolate (Tofranil PM) is available in a single bedtime dose for adults. *Amitriptyline* (Elavil and Endep) preferentially potentiates serotonin and exerts the greatest anticholinergic and antianxiety effects among the tertiary amine TCAs. Amitriptyline is sedating and is often prescribed to be taken at bedtime to enhance sleep. Amitriptyline is also available in a parenteral form and in a fixed-dose combination with the antipsychotic drug perphenazine (Triavil).

Doxepin (Sinequan) is a widely used TCA that potentiates serotonin preferentially. Doxepin is sedating, has significant anticholinergic activity, and is often touted as a drug that effectively enhances sleep and reduces anxiety. Doxepin has often been recognized as a compound well tolerated among cardiac patients; however, there is no substantial evidence to show that doxepin is superior to other tertiary (or secondary amine) TCAs.

Trimipramine (Surmontil) is a TCA that theoretically potentiates serotonin; however, this effect has not been clearly established. Trimipramine, like the other tertiary amine TCAs, is quite sedating and has moderate anticholinergic effects.

Secondary amines. Secondary amine TCAs are represented by *desipramine* (Norpramin and Pertofrane), a widely used TCA that potentiates norepinephrine preferentially. Desipramine is a naturally occurring metabolite of imipramine, and many clinicians have noted its utility in depressed elderly patients sensitive to anticholinergic effects and in elderly individuals with open-angle glaucoma or prostatic hypertrophy, because of its low incidence of anticholinergic effects. This drug is also considered less sedating than other tricyclics and therefore is sometimes referred to as an "activating" antidepressant agent.

Nortriptyline (Aventyl and Pamelor) is a TCA often preferred because it has a lower potential for sedating and anticholinergic effects than other TCAs. It is a natural metabolite of amitriptyline, and because of the reliability of its measured serum levels, it is often used in patients for whom toxicity or compliance is an issue.

Protriptyline (Vivactil) is different from other TCAs in that it is quite stimulating. Protriptyline may produce a greater incidence of tachycardia and cardiovascular problems than other tricyclics and certainly has a high potential for anticholinergic side effects. Because some depressed patients have hypersomnia rather than insomnia, protriptyline may enable these individuals to reduce their amount of sleep.

Heterocyclics. *Maprotiline* (Ludiomil) represents a tetracyclic antidepressant. It potentiates norepinephrine, has a relatively mild potential for anticholinergic effects, and is sedating. Its neurochemical effects are similar to those of desipramine. Dosage increases are generally made more slowly than with the tertiary amine TCAs because this drug is almost twice as potent.

Amoxapine (Asendin), a secondary amine, is a relatively recent drug but not specifically a tricyclic antidepressant. It is a metabolite of the antipsychotic drug loxapine and also blocks dopamine receptors. Amoxapine potentiates norepinephrine preferentially and, perhaps because of its neuroleptic effects, has a faster rate of onset of action than other antidepressants. However, extrapyramidal and other side effects often noted with the antipsychotic agents have been reported with amoxapine and are no doubt related to the dopamine-blocking properties.

In addition to amoxapine and maprotiline, *trazodone* (Desyrel) represents the other heterocyclic that was introduced after the TCAs. Trazodone potentiates serotonin and is prescribed often because of its virtual lack of anticholinergic effects and low potential for cardiac effects. Trazodone's absorption is increased by 20%—an unusual reaction—when it is taken with a meal. Another unusual adverse reaction to this drug is priapism, that is, prolonged penile erection. Emergency or surgical intervention has been required in a small percentage of affected men. If priapism occurs, the patient should stop the medication and seek immediate medical advice.

NEWER ANTIDEPRESSANT AGENTS

Among the newer agents *bupropion* (Wellbutrin), *nefazodone* (Serzone), and the SSRIs, *fluoxetine* (Prozac), *sertraline* (Zoloft), *paroxetine* (Paxil), and *fluvoxamine* (Luvox) have been introduced. The SSRIs are a relatively new class of antidepressants, with unique pharmacologic, therapeutic, and side effect profiles. The SSRIs are now considered by most experts to be the first choice in antidepressant therapy. The SSRIs lack cholinergic, histaminergic, and adrenergic adverse effects. More frequent side effects include gastrointestinal complaints, anxiety, agitation, insomnia, somnolence, and sexual dysfunction. The SSRIs differ in chemical structure, pharmacokinetics, and pharmacodynamics, resulting in subtle differences in side effects. Patients who discontinue one SSRI because of side effects can be treated successfully with another (Brown and Harrison, 1995). However, the similarities among SSRI effects and side effects were greater than their differences (Table 5-6). Sexual dysfunction, that is, decreased libido, reduced sexual arousal, and impaired orgasmic function may be associated with depression. However, the SSRIs may also impair sexual function to a greater extent than do the TCAs, heterocyclics, or MAOIs. In perhaps up to one third of patients, SSRI antidepressants reduce libido, arousal, or orgasmic function. Dosage reduction, drug holiday, or a switch to bupropion or nefazodone, which both have a low incidence of sexual side effects, can be employed. The addition of bupropion 75 to 150 mg in the morning, cyproheptadine 4 to 12 mg in the evening, or buspirone 5 to 10 mg three times a day may offset sexual side effects. However, the strategies are not consistently effective. Other agents, including bethanechol, amantadine, and yohimbine, have been reported to be useful in reversing anorgasmia (Rothschild, 1995; Segraves, 1994). Interestingly, many individuals experience robust orgasmic function with SSRIs, and SSRIs in low doses have been used to treat premature ejaculation.

Table 5-6 Summary of Adverse-Effect Profiles of Paroxetine, Sertraline, Fluvoxamine, and Fluoxetine*

Adverse Effect	Paroxetine (*N*+2683)	Sertraline (*N*+861)	Fluvoxamine (*N*=24,624)	Fluoxetine (*N*+1034)
Nausea	27.0	26.1	15.7	24.3
Headache	19.0	20.3	4.7	10.4
Sedation	21.0	13.4	6.9	10.1
Insomnia	14.0	16.4	4.5	15.0
Dry mouth	18.0	16.3	4.6	11.2
Constipation	13.0	8.4	2.9	5.4
Diarrhea	11.0	17.7	2.2	12.6
Tremor	10.0	10.7	3.3	10.1
Dizziness	12.0	11.7	3.8	10.0
Weakness or fatigue	15.0	10.6	6.2	10.1
Increased sweating	12.0	8.4	1.7	8.4
Anxiety or agitation	8.0	5.6	1.4	15.3
Vision disturbances	5.0	4.2	—	4.7
Sexual dysfunction†	3.0	17.2	<0.1	—
Vomiting	2.0	3.8	3.2	—
Anorexia	4.0	2.8	2.1	11.7
Taste perversion	2.0	1.2	—	4.9
Urinary disturbances	2.0	1.4	—	0.6

* Percentage of patients reporting adverse effect per manufacturer's labeling.
† Sexual dysfunction is generally underreported.

Less common side effects of the SSRIs include rash, lymphadenopathy, swollen joints, and other types of allergic phenomena. Dystonia and dyskinesias, including nocturnal myoclonus, have been reported. The effects usually require discontinuation. *Serotonin syndrome,* potentially fatal, can be a serious adverse effect of all SSRIs or of venlafaxine and clomipramine when combined with an MAOI. Tachycardia, confusion, and a manic-like state develops as shown in Box 5-5. The final common pathway is very similar to neuroleptic malignant syndrome, with hyperthermia, profuse sweating, and cardiovascular collapse. The syndrome develops so rapidly that patients often die before physicians can intervene.

Generally the SSRIs have a broad spectrum of application in depression, from the atypical to the more severely depressed. Other applications include anxiety disorders, especially obsessive compulsive disorder, bipolar depression, eating disorders, and panic. Aside from sexual side effects, SSRIs are well tolerated for both long- and short-term therapy. They have a low lethality with overdose and have a low risk of seizures.

Interactions. The effect of SSRIs on hepatic isoenzymes represents an important characteristic among the SSRIs, as well as other antidepressant agents. SSRIs can inhibit specific P-450 isoenzymes. The inhibition is competitive and reversible and depends on the affinity of the SSRI and its concentration in relation to another substrate, for example, another drug. Drug interaction therefore may occur, resulting in marked elevations in drug concentrations and reduction in drug clearance (Preskorn and Magnus, 1994). Toxic effects of a variety of coadministered drugs can occur (Table 5-7 and Box 5-6). Coadministration of the SSRIs with TCAs or

Box 5-5 Drug Interactions of SSRIs Caused by Excess CNS Serotonin

Serotonin syndrome likely to occur if SSRI combined with:
- MAO inhibitors—phenelzine, tranylcypromine
- MAOI (selective)—selegiline, moclobemide
- Tryptophan (serotonin precursor)

Signs and symptoms of serotonin syndrome (most to least frequent):
- Mental status changes, including confusion or hypomania
- Restlessness or agitation
- Myoclonus
- Hyperreflexia
- Diaphoresis
- Shivering (or shaking chills)
- Tremor
- Diarrhea, abdominal cramps, nausea
- Ataxia or incoordination
- Headaches

trazodone can result in potentially toxic blood levels, as much as a tenfold increase (Preskorn et al, 1994). The extent and duration of effect on drug metabolism will depend on the potency of cytrochrome P-450 inhibition, the half-life of the drug, and its dose and duration of administration. Short half-life agents, for example, sertraline relative to fluoxetine, are less active inhibitors of metabolism of a coadministered drug. Also, inhibition becomes insignificant within a few days with short half-life SSRIs compared with fluoxetine, which may persist for a month after it is stopped. This switching from fluoxetine to a TCA may result initially in adverse or toxic effects or lead to a modest overdose of the tricyclic antidepressant. Because of its long half-life, this drug has the potential to interact with MAOIs for as long as 4 to 6 weeks after its discontinuation. Therefore the use of MAOIs during that interval after discontinuation or concomitantly is strictly forbidden. SSRIs should be used cautiously with CNS-active drugs. SSRIs are highly bound to plasma proteins, and combining these drugs with another tightly bound drug could cause a displacement in one or the other and the occurrence of potential adverse effects.

Patient education. Patients and their families should be instructed as follows concerning SSRIs:

- Although it is not clear that combining alcohol or over-the-counter medications with SSRIs is harmful, the patient should be cautioned against doing so and encouraged to discuss such decisions with the physician or nurse. An exception to over-the-counter drugs is dextromethorphan, an agent found in cough syrup. This combination could trigger the serotonin syndrome.
- When sedation results from taking these drugs, driving or operating hazardous machinery should be avoided.
- Pregnancy or breast-feeding should be discussed with the primary health care provider, because the harmful effects of SSRIs during these developmental stages are not clear.

Box 5-6 Drug Interactions of SSRIs Caused by Cytochrome P-450 Inhibition (SSRIs: Fluoxetine, Fluvoxamine, Paroxetine)

Blood levels and adverse effects of the following are increased:

- Antidepressants—tricyclics and trazodone
- Barbiturates
- Benzodiazepines—except lorazepam and oxazepam
- Carbamazepine
- Narcotics—particularly pentazocine, dextromethorphan, and meperidine
- Neuroleptics
- Nifedipine
- Phenytoin
- Valproate
- Verapamil

Venlafaxine

Venlafaxine (Effexor), a relatively new compound, is a structurally novel antidepressant that causes clinically significant inhibition of serotonin and norepinephrine reuptake. It is unique both in that it has a rapid onset of noradrenergic subsensitivity and it acts as an atypical serotonin reuptake inhibitor. Venlafaxine has no impact on alpha-adrenergic, histaminergic, or cholinergic receptors (Cunningham, 1994).

Venlafaxine is absorbed rapidly and is 98% bioavailable. Food delays absorption but does not change the overall absorption. Half-life and protein binding are shorter and lower respectively (Table 5-8). It is metabolized to O-desmethylvenlafaxine, which possesses similar biochemical and clinical properties and has a half-life of about 11 hours.

Because venlafaxine lacks affinity for histaminergic, cholinergic, and alpha-adrenergic receptors, common side effects associated with TCAs do not occur. The most common side effect is nausea, which may be severe and persistent. However, most patients build their tolerance to venlafaxine over a few weeks and are tolerant to the drug. Other side effects include somnolence, dry mouth, dizziness, constipation, nervousness, sweating, and ancrexia. Elevation in blood pressure in some patients ($\leq$ 5%) has occurred, especially at higher dosages, for example, 200 mg or greater; hence, patients should be monitored and screened before starting this drug. Venlafaxine is not a potent inhibitor of cytochrome P-450 enzymes. This property, together with low protein binding, reduces the potential for drug interaction. Venlafaxine has little effect on lithium, benzodiazepines, or ethanol and is much less likely than the SSRIs to interfere with hepatic enzymes.

Venlafaxine is reported to have a more rapid onset of action once therapeutic dosages are achieved (Guelfi, White, and Magni, 1992; Mendels et al, 1993). However, efficacy is similar to other antidepressants. It is effective in a broad range of depressive illnesses but particularly in the more treatment-resistant, chronically depressed patients (Keltner, 1995). Venlafaxine may not have as many drug interactions as the SSRIs, although the side effects associated with it are similar to those associated with the SSRIs. Other side effects most likely stem from its noradrenergic properties.

Table 5-7 Antidepressants and Cytochrome P-450 Enzyme Involvement

Cytochrome	Polymorphism	Substrates	Inhibitors	Potentially significant interactions between inhibitors (and substrates)
IA2 (P448‡)	Possible	Phenacetin, caffeine, theophylline, demethylation of TCAs, haloperidol*	Fluvoxamine	Fluvoxamine (haloperidol, phenytoin, theophylline, caffeine)
II9	Yes:2%-3% of Caucasians; 15%-25% of Asians	Diazepam, demethylation of TCAs, warfarin,§ tolbutamide,§ phenytoin§	Fluvoxamine, fluoxetine,§ sertraline§	Fluvoxamine, fluoxetine, (phenytoin) Sertraline (diazepam, tolbutamide)

IID6 (Debrisoquin hydroxylase‡; sparteine hydroxylase‡)	Yes:5%-8% of Caucasians; lower in Asians and African Americans	Haloperidol,* thioridazine, perphenazine, clozapine, risperidone, hydroxylation of nortriptyline & desipramine; paroxetine, venlafaxine, codeine, beta blockers, timolol, metroprolol, propranolol†; Type IC antiarrhythmics; encainide, flecanide, propafenone; verapamil	Quinidine, fluphenazine, levopromazine, fluoxetine, norfluoxetine, paroxetine, sertraline	Fluoxetine, sertraline, paroxetine (TCAs, type 1C antiarrhythmics, some antipsychotics)
IIIA4	Possible	Demethylation of TCAs, triazolam, midazolam, alprazolam, carbamazepine,§ cyclosporin, [terfenadine], [astemizole], quinidine, erythromycin, lidocaine [cisapride]	Ketoconazole, sertraline,§ fluoxetine,§ fluvoxamine, nefazodone	Fluoxetine, sertraline, (carbamazepine) Nefazodone (alprazolam, triazolam)

From DeVane CL: Pharmacokinetics of the newer antidepressants: clinical relevance, *Am J Med* 97(suppl 6A):19S. Used with permission.
* Evidence based on significant elevation of haloperidol concentrations during concomitant fluvoxamine administration.
†Catalyzes a minor pathway of reversible metabolism.
‡ Additional name for the same enzyme.
At least partially oxidized through this enzyme.
Evidence based on significant inhibition of alprazolam/triazolam metabolism.
§Suspected but not confirmed.
(Material in brackets indicates that elevated levels have been associated with cardiac irregularities.)

Table 5-8 Pharmacokinetic Profiles of Venlafaxine and Selective Serotonergic Compounds*

Characteristic	Venlafaxine	Fluoxetine	Paroxetine	Sertraline
Serum half-life (h)	5	48-72	21	26
Serum half-life active metabolite	11	168-216	0	48-98
Time to steady-state (d)	3	21-50	5-7	7-10
Protein-binding (%)	27	94	95	98

From Feighner JP: The role of venlafaxine in rational antidepressant therapy, *J Clin Psychiatry* 55:9(suppl A), 1994.
*Data on file, Wyethe-Ayerst Laboratories, Philadelphia, Pa.

Bupropion

Bupropion (Wellbutrin) is a novel antidepressant agent that is neither a TCA, an SSRI, nor an MAOI. Clinical tests indicate that orthostatic hypotension, cardiovascular conduction problems, anticholinergic effects, daytime sedation, and other typical effects of tricyclics are not seen with this compound. However, this drug is "activating," and agitation is sometimes produced. Bupropion is often prescribed as a second-line agent. It is useful in bipolar depression and in patients with comorbid attention disorder. Bupropion is contraindicated in patients with seizure disorders or in patients for whom a prior diagnosis of either bulimia or anorexia may exist. Bupropion, as with the other antidepressants, should not be given in combination with the MAOIs because of the potential for drug interaction and hypertensive crisis.

Bupropion's exact mechanism of action is unknown, although norepinephrine and serotonin systems are indirectly affected and dopamine reuptake is directly inhibited. Bupropion is rapidly absorbed, with a half-life of about 8 hours. Several metabolites are active. More common side effects include agitation, insomnia, gastrointestinal upset, and headache. The incidence of sexual side effects are low with bupropion. As previously mentioned, low doses are sometimes effective in controlling sexual side effects secondary to SSRIs. Dosing is twice a day or three times a day, with no more than 450 mg per day or 150 mg per dose, to avoid adverse effects. Initial dosing is 100 mg twice daily, with most patients responding to 300 to 450 mg. Elderly and debilitated patients may require reduced doses and should be titrated conservatively. Overdosage may result in grand mal/generalized seizures, hallucinosis, tachycardia, and signs of neurotoxicity.

Nefazodone

Nefazodone (Serzone), one of the newer antidepressants, is chemically related to trazodone but lacks the alpha-adrenergic blockade that accounts for trazodone's orthostasis, priapism, and certain cardiovascular effects. Thus nefazodone has less potential to cause priapism; it is also less sedating. Nefazodone is a selective 5-HT_2 receptor antagonist and also inhibits presynaptic reuptake of serotonin and norepinephrine. Nefazodone has a pharmacologic profile that is distinct from SSRIs, TCAs, MAOIs, and venlafaxine. The potent blockade of 5-HT_{2A} receptors is the most distinct difference between nefazodone and other new antidepressants. Nefazodone does not significantly bind to histaminergic, cholinergic, or alpha-adrenergic receptors and is not associated with TCA-like side effects.

Nefazodone is rapidly absorbed and extensively metabolized and has an active metabolite. Twice daily dosing gives a steady state within 5 days. Initially dosing is at 100 mg twice daily for the first week, with titrations to 150 mg twice daily or 300 mg per day. Most patients respond with 300 to 500 mg daily. The amount of nefazodone can be increased up to 600 mg per day, but a nonlinear plasma concentration results; thus, titrations should be conservative. Elderly and debilitated patients usually require only half the dosage. Nausea is the most common side effect, with dizziness, insomnia, asthenia, and agitation occurring in a small percentage of cases.

Nefazodone has been shown to be equally efficacious compared with imipramine (Rickels et al, 1994). Significant improvements with anxiety and sleep may occur in the first 2 weeks of therapy. Nefazodone has novel effects on sleep, reducing insomnia and nighttime awakenings. Full antidepressant response occurs after several weeks, which is similar to other antidepressants. Tolerability is usually excellent. The incidence of sexual dysfunction in men and women is comparable to that seen with placebo.

Nefazodone potently inhibits P-450 IIIA4 (Table 5-8). Hence drugs that affect IIIA4, for example, ketoconazole, may alter nefazodone metabolism, and drugs that induce IIIA4, for example, carbamazepine, may reduce plasma levels of nefazodone. Nefazodone, through inhibition of IIIA4, can increase levels of terfenadine (Seldane) and astemizole (Hismanal). Because of their potential for cardiotoxicity, these drugs are contraindicated with nefazodone. Also, alprazolam and triazolam concentrations may be increased twofold to threefold, and a 50% reduction in dosage of these drugs is warranted when coadministered with nefazodone. Coadministration of MAOIs is contraindicated. Other drugs that may be affected include antihypertensives but not propanolol, haloperidol, or lorazepam. Nefazodone is very safe with overdosage. Symptoms include nausea, vomiting, and somnolence. Overall, nefazodone is a novel antidepressant. It has a low incidence of side effects. It has a distinctly different profile from those of SSRIs, including a lack of sexual side effects, nervousness, and insomnia. Thus it should be considered a first-line agent for the treatment of depression (Ayd, 1995).

Other New Antidepressants

Other antidepressants currently under investigation include moclobemide and mirtazapine. Moclobemide will be discussed in the next section on MAOIs. Mirtazapine selectively blocks serotonin 5-HT_2 and 5-HT_3 receptors, which, as with 5-HT_2 receptor blockade by nefazodone, may suppress serotonergic side effects such as agitation while allowing antidepressant effects putatively associated with 5-HT_{1A} to predominate (Bender, 1995).

Mirtazapine enhancement of noradrenergic and serotonergic neurotransmission is comparable to that of tricyclic antidepressants (TCAs) but is not accompanied by TCA-associated anticholinergic or $alpha_1$-adrenolytic effects. Mirtazapine does exert antihistamine properties, and related somnolence occurred in 62% of 42 treated patients in 1 trial compared with 4% of 40 patients receiving placebo (Claghorn and Lesem, 1995).

MONOAMINE OXIDASE INHIBITORS

Monoamine oxidase inhibitors, another class of antidepressant, are almost always prescribed after SSRIs or other agents have been tried. An argument can be made that MAOIs are particularly effective in treating atypical depression, for example, depression characterized by mood reactivity, interpersonal hypersensitivity, hypersomnia, and compulsions such as excessive eating. MAOIs may also be useful in treating certain types of anxiety syndromes, for example, panic or agoraphobia associated with depression. The second-class status afforded the MAOIs is generally related to their potential for serious adverse reactions. Although many expert clinicians think the fear of MAOIs is unwarranted, the reluctance to use them seems to be the norm (Folks, 1982).

As a general rule the MAOIs can be divided into hydrazines, for example, phenelzine; nonhydrazines, for example, tranylcypromine; and atypical MAOIs, for example, selegiline and moclobemide (Figure 5-2 and Table 5-9). These drugs block

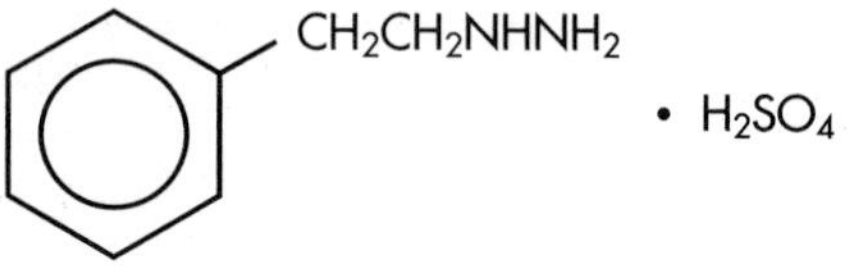

$CH_2CH_2NHNH_2$ • H_2SO_4

Phenelzine

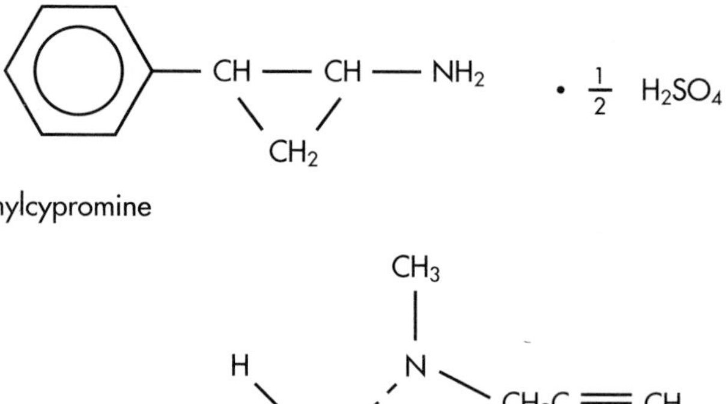

CH — CH — NH_2 • $\frac{1}{2}$ H_2SO_4

CH_2

Tranylcypromine

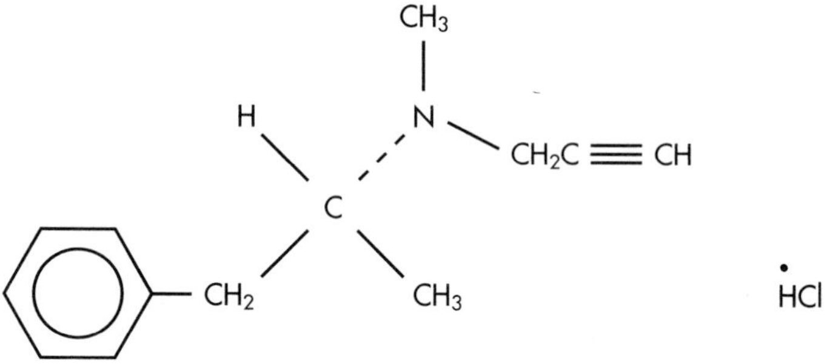

CH_3

H N $CH_2C \equiv CH$

C

CH_2 CH_3 • HCl

Selegiline

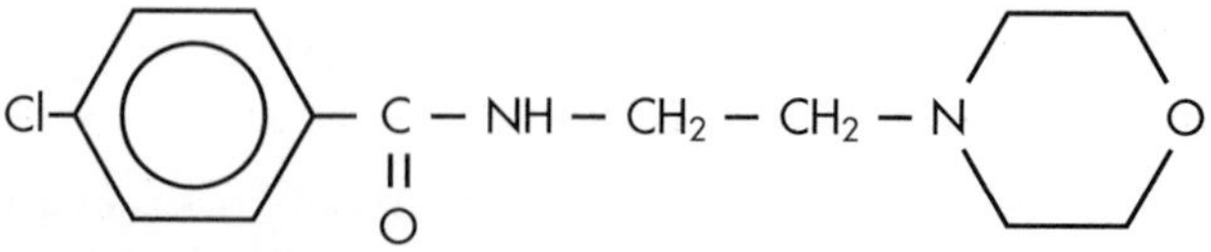

Cl– C – NH – CH_2 – CH_2 – N O

O

Moclobemide

Figure 5-2 Chemical structures of MAO inhibitors.

Table 5-9 Monoamine oxidase inhibitors*

Drug	Class	Dosage range (mg/day)	MAOI diet	Special characteristics
Phenelzine (Nardil)	Nonselective (hydrazine)	30-90	Yes	Atypical depression; anxious, phobic, obsessional patients Effect may be enhanced when combined with TCAs or lithium
Tranylcypromine (Parnate)	Nonselective (nonhydrazine)	20-60	Yes	Direct stimulant effect, often rapid onset Useful in fatigued, anergic patients Effect may be enhanced when combined with TCA or Li
Selegiline (Eldepryl)	Selective MAO-B (nonselective)	5-15 20-50	No Yes	20 mg/day or more requires dietary restriction Stimulant, energizing properties; tolerated and effective in some who cannot take other MAOIs
Moclobemide	Selective MAO-A (reversible [RIMA])	300-600	No	Minimal hypotension, excitation, and sexual effects Efficacy similar to that of other MAOIs but terminates more rapidly after discontinuation

From Bernstein JG: *Handbook of drug therapy in psychiatry,* ed 3, St. Louis, 1995, Mosby.
*It must be noted that none of these MAOIs can be safely combined with clomipramine or any SSRI.

monoamine oxidase, the major enzyme involved in the metabolic decomposition and thus the inactivation of norepinephrine, serotonin, and dopamine. The increased level of these neurotransmitters in the peripheral and the central nervous systems can be dramatic. According to the biogenic amine theory of depression, depressed individuals have a deficiency of these neurotransmitters. MAOIs help achieve the "normal" amount of neurotransmitters by slowing the deactivation of these enzymes. This mechanism is in contrast to mechanisms of TCAs and other agents, which achieve the "normal" level or restore the relative deficiency by preventing the reuptake of amines or by directly affecting the postsynaptic receptor. Generally a period of 10 days to 4 weeks is required for the antidepressant effects of the MAOIs to occur but, as with the other antidepressants, the physiologic action, that is, the inhibition of monoamine oxidase, occurs immediately. This phenomenon suggests that factors other than low levels of specific neurotransmitters are involved in the pathogenesis of depression.

Pharmacokinetics

Monoamine oxidase inhibitors are well absorbed from the gastrointestinal tract and are given orally. They are metabolized in the liver, and metabolites are excreted in the urine. They have long half-lives. Table 5-9 gives the usual doses for these drugs.

Side Effects

Monoamine oxidase inhibitors induce central nervous system, cardiovascular, and anticholinergic side effects.

Peripheral nervous system effects. In the peripheral nervous system the slow release of norepinephrine causes decreased heart rate, decreased vasoconstriction, and hypotension. Monoamine oxidase inhibitors also inhibit monoamine oxidase in the liver, which may lead to elevated levels of other drugs that are normally metabolized in the liver by a monoamine oxidase.

Hypotension is the most common nontherapeutic effect. Interestingly, pargyline (Eutonyl) is an MAOI that is not used as an antidepressant but rather as an antihypertensive agent. The slowdown in the release of norepinephrine is the presumed mechanism of action. Unlike the effect of tricyclic antidepressants, a reflex tachycardia does not occur. Because of the slowed release of norepinephrine experienced by the adrenergic system, the heart rate does not reflexively speed up. Thus hypotension combined with the failure of compensatory increased heart rate may lead to heart failure in predisposed individuals. Monoamine oxidase inhibitors may also cause anticholinergic effects such as dry mouth, blurred vision, urinary hesitancy, and constipation, although constipation occurs to a lesser extent than observed with TCAs. Hepatic and hematologic dysfunctions may rarely occur and are potentially serious. Blood cell counts and liver function tests should be obtained before therapy begins; symptoms indicating bone marrow suppression or liver dysfunction should be investigated.

Central nervous system effects. Because MAOIs increase the availability of biogenic amines in the brain, CNS hyperstimulation may also occur, causing agitation, acute anxiety, restlessness, insomnia, and euphoria. Full schizophrenic episodes may also develop in individuals with quiescent schizophrenia as a response to MAOIs. Hypomania (less than full mania) is also a common effect.

Specific Interactions

Monoamine oxidase inhibitors have a number of serious interactions. Potentially lethal interactions may occur with both drugs and foods and are listed in Boxes 5-7 and 5-8 and in Table 5-10. Drug and food interactions should be considered, particularly with compounds that have the potential to cause hypertension, anticholinergic effects, or sympathomimetic effects. Sympathomimetic drugs are classified as direct acting, indirect acting, and mixed acting, that is, having both direct and indirect properties. Indirect-acting and mixed-acting sympathomimetics may cause serious and sometimes fatal hypertension. Direct-acting sympathomimetics act by adding new norepinephrine to the body, whereas indirect agents release existing epinephrine or norepinephrine from the neuron. Because MAOIs increase the amount of stored norepinephrine in the peripheral nervous system, the potential for these indirect or mixed-acting sympathomimetics to release relatively large amounts of norepinephrine makes crucial the avoidance of these interacting drugs. Even small amounts may trigger a hypertensive crisis. Typical indirect-acting and mixed-acting sympathomimetics include amphetamines, cocaine, methylphenidate, dopamine, metfenturomine, and ephedrine. Over-the-counter weight-loss and stimulant products such as phenylephrine, phenylpropanolamine, and pseudoephedrine, which are mixed or indirect-acting sympathomimetics, should be avoided altogether. Direct-acting sympathomimetics, that is, norepinephrine, epinephrine, and isopropeterenol, theoretically should not trigger the release of existing norepinephrine. As previously noted, MAOIs should not be given in combination with TCAs except in unusually refractory cases of depression, in hospitalized patients, or in patients who are closely monitored. Use with other antidepressants, that is, SSRIs, venlafaxine, bupropion, and nefazodone should be avoided.

Box 5-7 Food-Drug Interactions with MAOIs

Sympathomimetic drugs should not be combined with MAOIs.
Tyramine-containing foods must not be ingested by the patient who is taking MAOIs.
MAOIs are contraindicated as follows:
- In the patient with a history of stroke or cardiovascular disease
- In the patient with a pheochromocytoma, a tumor that secretes pressor substance
- In the patient undergoing elective surgery (because of the hypotensive potential of combined MAOIs and anesthesia)

MAOIs should not be given in combination with the following:
- Other MAOIs
- TCAs
- Meperidine (Demerol)

Hypertensive crisis is a major concern. If it occurs, the nurse should respond as follows:
- Discontinue MAOIs and contact the physician
- Know that therapy to reduce the blood pressure is warranted, and know that phentolamine (Regitine) 5 mg intravenously is the appropriate drug
- Manage fever by external cooling
- Institute supportive nursing care as indicated

Box 5-8 Tyramine-rich Foods to Avoid While Taking MAOIs

Alcoholic beverages
Beer and ale
Chianti and sherry wine

Dairy products
Cheese: cheddar, blue, brie, and mozzarella
Sour cream
Yogurt

Fruits and vegetables
Avocados
Bananas
Fava beans
Canned figs

Meats
Bologna
Chicken liver
Fish, dried
Liver
Meat tenderizer
Pickled herring
Salami
Sausage

Other foods
Caffeinated coffee, colas, and tea (large amounts)
Chocolate
Licorice
Soy sauce
Yeast

The initial symptoms of hypertensive crisis are palpitation, tightness in the chest, stiff neck, and a throbbing, radiating headache. Extremely high blood pressure with elevation of heart rate is common. Cardiovascular consequences have included myocardial infarctions, cerebral hemorrhage, myocardial ischemias, and arrhythmias; diaphoresis and pupillary dilation are also prominent signs.

Anticholinergic effects may be present to a greater extent when other anticholinergic drugs are given in concert with the MAOIs. Typical anticholinergic side effects are similar to those for the TCAs.

Because MAOIs inhibit monoamine oxidase in the liver, some drugs, particularly central nervous system depressants, are not metabolized there; with these drugs, serum levels may be achieved more rapidly and may be high enough to seriously depress the central nervous system. Meperidine (Demerol) is specifically contraindicated; a marked potentiation of this drug can occur.

Hypotensive drugs are also potentiated by the MAOIs; hence these are relatively contraindicated. Food-drug interactions center on the amino acid tyramine, a precursor to dopamine, norepinephrine, and epinephrine. Tyramine is found in many foods commonly consumed in a North American diet; in fact, all high-protein foods that have undergone protein breakdowns by means of aging, fermentation, pickling, or smoking should be avoided. Hypotension and hypertensive crisis can develop from these food-drug combinations by the mechanism previously discussed.

Implications

Therapeutic versus toxic levels. As with the TCAs, an intensification of the effects already discussed may occur with overdosage of MAOIs. A lethal

Table 5-10 Drugs to Avoid While Taking MAOIs

Drugs	Interaction
Anticholinergic drugs	Compound anticholinergic response
Anesthetics (general)	Deepen CNS depression
Antihypertensives (diuretics, β blockers, hydralazine)	Compound hypotensive effect
CNS depressants	Intensify CNS depression
Meperidine	CNS depression; deaths have occurred
Guanethidine, methyldopa, reserpine	Produce severe hypertension
Sympathomimetics (mixed and indirect-acting) Amphetamines, methylphenidate, dopamine, phenylpropanolamine (in many over-the-counter medications)	Precipitate hypertensive crisis, cardiac stimulation, arrhythmias, cerebrovascular hemorrhage
Sympathomimetics (direct-acting) Epinephrine, norepinephrine, isoproterenol	Same as for mixed and indirect-acting sympathomimetics but theoretically should not produce as severe a reaction
Cyclic and newer antidepessants	Less likely to cause problems
	Same as for epinephrine, norepinephrine, isoproterenol

dose of MAOIs may be achieved at only 6 to 10 times the usual daily dose. Careful monitoring should occur when medications are being ingested. As noted with the antipsychotic agents, cheeking and hoarding of these drugs could be disastrous, and these possibilities should be considered in individuals at risk. When an MAOI overdose is suspected, the following should be performed:

1. Emesis and gastric lavage, which are particularly helpful if performed early
2. Monitoring of vital signs
3. External cooling, which is particularly warranted when high fever occurs
4. Standard treatment of hypotension

Use in pregnancy. Monoamine oxidase inhibitors should be given during pregnancy only when the anticipated benefit justifies the potential risk to the fetus and should be avoided altogether in the first trimester.

Side effects. Several important side effects associated with MAOIs and appropriate interventions are listed in Box 5-9.

Interactions. As previously discussed, drug-MAOI and food-MAOI interactions are significant. General guidelines for these interactions include the following: (1) *Sympathomimetic* drugs should not be combined with MAOIs. (2) *Tyramine-containing* foods should not be ingested by the patient taking MAOIs. (3) Do not give MAOIs in combination with another MAOI or with a TCA except in unusually refractory patients and then under close supervision. (4) Avoid MAOIs in

Box 5-9 Side Effects and Nursing Interventions for MAOIs

Central nervous system hyperstimulation
Reassure the patient. Assess for developing psychosis, hypomania, or seizures. When symptoms warrant, withhold the drug and notify the physician.

Hypotension
Monitor blood pressure frequently and intervene to prevent falls and injuries; having patient lie down may help return blood pressure to normal.

Anticholinergic effects
See the section on TCA side effects for appropriate nursing interventions.

Hepatic and hematologic dysfunction
Blood cell counts and liver function tests should be performed. When dysfunction is apparent, MAOI should be discontinued.

combination with meperidine. (5) If a hypertensive crisis is suspected, the following measures should be instituted:

- Discontinue the MAOI.
- Have phentolamine (Regitine) available. Phentolamine 5 mg intravenously reduces blood pressure.
- Manage fever by external cooling.
- Provide supportive care as indicated.

Patient education. Because combining MAOIs with a variety of interactants is a serious matter, it is important to be consistent in teaching both the patient and his or her family about these drugs (Table 5-10 and Boxes 5-7 and 5-8). Although in current thinking these interactions are not regarded quite as pessimistically as they were by the clinicians of a few years ago, appropriate education remains important. Teaching should include the following general points:

- A "lag time" of 10 days to 4 weeks occurs before a full therapeutic effect is experienced.
- Driving should be avoided if sedation is pronounced.
- The patient should inform all medication prescribers when he or she is taking MAOIs.
- High tyramine-containing foods should be avoided.
- Headaches, palpitations, and stiff neck should be reported immediately.

SPECIFIC MONOAMINE OXIDASE INHIBITORS

Three MAOIs are used to treat depression (Figure 5-2 and Table 5-9). *Isocarboxazid* (Marplan) is no longer generally available. It is considered the mildest MAOI; a clinical response may not be noticed for 4 weeks or longer after therapy is initiated. *Phenelzine* (Nardil) has been found to be the most effective in depressed individuals who are characterized as atypical on clinical examination. Phenelzine is considered the most effective MAOI and is the most sedative. A clinical response is generally experienced or begins to be experienced in about 4 weeks. *Tranylcypromine* (Parnate) seems to be the most effective MAOI for treatment of severe or endogenous depression. A clinical effect may be experienced rapidly, in about 10 days, which is quicker than with the other MAOIs. Tranylcypromine is the most stimulating MAOI. As mentioned previously, pargyline is not used as an antidepressant.

Phenelzine and tranylcypromine are irreversible, nonselective inhibitors of MAO A and MAO B. MAO A is primarily serotonergic. Selective inhibition of MAO B occurs with selegiline at doses less than 20 mg, that is, allows the drug to be used without dietary restriction (Yu et al, 1994). Moclobemide and brofasamine, both of which are investigational drugs, also do not require dietary restriction. The drugs, known as RIMAs, are reversible, selective inhibitors of MAO A. However, these agents cannot be combined with SSRIs, as they may result in adverse effects, such as serotonin syndrome.

Selegiline, or L-deprenyl, is a selective MAO B inhibitor at doses of 10 to 15 mg. It is metabolized to three active compounds, including amphetamine and methamphetamine, which may account for its therapeutic action. A favorable antidepressant response may occur at these smaller doses, although a more robust response occurs at larger doses of 30 to 50 mg (where the selective MAO B inhibition is lost and dietary restrictions are needed). Patients with anergic depression and bipolar depression may be particularly responsive to low-dose therapy. Fluoxetine should be discontinued 5 weeks before starting this drug.

Moclobemide (Aurorex) is not yet available in the United States. It is a reversible inhibitor of MAO A, with antidepressant efficacy similar to fluoxetine (Williams et al, 1993). Fewer adverse effects, for example, hypotension and sexual dysfunction, and hypertensive reactions occur. Divided doses of 300 to 600 mg are usually therapeutic. Brofaromine is similar to moclobemide but also inhibits reuptake of serotonin. These drugs show promise but are still under investigation in the United States (Bernstein, 1995).

TREATMENT ISSUES AND CAVEATS

SSRIs generally have a flat-dose response, that is, the starting dose is usually therapeutic, and few titrations are necessary. The drugs are conveniently dosed at one daily, usually in the morning. Other antidepressants are administered in doses divided throughout the day. The patient can gradually accommodate unwanted side effects, and the dosage is titrated upward until the desired clinical effect is achieved. Once an optimal dose is achieved or a therapeutic response experienced, the patient who is tolerating the medication satisfactorily may be given a single dose of tricyclic or heterocyclic agents with equal therapeutic efficacy. However, trazodone, nefazodone, bupropion, and venlafaxine are continued on a twice daily or possibly three times daily regimen. A short half-life or an ongoing potential for adverse effects prompts the divided dosing schedule. A single bedtime dose may not be desirable in elderly patients or in patients sensitive to the adverse effects of the antidepressant who may better tolerate the drug when the dose is divided throughout the day (Bernstein, 1995). With more sedating agents, patients may benefit from a similarly divided dosage scheduled to alleviate anxiety without the need to add an anxiolytic medication to the regimen. Coadministration of antianxiety or antipsychotic agents may sometimes be necessary while awaiting the therapeutic response of an antidepressant (Robertson and Trimble, 1982; Folks, 1990). In the event that a benzodiazepine is used concurrently, short- to intermediate-acting agents are the best choice, for example, lorazepam or alprazolam (see Chapter 6, Anxiety Disorders).

For patients with paranoid ideation and delusional thinking, concomitant treatment with the institution of a potent antipsychotic agent, for example, haloperidol, is preferable (see Chapter 4, Schizophrenia and Other Psychoses). Low-potency agents are unlikely to be useful and should be avoided where postural hypotension may result from the combination of an antidepressant and antipsychotic. Amoxapine has been found to be effective in treating psychotic depression without the need for simultaneous administration of a neuroleptic drug (Anton, Hitri, and Diamond, 1986).

Two common problems with antidepressant medications are the prescription of inadequate doses and the discontinuation of drug treatment before the patient has recovered from the immediate depressive symptoms. Prophylaxis, and therefore guarding against recurrence of the depression, can more likely be achieved if these two problems are avoided (Prien and Kupfer, 1986).

Another continuing problem in achieving a prompt, satisfactory response to antidepressant drugs is the inability to predict which patient will respond optimally to which type or class of antidepressant agent. Several reports have employed the use of stimulant drugs, that is, dextroamphetamine or methylphenidate, as predictors of antidepressant responsiveness (Goff and Jenike, 1986). Most commonly methylphenidate 5 to 20 mg, as a single or divided dose, is prescribed. Patients who experience a prompt mood improvement after stimulant drug administration are often responsive to a noradrenergic antidepressant such as desipramine (Sabelli, Fawcett, and Javaid, 1983). Patients who experience a dysphoric response to the stimulant test may, generally speaking, not respond well to noradrenergic antidepressants but more often are observed to achieve a favorable therapeutic response to "serotonergic" drugs, for example, amitriptyline (Van Kammen and Murphy, 1978).

The routine measurement of plasma concentration is generally not necessary for effective therapy. However, if the patient fails to respond and is, indeed, taking the medication, it is generally appropriate to increase the dose and evaluate the response. Most evidence, with the exception of the SSRIs, supports a linear relationship between plasma concentration and therapeutic response, although a therapeutic window for nortriptyline and, possibly, desipramine has been suggested in the literature (Bernstein, 1995). Table 5-5 suggests some generally accepted ranges of plasma levels of older agents (Risch, Janowsky, and Hyey, 1981). Because they may fail to take their medication appropriately or are noncompliant, patients of any age who fail to respond to standard antidepressant therapy may benefit from the measurement of plasma concentrations. Monitoring the plasma level may help to point out to the noncompliant patient the reason for nonresponse and give added emphasis to restructuring of a therapeutic relationship. Inadequate data exist to support reliable statements regarding the correlation of therapeutic response and plasma levels for newer agents such as amoxapine, trimipramine, trazodone, nefazodone, fluoxetine, sertraline, paroxetine, fluvoxamine, bupropion, and venlafaxine.

Patients who do not respond easily or quickly to antidepressant medication may not do so because of inadequate dosage or duration of treatment. However, treatment-resistant depression does exist. Nierenberg (1994) estimates that 10% to 15% of cases will show treatment resistance, yet only limited data exist to guide treatment in such instances. In these cases, an alternative agent or adjunct should be considered. Atypical depression probably responds best to an SSRI or MAOI. Augmentation or potentiation with adjunctive drugs can be useful. Lithium may potentiate a response in a matter of days to weeks, usually at levels of 0.5 to 0.9 mEq/L (Pope, McElroy Jr., and Nixon, 1988). T_3 (triiodothyronine [Cytomel]) appears to be more effective than T_4 (thyroxine [Synthroid]), including cases where "stable" thyroid disease exists (Joffe and Singer, 1991). Combination therapy with buspirone or pindolol may also be useful. These drugs tend to stimulate 5-HT_{1A} receptors (Joffe and Schuller, 1993; Blier and Bergeron, 1995). Psychostimulants, for example, methylphenidate, dextroamphetamine, or pemoline, may also be a useful adjunct. For example, methylphenidate in doses of 10 mg twice daily is started and titrated up to 30 mg twice daily in divided dosages given early in the day. Another strategy is the use of low-dose heterocyclics, for example, desipramine 10 to 25 mg or trazodone 50 to 100 mg combined with an SSRI (Zajecka, Jeffriess, and Fawcett, 1995) or with an MAOI (Schmauss et al, 1986). As mentioned previously, some patients will respond to an alternative SSRI or venlafaxine. Finally electroconvulsive therapy may be a very effective strategy for treatment-resistant depression, especially in cases of psychotic or endogenous depression. Some nonpsychotic depressed patients have a more favorable response when a low-dose neuroleptic is added to the antidepressant regimen (Stern and Mendels, 1981).

Premature discontinuation of antidepressant medication is a common cause for relapse in depressed patients (Prien and Kupfer, 1986). Although a 4-month course of medication may be appropriate with the first episode of depression, it is more reasonable to plan for a 6- to 12-month course followed by cautious tapering, particularly in an individual with a previous episode or a positive family history. As previously discussed, antidepressant medication should not be withdrawn abruptly, and the dosage should be tapered, preferably over several weeks. Depressed individuals with recurrent episodes of depression, even in the absence of mania, may also benefit from maintenance doses of lithium alone or lithium in conjunction with an appropriately chosen medication, in addition to the use of full-dose maintenance antidepressant drugs.

ANTIMANIC AND MOOD-STABILIZING DRUGS

LITHIUM

Lithium was discovered in 1817 by Arfwedson, who named the drug after the Greek word for stone. Lithium was touted as a cure for epilepsy, gout, and other problems. In the 1940s lithium was used as a salt substitute for cardiac patients in the United States. However, it was removed from the market after some of these individuals died of toxic effects of lithium.

John Cade, an Australian physician, employed lithium urate in his investigation of toxicity of urea in guinea pigs and found that the animals developed extreme lethargy while remaining fully conscious. Cade had been involved in this work in connection with his search for a toxin in the urine of patients with mania. He then employed lithium salts experimentally in an attempt to produce sedation in these patients; he also used lithium preparations in persons with epilepsy because of the apparent anticonvulsant action of the preparations (Cade, 1949).

Employing lithium to treat mental illness spread to England and Denmark and then throughout Europe before eventually coming to the United States, which became the last country to authorize the therapeutic use of lithium.

Precisely how lithium achieves its normalizing effects in mania is not known; however, what is known is that the lithium ion substitutes for the sodium ion, thereby compromising the ability of neurons to release, activate, or respond to neurotransmitters. Although indicated only for the treatment of mania and for maintenance in patients with a history of mania, lithium usage in a variety of other psychiatric illnesses has been noted throughout the world. These other uses of lithium remain controversial, despite an expanding body of literature supporting a therapeutic efficacy broader than simply the treatment and prophylaxis of mania.

Pharmacokinetics

Lithium is well absorbed from the gastrointestinal tract and is normally given in oral tablets, capsules, or concentrates. Peak blood serum levels are reached in 1 to 4 hours. More than 95% of the amount ingested is excreted by the kidneys; that is, it is not metabolized. The plasma half-life is approximately 24 hours. Renal insufficiency or disease lengthens the half-life, necessitating reduction in dosage. Absorption and excretion of lithium are closely linked to those of sodium. When dietary sodium intake increases, serum levels of lithium are likely to drop, because lithium is excreted more rapidly. Conversely, when sodium in the diet decreases or when sodium is lost in ways other than through the kidney, for example, sweating or diarrhea, lithium serum levels increase. Since a therapeutic serum level of lithium is not much lower than a toxic serum level, such considerations are significant. Diet and activity levels should not change abruptly.

Lithium is manufactured primarily in 300-mg capsules or tablets (lithium carbonate). A 450-mg, sustained-release capsule is available. Lithium is effective in as many as 80% of cases; however, it takes 1 to 2 weeks to achieve a clinical response. Lithium dosage is based on both the clinical response and lithium serum levels. The typical dosage for acute mania is 600 mg 3 times per day, usually producing a serum level of 1.0 to 1.5 mEq/L. Desirable serum levels for maintenance are 0.6 to 1.2 mEq/L, which can be maintained on an average dose of 900 to 1200 mg per day. Lithium serum levels over 1.5 mEq/L are usually toxic.

Although there is no consensus regarding the antidepressant efficacy of lithium carbonate, some studies have indicated its beneficial effect in patients with depressed mood (Ortiz, Dabbagh, and Gershon, 1984). Lithium carbonate in conjunction with TCAs or MAOIs may be quite useful in many patients who have not responded to adequate trials of antidepressants. Controlled studies have confirmed the ability of lithium to augment a therapeutic response (Heninger, Charney, and Sternberg, 1983; Price, Charney, and Heninger, 1985). Carbamazepine may also improve depressed mood when used alone or in combination with a heterocyclic or an MAOI-type antidepressant (Folks, 1982). A patient who has not responded to an adequate trial of antidepressant may benefit.

The efficacy of lithium to treat acute mania has been well documented (Jefferson et al, 1987). Lithium requires a cooperative patient who will take daily oral medication, whereas neuroleptic drugs may also be given orally or intramuscularly as required. Perhaps the major disadvantage of lithium in the treatment of acute mania is that improvement is gradual. It may take up to 3 weeks to adequately control manic symptoms. Thus haloperidol or other antipsychotic agents or potent benzodiazepines such as lorazepam or clonazepam may be used alone or in combination, with dramatic and rapid impact in controlling behavior in patients with mania. Although low-potency agents such as chlorpromazine or thioridazine may produce considerable sedation, these drugs do little to alter qualitatively the underlying manic symptoms (Shopsin et al, 1975).

Lithium serum levels ideally should be measured approximately 12 hours, plus or minus 2 hours, after administration of the last dose of lithium (Jefferson et al, 1987). Clinical observations and well-documented compliance should coincide with this practice.

Considerable evidence supports the beneficial effect of lithium and the prophylaxis of recurrent depression in persons with bipolar illness. Lithium may also be beneficial in the treatment of recurrent depression in patients who do not have a manic component to the mood disorder (Quitkin et al, 1976). Perhaps the most interesting and important application of lithium in depression is its apparent ability, as previously noted, to facilitate a therapeutic response to a conventional antidepressant (Nelson and Majore, 1986).

Side Effects

Lithium, an ion interchangeable with sodium, has a variety of physiologic and pathophysiologic actions in various organ systems. Thus it is important to ascertain whether the patient is in good health, has any medical contraindications to lithium, and has sufficient renal function to clear the ion adequately so that lithium intoxication may be prevented (Jefferson et al, 1987). Serum creatinine or blood urea nitrogen levels should be obtained. For patients on a low-salt diet or diuretics, electrolyte values should also be determined. A baseline electrocardiogram (ECG) is necessary, because lithium often produces repolarization (ST segment and T wave) changes in the ECG, and about 20% of patients taking lithium have a T-wave flattening or inversion at therapeutic blood levels that does not indicate underlying heart disease (Jefferson et al, 1987; Bucht et al, 1984). Patients who have lithium intoxication may show a variety of cardiovascular abnormalities, including arrhythmia, conduction disturbance, and hypotension (Mitchell and MacKenzie, 1982). Because lithium may be associated with the development of a euthyroid goiter, hyperthyroidism with or without thyroid gland enlargement or abnormalities in serum determinations of thyroid function warrant baseline measurements of thyroid function. Also, because lithium administration is frequently associated with weight gain, partially related to fluid retention, and to increased caloric intake, the patient should be considered at risk for this nontherapeutic effect.

Lithium frequently produces benign reversible leukocytosis; white blood cell counts of 12,000 to 15,000 cells/mm^3 are frequently seen during therapy. This condition does not indicate any hematologic disease, and lithium usage need not be discontinued (Jefferson et al, 1987).

Because lithium is a simple ion whose entry into the body is governed by the same physiologic mechanisms as sodium, lithium reaches virtually all body tissues. Lithium's side effects, however, are linked primarily to serum blood levels. Blood levels greater than 1.5 mEq/L can be toxic, and generally levels above 2.0 mEq/L induce toxic signs and symptoms. Common side effects include nausea, dry mouth, diarrhea, and thirst. Drowsiness, mild hand tremor, polyuria, weight gain, a bloated feeling, sleeplessness, and headaches are other relatively common side effects.

A lithium tremor tends to be irregular in rhythm and amplitude, affecting the fingers. Jerky motions of the flexion and extension of fingers are also commonly associated with lithium therapy (Tyrer, Lee, and Trotter, 1981). These tremors often disappear spontaneously when the dose is held constant for the first 2 to 3 weeks of lithium treatment. Sometimes reducing the dose of lithium or advising the patient to take smaller dosages several times throughout the day alleviates this unwanted effect. However, when the tremor is persistent and severe enough to cause inconvenience to the patient in daily activities, propranolol, metaprolol, and nadolol, all of which are beta-adrenergic blocking agents, are highly effective in controlling it (Zubenko, Cohen, and Lipinski, 1984). The use of slow-release lithium preparations may reduce the severity of lithium tremor by reducing serum blood level peaks.

Side effects unrelated to serum levels include weight gain, a metallic taste, headache, edema of the hands and ankles, and pruritus. Lithium, even in therapeutic levels, can affect thyroid gland function. In some patients thyroid hormone therapy may be required. Lithium may also impair the mental or physical capabilities required for driving.

Polyuria and polydipsia develop in many patients taking lithium. These symptoms are generally benign and are not indicative of renal or metabolic disease. Of the patients studied and reported in the literature who have renal changes in association with therapeutic doses of lithium, none has been reported to have renal failure (Bernstein, 1995). To prevent kidney damage, lithium should not be prescribed unless there is both a reasonable clinical indication of its necessity and the likelihood that it will benefit the patient therapeutically. It may add somewhat to the safety of long-term lithium management and provide reassurance to the patient and the clinician to measure urine osmolality once or twice yearly, after a 12-hour period of fasting. This practice is, of course, in addition to periodic determinations of lithium serum levels, which should be monitored.

During lithium treatment, patients with edema of the ankle or lower legs generally do have normal renal, cardiovascular, and hepatic function. This edema may disappear spontaneously or may respond favorably to 25 to 50 mg twice a day of spironolactone, a specific aldosterone inhibitor that perhaps attempts to normalize tubular reabsorption of sodium, which has some role in the edema formation (Demers and Heninger, 1970). Additionally, patients who have edema may also respond favorably to an intermittent dose of a thiazide diuretic, for example, hydrochlorothiazide 50 mg daily or every other day. If hydrochlorothiazide is administered regularly, serum potassium and supplemental oral potassium levels should be monitored as with any patient simultaneously receiving a thiazide diuretic and lithium.

Although weight gain is common in patients receiving lithium, and may in part be due to the fluid retention described previously, variable changes in glucose metabolism may be an important mechanism in weight gain (Jefferson et al, 1987). Patients should be educated about this possibility and taught to maintain adequate fluid and salt intake during the course of any rapid weight loss. Moreover, it is often appropriate to measure lithium serum concentration more frequently in individuals who may be on a weight-reducing diet.

Lithium therapy may be associated with the development of goiter in the presence of normal thyroid function tests and a euthyroid state. This condition is usually associated with an increased thyroid-stimulating hormone level and an enlarged thyroid gland as it attempts to maintain the euthyroid state. Hypothyroidism may also be induced by lithium treatment. This occurrence does not indicate that the dosage needs to be changed or the medication discontinued; however, proper evaluation and replacement therapy with an appropriate thyroid hormone regimen may be necessary in conjunction with lithium treatment (Myers et al, 1985).

Dermatologic reactions may occur with lithium (Folks and Kinney, 1991). Acne may worsen. Lithium has also been reported to exacerbate psoriasis. Occasionally a maculopapular rash, with or without pruritus, may emerge during the course of lithium treatment. Hair loss may also occur and may be limited to the scalp or may affect other body regions.

Many patients taking lithium have gastrointestinal tract complaints, most commonly upper gastric burning sensations and persistent indigestion. Taking lithium at mealtime or with a snack often alleviates these symptoms. Mild diarrhea is also occasionally associated with conventional therapeutic doses and serum levels of lithium but is more apt to occur in the presence of excessive lithium serum concentration. Vomiting is a major risk because it contributes to dehydration, which, in turn, may worsen any lithium intoxication. Patients who have nausea, vomiting, or other flulike symptoms during lithium therapy should be advised to discontinue lithium and maintain adequate fluid intake for a short time.

Lithium intoxication is a common problem; when it is suspected, the drug should be discontinued and blood samples sent for determinations of lithium serum concentration and serum creatinine and electrolyte levels. Specific interventions include adequate hydration, antiemetics as necessary, and monitoring of serum levels of electrolytes, lithium, and creatinine, which, in turn, can guide the rate and nature of fluid replacement. An ECG should also be obtained, because the possibility of cardiac arrhythmia is always present. A patient with lithium intoxication may also have a variety of central nervous system effects, including confusion, stupor, and the potential for seizure (Sansone and Zeigler, 1985; Himmelhoch et al, 1980).

Implications

Therapeutic versus toxic levels. Therapeutic lithium serum levels are 0.6 to 1.2 mEq/L. At serum levels above 1.5 mEq/L adverse reactions can occur. Typically the higher the serum levels, the more severe the reaction. Mild to moderate toxic reactions occur at levels of 1.5 to 2.5 mEq/L, and moderate to severe reactions at 2.0 to 2.5 mEq/L. Diarrhea, vomiting, drowsiness, muscular weakness, and lack of coordination can be early signs of lithium intoxication. At higher levels ataxia, giddiness, tinnitus, blurred vision, and a large output of dilute urine may be seen. At serum levels above 3 mEq/L multiple organs and organ systems may be involved, leading to coma and death (Sugarman, 1984). Patients with serum levels as high as 10 mEq/L have survived. Serum levels should be monitored and should not be allowed to exceed 2 mEq/L.

There is no antidote for lithium poisoning. When supportive intervention is available, discontinuing the drug may be enough. In acute overdose, gastric lavage has been used successfully. Parenteral normal saline solution infused over 6 hours (1 to 2 L) may provide enough volume to prevent hypovolemia and restore blood pressure and enough sodium to counteract lithium's ill effects, enhancing renal excretion for serum levels below 2.5 mEq/L. Forced diuresis may be necessary for patients with lithium poisoning, and mannitol may be used. Acetazolamide, which alkalinizes the urine, may also be given to increase lithium excretion in case of an acute overdose. In some severe cases hemodialysis has been found to be helpful.

Use in pregnancy. Cessation of lithium during pregnancy is suggested because of its relationship to Ebstein's anomaly and other teratogenic effects in the first trimester. If antimania treatment is essential during this time, treatment with thioridazine or, perhaps, carbamazepine or valproate, may be beneficial. These drugs, when used instead of lithium, also carry unknown risks when prescribed in the second and third trimesters. Doses should be reduced as much as 50% before the delivery because of the potential for neonatal intoxication resulting from high maternal serum levels of lithium (Cohen, 1989).

Side effects. Because lithium has a narrow therapeutic index, lithium serum levels should be determined frequently. Levels are determined daily in some acute-treatment units. Once the patient's condition is stabilized, monthly serum level determinations are usually adequate. Blood is usually drawn before administration of the first dose of lithium in the morning (usually 8 to 12 hours after the last dose). However, do not rely on laboratory tests alone but rather continue to evaluate the patient.

Interactions. Familiarity with the drugs that can elevate lithium serum levels is essential. Diuretics, with the exception of acetazolamide, increase sodium excretion, thereby elevating serum lithium levels. Indomethacin and other nonsteroidal antiinflammatory agents, for example, ibuprofen, increase serum levels of lithium by reducing renal elimination. Switching to a low-salt diet also elevates lithium serum levels.

Some drugs decrease serum lithium levels and pose problems of inadequate treatment and symptom exacerbation. This decrease may occur in one of two ways: by increasing lithium excretion or by decreasing lithium absorption. Drugs that increase lithium excretion include acetazolamide, caffeine, and alcohol.

Lithium and antipsychotic or anxiolytic drugs are frequently combined. Antipsychotics are prescribed with lithium because lithium's clinical response time is delayed to 1 to 2 weeks. Antipsychotic agents are prescribed to produce an immediate neuroleptic or antipsychotic effect (see Chapter 9, Acute Psychoses and the Violent Patient). A potential problem with this combination that has not been previously mentioned is that the antiemetic properties of the antipsychotic agent can potentially mask the early signs of lithium intoxication, that is, nausea and vomiting. Moreover, there are some concerns that the specific combination of lithium and haloperidol has a greater-than-normal potential for neurotoxicity. This possibility, however, seems to be primarily a matter of drug interaction and should be a concern with any combination of lithium and an antipsychotic agent. Lithium also prolongs the paralyzing effect of some neuromuscular-blocking agents that may be given before surgery or used during ECT. Appropriate measures should be taken in these cases.

Patient education. The patient and family alike must be familiar with the nontherapeutic effects of lithium and the symptoms of minor and major toxic effects (Box 5-10). Side effects associated with lithium should be reviewed, and in individuals of child-bearing age appropriate measures should be taken to avoid conception during lithium treatment because of its definitive ability to harm the fetus. Avoidance of driving until the patient is stabilized on a regimen of lithium is a reasonable expectation. The interventions outlined in Box 5-11 should also be considered in applicable cases.

ALTERNATIVE ANTIMANIC AND MOOD-STABILIZING DRUGS

Valproic Acid

Sodium valproate, valproic acid, and related compounds such as divalproex (Depakote) have been used since the 1960s as antiepileptic agents. More recently divalproex has been studied using controlled trials with placebo and lithium in the treatment of bipolar disorder (Box 5-12), particularly its antimanic properties (Bowden et al, 1994). Divalproex has received FDA approval and is indicated for the primary treatment of mania (Box 5-13).

Moreover, divalproex showed significantly better response in cases with clinical presentations of mixed mania (Box 5-14) and rapid cycling (Box 5-15). Valproate, along with carbamazepine (Tegretol), is effective in treating mania secondary to general medical conditions, that is, secondary mania (Box 5-16). The advantages and disadvantages of valproate and lithium are compared in Boxes 5-17 and 5-18.

The various formulations of valproate differ with respect to absorption and potential side effects. Valproic acid formulations are rapidly absorbed. Divalproex in the form of an enteric-coated or sprinkle tablet is more slowly absorbed, that is, 2 versus 4 hours. Common side effects of valproate include gastrointestinal upset, somnolence, tremor, and dizziness. These dose-related side effects can be avoided or reduced by using the enteric-coated fomulations. Other possible adverse effects are shown in Box 5-17.

Box 5-10 Patient Guidelines for Taking Lithium

To achieve a therapeutic effect and prevent toxic effects of lithium, patients taking lithium should be advised of the following:

1. Lithium must be taken on a regular basis, preferably at the same time daily. If a patient is taking lithium, for example, on a three-times-daily schedule and forgets a dose, he or she should wait until the next scheduled time to take the lithium but should not take twice the amount at that time, because lithium intoxication could occur.
2. When lithium treatment is initiated, mild side effects such as a fine hand tremor, increased thirst and urination, nausea, anorexia, and diarrhea or constipation may develop. Most of the mild side effects are transient and do not represent toxic effects of lithium. Also, in some patients who are taking lithium some foods such as celery and butter have an unappealing taste.
3. Serious side effects of lithium that necessitate its discontinuance include vomiting, extreme hand tremor, sedation, muscle weakness, and vertigo. If any of these occur, the prescribing clinician should be notified immediately.
4. Lithium and sodium compete for elimination from the body through the kidneys. An increase in salt intake increases lithium elimination, and a decrease in salt intake decreases lithium elimination. Thus it is important that the patient maintain a balanced diet and salt intake. If the patient wishes to alter his or her diet, he or she should first consult with the prescribing clinician.
5. Various situations can require an adjustment in the amount of lithium administered to a patient, for example, the addition of a new medication to the patient's drug regimen, a new diet, or an illness with fever or excessive sweating.
6. Blood should be drawn in the morning for determination of lithium levels, approximately 10 to 14 hours after the last dose was taken.

Box 5-11 Nursing Interventions for Patients Taking Lithium

Prepare the patient for expected side effects in a nonanxious manner.

Discuss which side effects should subside (nausea, dry mouth, diarrhea, thirst, mild hand tremor, weight gain, bloatedness, insomnia, and lightheadedness).

Identify the side effects that require immediate notification of the physician (e.g., vomiting, severe tremor, sedation, muscle weakness, and vertigo).

Suggest taking lithium with meals to reduce nausea.

Suggest drinking 10 to 12 8-oz (240 ml) glasses of water per day to reduce thirst and maintain normal fluid balance.

Advise patient to elevate feet to relieve ankle edema.

Advise patient to maintain a consistent dietary sodium intake but to increase sodium if there is a major increase in perspiration.

Box 5-12 Valproate: Role in Bipolar Illness

Acute mania or hypomania
Lithium refractoriness/intolerance/noncompliance
Bipolar subtypes known to be poorly responsive to lithium:
- Mixed mania
- Rapid cycling
- Secondary mania
- Comorbid substance abuse

Augmentation of response to other mood stabilizers

Box 5-13 Divalproex: Rapid Titration

For a 70-kg person*

Day 1	250 mg three times a day
Day 2	250 mg three times a day and 500 mg at bedtime
Day 3	500 mg three times a day
Day 5	check plasma level

*20 mg per kg per day after titration.

Box 5-14 Mixed Mania

Symptoms of mania and depression occur every day for at least 1 week to a degree that meets the criteria (except for duration) of a major episode of each.
Mood: Usually depressed
Activity: Usually increased
Thinking: Characteristic of depression or mania or both
Common features: History of substance abuse or neurologic disorder.
Poor response to lithium
Incidence: Up to 50% of bipolar patients
Women may be at greater risk

Box 5-15 Rapid Cycling Bipolar Disorder

At least four affective episodes per year
10% to 15% of all bipolar patients
Depressive episode initiates rapid cycling
More common for patients with the following traits:
- Long-term illness
- Females
- Controlled and uncontrolled hyperthyroidism

Poor response to lithium
May be triggered by use of TCAs

Box 5-16 General Medical Conditions that Cause Secondary Mania

Anoxia	Stroke
Hyperthyroidism	Brain tumor
Hemodialysis	Multiple sclerosis
Lyme disease	Normal pressure hydrocephalus
Hypercalcemia	Medications
AIDS-related	Other neurologic disorders

Box 5-17 Valproate

Advantages	**Disadvantages**
Rapid onset	Transient hair loss
Can be used as initial treatment	Weight gain
High quality of clinical studies (acute mania)	Tremors, GI upset
Divalproex formulation well tolerated; minimal effects on cognition	Dose-related thrombocytopenia
Effective in bipolar disorder subtypes	Rare hepatotoxicity, pancreatitis

Box 5-18 Lithium

Advantages	Disadvantages
More than 40 years of clinical experience	Nonresponse in 30% to 50% of cases
Most effective for euphoric mania and hypomania	Narrow therapeutic index
Can reduce mortality by decreasing suicide	Slow onset of action
Inexpensive	Side effects very common
	High rate of noncompliance
	Less effective in bipolar subtypes

The bioavailability of valproate is 100% at therapeutic concentrations, with up to 95% protein binding. Unbound (active) drug may be displaced by other drugs, for example, carbamazepine or coumadin, causing toxicity or side effects. Metabolism of valproate is complex, with several active metabolites. Divalproex has a half-life of 16 hours and reaches steady state in 2 to 5 days. Induction of microsomal enzymes, for example, P-450, may lead to lower plasma concentrations, as occurs with coadministration of phenobarbital or carbamazepine. These drugs, along with phenytoin (Dilantin) and alcohol, represent the more significant drug interactions. Compared with lithium and carbamazepine, the potential for drug interaction is relatively more favorable (Box 5-19).

Valproate, or divalproex, is initially dosed at 250 mg twice daily or three times a day and titrated at 250 to 500 mg every 3 days. A more rapid onset of effect occurs with valproate than with lithium when therapeutic concentrations of 50 to 120 μg/mL are achieved. Oral loading of valproate at 20 mg per kg per day (in divided doses) has resulted in a rather quick response in some cases, that is, 5 to 7 days (Keck et al 1993). A rapid titration using this technique is depicted in Box 5-13.

Lithium and valproate are highly effective, are generally safe, and produce a tolerable level of side effects in the great majority of patients. However, when lithium or valproate are not tolerated or when response does not occur, alternative agents may be required. Alternative antimanic and mood-stabilizing drugs are currently marketed for treatment of other conditions and are not at this writing approved by the FDA for use in mood disorders.

Box 5-19 Drug Interactions

Carbamazepine	Lithium
Erythromycin	Thiazides
Isoniazid	NSAIDs
Oral contraceptives	Digoxin
Theophylline	Methyldopa
Divalproex	Verapamil
Cimetidine	Neuroleptics
Fluoxetine	ACE inhibitors

Carbamazepine

Carbamazepine (Tegretol) is perhaps the best alternative treatment for manic episodes when lithium or valproate are ineffective, contraindicated, or not tolerated (Table 5-11, Box 5-20). Carbamazepine is chemically related to the tricyclic antidepressants. Patients with rapid-cycling bipolar disorder or secondary mania may respond especially well to carbamazepine, and at times carbamazepine may be given in combination with lithium and/or valproate (Folks et al, 1982). Although the mechanism of the antimanic action of carbamazepine is unknown, early work focused on its ability to inhibit kindling (Post et al, 1982).

Carbamazepine is absorbed erratically, with bioavailability of 75% to 85%. Although plasma concentrations of carbamazepine correlate to its anticonvulsant effect, the relationship of blood level to antimanic activity is less clear (Jefferson et al, 1987). Initial doses of 250 mg twice daily or three times daily are titrated slowly to achieve levels of 8 to 12 μg/mL (Ballenger, Post, and Bunney, 1982).

Table 5-11 Comparison of Side Effects Profiles for Lithium and Carbamazepine

Lithium* (0.7-1.2 mEq/L)	Frequency (%)	Carbamazepine† (5-12 μg/ml)
Memory disturbances‡	—	?
Thirst and polyuria	50-70	—
Tremor	30-50	—
Weight gain‡	10-30	?
Diarrhea	10-20	—
Hypothyroidism	5-10	Essentially absent
Psoriasis	1	—
	—	Blood dyscrasias
	—	Hepatitis
	—	Dizziness and ataxia
	—	Water intoxication

*Vestergaard P, Shou M: The effect of age on lithium requirements, *Pharmacopsychiatry* 17:199, 1984.
†Post RM et al: Selective response to the anticonvulsant carbamazepine in manic-depressive illness: a case study, *J Clin Psychopharmacol* 4:178, 1984.
‡Reasons for noncompliance. (From Jamison KR, Akisal HS: Medication compliance in patients with bipolar disorder, *Psychiatr Clin North Am* 6:175, 1983.)

Box 5-20 Carbamazepine

Advantages	Disadvantages
More rapid onset than lithium	Stimulates own oxidative metabolism (autoinduction)
May be effective in difficult-to-treat cases	Complex drug interactions
May be effective as adjunctive therapy in acute mania	Sedation, poor coordination
Generally well tolerated	Blood dyscrasias, skin reactions
	Hyponatremia (poorly tolerated by elderly)

Nausea, anorexia, and occasional vomiting may occur with carbamazepine, particularly when the drug is administered on an empty stomach or when relatively high doses are used. Sedation and drowsiness are other common side effects, which may be minimized by lowering initial doses and by slower titrating and use of a three times or four times a day regimen. As with valproate, the sedative effects of carbamazepine may be useful in managing insomnia and agitation in some patients with mood disturbances (see Chapter 9, Acute Psychoses and the Violent Patient).

The most serious and rare side effect of carbamazepine is its potential to produce agranulocytosis (Jefferson et al, 1987; Folks et al, 1982). Mild to moderate leukopenia, anemia, and thrombocytopenia may also occur. Complete blood cell counts and examination of the blood smear should be performed weekly during the first month of therapy and may be performed at progressively longer intervals during the course of treatment. Complete blood cell counts and other appropriate laboratory tests in patients receiving maintenance therapy with carbamazepine should be monitored every 3 to 4 months during treatment. For patients who benefit greatly from taking carbamazepine but who have mild leukopenia, anemia, or thrombocytopenia, periodic monitoring may be acceptable and tolerated. In addition to its antimanic effect, carbamazepine has been shown to possess antidepressant actions when employed alone or in conjunction with other antidepressant drugs (Post et al, 1986).

Toxic effects of carbamazepine, as well as drowsiness, may occur with coadministration of erythromycin; neurotoxic effects may result from the ability of this antibiotic to inhibit carbamazepine metabolism. When given alone or in combination with other antiepileptic drugs, for example, phenobarbital, carbamazepine may induce its own metabolism through microsomal induction (Figure 5-3). Carbamazepine may also increase serum lithium concentration and decrease serum concentrations of a number of drugs, including valproate and neuroleptics. Neurotoxic effects may occur when carbamazepine is combined with calcium channel blockers, for example, verapamil or angiotensin-converting enzyme (ACE) inhibitors (Bernstein, 1995).

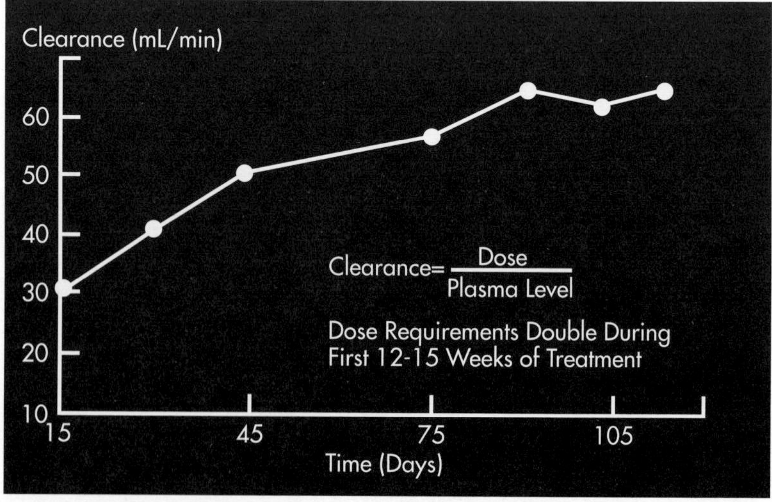

Figure 5-3 Carbamazepine autoinduction after initiation of treatment.

Benzodiazepines

Clonazepam (Klonopin) is a benzodiazepine with potent anticonvulsant properties (see Chapter 7, Seizure Disorders) and is used as a treatment or as an adjunct for the treatment of mania. Clonazepam has been shown to have an acute therapeutic effect in manic patients (Chouinard, Young, and Annable, 1983; Chouinard, 1985). This drug may obviate or reduce the need for the adjunct use of haloperidol or other neuroleptic agents; except for considerable drowsiness, minimal adverse effects are seen in patients receiving clonazepam in doses of 2 to 16 mg per day (Chouinard, Young, and Annable, 1983; Victor et al, 1984; Chouinard, 1985).

Clonazepam may be used as a maintenance drug to treat bipolar affective disorder in conjunction with lithium, valproate, or carbamazepine. Clonazepam is useful in patients for whom neuroleptic drugs cannot be employed, such as patients with Parkinson's disease. Similarly, *lorazepam* (Ativan) in doses of 3 to 20 mg daily has been employed (Modell, Lenox, and Weiner, 1985) as an adjunct in lieu of neuroleptic drugs. Lorazepam is the only benzodiazepine that is reliable when administered intramuscularly. Lorazepam may also minimize the acute extrapyramidal side effects of high-potency antipsychotic drugs used to treat acute psychosis (see Chapter 9, Acute Psychoses and the Violent Patient).

Miscellaneous Agents

Several investigators have discussed the use of calcium channel blockers, specifically, verapamil and nimodipine, to exert a clinically significant antimanic effect (Pollack, Rosenbaum, and Hyman, 1987). Further investigation of the psychotropic effects of this class of drug is needed. One study has shown no improvement in manic symptoms (Barton and Gitlin, 1987). Moreover, there have been reports of patients receiving calcium channel blockers, including verapamil, diltiazem, and nifedipine, in whom symptoms of depression or dysphoria emerged as a possible side effect (Bernstein, 1995).

REFERENCES

American Psychiatric Association: *Diagnostic and statistical manual of mental disorders,* ed 4, revised, Washington, DC, 1994, The Association.

Anton RF, Hitri A, Diamond BI: Amoxapine treatment of psychotic depression: dose effect and dopamine blockage, *J Clin Psychiatry (Monogr Ser)* 4:32, 1986.

Ayd FJ Jr: Lexicon of psychiatry, neurology and the neurosciences, Baltimore, 1995, Wiliams & Wilkins.

Baldesserini RJ: *Chemotherapy in psychiatry,* Cambridge, Mass, 1985, Harvard University.

Ballenger JC, Post RM, Bunney WE: Carbamazepine in manic-depressive illness: a new treatment, *Am J Psychiatry* 139:115, 1982.

Barton BM, Gitlin MJ: Verapamil in treatment-resistant mania: an open trial, *J Clin Psychopharmacol* 7:101, 1987.

Bender KJ: Novel antidepressant, antipsychotics progress in developmental pipeline, *Psychiatr Times* 13-14, Dec 1995.

Bernstein JG: *Handbook of drug therapy in psychiatry,* ed 3, St. Louis, 1995, Mosby.

Blier P, Bergeron R: Effectivenss of pindolol with selected antidepressant drugs in the treatment of major depression, *J Clin Psychopharmacol* 15:217-22, 1995.

Bowden CL, Brugger AM, Swann AC et al: Efficacy of divalproex vs lithium and placebo in the treatment of mania, *JAMA* 271:918-24, 1994.

Brown WA, Harrison W: Are patients who are intolerant to one serotonin selective reuptake inhibitor intolerant to another? *J Clin Psychiatry* 56:1, 30-4, Jan 1995.

Bucht G et al: ECG changes during lithium therapy: a prospective study, *Acta Med Scand* 216:101, 1984.

Cade JFJ: Lithium salts in the treatment of psychotic excitement, *Med J Aust* 2:349, 1949.

Chouinard G: Antimanic effects of clonazepam, *Psychosomatics* 26(12):7-12, 1985.

Chouinard G, Young SN, Annable L: Antimanic effects of clonazepam, *Biol Psychiatry* 18:451, 1983.

Claghorn JL, Lesem MD: A double-blind placebo-controlled study of ORG 3770 in depressed outpatients, *J Affect Disord* 34:165-71, 1995.

Cohen LS: Psychotropic drug use in pregnancy, *Hosp Community Psychiatry* 40:566, 1989.

Cunningham LA et al: A comparison of venlafaxine, trazodone, and placebo in major depression, *J Clin Psychopharmacol* 14(2):99-106, 1994.

Demers R, Heninger G: Pretibial edema and sodium retention during lithium carbonate treatment, *JAMA* 214:1845, 1970.

Folks DG: Clinical approaches to anxiety in the medically ill elderly, *Drug Ther Suppl* p 72, August 1990.

Folks DG, Kinney FC: Dermatology. In Stoudemire A, Fogel BS, editors: *Medical psychiatric practice,* vol 1, Washington, DC, 1991, American.

Folks DG et al: Carbamazepine treatment of selected affectively disordered inpatients, *Am J Psychiatry* 139:115, 1982.

Ford CV: *The somatizing disorders: illness as a way of life,* New York, 1983, Elsevier Biomedical.

Freud S: Mourning and melancholia. In *The complete psychological works of Sigmund Freud,* London, 1957, Hogarth.

Goff DC, Jenike MA: Treatment-resistant depression in the elderly, *J Am Geriatr Soc* 34:63, 1986.

Goodman WK, Charney DS: Therapeutic applications and mechanisms of action of monoamine oxidase inhibitor and heterocyclic antidepressant drugs, *J Clin Psychiatry* 46(10, sec 2):6, 1985.

Goodwin DW, Guze SB: *Psychiatric diagnosis,* New York, 1984, Oxford University.

Guelfi JD, White C, Magni G: A randomized double-blind comparison of venlafaxine and placebo in inpatients with major depression and melancholia, *Clin Neuropharmacol* 15(suppl 1):323b, 1992.

Guze SB, Robins E: Suicide and primary affective disorders, *Br J Psychiatry* 117:437, 1970.

Harsch HH, Holt RE: Use of antidepressants in attempted suicide, *Hosp Community Psychiatry* 39:990, 1988.

Heninger GR, Charney DS, Sternberg DE: Lithium carbonate augmentation of antidepressant treatment: an effective prescription for treatment-refractory depression, *Arch Gen Psychiatry* 40:1335, 1983.

Himmelhoch JM et al: Age, dementia dyskinesias, and lithium response, *Am J Psychiatry* 137:941, 1980.

Jamison KR, Akisal HS: Medication compliance in patients with bipolar disorder, *Psychiatr Clin North Am* 6:175, 1983.

Jefferson JW et al: *Lithium encyclopedia for clinical practice,* Washington, DC, 1987, American Psychiatric Association.

Joffe RT, Schuller DR: An open study of buspirone augmentation of serotonin reuptake inhibitors in refractory depression, *J Clin Psychiatry* 54(7):269-71, 1993.

Joffe RT, Singer W: Thyroid hormone potentiation of antidepressants. In Amsterdam JD, editor: *Refractory depression: advances in neuropsychiatry and psychopharmacology,* vol 2 New York, 1991, Raven Press.

Keck PE et al: Valproate oral loading in the treatment of acute mania, *J Clin Psychiatry* 54(8)305-8, 1993.

Keltner NL: Venlafaxine: a novel antidepressant. Update on Psychopharmacology, *J Psychosoc Nurs Ment Health Serv* 33:1:51-C3, 1995.

Keltner NL: Drugs for treatment of depression and mania. In Shlafer M, Marieb E, editors: *The nurse, pharmacology, and drug therapy,* Menlo Park, Calif, 1989, Addison-Wesley.

Keltner NL, Folks DG: Alternatives to lithium in the treatment of bipolar disorder, *Perspect Psychiatr Care* 27(2):36, 1991.

Keltner N: Serotonin syndrome: a case of fatal SSRI/MAOI interaction, *Perspect Psychiatr Care* 30:4, 26-31, Oct-Dec 1994.

Kerr TA, Schapira K, Roth M: The relationship between premature death and affective disorders, *Br J Psychiatry* 115:1277, 1969.

Meador-Woodruff JH: Psychiatric side effects of tricyclic antidepressants, *Hosp Community Psychiatry* 41:84, 1990.

Mendels J et al: Efficacy and safety of b.i.d. doses of venlafaxine in a dose-response study, *Psychopharmacol Bull* 29:169-74, 1993.

Mitchell JE, MacKenzie TB: Cardiac effects of lithium therapy in man: a review, *J Clin Psychiatry* 43:47, 1982.

Modell JG, Lenox RH, Weiner S: Inpatient clinical trial of lorazepam for the management of manic agitation, *J Clin Psychopharmacol* 5:109-13, 1985.

Myers DH et al: A prospective study of the effects of lithium on thyroid function and on the prevalence of antithyroid antibodies, *Psychol Med* 15:55, 1985.

Nelson JC, Majore CM: Lithium augmentation in psychotic depression refractory to combined drug treatment, *Am J Psychiatry* 143:363, 1986.

Nierenberg AA: Treatment-resistant depression in the age of serotonin, *Psychiatr Ann* 24:5, 1994.

Ortiz A, Dabbagh M, Gershon S: Lithium: clinical use, toxicology, and mode of action. In Bernstein JG, editor: *Clinical psychopharmacology,* ed 2, Boston, 1984, John Wright–PSG.

Pollack MH, Rosenbaum JF, Hyman SE: Calcium channel blockers in psychiatry, *Psychosomatics* 28:356, 1987.

Pope HG, Jr, McElroy SL, Nixon RA: Possible synergism between fluoxetine and lithium in refractory depression, *Am J Psychiatry* 145:1292-4, 1988.

Post RM et al: Kindling and carbamazepine in affective illness, *J Nerv Ment Dis* 170:717, 1982.

Post RM et al: Selective response to the anticonvulsant carbamazepine in manic-depressive illness: a case study, *J Clin Psychopharmacol* 4:178, 1984.

Post RM et al: Antidepressant effects of carbamazepine, *Am J Psychiatry* 143:29, 1986.

Preskorn SH, Alderman J, Chung M et al: Pharmacokinetics of desipramine coadministered with sertraline and fluoxetine, *J Clin Psychopharmacol* 14:90-98, 1994.

Preskorn SH, Magnus RD: Inhibition of hepatic P-450 isoenzymes by serotonin selective reuptake inhibitors: In vitro and in vivo findings and their implications for patient care, *Psychopharmacol Bull,* 30:251-9, 1994.

Price LH, Charney DS, Heninger GR: Efficacy of lithium-tranylcypromine treatment in refractory depression, *Am J Psychiatry* 142:619, 1985.

Prien RF, Kupfer DJ: Continuation of drug therapy for major depressive episodes: how long should it be maintained? *Am J Psychiatry* 143:18, 1986.

Quitkin F et al: Prophylaxis in unipolar affective disorder, *Am J Psychiatry* 133:1091, 1976.

Rickels K et al: Nefazodone and imipramine in major depression: a placebo-controlled trial, *Br J Psychiatry* 164:802-5, 1994.

Risch SC, Janowsky DS, Hyey LY: Plasma levels of tricyclic antidepressants and clinical efficacy. In Enna SJ, Malick JB, Richelson E, editors: *Antidepressants: neurochemical, behavioral, and clinical perspectives,* New York, 1981, Raven.

Robertson MM, Trimble MR: Major tranquilizers used as antidepressants, *J Affective Disord* 4:173, 1982.

Rothschild AJ: Selective serotonin reuptake inhibitor-induced sexual dysfunction: efficacy of a drug holiday, *Am J Psychiatry* 152:10, 1514-16, Oct 1995.

Sabelli HC, Fawcett J, Javaid JI: The methylphenidate test for differentiating desipramine-responsive from nortriptyline-responsive depression, *Am J Psychiatry* 140:212, 1983.

Sansone MEG, Ziegler DK: Lithium toxicity: a review of neurologic complications, *Clin Neuropharmacol* 8:242, 1985.

Schmauss M, Kapfhammer HP, Meyr P et al: Combined MAO-inhibitor and tri(tetra)cyclic antidepressant in therapy resistant depression: a retrospective study, *Pharmacopsychiatry* 19:251-2, 1986.

Segraves RT: Treatment-emergent sexual dysfunction in affective disorder: a review and management strategies, *J Clin Psychiatry (Update Monogr)* 1:1, Nov 1994.

Shopsin B et al: Psychoactive drugs in mania, *Arch Gen Psychiatry* 32:34, 1975.

Stern SI, Mendels J: Drug combinations in the treatment of refractory depression: a review, *J Clin Psychiatry* 42:368, 1981.

Sternberg DE, Jarvik ME: Memory functions in depression, *Arch Gen Psychiatry* 33:219, 1976.

Stone T, Folks DG: Somatization in the elderly. In Hall RCW, editor, *Psychiatric medicine,* 1992.

Sugarman JR: Management of lithium intoxication, *Fam Pract* 18:347, 1984.

Tyrer P, Lee I, Trotter C: Physiological characteristics of tremor after chronic lithium therapy, *Br J Psychiatry* 139:59, 1981.

Van Kammen DP, Murphy DL: Prediction of imipramine antidepressant response by a one-day *d*-amphetamine trial, *Am J Psychiatry* 135:1179, 1978.

Vestergaard P, Shou M: The effect of age on lithium requirements, *Pharmacopsychiatry* 17:199, 1984.

Williams R et al: A double-blind comparison of moclobemide and fluoxetine in the treatment of depressive disorders, *Int Clin Psychopharmacol* 7:155-8, 1993.

Winokur G: Types of depressive illness, *Br J Psychiatry* 120:265, 1972.

Yu PH, Boulton AA: Clinical pharmacology of MAO-B inhibitors. In Kennedy SH, editor: *Clinical advances in monoamine oxidase inhibitor therapies,* Washington DC, 1994, American Psychiatric Press.

Zajecka JM, Jeffriess H, Fawcett J: The efficacy of fluoxetine combined with a heterocyclic antidepressant in treatment-resistant depression: a retrospective analysis, *J Clin Psychiatry* 56(8)338-43, 1995.

Zubenko GS, Cohen BM, Lipinski JF: Comparison of metroprolol and propranolol in the treatment of lithium tremor, *Psychiatry Res* 11:163, 1984.

CHAPTER 6

Anxiety Disorders

Historical Considerations

Anxiety and insomnia (see Chapter 8, Sleep Disorders) are among the most common symptoms for which drug therapy is prescribed (Folks, 1990). Anxiety may occur in association with a variety of medical or psychiatric illnesses. The onset, course, and symptoms associated with anxiety syndromes vary significantly. Anxiety may occur suddenly, with or without a precipitating cause, or may develop in a rather subtle course. Anxiety may be associated with a clearly definable stress or stressors or may accompany problems within the family or psychosocial constellation. Anxiety may also occur when manifest symptoms are primarily somatic, may be secondarily associated with a significant medical or surgical problem, or may even be induced by medication or dietary substances.

Regardless of the course or circumstances surrounding the onset, anxiety requires intervention when it is disabling with respect to daily activities, social or occupational functioning, or relationship functioning. Intervention, of course, must always be preceded by adequate assessment to consider underlying emotional, family, biologic, or other factors that may respond to a specific intervention. As with depression, the use of anxiolytic medications is ideally combined with psychotherapeutic approaches, behavioral therapy techniques, or other adjunctive interventions that promote compliance and increase the likelihood of both an initial and a sustained response.

Drugs historically used to treat anxiety, referred to as *antianxiety* or *anxiolytic* agents, include those listed in Box 6-1. Clearly alcohol is the oldest known agent to be used both medically and nonmedically. Alcohol is still the most frequently *self-prescribed* treatment for anxiety. The development of anxiolytic compounds has improved safety and efficacy, yet the dangers of dependency and the complications associated with anxiolytic treatment persist. The risks and adverse effects of alcohol have been documented in sources as old as the first book of the Old Testament, which declares that Noah "drank of the wine, was drunken and uncovered within his tent."

After the widespread use of alcohol through the ages as a sedative and an anxiolytic medicine, a variety of other compounds, presumably safer and more effective, were developed (Table 6-1). Many of these historical compounds were neither safe nor effective in long-term treatment. For example, in the early 1900s the bromo seltzers were proclaimed efficacious, but bromide dependency became a significant problem, and these products were withdrawn from the market (Harvey, 1985). Subsequently the barbiturates were developed and were seen as another potentially safe class of drugs; again their development was followed by the recognition of adverse effects, including seizures and the potential for addiction, dependence, and withdrawal symptoms. These compounds, as well as the opiates and tincture of belladonna, were indeed fraught with problems.

Perhaps the first major advance after the development of barbiturates was the development of meprobamate in the mid-1950s. This drug was initially heralded as an effective and addiction-free agent that did not possess the disadvantages of the bar-

Box 6-1 Historical and Contemporary Anxiolytic Drugs

- Alcohol
- Opiates
- Belladonna
- Barbiturates
- Meprobamate
- Phenothiazines
- Antihistamines
- Beta blockers
- Benzodiazepines
- Monoamine oxidase inhibitors
- Cyclic antidepressants
- Buspirone

Table 6-1 Historical Anxiolytics

Agent	Trade name	Comments
Alcohols, aldehydes, and propanediols		
Ethanol	Generic	Not recommended*
Ethchlorvynol	Placidyl	Not recommended*
Chloral hydrate	Generic	1-2 gm for sleep
Paraldehyde	Generic	Not recommended*
Meprobamate	Equanil, Miltown, generic	Not recommended*
Tybamate	Tybatran, Solacen, generic	Not recommended*
Barbiturates		
Amobarbital	Amytal, generic	100-800 mg/hr, intravenously in diagnosis, or parenterally for emergency sedation
Methohexital	Brevital	10 mg/5 sec intravenously (average dose = 70mg) for ECT only
Pentobarbital	Nembutal, generic	Can be used for withdrawal in most sedative addictions†‡
Phenobarbital	Luminal, generic	30-90 mg/day†‡
Secobarbital	Seconal, generic	Not recommended†
Structural relatives of barbiturates (nonbarbiturates)		
Glutethimide	Doriden	Not recommended*
Methyprylon	Noludar	Not recommended*
Methaqualone	Quaalude, Sopor, generic	Not recommended*
Antihistamines		
Diphenhydramine	Benadryl	25-50 mg parenterally for dystonia
Hydroxyzine	Atarax, Vistaril	Not recommended*
Promethazine	Phenergan, generic	Not recommended*

Modified from Baldessarini RJ: *Chemotherapy in psychiatry,* Cambridge, Mass, 1985, Harvard University.

*These agents are not recommended for routine use.

†Short-acting barbiturates are prescribed for sleep because of their low cost; phenobarbital is inexpensive and not often abused.

‡Pentobarbital and phenobarbital are used to treat addiction to and dependence on the sedative-hypnotic class of drugs.

biturates. However, with widespread initial use of meprobamate a number of individuals using the drug over an extended period began to have problems. Symptoms of addiction and withdrawal and grand mal seizures were observed and were similar to those associated with the barbiturates.

After meprobamate the first benzodiazepine, chlordiazepoxide (Librium), appeared on the scene in the 1960s (Figure 6-1). Again, this drug was introduced

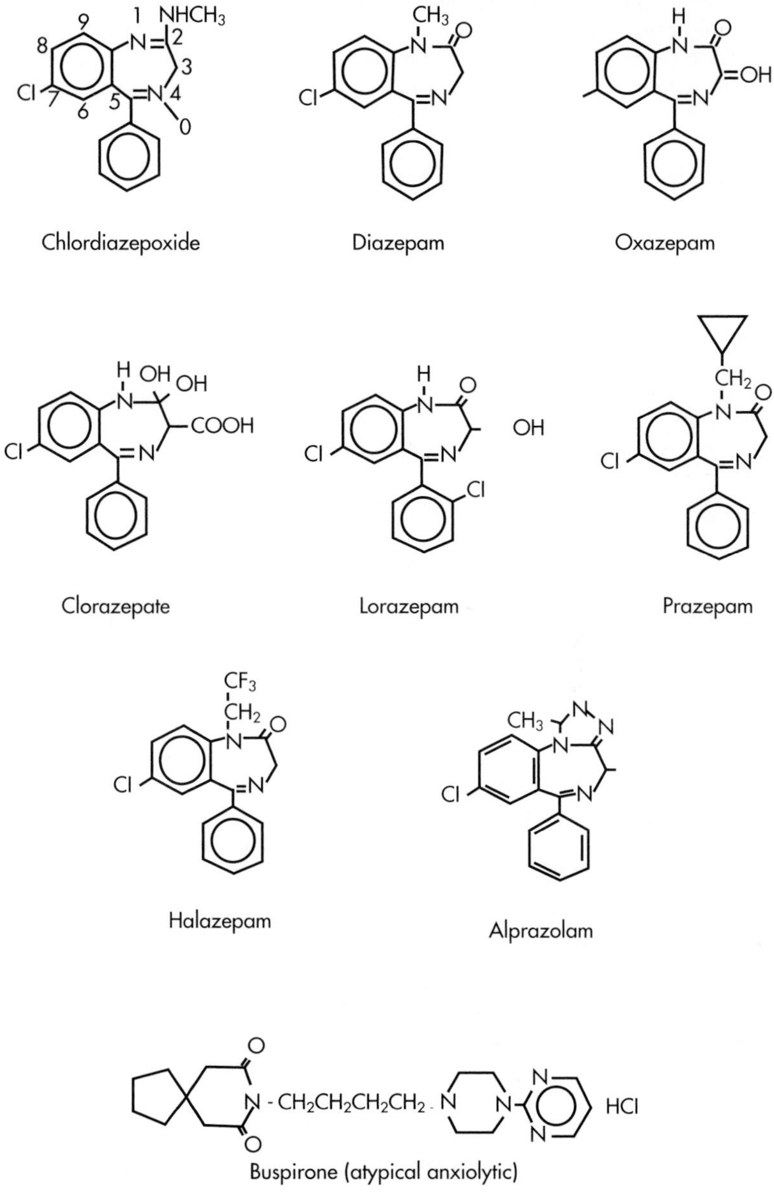

Chlordiazepoxide

Diazepam

Oxazepam

Clorazepate

Lorazepam

Prazepam

Halazepam

Alprazolam

Buspirone (atypical anxiolytic)

Figure 6-1 Chemical structures of benzodiazepines and buspirone.

with the promise of efficacy and safety and a specific lack of risk for addiction, dependency, and withdrawal. As greater experience was gained, however, this compound and related compounds such as diazepam were associated with drug withdrawal symptoms similar to those seen with meprobamate and the barbiturates.

In 1986 buspirone, a structurally unique nonbenzodiazepine antianxiety drug, was introduced; this drug appears not to have the tolerance, dependency, or withdrawal symptoms associated with its predecessors (Figure 6-1). Compounds currently being investigated within this class and others hold promise that, indeed, anxiolytic compounds will someday be available without some of the adverse effects that have been so typical of the sedative-hypnotic class of these compounds.

DIAGNOSTIC CONSIDERATIONS

The clinical picture of anxiety suggests that a variety of symptomatic presentations exist. Anxiety may represent a symptom, a syndrome, or a disorder or may simply be part of another underlying psychiatric disorder, for example, depression. Therefore a uniform clinical approach to the diagnosis and treatment of anxiety does not exist. Anxiety may be conceptualized in a variety of ways. For example, in the early psychoanalytic period, anxiety was described as either signal anxiety, separation anxiety, or castration anxiety. Moreover, the current nomenclature suggests that anxiety may be experienced in anticipation of an unpleasant or stressful experience *(anticipatory anxiety),* may be experienced as a component of a *phobia,* in which excessive anxiety or apprehension is associated with a specific external situation or object, or may be quite severe and discrete, as with *panic anxiety,* in which severe episodes exist and may occur without an apparent external cause. *Obsessive-compulsive disorder* has emerged as a specific type or subtype of anxiety in which intrusive thoughts and compulsive rituals result in social, occupational, and relationship dysfunction. Other more generalized or *mixed syndromes* include mixed anxiety-depression and *posttraumatic stress disorder* (PTSD), in which symptoms follow a psychologically distressing event such as fear, terror, or helplessness. *Generalized anxiety* may be present when the essential features are associated with unrealistic or excessive anxiety and worry focused on two or more life circumstances. In this chapter the treatment approach to generalized and syndromal forms of anxiety and specific interventions that are currently applied to anxiety are discussed, as well as panic disorder, phobic disorders, and obsessive-compulsive disorder. Symptoms of anxiety may be generally described as psychologic, behavioral, or somatic (Boxes 6-2 through 6-4).

Anticipatory Anxiety

Anticipatory anxiety is a relatively common pathologic state and is generally less incapacitating than other forms of anxiety. Anxiety as an emotion most often does not require pharmacologic intervention, although the intermittent use of drugs such as benzodiazepines may be necessary when precipitating stress or situational factors are disabling.

Posttraumatic Stress Disorder

In contrast to anticipatory anxiety, posttraumatic stress disorder generally follows exposure to a catastrophic event.

Box 6-2 Psychologic Symptoms of Anxiety

Anxious
Apprehensive
Fearful
Feeling of dread
Irritable
Frustrated
Intolerant
Nervous
Overconcerned
Sensitive to shame
Worried

From Rosenbaum JF, Pollack MH. In Hackett TP, Cassem NH, editors: *Massachusetts General Hospital handbook of general hospital psychiatry,* ed 2, Littleton, Mass, 1987, PSG Publishing.

Box 6-3 Behavioral Symptoms of Anxiety

Amotivational
Compulsive
Distractable
Frightened
Judgment impairment
Panicky
Phobic
Preoccupied
Reactive
Repetitive motor acts
Rigid
Threatened
Wound up

From Rosenbaum JF, Pollack MH. In Hackett TP, Cassem NH, editors: *Massachusetts General Hospital handbook of general hospital psychiatry,* ed 2, Littleton, Mass, 1987, PSG Publishing.

Box 6-4 Somatic Signs and Symptoms of Anxiety

Anorexia
Backache
"Butterflies" in stomach
Chest discomfort
Diaphoresis
Diarrhea
Dizziness
Dyspnea
Dry mouth
Faintness
Fatigue
Flushing
Headache
Hyperventilation
Light-headedness
Muscle tension
Nausea
Pallor
Palpitations
Paresthesia
Sexual dysfunction
Shortness of breath
Stomach pain
Sweating
Tachycardia
Tremulousness
Urinary frequency
Vomiting

From Rosenbaum JF, Pollack MH. In Hackett TP, Cassem NH, editors: *Massachusetts General Hospital handbook of general hospital psychiatry,* ed 2, Littleton, Mass, 1987, PSG Publishing.

PTSD is characterized by anxiety that is *persistently experienced* in one of the following ways:

Recurrent or intrusive distressing recollections of the event

Recurrent distressing dreams of the event or other sleep disturbances

Sudden acting or feeling as if the traumatic event were recurring, that is, flashback episodes, hallucinations, or illusions

Intense psychologic distress upon exposure to events that symbolize or reassemble an aspect of the trauma, including an anniversary reaction (Bernstein, 1995)

Mixed Anxiety-Depression

Especially noteworthy in primary care and ambulatory outpatient facilities are individuals who manifest mixed symptoms of anxiety and depression. These individuals often do not meet conventional diagnostic criteria for a mood or anxiety disorder but nonetheless come to medical attention with a mixed picture of mood and anxiety symptoms in an aggregate that appears to cause clinically significant impairment or distress, or both, and deserves recognition as a mental disorder. This subthreshold disorder may be particularly important in choosing of a pharmacologic agent. This syndrome may also be a promising subject of further research. Specific symptoms of anxiety as target symptoms for treatment with newly developed pharmacologic agents have been considered worthwhile areas of study (Table 6-2).

Generalized Anxiety

As stated previously, generalized anxiety disorder is manifested by unrealistic or excessive anxiety and worry about two or more life circumstances, for example, misfortune occurring to one's child or worry about finances, which persists for 6 months or longer. Diagnostic features are listed in Box 6-5. The symptoms of generalized anxiety may vary and are distinct from the types of anxiety associated with mood or psychotic disorders. Patients with generalized anxiety have a variety of autonomic or somatic signs and symptoms. Symptoms generally include psychologic and physical complaints that disturb concentration, result in irritability or sleep disturbance, and, if they persist, result in "chronic" anxiety. Essentially the anxiety and worry are excessive. The worry is pervasive and uncontrollable. The person finds it

Table 6-2 Mixed Symptoms of Anxiety-Depression

Symptom	Example
Affective	Dysphoria
Motor	Fears, worry, agitation, restlessness
Somatic	Insomnia, appetite disturbance, loss of libido, neuromuscular symptoms, cardiorespiratory symptoms, gastrointestinal tract symptoms
Psychologic	Concentration difficulty, memory complaints, indecisiveness, guilt, suicide*

*Suicide, although more likely to occur with depression, may also be likely to occur with anxiety, especially panic or obsessional anxiety.

Box 6-5 Diagnostic Features of Generalized Anxiety

Excessive worry and apprehension
Difficulty controlling worry
Associated symptoms*
1. Restlessness/nervousness
2. Fatigue
3. Concentration difficulties
4. Irritability
5. Tension
6. Sleep disturbance

*Three or more are needed to meet current diagnostic criteria.
Modified from American Psychiatric Association: *Diagnostic and Statistical Manual of Mental Disorders,* ed 4, Washington, DC, 1994, The Association.

Table 6-3 Drug-Induced Anxiety*

Drug	Example
Stimulants	Caffeine
Anorectics	Fenfluramine
Analgesics	Salicylates
Anticholinergics	Diphenhydramine
Hallucinogens	Cannabis
Sympathomimetics	Ephedrine
Neuroleptics (akathisia)	Haloperidol
Diuretics	Acetazolamide

*Anxiety may emerge acutely or with long-term treatment.

difficult to focus his or her attention on the tasks at hand because worry and energies are directed toward seeking relief.

Nonpsychiatric Anxiety

Anxiety may be present as a result of a general medical condition, that is, an "organic" anxiety, which may also be induced by specific substances. It is often difficult to determine whether the anxiety exists primarily or secondarily; despite the presence of a general medical condition or substance use disorder, anxiety often becomes or needs to be a focus of treatment (Table 6-3 and Box 6-6).

TREATMENT

The treatment approach to anxiety (as noted for depression in Chapter 5, Mood Disorders) ideally should combine pharmacotherapy, psychotherapy, and behavioral techniques in the context of medical and physiologic management. Adjunctive interventions may be essential to the therapeutic process. Despite the popularity of

Box 6-6 General Medical Causes of Anxiety

Cardiovascular disorders
Arrhythmias, especially paroxysmal
Atrial tachycardia
Angina pectoris
Mitral valve prolapse
Orthostatic hypotension
Myocardial infarction

Endocrine disorders
Hyperthyroidism
Hypothyroidism
Pheochromocytoma
Hypoglycemia
Carcinoid syndrome
Hypoparathyroidism
Insulinoma
Cushing's syndrome
Acute intermittent porphyria

Respiratory disorders
Chronic obstructive respiratory disease
Hypoxia resulting from any cause
Pulmonary embolism
Asthma

Neurologic disorders
Aura of migraine
Early dementia
Cerebral neoplasia
Delirium
Partial complex seizures
Demyelinating disease
Vestibular disturbance
Postconcussive syndrome
Withdrawal from sedative-hypnotics, caffeine, or nicotine

From Rosenbaum JF, Pollack MH. In Hackett TP, Cassem NH, editors: *Massachusetts General Hospital handbook of general hospital psychiatry,* ed 2, Littleton, Mass, 1987, PSG Publishing.

the sedative-hypnotic class of agents and, more specifically, the benzodiazepines, these drugs are too often prescribed in a universal or cavalier fashion. Providing the patient with quick relief may serve to alleviate distress but also may diminish the patient's awareness. This diminished level of consciousness may interfere with the patient's ability to adapt, adjust his or her lifestyle, or improve coping behaviors.

A haphazard pharmacologic approach may also simply serve as a substitute for the time required to assist an anxious or unhappy individual to discover and modify the sources of his or her psychic pain. Of course, investigations for new methods of treating anxiety, including novel agents that may be nontranquilizing or that may enhance the processes of improved coping and lifestyle adjustment, are under way. Perhaps buspirone (BuSpar) represents the first of a new generation of anxiolytic compounds that fall conceptually within this subtype of nonbenzodiazepine anxiolytics.

Of the anxiolytics that are most effective and that are frequently recommended for treating anxiety, the benzodiazepines, buspirone, and antidepressant agents are the most efficacious. Additionally, beta blockers represent a class of drug that is useful in treating somatic anxiety, because an anxious patient may feel uncomfortable and nervous and may have prominent physical signs and symptoms (Box 6-4). In fact, severe anxiety is usually accompanied by a variety of somatic or autonomic nervous system manifestations, including dry mouth, tachycardia, palpitations, irregular heart rhythm, dizziness, diarrhea, abdominal pain, headache, and other neuromuscular symptoms. These physiologic, somatic, and autonomic manifestations may be present in each of the various types of anxiety that have been discussed previously. These symptoms are less likely to be fully responsive to benzodiazepines or other conventional anxiolytic compounds. However, beta-adrenergic blocking drugs, for example, propranolol, metoprolol, atenolol, and pindolol, may dramatically inhibit these physiologic manifestations of anxiety when administered alone or in conjunction with modest doses of an anxiolytic compound (Noyes et al, 1984). This ability to inhibit physiologic anxiety has made beta blockers a popular "stage fright" antidote.

Patients with anxiety symptoms require assessment and ideally are assigned a specific diagnosis. This diagnosis helps identify those individuals who may have a specific anxiety subtype (discussed later in this chapter) for which a monoamine oxidase inhibitor (MAOI), tricyclic antidepressant (TCA), selective serotonin reuptake inhibitor (SSRI), or other novel compound is primarily indicated. The practitioner should also consider whether the patient might benefit from a nonbenzodiazepine and nonsedative agent such as buspirone. Although buspirone appears to have no specific antipanic or antiphobic effects, it may be effective and useful in patients with generalized syndromes, obsessive-compulsive disorder, or mixed anxiety-depression (Rakel, 1990).

ANXIOLYTICS

BENZODIAZEPINES

Despite the lengthy history of the use of barbiturates and extensive experience with benzodiazepines and a variety of other sedative-class medications, the mechanisms of action of anxiolytics are not fully understood. Among anxiolytics the benzodiazepines have dominated recent clinical practice and are emphasized in the following discussion. The structures of most of the readily available agents are shown in Figure 6-1. The clinical characteristics and pharmacologic doses of these agents are provided in Table 6-4. Compounds used frequently before 1964 that are still used include several barbiturates and related agents, compounds that share structural and pharmacologic properties with alcohol, and the sedative antihistamines, diphenhydramine (Benadryl) and hydroxyzine (Vistaril) (Table 6-1). Most of these agents are used infrequently and are not recommended because of their inferior effects or their potentially dangerous pharmacologic and toxicologic properties.

Pharmacologic Effect

Many benzodiazepine agents used to treat anxiety are helpful in inducing sleep and exert a general depressing effect on the central nervous system (CNS) that is dose-related (see Chapter 8, Sleep Disorders). Benzodiazepines compete for gamma-aminobutyric acid (GABA) receptors in the brain and for specific benzodiazepine receptors responsible for the selective actions of these drugs on neuronal pathways throughout the CNS. The anxiolytic potency of the various benzodiazepines correlates with their affinity for benzodiazepine receptors.

Gamma-aminobutyric acid increases the affinity of benzodiazepines for their specific receptor sites; it is a naturally occurring inhibitory neurotransmitter. Benzodiazepines increase the frequency with which anion channels open in response to GABA (Enna, 1984). The relationship of GABA to specific anxiolytic effects of benzodiazepines is not definitively proven; however, the gabaminergic action of benzodiazepines may at least partially account for their anticonvulsant and muscle relaxant effects. There is also evidence that benzodiazepines may decrease norepinephrine and serotonin turnover rates. This mechanism may partially account for the antianxiety and hypnotic effects of the benzodiazepines.

Table 6-4 Pharmacologic Doses and Clinical Characteristics of Benzodiazepines and Buspirone

Nonproprietary name	Trade name	Usual daily dose (mg)[a]	Extreme daily dose (mg)	Rapidity of absorption[b]	Half-life (hr)[c]	Metabolites[d]
Anxiolytic benzodiazepines						
Alprazolam	Xanax	0.75-4	0.5-10	+++	12	Minor
Chlordiazepoxide	Libritabs	15-60	10-100	+++	18	Yes
Chlordiazepoxide hydrochloride[e]	Librium, A-poxide	15-60	10-100	+++	18	Yes
	SK-lygen	50-100 (IV per dose)	300 (IV)			
Clorazepate dipotassium[f]	Tranxene	30	7.5-90	++++	100	Yes
Diazepam[f,g]	Valium	4-40; 2-20 (IV per dose)	2-60	+++++	60	Yes
Halazepam	Paxipam	60-160	20-160	+++	14	Yes
Lorazepam[g]	Ativan	2-4; 2-4 (IM or IV per dose)	1-10	+++	15	No
Oxazepam	Serax	30-60	10-120	++	8	No
Prazepam	Centrax	20-40	5-60	+	100	Yes

Anticonvulsant benzodiazepine						
Clonazepam[h]	Klonopin	1.5-10	0.5-20	++	34	Yes
Anxiolytic non-benzodiazepine						
Buspirone[i]	BuSpar	15-40	10-60	Not applicable	7	Minor

Modified from Baldessarini RJ: *Chemotherapy in psychiatry,* Cambridge, Mass, 1985, Harvard University.

a. The daily doses are given as total milligrams per day, assuming doses are divided into two to four portions per day.

b. Ranked from 5+ (fastest: diazepam, <1 hour) to 1+ (slowest; prazepam, about 6 hours).

c. Elimination half-life is an estimated average, including active metabolites.

d. Most include desmethylated products, notably the long-acting nordiazepam; alprazolam has some active desmethylated and hydroxylated products that do not greatly prolong elimination.

e. Chlordiazepoxide is also available in combination with clidinium bromide (Librax and Clipoxide) or amitriptyline (Limbitrol).

f. Clorazepate dipotassium is also available as slow-release tablets (Tranxene-sd) containing either 11.25 or 22.5 mg to be taken once daily. Diazepam is also available as slow-release capsules (Valrelease) containing 15 mg.

g. Parenteral preparations are available only for chlordiazepoxide hydrochloride, diazepam, and lorazepam; intramuscular administration is not advisable, except with lorazepam (which is also very active sublingually); for details concerning intravenous use, see the manufacturer's instructions.

h. Clonazepam, while used primarily as an anticonvulsant for petit mal epilepsy and other non-grand mal seizure disorders, has been reported to have antimanic and antipanic activity as well.

i. Buspirone should be given in 2 to 4 daily divided doses with food or a snack.

The structural and pharmacologic properties of buspirone are unrelated to those of the benzodiazepines (Figure 6-1). Buspirone is not a CNS depressant, nor does it produce significant sedation, yet it alleviates many symptoms of generalized anxiety. Because this drug does not cross-react with the benzodiazepines, it theoretically does not protect against benzodiazepine withdrawal symptoms; it does not appear to produce tolerance or dependency. Its utility in treating substance abuse is discussed in a later chapter. A comparison of buspirone and the benzodiazepine diazepam and the antipsychotic haloperidol is presented in Table 6-5. An expanded discussion of buspirone appears later in the chapter.

Pharmacokinetics

Benzodiazepines differ from one another in pharmacokinetic profile and metabolism. Diazepam (Valium) is a rapidly absorbed benzodiazepine, reaching peak plasma levels in less than half an hour after oral administration; clorazepate (Tranxene) is also rapidly absorbed. Intravenously administered diazepam has an almost immediate effect, but with the possible exception of lorazepam (Ativan), diazepam and other benzodiazepines are absorbed unpredictably when injected intramuscularly. Benzodiazepines that have high potency and are rapid acting may perhaps be the most likely to be abused or to induce intoxication. However, most benzodiazepines are absorbed at an intermediate rate, with peak plasma levels appearing between 1 and 3 hours after administration. The relative rates of absorption, the approximate half-life, the presence of active metabolites, and usual daily doses of benzodiazepines and buspirone are summarized in Table 6-4.

Benzodiazepines are lipophilic and highly bound to plasma membranes, 85% to 90%. Pharmacokinetics of benzodiazepines are often complex, because many of these agents have active metabolites that dominate the course of their activities. Agents with slowly eliminated active metabolites have prolonged clinical actions and an elimination half-life from plasma in excess of 2 days (long-acting benzodiazepines). Plasma levels twice the level considered effective and safe may be associated with undesirable degrees of sedation or may result in toxicity. Thus long-acting benzodiazepines should be given in two to four single daily doses that are small. Shorter-acting agents are best given in two to four small portions as well, particularly for the treatment of daytime anxiety, in which a minimal risk of oversedation is desirable.

Table 6-5 Comparative Properties of Buspirone in Humans

Property	Diazepam	Haloperidol	Buspirone
Anxiolytic	++	0	++
Antipsychotic	0	++	0
Extrapyramidal	0	++	0
Sedation	++	+	+−
Muscle relaxant	++	0	0
Physical dependence	+	0	0
Anticonvulsant	++	−	0

From Neppe VM: *Innovative psychopharmacotherapy,* New York, 1989, Raven.
++ = Marked effect; + = mild effect; 0 = no effect; − = mild effect against; +− = dubious effect.

Lorazepam, oxazepam (Serax), and, alprazolam (Xanax) are exceptional benzodiazepines in that they have virtually no important pharmacologically active metabolites. However, all three agents ultimately rely on conjugation with glucuronic acid to form inactive metabolites. Because benzodiazepines rely heavily on hepatic mechanisms, they should be used cautiously in patients with liver disease, whose ability to eliminate these agents may be reduced significantly. Oxazepam, lorazepam, and, possibly, alprazolam may represent the safest benzodiazepine agents for patients with inefficient hepatic functioning.

Side Effects

The most commonly encountered nontherapeutic side effects of the benzodiazepines are sedation with drowsiness, decreased mental acuity, and some decrease in coordination, occupational efficiency, and productivity, with increased risk of accidents. Combining the drugs with alcohol increases these risks.

Autonomic side effects, anticholinergic side effects, and extrapyramidal side effects are rarely encountered. Liver damage, blood dyscrasias, and other end organ toxic effects are also rare. Benzodiazepines are frequently associated with dysphoria, irritability, agitation, or otherwise "disinhibited" behavior. These reactions seem to be more characteristic of benzodiazepines than of barbiturates or meprobamate (Baldessarini, 1985). Some nonspecific side effects of benzodiazepines, including weight gain, skin reactions, headaches, impairment of sexual function, and menstrual irregularity, have been described in the literature. However, it is often difficult to determine whether these are symptoms or side effects of anxiety. Additionally, when doses are temporarily discontinued or dosage reduction occurs rapidly, it is sometimes difficult to determine whether the patient is having a resurfacing of anxiety symptoms or a mild withdrawal reaction.

Perhaps the most serious unwarranted effect of the benzodiazepines and other sedative hypnotics is their relative tendency to produce tolerance, physiologic dependence, and psychologic habituation. Tolerance can contribute to innocent self-medication and dose escalation. Further, these drugs, because of their ability to produce euphoria or intoxication, may have street value. The probability of becoming physiologically dependent or of developing tolerance depends largely on the daily dose and the duration of use. Physical dependence on the benzodiazepines chlordiazepoxide and diazepam has been studied extensively; however, the greatest risks of tolerance and dependence may be more significant with the new, shorter-acting benzodiazepines, especially those of high potency, that is, alprazolam and lorazepam.

Implications

Therapeutic versus toxic levels. Therapeutic levels of benzodiazepines have a comfortable margin of safety compared with those of other sedatives. However, overdoses equivalent to approximately twice a monthly supply, or even less, when taken with alcohol, have led to death. Moreover, the use of long-acting benzodiazepines, as well as the use of intravenous diazepam to control seizures or cardiac arrhythmias, is occasionally complicated by respiratory depression, apnea, ventricular arrhythmias, or even cardiac arrest. Most deliberate overdoses seem to involve more than one agent; typically alcohol is involved. Thus it is difficult to assess or determine what supply of benzodiazepines would be considered safe. The continued use of benzodiazepines for longer than several weeks should be applied in the context of the critical appraisal of risks and benefits in individual cases.

Use in pregnancy. The safety of sedative tranquilizer use in pregnancy is not established. There is inconclusive evidence that benzodiazepines may be teratogenic, causing cleft lip and palate in the first trimester. The level of risk involved is probably below the overall level of risk for birth defects, and in general the risk of toxic effects of benzodiazepines is low.

Side effects. The most common side effects of benzodiazepines are related to mental alertness. The patient should be cautioned about driving or operating hazardous machinery. Tolerance to most side effects develops quickly. The blood pressure of inpatients should be monitored routinely, and a drop in pressure of 20 mm Hg (systolic) on standing warrants withholding the drug and notifying the prescriber.

Interactions. Benzodiazepines tend to have "minimal true" pharmacokinetic interactions with most other drugs, with the possible exception of the MAOIs, which potentiate the sedating effects of the benzodiazepines and nefazodone, which inhibits the metabolism of alprazolam and triazolam. Unlike phenobarbital, the benzodiazepines have a relatively minor ability to induce their own hepatic metabolism. Also, in contrast to the barbiturates, benzodiazepines have less potential for tolerance building and dose escalating. In other words, in contrast to the barbiturates and most traditionally prescribed sedatives, to obtain a sustained antianxiety or hypnotic effect, steadily increasing doses of benzodiazepines are not usually required. However, a degree of tolerance to the sedating effects and habituation can develop. Marked withdrawal symptoms are usually indicative of prolonged use at high doses.

Recently developed benzodiazepines of high potency and relatively short duration of action may present an increased risk of habituation and minor symptoms of withdrawal, warranting the slow tapering of doses of these agents. Such risks are lessened or at least delayed with the use of long-acting benzodiazepines.

Interactions between benzodiazepines and other agents occur. Phenytoin and digitalis preparations, when combined with the benzodiazepines, can result in increased plasma levels via hepatic metabolic interactions. Antacids and agents with anticholinergic activity, especially clorazepate, chlordiazepoxide, and diazepam, may decrease the absorption of benzodiazepines. Alcohol and the MAOIs may increase the intoxication potential. Disulfiram and cimetidine, but apparently not other H_2-receptor blockers, increase the plasma levels of long-acting benzodiazepines such as chlordiazepoxide but not short-acting benzodiazepines, particularly those metabolized exclusively by conjugation, that is, oxazepam and lorazepam. In addition, the interaction between benzodiazepines and food may produce a differential effect on absorption. These effects may include an initial decrease in absorption, followed by a gradual increase, particularly with diazepam (Baldessarini, 1985).

Patient education. Benzodiazepines have a great potential for abuse. Consequently it is important to teach the patient and his or her family about these drugs. The clinician must instruct the patient and the family as follows:

Benzodiazepines are not used in response to the minor stresses of everyday life.
Over-the-counter drugs may potentiate the actions of benzodiazepines.
Driving should be avoided until tolerance develops.
Alcohol and other CNS depressants potentiate the effects of benzodiazepines.
Hypersensitivity to one benzodiazepine may mean hypersensitivity to another.
Benzodiazepine use should not be discontinued abruptly.

Clinical implications and treatment issues. Diazepam and, possibly, other benzodiazepines have been known to result in disinhibition, a phenomenon characterized by increasing agitation leading to violence or terror (Hall, 1981). This loss of behavioral control sometimes associated with explosive or violent behavior may occur during the course of benzodiazepine treatment. Some evidence suggests that oxazepam is least likely to have a disinhibiting effect (Gardos et al, 1968).

Alprazolam and triazolam (discussed in Chapter 8, Sleep Disorders) are structurally unique among the benzodiazepines, with a triazolo ring bearing a somewhat similar configuration to the TCAs (Figure 6-1). Thus it is not surprising that studies have shown the specific antidepressant and antipanic effects of alprazolam (Feighner et al, 1983; Liebowitz et al, 1986). Loss of behavioral control may emerge in patients receiving alprazolam and may be connected with the antidepressant action or may simply parallel the disinhibiting effect of other benzodiazepines (Bernstein, 1987). Moreover, alprazolam has recently gained FDA approval for use in treating panic disorder (discussed later in this chapter). Not surprisingly, alprazolam has been reported to induce mania. By contrast, clonazepam, differing somewhat in structure and having only partial agonist effects, may actually have an antimanic effect (Goodman and Charney, 1987).

Benzodiazepines have well-known amnestic properties. This phenomenon has been observed during the treatment of patients and in various studies assessing the anesthetic use of benzodiazepines. Diazepam, for example, selectively impairs anterograde episodic memory and attention while sparing access to information in long-term memory (Liebowitz et al, 1987; Kumar et al, 1987). Amnestic properties of triazolam are discussed in Chapter 8, Sleep Disorders.

The use of benzodiazepines in a manner conducive to the development of addiction is of great concern to patients and clinicians alike. Treatment should not be discontinued suddenly in patients who have used these drugs excessively or at high doses. Obviously the same applies to patients who are taking other hypnotic agents such as barbiturates, meprobamate, and chloral hydrate. Occasionally barbiturates, for example, phenobarbital, are employed to alleviate anxiety. This use may be particularly important in psychotic patients who are receiving optimal doses of antipsychotic medication but in whom persistent agitation occurs. Meprobamate has also been cautiously employed to provide sedation, improving both anxiety and insomnia, in nonpsychotic individuals. Obviously, recognizing the potential risks of dependency associated with the long-term use of these agents and the benzodiazepines is important. In chronically anxious patients who need prolonged drug therapy, other agents are worthy of consideration, for example, buspirone.

Patients with discrete panic attacks, phobic anxiety, or obsessive-compulsive disorder (OCD) benefit primarily from different classes of drugs, that is, the antidepressants (discussed later). Antidepressants that have significant sedating effects may have some advantage in treating anxiety, for example, TCAs and trazodone. Antipsychotic and neuroleptic drugs also have been both recommended and condemned for use in treating chronic anxiety. Obviously those agents with strongly sedating properties are preferable, for example, thioridazine, at a regimen in the range of 10 to 50 mg, 1 to 4 times per day. Of course, choosing these agents to treat chronic anxiety avoids the risks of drug dependency. However, concern about the potential development of tardive dyskinesia is well established. With the development of new-generation anxiolytics, that is, buspirone, the use of antipsychotics and neuroleptics should be avoided, or these agents should be prescribed in the context of a risks-versus-benefits approach.

A variety of sedating antihistamines have been used for the management of anxiety and insomnia (Carruthers et al, 1978). These compounds exert some anticholinergic and other nontherapeutic effects. Hydroxyzine, diphenhydramine, and promethazine are examples. Recently hydroxyzine, a moderately sedating nonphenothiazine antihistamine, has perhaps been the most popularly used, in a regimen of 10 to 25 mg, 1 to 4 times daily. However, these drugs primarily exert antianxiety effects through sedation and are not recommended.

BUSPIRONE

Buspirone (BuSpar), which belongs to a chemical subgroup, the azapirones, is the first in a class of pure anxioselective agents (Figure 6-1). Differing substantially in both clinical and pharmacologic characteristics from the benzodiazepines, buspirone does not cause the sedation, hypnosis, anticonvulsant effects, and muscle relaxant effects of the benzodiazepines; 3 to 6 weeks are required for buspirone to achieve maximal anxiolytic effects. Consequently, improvement in target symptoms, such as decreased agitation, improved concentration, and improved function, should be sought during its first week of administration. On chemical analysis the mechanism of buspirone's anxiolytic effect is uncertain but probably relates to its partial agonist effects at the serotonin 1A receptor. At high doses intrinsic dopaminergic activity occurs hypothetically at cerebral, cortical, and midbrain levels. However, the drug primarily affects presynaptic dopamine, with no significant neuroendocrine effects or consequential antipsychotic effects.

The anxiolytic action of buspirone also may be due in part to an active metabolite, 1-2 pyrimidinyl piperazine (1PP). This compound is particularly useful in treating anxiety or mixed anxiety-depression because it poses few of the disadvantages associated with benzodiazepines, such as physical or psychologic dependence, and does not significantly interact with other compounds, with the exception of the MAOIs and haloperidol. Anxiety control is distinguished from sedative and euphoric actions of older anxiolytic drugs. In particular, symptoms of worry, apprehension, irritability, difficulty with concentration and cognition, and an inability to cope are the focus of treatment. Patients on regimens of buspirone frequently become less fearful, have fewer somatic symptoms, and are more interpersonally responsible than before treatment.

Pharmacokinetics

Buspirone is extensively metabolized, and after the first pass as little as about 1% becomes bioavailable. The main metabolite 1PP is also present and reaches relatively higher concentrations in the brain than does the parent compound buspirone itself. However, 1PP has only 1% to 20% of the potency of buspirone (Riblett et al, 1982). The distribution half-life of 1PP is four times longer than that of buspirone: the distribution half-life of buspirone is short and difficult to fully establish. Food increases its bioavailability by decreasing first-pass metabolism, and buspirone is rapidly and completely absorbed and widely distributed to all tissues. The drug is excreted almost exclusively as metabolites. Because of the large amount of hepatic metabolism of this lipid-soluble compound, one would expect this drug to antagonize effectively the cytochrome P-450 enzyme system in the liver (Gammans, Mayol, and LaBudde, 1986).

Target symptoms in response to buspirone may begin to improve within days of initiation of an adequate dose, with the full effect occurring at 3 to 6 weeks. The average daily dose is 20 to 30 mg given in divided doses, with a range of 15 to 60 mg per day. Buspirone may be particularly effective in mixed anxiety-depression or when cognitive and interpersonal problems exist (Rickels et al, 1982; Feighner et al, 1983).

Implications

Therapeutic versus toxic levels. The most remarkable aspect of buspirone is its safety. There have been no reports of deaths resulting from the overdosage of buspirone when it is taken alone. Early studies in which doses of up to 2400 mg per day were used in patients with schizophrenia revealed no major untoward side effects.

Use in pregnancy. Buspirone can be administered with most medications; however, there are no data regarding the use of the drug during pregnancy. A comparison of the properties of buspirone, diazepam, and haloperidol in humans is given in Table 6-5.

Side effects. Common side effects associated with buspirone include headache, dizziness, light-headedness, and nausea, each of which can occur in 3% to 12% of patients (Domantay and Napoliello, 1989). These side effects can be treated as symptoms when they occur. Compared with the benzodiazepines, sedation seldom occurs with buspirone. In addition, objective measures of motor impairment are far more common with the benzodiazepines, and the addictive effects seen when benzodiazepines are combined with alcohol are not observed with buspirone (Shuckit, 1984). Nonetheless, precautions against falls or driving are important should a sedative response occur with buspirone.

Interactions. As previously mentioned, drug interactions with buspirone are not observed; however, haloperidol does interact with buspirone in as much as serum levels of haloperidol increase. Cimetidine has been reported to increase the 1PP metabolite by 30% (Gammans, Mayol, LaBudde, 1986; Domantay and Napoliello, 1989). Interaction with MAOIs, resulting in a hypertensive reaction, has also been reported (Bristol-Myers Squibb, 1991).

Patient education. Buspirone has little potential for abuse; however, issues of safety and effective usage should be considered when this agent is discussed with the patient. Patients should be taught the following:

- To avoid alcohol use and to inform the prescriber about prescriptive and nonprescriptive drugs he or she is taking
- To discuss pregnancy and breast-feeding with the prescriber
- To avoid driving or operating hazardous machinery, if buspirone causes drowsiness, light-headedness, or dizziness

Implications. An important clinical implication is that buspirone cannot be substituted immediately for benzodiazepines, that is, their pharmacologic characteristics are dissimilar, and in clinical practice buspirone takes many weeks to become fully therapeutic. Hence benzodiazepines must be gradually tapered while buspirone therapy is being initiated. Higher than usual doses of buspirone may be necessary for positive responses in patients who are not benzodiazepine naive (Kranzler, 1989). The common complaint of insomnia, which may be present in patients with mixed anxiety-depression, may be appropriately treated with trazodone, trimipramine, chloral hydrate, or other sedating compounds. Given the entirely different clinical and pharmacologic profiles of buspirone and benzodiazepines, buspirone and newly developed agents in this class require a shift of thinking with respect to anxiolytics (Neppe, 1989).

Because of the serotonergic effects and selectivity of buspirone, the potential for its use in treating panic disorders, as previously noted, aggression (discussed in Chapter 9, Acute Psychoses and the Violent Patient), and the affective spectrum disorders is noteworthy. Thus buspirone is effective in patients with mixed anxiety-depression but is as potent as diazepam for the control of psychic anxiety. Somatic anxiety may also be indirectly affected (Neppe, 1989).

The anxioselectivity of buspirone, without antipsychotic effects, extrapyramidal side effects, and the like, implies that it cannot induce tardive dyskinesia, despite its dopamine-related effects. Indeed, its serotonin-modulating effects, its intrinsic dopaminergic activity, and its presynaptic action may help to alleviate tardive dyskinesia in patients with chronic psychosis on long-term regimens of neuroleptics (Neppe, 1989). Buspirone causes little sedation, is safe, and has no dependence-inducing properties. These features should diminish social stigma, but as a psychotropic agent it remains an unscheduled prescription drug. In contrast to the benzodiazepines, which impair cognitive and motor functioning and may compromise concentration, motivation, and functioning, buspirone acts on pathologic rather than normal anxiety while the patient is retaining concentration, motivation, and adequate functioning. The therapeutic relationship is critical to successfully implementing buspirone treatment. As aforementioned, a shift in thinking must be considered with buspirone in terms of patient education and compliance (Neppe, 1989).

SPECIFIC ANXIETY DISORDERS AND MIXED SYNDROMES

A number of specific anxiety disorders outlined earlier in this chapter have been identified as distinct entities; these disorders appear to be individualized expressions of related biochemical and physiologic disturbances of brain function. These include panic, obsessive-compulsive disorder (OCD), phobias, posttraumatic stress disorder (PTSD), and perhaps other syndromes that represent subthreshold syndromes or fall within the spectrum of affective disorders. Patients with panic, phobias, OCD, or other similar conditions previously were viewed as having unresolved psychologic conflicts; this point of view is clearly no longer tenable.

PANIC DISORDER

Patients with panic disorder have discrete episodes of intense fear, discomfort, or anxiety that may vary considerably in frequency and severity. During an attack patients most commonly complain of shortness of breath, dizziness, palpitations, and sweating, as noted in Box 6-7. During a panic attack patients may have a sense of impending doom, a fear of "going crazy," and a profound loss of control. Sometimes these feelings are accompanied by feelings of depersonalization and derealization. Panic may be complicated by anticipatory anxiety, dependency, or agoraphobia.

The patient with panic must be reassured that this condition is not his or her fault and that, in fact, the condition is a biologic syndrome. The pharmacologic treatment alternatives for panic disorder are often best combined with other approaches, including behavioral techniques, psychotherapeutic intervention, and an attempt to identify any medical or physiologic contributors. Supportive psychotherapy, along with pharmacotherapy, may be beneficial, particularly with an emphasis on patient education about the disorder. Caffeine and other contributors to attacks

Box 6-7 Clinical Features of Panic Disorder

- Discrete and intense period of anxiety, apprehension, and distress
- Associated symptoms

Palpitations	Dizziness or light-headedness
Sweating	Depersonalization or derealization
Trembling	Fear of going insane
Dyspnea or a choking sensation	Fear of dying
Chest pain or discomfort	Parethesias
Gastrointestinal upset	Chills or hot flashes

- Agoraphobia may occur with or without panic or vice versa

can be identified and discussed with the patient (Charney, Heninger, and Breier, 1984).

Currently the biologic component of panic disorder is hypothesized to be increased sensitivity to augmented noradrenergic function with an impaired presynaptic noradrenergic regulation (Charney, Heninger, and Breier, 1984). An association between the occurrence of mitral valve prolapse and panic disorder has also been made (Liberthson et al, 1986). A subset of patients with atypical panic disorder may show hostility, irritability, severe derealization, and social withdrawal (Edlund, Swann, and Clothier, 1987). These patients may or may not show clear evidence of partial complex seizure disorder but typically exhibit temporal lobe abnormalities on electroencephalogram and may show a therapeutic response to carbamazepine and to the conventional treatments discussed in the following section.

Treatment

Four classes of drugs have proven therapeutically effective in managing panic disorder: benzodiazepines; TCAs or heterocyclics; SSRIs; and the MAOIs. Each class has advantages and disadvantages based on their therapeutic and side effect profiles. The two benzodiazepines alprazolam and clonazepam have the potential to produce excessive drowsiness, tolerance, and physical dependence. Cyclic antidepressants, the SSRIs, and MAOIs are reviewed in Chapter 5, Mood Disorders. Compared with placebo in patients with panic disorder, each of these classes of drugs can result in considerable benefit. Variations in efficacy between one drug and another may be evident between individuals. The SSRIs are perhaps the safest and most effective treatment for panic *in the long term* and *for prophylaxis* (Solyom, Solyom, and Ledwidge, 1991; Black et al, 1993). Low doses, for example, sertraline 25 mg daily or fluoxetine 10 mg every other day, are generally effective. Higher doses of SSRIs, more often prescribed for mood disorders, may exacerbate panic but may be required for a therapeutic effect. For a full response, 2 to 6 weeks are required. Therefore these agents are initially combined with benzodiazepines, usually clonazepam, lorazepam, or alprazolam. If low doses of SSRIs are ineffective, then cautious titration can occur.

Treating panic disorder with a benzodiazepine, either alprazolam or clonazepam, may be quite effective and likely to provide immediate relief (Beauclair et al, 1994; Jonas, 1993). Clonazepam has been used for a number of years as an anticonvulsant or an antiepileptic drug adjunct and is now employed effectively to treat anxiety disorders (Spier et al, 1986). The side effects and risks of benzodiazepines in general have been discussed. Liver enzyme abnormalities have been reported during treatment with clonazepam, and periodic liver function tests should be considered when high doses or long duration of administration is employed. Alprazolam has received FDA approval for use in patients with panic and has been effective in a number of controlled studies. However, clonazepam is probably equal or superior to alprazolam for treating panic disorder. Clonazepam, particularly with its longer half-life and slower clearance, may be less likely than alprazolam to result in a withdrawal syndrome upon abrupt discontinuation of the drug after several weeks of treatment. However, the longer half-life and slower clearance of clonazepam may produce a greater cumulative effect, which must be considered in each individual case (Herman, Rosenbaum, and Brotman, 1987).

Clonazepam is likely to be twice as potent as alprazolam and can therefore be administered in smaller daily doses and can be taken once or twice daily, as opposed to the regimen of three or four doses per day for alprazolam. The average antipanic dose of alprazolam is approximately 3 mg per day, but 6 to 8 mg per day may be required to achieve a favorable response. Clonazepam exerts its antipanic effect at a daily dose of approximately 1.5 mg, although patients may require up to 4 to 6 mg daily. With either drug a low dosage should be used initially, with gradual upward titration as tolerated by the patient and as required to achieve symptom control. Alprazolam treatment may be started at a dosage of 0.25 mg 3 times per day, titrating at 0.25-mg doses every 1 to 3 days. Clonazepam treatment may be started at a dosage of 0.25 mg twice per day, with dosage increments of 0.25 mg every 1 to 2 days as tolerated. Because these benzodiazepines may produce drowsiness and impair performance, patients whose dosage is being titrated should be advised against driving, operating machinery, and the like until a stable dosage is established, at which time the patient is free of significant impairment.

Tricyclic and heterocyclic antidepressants have been effectively used to treat panic disorder. Imipramine and, to a lesser extent, desipramine have been commonly used in the United States to treat panic. Other heterocyclic antidepressants, including amitriptyline and trazodone, have also been reported to have antipanic effects (Mavissakalian et al, 1987; Ballenger, 1986). The dosages of tricyclic and heterocyclic agents generally employed to treat panic are comparable to those used to manage depressive illness (see Chapter 5, Mood Disorders). However, a lower dosage should be initiated with careful titration, because a paradoxic effect may be observed in some individuals (Klein et al, 1980).

Clinical studies and extensive experience support the use of MAOIs to treat panic. Phenelzine, isocarboxazid, and tranylcypromine have all been used effectively to manage panic (Sheehan, 1984). Phenelzine is preferred, because it is a hydrazine compound and has less propensity to produce hepatic dysfunction than does isocarboxazid. The nonhydrazine compound, tranylcypromine, does not represent a hepatotoxic risk and is equally effective. In treating panic with MAOIs, heterocyclics, tricyclics, and benzodiazepines alike, 1 to 3 weeks of pharmacotherapy are often required before significant reduction of panic symptoms is achieved.

When MAOIs are employed, it is extremely important that the patient be educated regarding the dietary and medication restrictions, as previously discussed (see Chapter 5, Mood Disorders). Patients should receive this education in a nonthreatening and nonfrightening way, because many potential candidates will be terrified of the restrictions and cautions. Nonetheless, patients should be advised to go to the nearest hospital emergency department for evaluation and treatment if they experience a hypertensive reaction. Patients must also be advised and warned about headache, dizziness, and other symptoms that may be secondary to postural hypotension produced by the MAOIs. The patient's ability to monitor blood pressure at home may also be helpful during the course of treatment or when the possibility of elevated blood pressure becomes a concern. It is, of course, important to measure each patient's blood pressure before initiating treatment with an MAOI and to monitor the blood pressure and pulse rate. A drop of 10 to 20 mm Hg in systolic pressure may occur in half to two thirds of patients receiving MAOIs (Davidson and Turnbull, 1986). In some cases, moderately severe symptomatic postural hypotension may be counteracted by increased salt intake. The cautious administration of the salt-retaining steroid fluorocortisone in low dosages of 0.05 to 0.1 mg once or twice daily may also be a useful technique.

PHOBIC DISORDERS

Phobic disorders have become more prominent with the increasing ability to provide treatment. The two most common phobic disorders seen in adult psychiatry are agoraphobia, which may occur in association with panic attacks, and social phobia. *Agoraphobia* comes to medical attention as a fear of being in places or situations from which escape may be difficult or embarrassing or in places where help may not be readily available. Agoraphobic patients are often frightened to be away from their homes and may remain in the home, avoiding occupational, social, and relationship interactions. Some agoraphobic patients have elaborate schemes such that they leave their homes only in company with a significant other. Many agoraphobic patients attempt to participate in normal life situations and endure intense anxiety in the process. However, the majority of severely agoraphobic patients are unable to travel on public transportation and experience great difficulty in stores, theaters, or other public places.

Agoraphobic patients, whether or not they experience panic attacks, may benefit from pharmacologic intervention. These patients, like patients with obsessive-compulsive disorder, which is discussed later, may also have depression as a comorbid disorder.

The pharmacologic responsiveness of panic, agoraphobia, depression, and obsessive-compulsive disorder (OCD), suggests that there may be some common denominators in these disorders with respect to underlying neurochemical disturbances. As discussed with panic disorder, patients with agoraphobia or social phobia may be significantly helped by behavioral techniques, including exposure and other types of interventions. These are particularly effective when combined with pharmacologic intervention (Mavissakalian and Michelson, 1986). In most instances, optimizing the medical and physiologic status of the patient enhances responsivity to pharmacologic intervention and may also be combined with psychotherapeutic interventions, including supportive or cognitive therapy.

Treatment

The pharmacologic approach to agoraphobia has generally included the use of benzodiazepines, SSRI antidepressants, TCAs, and MAOIs. As with panic, alprazolam at relatively high doses (between 3 and 6 mg per day) may be effective. Imipramine alone or in combination with behavioral techniques has been reported to be highly beneficial in treating agoraphobia (Mavissakalian and Perel, 1985).

Whereas patients with panic may be responsive to low doses of TCAs or may require higher doses, patients with agoraphobia may also respond to low doses, but conventional doses of tricyclic or heterocyclic drugs are usually required, for example, between 150 and 200 mg per day. Heterocyclic antidepressants that are strongly serotonergic, for example, clomipramine, amitriptyline, and trazodone, as well as the SSRIs, are effective in patients with agoraphobia (Sheehan, 1984; Gloger et al, 1981).

MAOIs, especially phenelzine, have demonstrated their utility in effectively treating of agoraphobia (Phol, Berchou, and Rainey, 1982). Phenelzine is the preferred agent when SSRIs or imipramine are ineffective. Bernstein (1995) suggested that MAOIs in agoraphobic patients may produce greater relief of symptoms than do other antidepressants or anxiolytics; however, the disadvantages of dietary and medication restrictions and the potential for postural hypotension must be considered carefully in each case.

Social phobia is a fairly common and limiting disorder characterized by persistent fear of situations in which one is exposed to the scrutiny of others; the patient with social phobia may be responsive to pharmacologic interventions with benzodiazepines, such as alprazolam, used alone or in combination with beta-blocking drugs. Generally, establishing an effective pharmacologic regimen and response should precede any encouragement or effort to return the patient to normal function in all spheres of life. Many patients are responsive to beta-blocking agents often prescribed in combination with antidepressants or benzodiazepines. Propranolol in dosages of 10 to 20 mg 3 to 4 times a day, metaprolol in dosages of 25 to 50 mg twice daily, or atenolol in dosages of 50 to 100 mg once daily have been effective (Liebowitz et al, 1987; Gorman et al, 1985). Obviously, a careful history and assessment of blood pressure, pulse rate, heart, and lungs should precede the use of beta-adrenergic blocking agents. The histories of congestive heart failure, cardiac arrhythmia, and chronic obstructive pulmonary disease with asthma pose contraindications to treatment with beta-adrenergic blocking drugs.

Benzodiazepines alone or in combination with antidepressants, for example, alprazolam and clonazepam, may be effective with social phobia (Davidson et al, 1993; Gerlernter et al, 1991). Low-dose therapy, for example, clonazepam 0.5 mg twice daily, may be initiated; this drug may be more effective than other benzodiazepines because of its serotonergic properties (Bernstein, 1995).

SSRIs also have been proven to be effective with social phobias (Den Boer et al, 1987; Sternbach, 1990). As with panic, low doses are initially used and may be effective at 2 to 3 weeks.

Several studies have documented the therapeutic efficacy of MAOIs, primarily phenelzine, in treating social phobia (Liebowitz et al, 1985). Phenelzine is usually more powerful in these cases. MAOIs used to treat social phobia should be given in conventional antidepressant doses, as previously discussed. Buspirone, which has proven effective in treating generalized anxiety and mixed anxiety-depression, is largely free of sedating or dependency-producing effects. However, buspirone has not been documented to be particularly effective in either panic, agoraphobia, or social phobia (Olajide and Lader, 1987). Nonetheless, this compound may be particularly useful in treating anticipatory anxiety or may be useful when the patient is being provided with behavioral therapy techniques, such as exposure or desensitization.

OBSESSIVE-COMPULSIVE DISORDER

Obsessive-compulsive disorder is now recognized as a frequently occurring disorder. Individuals with OCD may experience both obsessions and compulsions, and either one may occur individually. Clinical features are shown in Box 6-8. In patients with OCD these symptoms worsen when coexisting symptoms of depression or other disorders develop (Table 6-6). OCD is thought to fall within the "affective

Box 6-8 Clinical Features of Obsessive-Compulsive Disorder

Obsessions

1. Unrealistic recurring or persistent thoughts, impulses, or images; intrusive or distressing
2. Attempt to neutralize or suppress the thoughts, images, or impulses
3. Impairment or interference with daily routine, functioning, or relationships

Compulsions

1. Repetitive behaviors in response to an obsession, rigidly applied
2. Behavior or actions that serve to prevent or reduce distress
3. Impairment or interference with daily routine, functioning, or relationships

Table 6-6 Coexisting Axis I Diagnoses in Primary OCD ($N=100$)

Diagnosis	Current %	Lifetime %
Major depressive disorder	31	67
Simple phobia	7	22
Separation anxiety disorder	—	21
Social phobia	11	18
Eating disorder	8	17
Alcohol abuse (dependence)	8	14
Panic disorder	6	12
Tourette's syndrome	5	7

From Rasmussen SA, Eisen JL: Clinical and epidemiologic findings of significance to neuropharmacologic trials in OCD, *Psychopharmacol Bull* 24(3):466-70, 1988, U.S. Public Health Service.

spectrum," similar to eating disorders, premenstrual dysphoria, and seasonal affective disorder, which are not addressed in this text. The effect of antidepressant drugs in treating OCD lends further support to the possibility that this condition shares some common neurochemical or neurobiologic disturbance with depression. In general, obsessions represent recurrent and persistent ideas, thoughts, impulses, or images that are experienced as intrusive or senseless.

Treatment

Clomipramine (Anafranil) and the SSRIs have emerged as the more effective drug treatments of OCD. Other TCAs and the MAOIs continue to be effective therapeutic agents. Buspirone is an alternative treatment that may be used alone or usually as an adjunct (Mavissakalian, 1985; Jenike, Armentano, and Baer, 1987; Pato, 1990). Alprazolam or clonazepam may also be useful in treating this condition (Tesar and Jenike, 1984). However, alprazolam and other benzodiazepines may significantly exacerbate the symptoms of OCD because the patient may feel uncomfortable with sedation and other side effects; patients with coexisting symptoms of depression are much more likely to benefit from the use of an SSRI or other antidepressant. Neuroleptic medications may be useful in treating psychotic features. Lithium has not been found to be significantly therapeutic alone or as an adjunct. Overall, conventional antidepressants remain the preferred pharmacologic agents.

Clomipramine (Anafranil) is the most serotonergic of the TCAs; at a dose of approximately 100 to 200 mg per day it is a potent antiobsessional agent. Clomipramine is a TCA and not a pure serotonin reuptake inhibitor. Its active metabolite desmethylclomipramine, a potent inhibitor of norepinephrine, may account in part for its clinical efficacy (Asberg, Thoren, and Bertilsson, 1982). Three carefully controlled, double-blind studies have shown clomipramine's preferential effectiveness in reducing obsessional symptoms (Montgomery, 1980; Ananth et al, 1979; Insel et al, 1983). Its effect may not be fully apparent until 5 to 10 weeks after treatment. Plasma level determinations may be helpful in avoiding doses that are too high or too low, both of which seem to be connected to poor outcome (Asberg, Thoren, and Bertilsson, 1982). Combining clomipramine with behavioral exposure treatment is desirable, and treatment is generally prolonged over several years. With the exception of dental problems that result from the reduced production of saliva (which can be avoided by careful oral hygiene), no serious long-term effects have been described with clomipramine. In any event, heterocyclics, with clomipramine being the drug of choice, are clearly indicated in a depressed patient with OCD.

SSRI therapy, including use of venlafaxine for OCD, is gaining in popularity and now represents a first-line approach. Fluoxetine and fluvoxamine are approved for use with OCD. However, sertraline, paroxetine, and venlafaxine all have shown significant effect and have some advantages as noted in Chapter 5, Mood Disorders (Jenike, 1992; Greist et al, 1995). Fluvoxamine is the most extensively studied and used (Rasmussen, Eisen, and Pato, 1993). Doses of 200 to 300 mg are generally used with good tolerability and response. With concomitant use of alprazolam or clonazepam, sertraline and venlafaxine may be advantageous and represent a lower risk for drug interaction and adverse effect. Incidentally, many patients with OCD require high doses of SSRI, perhaps two to three times the dosage required for depression.

There are no controlled studies using MAOIs in patients with OCD. However, many case reports have alluded to a favorable response (Jenike, Baer, and Minichiello, 1986). Generally the MAOIs may be particularly effective in patients with OCD who have associated panic or severe anxiety.

Some patients with OCD have been reported to be responsive to lithium and in fact may have an underlying cyclothymia or manic depressive illness (Stern and Jenike, 1983). However, controlled trials have not been supportive of its use (McDougle et al, 1990). Likewise, antipsychotic agents may be useful in patients with psychotic symptoms. However, anxiolytic agents, in particular, alprazolam, possibly in part because of its antidepressant effects, may be successful in some patients with mixed anxiety-depression. Furthermore, as suggested for panic, patients may also be responsive to alprazolam because it acts as an anticonvulsant. However, as with lithium and antipsychotic agents, anxiolytics have not been extensively studied.

Electroconvulsive therapy is generally regarded as not useful in treating OCD. Although a link between depression and OCD may be present, ECT has not been found to be effective, and there are no reports of success in patients who have classic OCD, that is, who exhibit rituals and the like. Many patients with OCD have had psychosurgery when severe illness is present, and multiple therapeutic approaches have failed. The results of surgical intervention are impressive. A discussion of this topic, however, is beyond the scope of this text.

REFERENCES

Ananth J et al: Clomipramine therapy for obsessive-compulsive neurosis, *Am J Psychiatry* 136:700, 1979.

Asberg M, Thoren P, Bertilsson L: Psychopharmacologic treatment of obsessive-compulsive disorder: clomipramine treatment of obsessive disorder, biochemical and clinical aspects, *Psychopharmacol Bull* 18:13, 1982.

American Psychiatric Association: *Diagnostic and statistical manual of mental disorders,* ed 4, Washington, DC, 1994, The Association.

Baldessarini RJ: *Chemotherapy in psychiatry,* Cambridge, Mass, 1985, Harvard University.

Ballenger JC: Pharmacotherapy of the panic disorders, *J Clin Psychiatry* 47(suppl 6):27, 1986.

Bernstein JG: Lithium and other mood-stabilizing drugs. In Hackett TP, Cassem NH, editors: *Massachusetts General Hospital handbook of general hospital psychiatry,* ed 2, Littleton, Mass, 1987, PSG Publishing.

Bernstein JG: *Drug therapy in psychiatry,* ed 3, Littleton Mass, 1995, PSG Publishing.

Black DW et al: A comparison of fluvoxamine, cognitive therapy, and placebo in the treatment of panic disorder, *Arch Gen Psychiatry* 50:44-50, 1993.

Bristol-Myers Squibb: Personal communication, 1991.

Carruthers SG et al: Correlation between plasma diphenhydramine level and sedative and antihistamine effects, *Clin Pharmacol Ther* 23:375, 1978.

Charney DS, Heninger GR, Breier A: Noradrenergic function in panic anxiety, *Arch Gen Psychiatry* 41:751, 1984.

Davidson JRT et al: Treatment of social phobia with clonazepam and placebo, *J Clin Psychopharmacol* 13:423-8, 1993.

Davidson J, Turnbull CD: The effects of isocarboxazid on blood pressure, *J Clin Psychopharmacol* 6:139, 1986.

Den Boer JA et al: Effect of serotonin uptake inhibitors in anxiety disorders: a double-blind comparison of clomipramine and fluvoxamine, *Int Clin Psychopharmacol* 2:21-32, 1987.

Domantay AG, Napoliello MJ: Buspirone for elderly anxious patients, *Int Med Certif* 3:1, 1989.

Edlund MJ, Swann AC, Clothier J: Patients with panic attacks and abnormal EEG results, *Am J Psychiatry* 144:508, 1987.

Enna SJ: Role of gamma-aminobutyric acid in anxiety, *Psychopathology* 17:15, 1984.

Feighner JP et al: Comparison of alprazolam, imipramine and placebo in the treatment of depression, *JAMA* 249:3057, 1983.

Folks DG: Clinical approaches to anxiety in the medically ill elderly, *Drug Ther Suppl* p 72, August 1990.

Gammans RE, Mayol RF, LaBudde JA: Metabolism and disposition of buspirone, *Am J Med* 80(suppl 3B):41, 1986.

Gardos G et al: Differential actions of chlordiazepoxide and oxazepam on hostility, *Arch Gen Psychiatry* 18:757, 1968.

Gerlernter CS et al: Cognitive-behavioral and pharmacological treatments of social phobias, *Arch Gen Psychiatry* 48:938-945, 1991.

Gloger S et al: Treatment of spontaneous panic attacks with clomipramine, *Am J Psychiatry* 138:1215, 1981.

Goodman WK, Charney DS: A case of alprazolam, but not lorazepam, inducing manic symptoms, *J Clin Psychiatry* 48:117, 1987.

Gorman JM et al: Treatment of social phobia with atenolol, *J Clin Psychopharmacol* 5:298, 1985.

Greist J et al: Double-blind parallel comparison of three dosages of sertraline and placebo in outpatients with obsessive-compulsive disorder, *Arch Gen Psychiatry* 52:289-293, April 1995.

Hall RCW, Zisook S: Paradoxical reactions to benzodiazepines, *Br J Clin Pharmacol* 11:995, 1981.

Harvey SC: Hypnotics and sedatives. In Gilman AG, Goodman LS, Rall TW, editors: *The pharmacological basis of therapeutics,* ed 7, New York, 1985, Macmillan.

Herman JB, Rosenbaum JF, Brotman AW: The alprazolam-to-clonazepam switch for the treatment of panic disorder, *J Clin Psychopharmacol* 7:175-8, 1987.

Insel TR et al: Obsessive-compulsive disorder: a double-blind trial of clomipramine and clorgyline, *Arch Gen Psychiatry* 40:605, 1983.

Jenike MA: Pharmacologic treatment of obsessive-compulsive disorders, *Psychiatr Clin North Am* 15(4):895-919, 1992.

Jenike MA, Armentano ME, Baer L: Disabling obsessive thoughts responsive to antidepressants, *J Clin Psychopharmacol* 7:33, 1987.

Jenike MA, Baer L, Minichiello WE: *Obsessive-compulsive disorders: theory and management,* St Louis, 1986, Mosby.

Jonas JM, Cohon MS: A comparison of the safety and efficacy of alprazolam versus other agents in the treatment of anxiety, panic, and depression: a review of the literature, *J Clin Psychiatry* 54(10):25-45, 1993.

Klein DF et al: *Diagnosis and drug treatment of psychiatric disorders: adults and children,* ed 2, Baltimore, 1980, Williams & Wilkins.

Kranzler HR: Buspirone treatment of anxiety in a patient dependent on alprazolam, *J Clin Psychopharmacol* 9:153, 1989.

Kumar R et al: Anxiolytics and memory: a comparison of lorazepam and alprazolam, *J Clin Psychiatry* 48:158, 1987.

Liberthson R et al: The prevalence of mitral valve prolapse in patients with panic disorders, *Am J Psychiatry* 143:511, 1986.

Liebowitz MR et al: Social phobia, *Arch Gen Psychiatry* 42:729, 1985.

Liebowitz MR et al: Alprazolam in the treatment of panic disorders, *J Clin Psychopharmacol* 6:13, 1986.

Liebowitz MR et al: Pharmacotherapy of social phobia, *Psychosomatics* 28:305, 1987.

Mavissakalian M, Michelson L: Two-year follow-up of exposure and imipramine treatment of agoraphobia, *Am J Psychiatry* 143:1106, 1986.

Mavissakalian M, Perel J: Imipramine in the treatment of agoraphobia: dose-response relationships, *Am J Psychiatry* 142:1032, 1985.

Mavissakalian M et al: Tricyclic antidepressants in obsessive-compulsive disorder: antiobsessional or antidepressant agents? *Am J Psychiatry* 142:572, 1985.

Mavissakalian M et al: Trazodone in the treatment of panic disorder and agoraphobia with panic attacks, *Am J Psychiatry* 144:785, 1987.

McDougle CJ, Goodman WK, Price LH et al: Neuroleptic addiction in fluvoxamine-refractory obsessive-compulsive disorder, *Am J Psychiatry* 147(5):652-4, 1990.

Montgomery SA: Clomipramine in obsessional neurosis: a placebo-controlled trial, *Pharmacol Med* 1:189, 1980.

Neppe VM: Buspirone: an auxioselective neuromodulator. In VM Neppe, editor: *Innovative psychopharmacotherapy,* New York, 1989, Raven.

Noyes R et al: Diazepam and propranolol in panic disorder and agoraphobia, *Arch Gen Psychiatry* 41:387, 1984.

Olajide D, Lader M: A comparison of buspirone, diazepam, and placebo in patients with chronic anxiety states, *J Clin Psychopharmacol* 7:148, 1987.

Pato MT: Treatment of obsessive-compulsive disorder with serotonergic agents, *Drug Ther Suppl,* p 122, August 1990.

Phol R, Berchou R, Rainey JM: Tricyclic antidepressants and monoamine oxidase inhibitors in the treatment of agoraphobia, *J Clin Psychopharmacol* 2:399, 1982.

Rakel RE: Mixed anxiety-depression, *Drug Ther Suppl,* p 137, August 1990.

Rasmussen SA, Eisen JL, Pato MT: Current issues in the pharmacologic management of obsessive-compulsive disorder. *J Clin Psychiatry* 54:(suppl 6):4-9, June 1993.

Rasmussen SA, Eisen JL: Clinical and epidemiologic findings of significance to neuropharmacologic trials in OCD, *Psychopharmacol Bull* 24(3):466-70, 1988.

Riblett LA et al: Pharmacology and neurochemistry of buspirone, *J Clin Psychiatry* 43:11, 1982.

Rickels K et al: Buspirone and diazepam in anxiety: a controlled study, *J Clin Psychiatry* 43:81, 1982.

Rosenbaum JF, Pollack MH. In Hackett TP, Cassem NH, editors: *Massachusettes General Hospital Handbook of general hospital psychiatry,* ed 2, Littleton, Mass, 1987, PSG Publishing.

Sheehan DV: The treatment of panic and phobic disorders. In Bernstein JC, editor: *Clinical psychopharmacology,* ed 2, Boston, 1984, John Wright–PSG.

Shuckit MA: Clinical studies of buspirone, *Psychopathology* 17(suppl 3):61, 1984.

Solyom L, Solyom C, Ledwidge B: Fluoxetine in panic disorder, *Can J Psychiatry* 36(5):378-80, 1991.

Spier S et al: Clonazepam in the treatment of panic disorder and agoraphobia, *J Clin Psychiatry* 47:238-242, 1986.

Stern TA, Jenike MA: Treatment of obsessive-compulsive disorder with lithium carbonate, *Psychosomatics* 24:671, 1983.

Sternbach H: Fluoxetine treatment of social phobia, *J Clin Psychopharmacol* 10:230-1, 1990 (letter).

Tesar GE, Jenike MA: Alprazolam as treatment for a case of obsessive-compulsive disorder, *Am J Psychiatry* 141:689, 1984.

CHAPTER 7

Seizure Disorders

Epilepsy is the most common seizure disorder, with an incidence somewhere between 1% and 3% among the U.S. population (Parks, Dostrow, and Noble, 1994). Worldwide as many as 50 million people are affected (Rogawski and Porter, 1990). According to McKenna, Kane, and Parrish (1985), about 7% of the patients diagnosed with epilepsy have a persistent psychosis. When this level of disorder (7%) is compared with the morbidity rate for schizophrenia in the general population (about 1%), it appears that a relationship exists between epilepsy and psychosis (Trimble, 1991). Extrapolating from this data, it is clear that perhaps hundreds of thousands of individuals suffer from both a psychosis and a seizure disorder. Because seizure disorders among a psychiatric population are common, antiepileptic drug information is an important part of both the mental health and the primary care clinician's resources.

EPILEPSY

Epilepsy is a condition in which abnormal electrical activity in the brain occurs. The abnormal electrical activity has varying effects, hence several distinguishable forms of epilepsy are recognizable. Onset is most common during childhood or after age 50; however, onset is not limited to these particular developmental stages. Epilepsies may be broadly categorized as either *acquired* or *idiopathic* (cause unknown). It should be noted that seizures and epilepsy are not synonymous (Engel and Starkman, 1994). Seizures are a symptom of epilepsy and can also occur because of alcohol withdrawal, hypoglycemia, anoxia, and fever, to name a few causes (Ramsey et al, 1993). The extent of genetic influence is not known, but even clinicians who are prone to look for environmental factors in other illnesses acknowledge a genetic predisposition for epilepsy. Treatment is aimed at controlling seizure activity, and for many individuals this entails a lifelong dependence on antiepileptic therapy.

Categories of Seizures

Epileptic seizures are grouped according to characteristic physical and neurologic signs (Box 7-1 and Table 7-1). Each subtype also has a characteristic electroencephalogram (EEG) pattern (Jallon, 1994). Seizures are divided into two broad categories: *partial seizures* and *generalized seizures.* If an aberrant electrical discharge is confined to a local area, the seizure is partial or focal. If the electrical aberration spreads from the focal areas to affect the entire cerebrum, it is a generalized seizure. The diagnosis of each of these seizure types can be refined to include several subtypes.

Partial seizures. Partial seizures are more common than generalized seizures, accounting for approximately 70% of all seizures in adults and 40% of all seizures in children (Delgado-Escueta, Treiman, and Walsh, 1983). As defined, partial seizures typically begin in a focal area. Abnormal brain activity can spread to other parts of

Table 7-1 Major Characteristics of Epileptic Seizures

Seizure type	Comments
Partial seizures (focal or local)	Most common seizure type (accounts for about 70% of adults and 40% of children with epilepsy); EEG changes initially are localized, may evolve into other seizure types
Simple partial seizures	Typically no loss of consciousness; motor symptoms (jacksonian); sensory symptoms (visual, auditory, gustatory, and hallucinations) and somatosensory symptoms (tingling); autonomic symptoms (pallor, sweating, vomiting, and flushing)
Complex partial seizures	Consciousness is impaired at onset of seizure or later, after onset of simple partial seizure
Partial seizures evolving to generalized tonic-clonic seizures	
Generalized seizures	Involve symmetric (both hemispheres) distribution of abnormal brain discharge; bilateral motor changes; consciousness may be totally impaired
Nonconvulsive seizures	
Absence seizures	Abrupt loss of consciousness, usually lasting <10 sec; usually begin in childhood, often stop spontaneously during teenage years; mild clonic component; atonic component; diminution of muscle tone; automatisms; autonomic components
Myoclonic seizures	Single or multiple jerks, typically lasting 3-10 sec; sudden, brief, shocklife contractions, generalized or confined
Atonic seizures	Sudden diminution of muscle tone ("drop attacks")
Convulsive seizures	
Clonic seizures	Occur mostly in childhood; generalized convulsive seizures lacking tonic component; characterized by clonic jerks; postictal phase typically short
Tonic seizures	Sustained contraction of large muscles; continuous tension of chest musculature impairs ventilation and causes pallor or more serious problems if prolonged
Tonic-clonic	Consciousness lost abruptly; series of muscle spasms lasting 3-5 min from onset to recovery; postictal state may last from a few minutes to about half an hour; often characterized by confusion, dizziness, sleepiness, and "glazed" look
Status epilepticus	Could apply to any prolonged or repetitive seizure but best applied to repetitive or fused tonic-clonic seizures; a medical emergency requiring immediate drug intervention to prevent brain damage or death resulting from impaired ventilation; only seizure for which there is no contraindication to drug use
Unclassified epileptic seizures	Includes all seizures that cannot be classified, whether because of inadequate or incomplete criteria or characteristics

Modified from Commission on Classification and Terminology of the International League Against Epilepsy: *Epilepsia* 22:489, 1981.

Box 7-1 Epilepsy Types Based on International Classification System

Partial seizures (generally involve one hemisphere of the brain at onset of seizure)

Simple (consciousness not impaired)

- With motor symptoms (jacksonian, adversive)
- With somatosensory or other special sensory symptoms
- With autonomic symptoms
- With psychic symptoms

Complex (consciousness impaired)

- Simple partial onset followed by impaired consciousness
- Impaired consciousness at onset

Secondarily generalized

- Simple partial seizures evolving to generalized tonic-clonic seizures
- Complex partial seizures evolving to generalized tonic-clonic seizures
- Simple partial seizures evolving to complex partial seizures, then to generalized tonic-clonic seizures

Generalized seizures (involve both hemispheres of the brain at onset, consciousness usually impaired)

Absence

- Typical
- Atypical

Myoclonic

Clonic

Tonic

Tonic-clonic

Atonic

Localization-related (focal)

Idiopathic

- Benign focal epilepsy of childhood

Symptomatic

- Chronic progressive epilepsia partialis continua
- Temporal lobe
- Extratemporal

Generalized epilepsy

Idiopathic

- Benign neonatal convulsions
- Childhood absence
- Juvenile myoclonic
- Other

Cryptogenic or symptomatic

- West syndrome (infantile spasms)
- Early myoclonic encephalopathy
- Lennox-Gastaut syndrome
- Progressive myoclonic epilepsy

Box 7-1 Epilepsy Types Based on International Classification System—cont'd

Special syndromes
Febrile seizures

Unclassified

From Commission on Classification and Terminology of the International League Against Epilepsy, *Epilepsia* 22:489, 1981; 30:389, 1989.

that cerebral hemisphere or even to the other hemisphere (Delgado-Escueta, Treiman, and Walsh, 1983). Partial seizure subtypes include simple partial seizures (no loss of consciousness), complex partial seizures (consciousness impaired), and partial seizures evolving to generalized tonic-clonic seizures.

Simple partial seizures. Simple partial seizures do not impair consciousness, and because electrical abnormality is localized, symptoms depend on the area affected. Motor symptoms include localized jerks, focal jerks that "march" to involve other muscles (sometimes referred to as *jacksonian seizures*), and speech involvement. Sensory symptoms (visual, auditory, gustatory, and hallucinations) and somatosensory symptoms, that is, tingling, also develop. Autonomic symptoms such as pallor, sweating, vomiting, flushing, tachycardia, hypotension, and hypertension are distressing to patients. Automatic behaviors can include lip smacking and repetitive movements.

Complex partial seizures. Complex partial seizures are also known as *psychomotor* or *temporal lobe epilepsy.* Consciousness is impaired, and violent behavior may be a major component of seizure activity. Complex partial seizures typically begin as a perceived aura. A number of cognitive, affective, perceptive, and psychomotor symptoms can occur. Deja vu, fear and anxiety, hallucinations, and automatic behaviors (automatism) are commonly present.

Generalized seizures. Generalized seizures involve a symmetric distribution of abnormal electrical activity in the brain. Generalized seizures include a number of nonconvulsive seizures, which primarily cause unresponsiveness and amnesia, and convulsive seizures, which cause unconsciousness and major convulsions. Nonconvulsive seizures include absence seizures, myoclonic seizures, and atonic seizures. Major motor tonic-clonic seizures and status epilepticus are major types of convulsive seizure.

Absence seizures. Absence seizures are characterized by a sudden loss of responsiveness. Often the loss of consciousness is so brief (10 seconds) that those around the person are unaware of a change. A variant of absence seizure is the true petit mal seizure, which produces a distinct three-per-second, spike-and-wave EEG pattern. These seizures typically start in childhood and remit during the teenage years (Norman and Browne, 1981).

Convulsive seizures. Tonic-clonic convulsions, also called *grand mal seizures,* are characterized by intense, repetitive tonic-clonic contractions of the whole body. Abnormal brain activity is symmetric, with most brain pathways involved. Seizures may typically last between 3 and 5 minutes, but prolonged seizure activity can result in brain hypoxia. A number of other physical consequences may result.

Status epilepticus is a seizure type in which tonic-clonic convulsions occur successively without intervals of restored consciousness or normal muscle movement. Brain damage can occur as a result of prolonged hypoxia. Status epilepticus is a medical emergency requiring immediate attention (Delgado-Escueta et al, 1982) and has a mortality rate of 6% to 20% (Borgsdorf and Caldwell, 1985). Published reports indicate a 60-minute window of time exists from the beginning of a status epilepticus "attack" until it is successfully controlled. Neuronal necrosis and permanent cerebral injury result from prolonged refractory status epilepticus (Jordan, 1994). Several drugs given intravenously have been used successfully to stop these seizures, including the benzodiazepines diazepam and lorazepam (Jordan, 1994).

ANTIEPILEPTIC DRUGS

The straightforward goals for antiepileptic treatment are as follows: (1) control seizure activity, (2) keep side effects of antiepileptic therapy to a minimum, and (3) attempt maintenance with a regimen of one drug (monotherapy), if possible. Unfortunately, between 20% and 30% of patients with epilepsy have intractable epilepsy, causing them numerous social and psychologic difficulties (Patsalos and Sander, 1994; Wilder, 1995). Five categories of antiepileptic drugs may be distinguished; when these are added to noncategorized drugs called "other antiepileptics," a substantial number of individual drugs are at the clinician's disposal. There are also several "new" antiepileptics that show both promise and potential for harm. Antiepileptics suppress the start of seizure activity or reduce the spread of seizure

Duration of Antiepileptic Therapy

Case study: Alice Smith is a 65-year-old woman nearing retirement. In the 1950s she experienced a grand mal seizure and was placed on phenytoin 100 mg tid. Now, 40 years later, she is still taking phenytoin and has never experienced another seizure. On the one hand, it could be argued that this antiepileptic strategy has worked, i.e., seizure control. On the other, given the side effect profile associated with phenytoin, this approach appears far too conservative.

The literature suggests that 25% of patients withdrawing from antiepileptics will relapse within one year. Discontinuing antiepileptic therapy has several advantages, including minimization of long-term adverse responses, financial savings, and lifestyle benefits. The important question concerns the variables that may enhance successful withdrawal from these agents. The following characteristics seem to affect the success of discontinuation:

Age at onset: Adolescent onset is associated with higher relapse
Seizure type: Complex partial and generalized seizures are associated with higher relapse
Abnormal EEG: Patients with abnormal EEGs are more likely to relapse
Treatment duration: The longer a patient is on a drug, the greater the risk of relapse

Berg AT, Shinnar S: Relapse following discontinuation of antiepileptic drugs: a meta-analysis, *Neurology* 44(4):601-608, 1994.
Borgsdorf LR, Caldwell JW: Clinical therapeutics: a disease-oriented approach to pharmacology and therapeutics, Bakersfield, Calif, 1985, Kern Medical Center.
Olin BR, editor: *Drug facts and comparisons,* St. Louis, 1995, Wolters Kluwer.

activity. The five major categories are the hydantoins, the long-acting barbiturates, the succinimides, the oxazolidinediones, and the benzodiazepines. The "other antiepileptics" group includes promising drugs such as carbamazepine, valproic acid, gabapentin, and lamotrigine; rarely used anticonvulsants such as lidocaine and paraldehyde; and drugs that cause serious adverse effects such as phenacemide and felbamate. Some of the drugs have rather broad indications; others have limited application. For instance, phenacemide is used only for complex partial seizures and then only after the disorder has proven refractory to safer drugs. Antiepileptic drugs may also be categorized according to their presumed mechanisms of action. Box 7-2 lists general rules for using antiepileptic drugs.

Careful medical evaluation is needed before an antiepileptic is prescribed. Based on an evaluation that includes an EEG, a specific seizure type may be identified and an antiepileptic drug selected (Table 7-2). The clinician chooses an antiepileptic drug based on the considerations listed in Box 7-3.

Based on information found in Table 7-2, it is obvious that more than one drug may control seizure activity. However, one drug may be preferred over another based on the criteria found in Box 7-3. Additionally, because more than one seizure

Box 7-2 General Rules for Using Antiepileptics

1. When possible (i.e., when there is not great urgency, as there is during status epilepticus), start with a low dose and gradually increase until a steady therapeutic blood level of the drug is reached. For example, an initial dose should be one fourth to one third the recommended therapeutic dose. This incremental approach is important with carbamazepine, valproic acid, and primidone and is less important with phenytoin and phenobarbital.
2. Give antiepileptics on time, to achieve a steady state and then to maintain the drug's therapeutic effect.*
3. Understand that drug dosage varies among individuals; accordingly each dosage must also be individualized.
4. Understand the patient's history, including baseline pretreatment laboratory test results.
5. When an antiepileptic is to be discontinued, do so gradually, to decrease the possibility of withdrawal-related seizures, i.e., status epilepticus.† Other caregivers should be made aware of the patient's drug regimen so that they may provide fully informed care of their own.
6. Monitor the patient's laboratory results, including serum drug levels, hematologic responses to drugs, and trough levels.‡ (Pellock, Willmore, 1991). Indications for drawing serum levels include therapeutic failure, noncompliance (may be as high as 50%), toxicity, and drug interactions. In general, serum drug level determinations are overused.
7. Attempt to use a single drug, if possible. Patients receiving combination therapy have twice as many adverse responses as patients who receive one antiepileptic, i.e., monotherapy.

*From Woodward ES: *J Neurosurg Nurs* 14:166, 1982.
†From Callaghan N, Garrett A, Goggin T: *New Engl J Med* 318(15):942, 1988.
‡From Pellock JM, Willmore LJ: *Neurology* 41(7):961, 1991.

Table 7-2 Seizure Types Matched with Appropriate Antiepileptic Agents

Antiepileptic agent	Seizure types amenable to drug (bold indicates first-line agent)
Hydantoins	
Phenytoin	**Tonic-clonic**
	Psychomotor (complex partial)
	Status epilepticus (second line)
Ethotoin	Tonic-clonic
	Psychomotor (complex partial)
Mephenytoin	Focal
	Jacksonian
Barbiturates	
Phenobarbital	**Tonic-clonic**
	Simple partial seizures
	Complex partial seizures
	Status epilepticus (second line)
Mephobarbital	Tonic-clonic
	Absence seizures
Barbiturate-like	
Primidone	Tonic-clonic (second line)
	Simple partial
	Complex partial
Succinimides	
Ethosuximide	**Absence seizures**
Methsuximide	Absence seizures (second line)
Phensuximide	Absence seizures
Oxazolidinediones	
Trimethadione	Absence seizures
Paramethadione	Absence seizures
Benzodiazepines	
Clonazepam	**Lennox-Gastaut seizures**
	Akinetic seizures
	Myoclonic
	Absence seizures
Clorazepate	Partial seizures
Diazepam	**Status epilepticus**
Other antiepileptics	
Carbamazepine	**Tonic-clonic**
	Psychomotor (complex partial)
	Mixed seizures
Valproic acid	**Absence seizures**
	Tonic-clonic
	Myoclonic
	Complex partial seizures
Gabapentin	Partial seizures
Lamotrigine	Partial seizures
Acetazolamide	Absence seizures

Continued

Table 7-2 Seizure Types Matched with Appropriate Antiepileptic Agents—cont'd

Antiepileptic agent	Seizure types amenable to drug (bold indicates first line agent)
Acetazolamide—cont'd	Tonic-clonic Myoclonic seizures
Lidocaine	Status epilepticus (last-resort agent)
Magnesium sulfate	Seizures related to magnesium deficiency, e.g. eclampsia
Paraldehyde	Alcohol withdrawal seizures
Phenacemide	Psychomotor (last-resort agent)
Felbamate	Withdrawn from the market

Box 7-3 Considerations in Initiating Antiepileptic Thereapy

1. Size of the patient
2. Expense of the drug
3. Allergic response to the drug, if any
4. Child-bearing potential
5. Tolerance to side effects

type may be present, determining whether a given drug might exacerbate a particular seizure pattern is a secondary consideration in selecting the correct antiepileptic.

In the following discussion a prototype drug from each of the five classes of antiepileptics will be highlighted, as well as significant drugs from the "other antiepileptics" group. Table 7-3 presents examples of antiepileptic agents and their proposed mechanism of action.

HYDANTOINS: PROTOTYPE DRUG, PHENYTOIN

Historically hydantoins have been considered the most effective antiepileptics. Hydantoins are particularly effective in treating tonic-clonic and complex partial seizures. Phenytoin (Dilantin) is the most widely used hydantoin, but two other hydantoins, ethotoin and mephenytoin, are available. Because hydantoins controlled seizures without causing sedation, it became apparent that central nervous system (CNS) depression was not a prerequisite for seizure control.

Pharmacologic Effects

The main site of action of hydantoins is in the motor cortex. Phenytoin inhibits the spread of abnormal brain electrical activity by normalizing abnormal fluxes of sodium across the nerve cell membrane during or after depolarization. This inhibition stabilizes a state of hyperexcitability. Hydantoins also decrease the activity of brain stem centers responsible for the tonic phase of grand mal seizures (Olin,

Table 7-3 Antiepileptic Drugs and Proposed Mechanism of Action

Drug	Mechanism of action
Phenytoin	1, 2
Phenobarbital	2, 5
Primidone	7
Ethosuximide	1, 3
Carbamazepine	1, 4
Valproic acid	5
Acetazolamide	6
Benzodiazepines	5

1 = Modifies Na^+, Ca^{++} conductances.
2 = Inhibits spread of abnormal brain electrical activity.
3 = Depresses neuronal activity; Raises seizure threshold.
4 = Reduces polysynaptic responses.
5 = Augments GABA-mediated synaptic inhibition.
6 = Carbonic anhydrase inhibitor.
7 = Mechanism unknown.
GABA = gamma-aminobutyric acid.

1995). Phenytoin also depresses cardiac electrical conduction, making it useful therapeutically for patients with arrhythmias.

Pharmacokinetics

Phenytoin is slowly absorbed from the gut after oral administration. The bioavailability can vary from as much as 10% to 90% among the different brands of phenytoin. Peak serum levels are reached in 1.5 to 3 hours when the promptly absorbed form is used; the extended-acting form reaches peak levels in 4 to 12 hours. The therapeutic serum level is 10 to 20 μg/mL (Penry and Newmark, 1979). Four to seven days of use are needed before a steady state is reached, because of the average half-life of 22 hours; however, the half-life is dose-dependent and has little clinical importance. Phenytoin is seldom administered by intramuscular injection because it is stored in tissue and released slowly. Absorption can take up to 5 days, which necessitates a 50% dosage adjustment when switching between oral and intramuscular routes of administration. When switching from oral to intramuscular modes, the dosage must be increased by 50%. When switching from intramuscular to oral routes, the dosage must be decreased by 50%. Table 7-4 compares the pharmacokinetics of the major antiepileptics.

Phenytoin is metabolized in the liver and excreted in the urine. A small amount (1% to 5%) is excreted unchanged. High serum levels can occur at "normal" doses when the patient has impaired liver function or congenital deficiencies in enzymes that break down phenytoin or when the patient is taking other drugs that interfere with phenytoin metabolism. Obviously, if the health care provider does not understand the difference between oral and parenteral forms of the drug, overdosing or underdosing can occur. Plasma protein binding is approximately 90%. Table 7-5 summarizes dosages for antiepileptic agents.

Oral administration. Phenytoin is available for oral administration in tablets, capsules, and suspensions and in pediatric and extended-acting forms. The extended-acting form is the only one available for once-per-day dosage. Oral therapy

Table 7-4 Pharmacokinetic Comparison of Major Antiepileptics

Agent	Time to steady state (days)	Therapeutic serum levels (μg/mL)	Toxic blood level (μg/mL)	Half-life (hr)	Protein-bound (%)
Hydantoin					
Phenytoin	7-10	10-20	>20	7-42†	≈90
Barbiturates					
Phenobarbital	16-21	15-40	>40	80 (before increased hepatic metabolism rate is induced)	40-60
Primidone*	1-5	5-12	>12	3-12	20-25
Succinimide					
Ethosuximide	5-10	40-100	>100	40-60 (adult); 30 (child)	0
Benzodiazepines					
Clonazepam	3-7	20-80 nanograms	>80 nanograms	18-60	80
Other antiepileptics					
Valproic acid	2-4	50-100	>100	6-16	90
Carbamazepine	2-4	4-12	>12	12-17	76

*When primidone is administered, phenobarbital levels must also be measured. With therapeutic primidone doses, phenobarbital levels should be 10-30 μg/mL.
†Half-life increases as serum level increases.

in adults usually begins with a dosage of 100 mg 3 times per day. However, a loading dose of 1 g (given over 4 hours) can be given to hospitalized patients with good hepatic functioning. See Table 7-5 for specific dosing information.

Parenteral administration. Intramuscular phenytoin is given to patients who cannot tolerate oral administration or when a risk of seizure is suspected during or soon after surgery. Intramuscular use is absolutely *not indicated* for status epilepticus because of the slow absorption of the route; thus careful attention to the appropriate dosage must be observed.

Intravenous (IV) use of phenytoin for status epilepticus is warranted in many situations; however, diazepam and lorazepam are first-line drugs for status epilepticus, whereas phenytoin is given only in combination with diazepam because of its slow onset of action (Jordan, 1994). Diazepam only aborts the seizure in progress and is not appropriate for continuous use as an antiepileptic. Close scrutiny of IV phenytoin is advised because of its narrow therapeutic index. Maintenance dosages of 100 mg every 6 to 8 hours to prevent breakthrough seizures are warranted. Other dosing information is found in Table 7-5.

Table 7-5 Dosage for Selected Antiepileptics

Drug and clinical indication	Dosage
Hydantoins	
Phenytoin (Dilantin)	
Tonic-clonic and complex partial seizures	*Oral:* Adults: 100-200 mg tid or qid; Dilantin Kapseals (extended form) can be given once daily. Children: 5 mg/kg/day; children > 6 yr may require minimum adult dose (300 mg/day).
Status epilepticus	*IV:* Adults: Give loading dose of 10-15 mg/kg; IV rate should not exceed 50 mg/min (or, in elderly patients, 25 mg/min); initial dose should be followed by maintenance dose of 100 mg orally or IV every 6-8h. Children: Give 15-20 mg/kg slowly (not more than 1-3 mg/kg/min). Use normal saline to avoid precipitation.
Mephenytoin (Mesantoin)	
Tonic-clonic, simple, and complex partial seizures	*Oral:* Adults: Initially, 50 to 100 mg/day. Maintenance dose is 200-600 mg/day. Children: 100-400 mg/day.
Ethotoin (Peganone)	
Tonic-clonic and complex partial seizures	*Oral:* Adult: Initially, 1000 mg or less in 4 to 6 doses. Maintenance dose is 2000-3000 mg/day given in 4 to 6 doses after eating. Children: Initially, 750 mg/day. 500-1000 mg/day given in 4 to 6 doses after eating is typical.
Long-acting barbiturates	
Phenobarbital (Luminal)	
Tonic-clonic and simple and complex partial seizures	*Oral:* Adults: 100-300 mg/day. Children: 3-5 mg/kg/day.
Status epilepticus	*IV:* Adults: 200-300 mg, repeating in 6 hours, if needed. Children: 15-20 mg/kg over 10-15 min; then 6 mg/kg every 20 min prn to maximum dose of 40 mg/kg in 24 hr.
Mephobarbital (Mebaral)	
Tonic-clonic and absence seizures	*Oral:* Adults: 400-600 mg/day. Children > 5 yr: 32-64 mg tid or qid. Children < 5 yr: 16-32 mg tid or qid.
Primidone (Mysoline)	
Tonic-clonic, simple, and complex partial seizures	*Oral:* Adults and children > 8 yr: Days 1 to 3, 100-125 mg hs; days 4 to 6, 100-125 mg bid; days 7 to 9, 100-125 mg tid; day 10, up to 250 mg tid or qid per day, if needed. Children < 8 yr: 50 mg hs at first, then gradually increase by Day 10 to 10-25 mg/kg/day in divided doses (125-250 mg tid), if needed.
Succinimides	
Ethosuximide (Zarontin)	
Absence seizures (petit mal)	*Oral:* Adults and children > 6 years: 500 mg/day at first, then increase by 250 mg/day every 4 to 7 days until seizures are satisfactorily controlled (40-100 μg/ml). Children 3-6 yr: 250 mg/day at first, then increase by 250 mg/day every 4 to 7 days. (20 mg/kg/day is typical optimal dose.) No person should receive > 1.5 g/day.

Table 7-5 Dosage for Selected Antiepileptics—cont'd

Drug and clinical indication	Dosage
Methsuximide (Celontin)	
Absence seizures (petit mal)	*Oral:* Adults: 300 mg/day at first, then weekly increases of 300 mg/day up to 1200 mg/day, if needed. Children: Same as for adults; however, increments are 150 mg.
Phensuximide (Milontin)	
Absence seizures (petit mal)	*Oral:* Adults and children: 500-1000 mg bid or tid; 1500 mg/day is average maintenance dose.
Oxazolidinediones	
Trimethadione (Tridione)	
Absence seizures (petit mal) refractory to other drugs	*Oral:* Adults: 900 mg/day at first, then increase by 300 mg/day every 7 days until seizures are controlled or until symptoms of toxic effects occur; maintenance dose usually 300-600 mg tid or qid; maximum dose is 2400 mg/day. Children: 300-900 mg/day in 3 or 4 divided doses.
Paramethadione (Paradione)	
Absence seizures (petit mal) refractory to other drugs	*Oral:* Adults: 900 mg/day at first, then increase by 300 mg/day every 7 days until seizures are controlled or until symptoms of toxic effects occur; maintenance dose usually 300-600 mg tid or qid; maximum dose is 2400 mg/day. Children: 300-900 mg/day in 3 or 4 divided doses.
Benzodiazepines	
Diazepam (Valium)	
Status epilepticus	*IM or IV (preferred route):* Adults: 5-10 mg, repeat every 10-15 min, if needed, up to a total dose of 30 mg; *must be given slowly.* May be repeated in 2 to 4 hours. Children > 5 yr: 1 mg every 2-5 min, up to 10 mg, repeated in 2 to 4 hours prn. Children from 1 mo to 5 yr: 0.2 to 0.5 mg slowly every 2-5 min, up to a total dose of 5 mg.
Clonazepam (Klonopin)	
Absence (petit mal), Lennox-Gastaut, and myoclonic seizures	*Oral:* Adults: 0.5 mg tid at first, then increase every 3 days by 0.5-1.0 mg until seizures are controlled; 20 mg/day is the maximum dose. Children < 10 yr: 0.01-0.03 mg/kg/day in divided doses at first, then increased by 0.25 to 0.5 mg every 3 days until seizures are controlled; usual dose is 0.1-0.2 mg/kg/day in 3 divided doses.
Clorazepate (Tranxene)	
Partial seizures (adjunctive)	*Oral:* Adults and children > 12 yr: up to 7.5 mg tid to start, then increase by no more than 7.5 mg every week: maximum dose is 90 mg/day. Children 9 to 12 yr: Up to 7.5 mg bid to start, then increase by no more than 7.5 mg every week; maximum dose is 60 mg/day. Not recommended for children < 9 yr.

Continued

Table 7-5 Dosage for Selected Antiepileptics—cont'd

Drug and clinical indication	Dosage
Other antiepileptics	
Valproic acid (Depakene)	
Absence, tonic-clonic, complex partial, and myoclonic seizures	*Oral:* Adults and children: 15 mg/kg/day at first, then increase weekly by 5-10 mg/kg/day up to a maintenance dose of 20-60 mg/kg/day in divided doses.
Carbamazepine (Tegretol)	
Tonic-clonic, complex partial, and mixed seizures	*Oral:* Adults and children > 12 yr: 200 mg bid at first, then increase by 200 mg/day every 7 days, if needed; maintenance dose usually 800-1200 mg/day in divided doses; adult dose rarely exceeds 1200 mg/day. Children 12-15 yr should not receive more than 1000 mg/day. Children 6-12 yr: 100 mg bid at first, then increase by 100 mg/day every 7 days, if needed; maintenance dose is usually 400-800 mg/day in divided doses; do not exceed 1000 mg/day.
Phenacemide (Phenurone)	
Complex partial seizures refractory to safer drugs	*Oral:* Adults: 250-500 mg tid to start; maintenance dose is typically 2000 to 3000 mg/day but may reach 5000. Children 5-10 yr: Half the adult dose at the same intervals as for adults.
Gabapentin (Neurontin)	
Adjunctive therapy for partial seizures	Adults and children > 12 yr: 300 mg by mouth on Day 1, 300 mg twice a day on Day 2, and 300 mg 3 times a day on Day 3. The dose on Day 1 should be given at bedtime to reduce somnolence or daytime dizziness. Dosage can be increased up to 1800 mg/day. Spacing should not exceed 12 hours between doses.
Lamotrigine (Lamictal) Adjunctive therapy for partial seizures	Adults taking an enzyme-inducing antiepileptic (carbamazepine, phenytoin, phenobarbital, primidone): 50 mg once daily for 2 weeks; then can increase to 50 mg twice a day for 2 more weeks; then weekly changes of 100 mg/day up to a maintenance dosage of 300 to 500 mg/day in 2 doses. If valproic acid is being taken in addition to an enzyme-inducing drug, the starting dose should be 25 mg qod for 2 weeks followed by 25 mg/day for 2 weeks. Then increase by 25 to 50 mg/day every 1 to 2 weeks up to a maintenance dosage of 100 to 150 mg/day in 2 divided doses. If valproic acid is given alone, the dosage of lamotrigine would no doubt be lower. Children and adolescents: Not recommended for children <16. (The Medical Letter, 1995.)

Side Effects

The most common side effects of phenytoin are those involving the CNS, that is, sluggishness, ataxia, nystagmus, confusion, and slurred speech (Table 7-6). Dizziness, insomnia, nervousness, and fatigue occur less frequently. Phenytoin is considered the least sedating antiepileptic.

Peripheral side effects include those involving the blood, the gastrointestinal (GI) tract, connective tissue, and the skin. Hematologic effects such as leukopenia, agranulocytosis, megaloblastic anemia, and coagulation deficits in newborns have been reported. Nausea, vomiting, and constipation are the major GI tract effects. Gingival hyperplasia (overgrowth of gums down over the teeth) is a fairly common side effect of phenytoin use in children and in those who do not engage in good oral hygiene. Psychiatric patients and individuals with developmental disabilities seem to be susceptible to gingival hyperplasia. Other connective tissue problems include enlarged lips, coarsened facial features, and excessive growth of body hair (hypertrichosis). Skin reactions can range from the embarrassing, such as worsening of acne in a teenager, to the potentially fatal exfoliative dermatitis. Other skin reactions are a mild measlelike (morbilliform) rash and lupus erythematosus. Other adverse responses include hepatitis and liver damage, hyperglycemia, edema, chest pain, numbness and paresthesia, photophobia, pulmonary fibrosis, osteomalacia caused by enhanced vitamin D metabolism, and lymphadenopathy (as severe as Hodgkin's disease).

Central nervous system side effects are particularly debilitating for elderly patients because of the high susceptibility to falls and a tendency to misjudge situations, that is, forgetting that a medication was taken and then ingesting an extra dose. Megaloblastic anemia can be countered with folic acid; however, excessive doses of folic acid can lower phenytoin serum levels to a subtherapeutic range. Discontinuance of phenytoin can reverse lymph node involvement.

Table 7-6 General Side Effects: Relative Frequency by Drug and Appropriate Interventions

Side effect (Drugs in which this side effect is common or a major concern are identified)	**Intervention**
CNS effects **(P, Pb, E, Cl, CBZ)**	Monitor for and prevent falls; caution against driving
Hematologic disorders (P, E, Cl)	Carefully assess for fever, sore throat, malaise, and bruises
GI symptoms (**E,** P, Pb, Cl, V, CBZ)	Give with meals
Gingival hyperplasia (**P,** E)	Encourage and supervise, if appropriate, meticulous oral hygiene
Skin rashes (**P,** Pb, E, Cl)	May indicate a serious skin disorder such as exfoliative dermatitis; discontinue drug
Acne in teenagers (P)	Medication should be changed, if possible

KEY: P = Phenytoin; Pb = Phenobarbital; E = Ethosuximide; Cl = Clonazepam; V = Valproic acid; CBZ = Carbamazepine; **Bold type = occurs commonly**

Implications

Therapeutic versus toxic levels. The typical therapeutic dose of phenytoin ranges from 300 to 600 mg per day given in several doses or, if the extended-acting form is used, once per day. Toxic serum levels can occur at normal dosage levels for a variety of reasons, for example, impaired liver function, enzyme deficiencies, or drug interactions. Therapeutic serum levels range from 10 to 20 μg/mL. A toxic level of phenytoin occurs at serum levels above 20 μg/mL. Symptoms can include far-lateral nystagmus, ataxia, dysarthria, tremor, slurred speech, and nausea and vomiting. Diminished mental capacity occurs at serum levels above 40 μg/mL. Serum levels above 50 μg/mL may cause seizures. At serum levels above 100 μg/mL the same symptoms are intensified, and hypotension, circulatory and ventilatory failure, coma, and death can occur. The estimated lethal dose in an adult is 2 to 5 g (Olin, 1995). Death is caused by respiratory and circulatory failure.

Treatment for overdose and toxic effects are driven by the principle of reducing further drug absorption. Induced emesis, repeated gastric lavage and suctioning, and activated charcoal are interventions useful in interrupting phenytoin absorption. Because there is no known antidote, supportive measures for respiratory and circulatory systems should be employed. Hemodialysis may be useful, because phenytoin is not completely bound to plasma proteins.

Use in pregnancy. Expectant women treated for epilepsy have a higher propensity for experiencing seizures caused by poor phenytoin absorption that occurs during pregnancy (Olin, 1995). Phenytoin has been implicated in congenital defects, that is, cleft lip, cleft palate, and heart malformations (Dalessio, 1985). In addition, children of women taking phenytoin are susceptible to coagulation defects caused by lower levels of vitamin K–dependent clotting factors, which can lead to hemorrhage. Prophylactic administration of vitamin K (phytonadione) to the mother at 1 month before delivery and to the newborn at birth (about 1 mg) can prevent the development of this hematologic disorder. Hematologic studies should be routinely acquired. Breast-feeding is not appropriate for women taking phenytoin because this drug is excreted in breast milk.

Side effects. Central nervous system symptoms are most troublesome for elderly patients. These individuals should be observed closely to prevent falls or other problems associated with impaired judgment. Evaluation of mood, affect, and memory provide data from which interventions can be formulated.

Hematologic disorders can be minimized through careful assessment for fever, sore throat, malaise, or bruises (Keltner, 1993). The patient should be instructed to self-assess for these signs and to report them. A contraindication for phenytoin use is the presence of bone marrow depression or a blood dyscrasia.

Nausea, vomiting, and other gastrointestinal problems are reduced when phenytoin is given with meals. Gingival hyperplasia, coarsening of facial features, and other connective tissue consequences of phenytoin therapy can cause a loss of self-esteem because of disfigurement. Thorough oral hygiene can reduce the severity of gingival hyperplasia.

Because skin rashes can range from mild, measlelike conditions to serious skin disorders such as exfoliative dermatitis and lupus erythematosus, phenytoin should be discontinued when a rash appears. Finally, acne is a frequent adverse reaction to phenytoin among teenagers and young adults, and its potential to lower self-esteem should not be underestimated by those responsible for care. If antiepileptic besides phenytoin will control seizures, a change is indicated.

Parenteral phenytoin can cause cardiovascular effects such as hypotension, circulatory collapse, depression of cardiac conductility, and cardiac arrest. Patients with a history of sinus bradycardia, sinoatrial or second- or third-degree atrioventricular block, or Adams-Stokes syndrome should not be given this drug. Monitoring the patient's blood pressure and respirations while giving phenytoin slowly IV (50 mg per minute) reduces the likelihood of triggering a cardiovascular response.

Interactions. Many drugs interact with phenytoin (Box 7-4). These interactions can be generally categorized as those that cause an increase or decrease in phenytoin serum levels, those that cause a decrease in the action of the interacting drug, and those interactants with unpredictable effects. Nonetheless, if phenytoin serum levels are closely monitored, multiple drug therapy is possible without serious consequences for the patient.

Drugs that increase phenytoin serum levels (potential toxic effects). Other drugs increase serum phenytoin by one of the following means: (1) inhibiting phenytoin metabolism or (2) displacing phenytoin from plasma protein-binding sites, thereby leading to excessive levels of free (and active) phenytoin. Interactants that inhibit metabolism include acute alcohol ingestion, allopurinal, benzodiazepines, H_1-receptor blocking antihistamines, disulfiram, isoniazid, phenacemide, phenylbutazone, succinimides, sulfonamides, and valproic acid. Diazepam and

Box 7-4 Drug Interaction for Most Antiepileptics

Drugs affecting antiepileptics

- Alcohol
- Antacids
- Aspirin
- Carbamazepine
- Cimetidine (Tagamet)
- Disulfiram (Antabuse)
- Erythromycin
- Fluoxetine (Prozac)
- Phenobarbital
- Phenytoin
- Propoxyphene (Darvon)
- Rifampin
- Valproate

Drugs affected by antiepileptics

- Folic acid
- Meperidine (Demerol)
- Oral anticoagulants
- Oral contraceptives
- Steroids
- Theophylline
- Vitamins D and K

Modified from Ramsey RE et al: *Clinical issues in the management of epilepsy,* Miami, 1993, University of Miami.

ethosuximide are antiepileptics that might be prescribed along with phenytoin, so a downward adjustment in the dose of phenytoin should be made. Disulfiram, a major drug treatment for chronic alcoholism, necessitates a low starting dose of phenytoin, monitoring of serum levels of phenytoin, and careful assessment of the patient. Drinking alcohol when taking phenytoin leads to higher serum levels of the drug because alcohol successfully competes for liver enzymes. Valproic acid and salicylates increase phenytoin serum levels by displacing phenytoin from plasma protein-binding sites.

Drugs that decrease phenytoin serum levels (potential seizure breakthrough). A number of drugs decrease the serum levels of phenytoin by means of the following distinct mechanisms: (1) increasing phenytoin metabolism or (2) decreasing its absorption. Barbiturates (including phenobarbital), theophylline, carbamazepine, chronic alcoholism (enzyme induction), and theophylline decrease phenytoin serum levels by increasing its breakdown in the liver. Antacids block phenytoin absorption. Folic acid, sometimes given prophylactically to prevent megaloblastic anemia, antineoplastics, influenza vaccine, and calcium gluconate decrease phenytoin serum levels by some unknown mechanism.

Interactant effects that are decreased by phenytoin. The effects of acetaminophen, corticosteroids, oral anticoagulants, oral contraceptives, quinidine, and vitamin D are all compromised by phenytoin. Dangers of these interactive patterns include decreased corticosteroid effect; increased blood clotting; pregnancy, spotting, and breakthrough bleeding; reduced antiarrhythmic action; and increased risk of osteomalacia, respectively. Assessment should address these issues. Increasing the level of estrogen in the contraceptive may improve efficacy, and instructing the patient to seek medical help should a pregnancy be expected is a prudent measure to ensure optimal benefit. Additionally, fluid retention lowers the seizure threshold; because retention occurs with the use of contraceptives, alternative birth control methods should be considered. Increasing quinidine dosage can maintain its antiarrhythmic quality, and encouraging more vitamin D in the diet can forestall skeletal problems.

Psychotropic drugs whose metabolism is enhanced by phenytoin include clonazepam, haloperidol, and methadone.

Interactants that behave unpredictably. Several drugs may either increase or decrease phenytoin serum levels. Two antiepileptics, phenobarbital and valproic acid, may cause phenytoin serum levels to rise or fall. Consequently, monitoring of laboratory data is important. Paradoxically phenytoin can have the same effect on these two drugs; that is, their effects may increase or decrease.

Patient education. Patient teaching should focus on helping the patient maximize the therapeutic benefits of phenytoin while preventing or minimizing its serious side effects. The patient should be familiar with the desired action of the drug, the importance of taking the drug on time and as prescribed (maintaining therapeutic serum levels), the difference in efficacy between oral and parenteral routes, and the need to notify the clinician when certain side effects occur. Side effects that must be punctually reported include sore throat, fever, malaise, petechiae, and bruising. The other major significant issues in patient teaching are meticulous oral hygiene (brushing and flossing) to reduce gingival hyperplasia, warnings against driving when CNS symptoms such as dizziness or sedation occur, care when rising (to reduce the risk of falls), avoidance of prescription drugs that interact with phenytoin (all health care providers should be aware of phenytoin therapy), and consumption of alcohol. Generally it is advisable for individuals taking antiepileptic drugs to wear a medical identification bracelet.

Young women should be made aware of the potential for congenital defects should they become pregnant, and those desiring to become pregnant should first talk with their physician. Individuals who have GI tract effects as a result of taking phenytoin should be encouraged to take the drug with their meals, because doing so enhances absorption and decreases GI tract upset.

Patients should be advised not to abruptly discontinue phenytoin, because of the potential for status epilepticus. As little as a 10% change in daily dose can result in a 50% change in serum concentration.

Related Hydantoins

The two hydantoins other than phenytoin that are successfully used to treat epilepsy are ethotoin (Peganone) and mephenytoin (Mesantoin). Ethotoin is indicated for the treatment of tonic-clonic and psychomotor seizures. It can be given alone or in conjunction with another antiepileptic. It is rapidly absorbed. Therapeutic serum levels of ethotoin are 15 to 50 μg/mL. Ethotoin is compatible with all antiepileptics except phenacemide (Phenurone). The combination of ethotoin and phenacemide has been reported to cause a paranoid syndrome. Ethotoin is *contraindicated* in patients with known hepatic abnormalities or hematologic disorders.

Mephenytoin is used to treat focal and jacksonian seizures but is not usually prescribed unless other, safer antiepileptics have been attempted first.

LONG-ACTING BARBITURATES: PROTOTYPE DRUG, PHENOBARBITAL

Barbiturates are relatively old drugs. Many individual drugs are available, but only long-acting barbiturates have antiepileptic potential. Phenobarbital (Luminal) is the prototypical long-acting barbiturate. Mephobarbital (Mebaral) and primidone (Mysoline) are related drugs.

Antiepileptic treatment is the only therapy for which long-term use of barbiturates is recognized. Although barbiturates have been used for nearly a century as sedatives, at subsedation doses a few have been found to possess antiepileptic qualities. All barbiturates have antiepileptic properties at high doses. It is phenobarbital's ability to inhibit seizures without inducing sedation that makes it and the related drugs beneficial.

Pharmacologic Effects

By altering ion movements across nerve membranes and inhibiting nerve transmission to the cerebral cortex, phenobarbital slows the response of nerves to seizure-causing stimuli and also slows the spread of abnormal electrical activity. The net effect is to raise the seizure threshold, that is, diminish the likelihood of a seizure. Oral phenobarbital is effective in treating tonic-clonic seizures and simple and complex partial seizures (Table 7-2). Parenteral phenobarbital is used to stop status epilepticus when diazepam or phenytoin is ineffective or unavailable. Phenobarbital can produce a paradoxic effect—excitement—in children.

Pharmacokinetics

Phenobarbital is usually given orally, absorbed in varying degrees, and uniformly distributed to all tissues (Table 7-4). Onset of action after an oral dose varies from 20 to 60 minutes. Phenobarbital is metabolized in the liver by the hepatic microsomal enzyme system, but 25% to 50% of its molecules are excreted unchanged in the urine. Nonetheless, phenobarbital has a dramatic effect on hepatic enzymes by increasing the synthesis of those enzymes (enzyme induction). The net effect is to expedite the metabolism of those drugs, including phenobarbital, that are metabolized by these liver enzymes. This mechanism produces tolerance to many effects and contributes to drug interactions. Tolerance to phenobarbital's antiepileptic activity and to its lethal effects is slight. Phenobarbital has the lowest lipid solubility and the longest duration of action of all barbiturates.

The therapeutic plasma level for phenobarbital is 15 to 40 μg/mL and takes 16 to 21 days to reach a steady state. It has a half-life of 80 hours (a range of 53 to 118 hours) initially, but that time is reduced after the aformentioned enzyme induction occurs. Phenobarbital is 40% to 60% bound to plasma proteins.

The low doses associated with phenobarbital therapy seldom produce physical dependence or withdrawal symptoms (Table 7-5). Phenobarbital is usually preferred over phenytoin to treat seizures in children because it does not cause gingival hyperplasia or the various skin problems associated with phenytoin. Elderly patients may require a reduced dosage. Patients who have status epilepticus or other acute seizures, for example, those caused by cholera, eclampsia, or meningitis, can be given IV phenobarbital (Table 7-5). Phenobarbital is not the first choice for these emergency situations (diazepam is a first-choice agent) because the high doses needed to stop these seizures can cause CNS, respiratory, and cardiovascular depression.

Oral administration. Phenobarbital is available in a variety of oral forms: tablets, capsules, and elixirs. Long-term antiepileptic therapy is typically accomplished by means of oral phenobarbital use.

Parenteral administration. Parenteral usage should be avoided unless oral administration is not feasible or a prompt antieptileptic response is needed. Parenteral phenobarbital is used to treat status epilepticus and other emergency convulsive states. Intramuscular phenobarbital should be injected into large muscles (gluteus maximus or vastus lateralis), where there is less risk of injecting into a peripheral nerve trunk or artery.

Intravenous injections are preferred over intramuscular injections and are typically reserved for emergency situations in which timely action is important. A vein must always be used because interarterial injection can lead to a gangrenous condition caused by vessel spasm. The drugs must be injected slowly, at a rate no faster than 50 mg per minute. The onset of action after IV injection is about 5 minutes. Again, parenteral phenobarbital is not the drug of choice for treating status epilepticus; diazepam or phenytoin is given.

Side Effects

Evidence of central nervous system depression, that is, drowsiness, ataxia, and sedation, is the most common side effect of phenobarbital (Table 7-6). However, because seizure control is a long-term, if not a lifetime, concern, many of the side effects associated with phenobarbital become tolerated by the patient. A history of porphyria (excessive hepatic formation of porphyrins) remains a contraindication to using phenobarbital because it induces the synthesis of porphyrins. Hypotension and respiratory depression are potential adverse responses to high oral doses or to rapid IV infusion.

Another major side effect of phenobarbital administration is the induction of hepatic microsomal enzymes. The effect of this induction phenomenon is the increased rate of metabolism of phenobarbital and other drugs metabolized in the liver. This effect leads directly to the development of tolerance mentioned in the preceding paragraph.

Vitamin D metabolism is stimulated by phenobarbital. The same concerns reviewed during the discussion of phenytoin pertain to phenobarbital. Barbiturates at low doses can cause excitability in children and elderly individuals.

Implications

Therapeutic versus toxic levels. The therapeutic serum phenobarbital level is 15 to 40 μg/mL. Serum phenobarbital levels of more than 40 μg/mL may be toxic. Although toxic doses vary among individuals, usually 1 g of phenobarbital taken orally can cause serious toxic effects and ingesting 2 to 10 g can be lethal.

A tolerance to many of the barbiturate effects, but not to the antiepileptic effects, develops with chronic use of phenobarbital. Therefore, although an increased amount of barbiturate may be needed for sedation, an increase is not required for continued seizure control nor does tolerance to lethal levels develop. At toxic levels respiratory and CNS depression, tachycardia, hypotension, hypothermia, and coma can occur. In cases of severe overdose, apnea, circulatory collapse, respiratory arrest, and death have been reported.

Treatment for overdose consists of maintenance of a patent airway and assistance with ventilation and oxygenation, if needed. Gastric lavage can be used to empty the stomach. Monitoring vital signs and fluid balance is important. When renal function remains normal, forced diuresis and alkalinizing of the urine help eliminate the phenobarbital.

Use in pregnancy. Phenobarbital has been implicated in congenital defects (Dalessio, 1985; Olin, 1995). Withdrawal symptoms can occur in infants born to mothers who took barbiturates in their last trimester, and a coagulation defect in infants has been associated with maternal barbiturate use.

Side effects. Central nervous system effects such as drowsiness can impair driving and put the patient at risk in many situations. Should an older patient or a child have paradoxic excitement after taking phenobarbital, precautions to prevent injury should be instituted. Patient assessment data should include information about a history of porphyria. Resuscitation equipment should be readily available when IV phenobarbital is given.

Interactions. Drugs that depress the CNS are the chief interactants with phenobarbital, so the patient who requires phenobarbital in conjunction with another CNS depressant should be carefully observed by physicians and nurses. Interactants can be categorized into two groups: drugs that increase the effects of barbiturates and drugs whose effects are decreased by barbiturates.

Drugs that increase effects of barbiturates (toxic effects). Central nervous system depressants such as sedatives, hypnotics, anesthetics, antihistamines, antipsychotics, and alcohol enhance the depressant effects of barbiturates. Alcohol and barbiturates should never be combined. Alcohol can reduce the antiepileptic effect of phenobarbital and dramatically increase the level of CNS depression. Many deaths each year are attributed to the combination of barbiturates and alcohol.

Other antiepileptic agents also interact with phenobarbital. Because multiple-drug therapy is common in treating seizure disorders, it is important to recognize potential problems and to develop protocols for evaluating them. Valproic acid, for example, interacts with phenobarbital through a mechanism referred to as *selective metabolism*. The hepatic microsomal enzyme system selectively metabolizes valproic acid, delaying the metabolism of phenobarbital. Phenobarbital serum levels may increase by 200%, clearly presenting a serious risk of toxic effects.

Drugs whose effects are decreased by phenobarbital. Many drugs are compromised by coadministration with phenobarbital. The induction of hepatic microsomal enzymes that more speedily metabolize these drugs is responsible for their shortened response in the body (Keltner, Schwecke, and Bostrom, 1995). Most notably reduced in effect are clonazepam, digitoxin, oral anticoagulants, oral contraceptives, and TCAs. Although the effect of phenobarbital on phenytoin is not precisely known, it is thought that phenytoin metabolism is accelerated and consequently renders the drug less effective. The concurrent use of these two antiepileptics is common, so frequent monitoring of serum levels of both drugs is appropriate. Other drugs whose effects are decreased include griseofulvin, quinidine, doxycycline, and monoamine oxidase inhibitors.

Patient education. Patient teaching focuses primarily on health and safety. Patients should be warned to avoid driving or operating hazardous machinery and to avoid combining phenobarbital, alcohol, and other CNS depressants. Other teaching concerns include the reporting of side effects and adverse responses. Although hematologic side effects are uncommon, symptoms such as sore throat, fever, and bleeding should be reported so that the development of blood dyscrasias can be prevented.

Related Barbiturates

One other barbiturate, mephobarbital, and a barbiturate-like drug, primidone, are effective antiepileptics.

Mephobarbital is used to treat both tonic-clonic and absence epilepsy. It has two major advantages over phenobarbital. First, mephobarbital can be used to treat absence seizure, whereas phenobarbital cannot. Second, mephobarbital causes less drowsiness and sedation in adults and less excitability in children than does phenobarbital. This second feature accounts for the predominant rationale for prescribing mephobarbital. Table 7-5 gives exact dosage guidelines.

Mephobarbital is sometimes used in combination with phenobarbital. When so used, the daily dose of both should be about half of what it would be if each were given alone, that is, 50 to 100 mg of phenobarbital and 200 to 300 mg of mephobarbital. Mephobarbital can also be given concurrently with phenytoin. In this combination, phenytoin should be reduced to about 230 mg per day, but mephobarbital can be given at its full dose.

Primidone is related to the barbiturates and is used alone or in conjunction with other antiepileptics to control tonic-clonic, simple partial, and complex partial seizures. Two metabolites of primidone, phenobarbital and phenylethylmalonamide, are responsible for the drugs's antiepileptic properties. When a barbiturate is indicated, primidone is not a first-line drug because it is responsible for consequential side effects, that is, ataxia, vertigo, GI tract upset, nystagmus, diplopia, impotence, and minor rashes. Emotional disturbances, including paranoid thinking and mood fluctuations, have also been reported in some patients. Some side effects, such as ataxia and vertigo, disappear after continued use. Adults and children are started on a regimen of primidone at modest doses (100 mg at bedtime and 50 mg at bedtime, respectively); then dosages are carefully elevated over the next 10 days to arrive at a therapeutic maintenance dose. Details on dosages are given in both Table 7-5 and the psychotropic drug profiles found in Part Two of this book. Adults are never given more than 2 g per day. Bioequivalence among brands of primidone is not supported by clinical experience, so switching products is not recommended.

SUCCINIMIDES: PROTOTYPE DRUG, ETHOSUXIMIDE

The succinimides are the third group of antiepileptic drugs discussed here. They are chemically distinct from the hydantoins and the long-acting barbiturates. The succinimides' contribution to the antiepileptic arsenal lies in their effectiveness in treating absence seizures (Table 7-2). The prototype drug of the succinimides is ethosuximide (Zarontin). The two related antiepileptics are methsuximide (Celontin) and phensuximide (Milontin).

Pharmacologic Effects

Ethosuximide decreases absence seizures by depressing the motor cortex and raising the threshold of the CNS to convulsive stimuli. The three-cycles-per-second, spike-and-wave EEG pattern associated with absence seizures is also effectively suppressed. Ethosuximide is not the first drug of choice for absence seizures in adults; valproic acid is. Nonetheless, ethosuximide remains an important drug and is much preferred over the oxazolidinediones (paramethadione and trimethadione), which may cause serious side effects.

Pharmacokinetics

Ethosuximide is readily absorbed in the GI tract, and peak serum levels are reached within 3 to 7 hours (Table 7-4). Ethosuximide, because of a long half-life of 60 hours in adults and 30 hours in children, can be given in once-per-day dosages. It is extensively metabolized to inactive metabolites and excreted in the urine.

Ethosuximide is available in oral forms (capsules and syrup). It can be used adjunctively with other antiepileptic agents in patients with seizures other than absence seizures; however, because ethosuximide can increase the risk of tonic-clonic seizure breakthrough, higher doses of the concurrent antiepileptic may be required. Used alone, ethosuximide can increase the risk of tonic-clonic seizures in some patients.

Side Effects

The common complaint associated with ethosuximide is GI tract upset. Nausea, vomiting, cramps, diarrhea, and anorexia are common but can be reduced by taking the medication with meals. Psychiatric and CNS symptoms (dizziness and drowsiness) can occur in some patients. Succinimides have been reported to cause abnormal hepatic and renal function in humans, so monitoring studies of these functions is consistent with good care. Giving ethosuximide to a patient with impaired liver functioning prolongs the already long half-life, increasing the risk of long-lasting toxic effects. Hematologic effects, which are infrequent but significant, and dermatologic effects occur in a few patients.

Implications

Therapeutic versus toxic levels. The therapeutic serum level of ethosuximide is 40 to 100 μg/mL. Toxic effects occur when the serum level is higher than 100 μg/mL. A state of overdose results in intensified GI tract, CNS, hematologic, and dermatologic side effects. Ataxia, lethargy, dizziness, and sedation are frequently the first signs of toxicity. The most severe reactions to overdose are myopia, vaginal bleeding, CNS depression, and systemic lupus erythematosus. Overdoses are treated symptomatically, and patient care is supportive.

Use in pregnancy. Although in general antiepileptic drugs are known to contribute to fetal abnormalities, ethosuximide seems to be a drug that can be given safely without the risk of significant defects in newborns. With appropriate monitoring, women have been able to take ethosuximide during pregnancy. This drug, as with most antiepileptics, is not recommended for use during lactation.

Side effects. Hepatic and renal studies should be performed before ethosuximide therapy is initiated. Thereafter, regularly scheduled testing is desirable so that deleterious effects to those organs can be evaluated or prevented. Because a few patients have had lethal blood dyscrasias, obtaining periodic blood cell counts is prudent. If the patient becomes depressed or aggressive, it may be necessary to withdraw ethosuximide.

Interactions. Ethosuximide does not interact in a significant way with any other drugs; however, excessive sedation could result from concurrent administration with a CNS depressant, for example, alcohol. Antipsychotic and antidepressant drugs lower the seizure threshold and increase the risk of seizure development when taken during ethosuximide therapy. Further, serum levels of hydantoins may increase and serum levels of primidone may decrease when given with succinimides.

Patient education. Patients who have any of the GI tract symptoms mentioned previously should be advised to take ethosuximide with food or milk. Because of the long half-life of ethosuximide and its once-a-day dosage pattern, patients who miss a day of medication should not take a double dose the next day. To do so could substantially raise the serum level of ethosuximide and, in turn, cause intensified side effects and toxic reactions.

Patients taking ethosuximide should be advised to avoid alcohol and to refrain from abrupt discontinuance of this drug. Abruptly ceasing use increases the risk of seizures. Because ethosuximide can cause drowsiness, driving a car or operating hazardous machinery should be limited until the drug is well tolerated. Patients should report symptoms that indicate blood dyscrasias to the physician.

Related Succinimides

The two related succinimides are methsuximide and phensuximide. Methsuximide is as effective as ethosuximide in treating absence seizures; however, it is slightly more toxic. Hence methsuximide is a second-choice antiepileptic. Typically an effort is made to prescribe the lowest effective dose of methsuximide to reduce the toxic effects. Methsuximide reaches peak serum levels within 4 hours and has a much shorter half-life (2 to 4 hours) than ethosuximide. Drowsiness, ataxia, and dizziness are the most frequent side effects of methsuximide. Toxicity occurs when serum levels exceed 40 μg/mL.

Phensuximide is thought to be slightly less effective than either ethosuximide or methsuximide. Peak serum levels of the drug are reached within 4 hours, and its half-life is about 8 hours. Significant genitourinary tract side effects not associated with the other succinimides, that is, urinary frequency, renal damage, and hematuria, have been reported to be caused by phensuximide. Also, a harmless urinary effect is pinkish, red, or red-brown urine. Regardless of patient age, the total daily dose may vary from 1 to 3 g.

OXAZOLIDINEDIONES: PROTOTYPE DRUG, TRIMETHADIONE

The oxazolidinediones are antiepileptics normally used only when other drugs have proven ineffective. The oxazolidinediones cause serious side effects and have been proven to be tetragenic.

Pharmacologic Effects

Trimethadione (Tridione) was introduced in 1946 and was the first drug developed to treat absence seizures. It is an effective antiepileptic agent, but because of its serious side effects, it is not a first-line drug of choice. Although the exact nature of trimethadione's antiepileptic effect is not known, it is thought that its antiepileptic properties may be associated with its ability to decrease synaptic stimulation to low-frequency impulses.

Pharmacokinetics

Trimethadione is rapidly absorbed from the GI tract. It is metabolized to an active metabolite, dimethadione, which is slowly excreted in the urine. Peak serum levels are reached within 30 to 60 minutes; the serum half-life of trimethadione is 16 to 24 hours and that of its active metabolite is 6 to 13 days. Table 7-5 provides dosage information.

Side Effects

Trimethadione causes several serious side effects, and occasionally patients on a regimen of trimethadione have died. Prominent among the adverse responses are hepatic impairment, nephrosis, blood dyscrasias, exfoliative dermatitis, systemic lupus erythematosus, lymphadenopathy, and a myasthenia gravis–like syndrome.

Less serious side effects include drowsiness early in the course of therapy, dose-related photophobia and hemeralopia (day blindness), and GI tract symptoms such as nausea, vomiting, anorexia, and weight loss. Acneform rashes, although usually innocuous, can also be indicative of an early stage of fatal exfoliative dermatitis.

Implications

Therapeutic versus toxic levels. Effective therapeutic serum levels for controlling absence seizures are about 700 μg/mL. Toxic levels of trimethadione cause drowsiness, nausea, dizziness, ataxia, and visual disturbances. Large overdoses can cause coma. Treatment for overdose includes general supportive care, monitoring of vital signs, gastric evacuation by emesis or lavage, and urinary alkalinzation to increase dimethadione excretion.

Use in pregnancy. Trimethadione is teratogenic, and of the available antiepileptics it *poses the greatest risk to the fetus.* Only when all other antiepileptics have proven ineffective and it has been established that the risk of nontreatment to the mother is substantial should trimethadione be prescribed.

Side effects. Because of the seriousness of some of the side effects of trimethadione, strict supervision of patients receiving the drug is required. If lymph node enlargement or other manifestations of lupus erythematosus occur, the drug should be withdrawn. Appearance of even mild or acneform rashes are suggestive of more serious skin disorders such as exfoliative dermatitis and warrant discontinuance of trimethadione. Even apparently benign rashes should be allowed to completely clear before the drug treatment is resumed. Jaundice or laboratory values consistent with hepatic dysfunction are cause for drug discontinuance. Patients with a history of hepatic problems ordinarily should not receive trimethadione. Because fatal nephrosis has occurred with oxazolidinediones, renal function should be monitored and should abnormalities, for example, proteinuria, occur, these agents should be withdrawn. Because depression of blood cell counts can occur, a complete blood cell count should be obtained before therapy begins and regularly thereafter. A marked depression of the blood cell count, especially a neutrophil count of less than 2500 cells per mm^3, requires discontinuance.

Interactions. Valproic acid elevates the blood level of trimethadione and causes a number of symptoms related to mild toxic effects. Other significant interactions with the oxazolidinediones have not been reported.

Patient education. Patients should be taught:

- To take oxazolidinediones with food, if GI tract problems occur
- To avoid abrupt discontinuance of these drugs because of the possibility of withdrawal seizures
- To avoid bright lights, if they have photophobia or hemeralopia
- To be cautious when driving because of the potential for drowsiness
- To notify caregivers when any of the preceding problems occur and when a sore throat, bleeding or bruising, a skin rash, or a pregnancy occurs

Related Oxazolidinedione

Paramethadione (Paradione) is related to trimethadione and is similar to that drug in most respects. The dosage for treating absence seizures is the same for both drugs, with the caveat that the liquid form, which has a high alcohol content, should be diluted before being given to children.

BENZODIAZEPINES: DIAZEPAM, CLONAZEPAM, CLORAZEPATE

The benzodiazepines are primarily prescribed for their antianxiety properties and are thoroughly reviewed in Chapter 6, Anxiety Disorders. However, three benzodiazepines are indicated for treating seizure disorders. The antiepileptic indications for benzodiazepines are briefly reviewed in this chapter.

Diazepam Indication: Treating Status Epilepticus

Diazepam (Valium) is the prototype benzodiazepine and is a drug of choice for treating status epilepticus. Diazepam is effective about 95% of the time in controlling these life-threatening seizures. Diazepam is also used adjunctively to treat other types of epilepsy.

A dose of 5 to 10 mg of diazepam given intravenously stops most seizures within 5 minutes. Because the serum levels fall rapidly, it may be necessary to repeat the dose to maintain a seizure-free state. Typically, repeated doses at 10- to 15-minute intervals may be required. No more than 30 mg of diazepam should be given to treat a single episode of status epilepticus (Olin, 1995). If a second episode of status epilepticus should occur within 2 to 4 hours, this protocol can be repeated (Olin, 1995). Because of residual metabolites of diazepam, caution should be used. All IV injections of diazepam must be administered slowly (no more than 5 mg per minute) to avoid thrombosis, phlebitis, and venous irritation. Children and infants have a significantly lower dosage restriction than do adults (Table 7-5).

Combination treatment. Because of the short-lived effect of diazepam, a phenytoin infusion (18 mg/kg or less at a rate no faster than 50 mg/min) can be hung to follow the first dose of diazepam, thereby avoiding repeated doses of diazepam.

If diazepam is used exclusively (up to 30 mg) and seizures are refractory to treatment, an IV phenytoin drip can be provided. A phenobarbital drip (at 100 mg/min) is the next option but should not follow diazepam because of the synergistic effect of these drugs in depressing respirations. For seizures still not controlled, a paraldehyde infusion should be considered. As a final resort, anesthesia coupled with a neuromuscular blocker can be administered to stop refractory status epilepticus.

Although the discussion of diazepam as a drug of choice for status epilepticus is informative, the real-life task of starting an IV line in a patient with this type of seizure is no easy matter. Should starting the IV line become impossible, an alternative is to inject the drug into a large muscle or to give a diazepam enema. These routes of administration are not as effective but decrease the seizures over time.

Diazepam can be given orally as an adjunct to chronic treatment of convulsive disorders (10 mg four times a day) when the possibility of withdrawal seizures is likely.

Because diazepam has a wide therapeutic index, when it is given alone, it is a safe drug. When mixed with other CNS depressants, however, diazepam can cause severe CNS depression. This fact is of slight clinical importance when diazepam is being used to treat the life-threatening emergency status epilepticus, but it becomes more significant when the drug is used adjunctively to treat other seizure forms. In either situation, support for ventilation and monitoring of blood pressure are critical precautions. Pharmacokinetics, side effects, and clinical implications for diazepam usage are discussed in Chapter 6, Anxiety Disorders.

Clonazepam Indication: Lennox-Gastaut

Clonazepam (Klonopin) is effective in treating Lennox-Gastaut syndrome, a variant form of absence seizure, akinetic, and myoclonic seizures. It may also be effective in treating absence seizures not responsive to the succinimides. Approximately one third of the patients taking clonazepam have breakthrough seizures, indicating a development of tolerance to this drug. Dosage adjustment can restore drug effectiveness. Therapeutic serum levels for clonazepam are 20 to 80 ng/mL. Clonazepam and valproic acid used concurrently can stimulate absence status epilepticus (prolonged absence seizures). Dosage information is found in Table 7-5.

Clorazepate Indication: Partial Seizures

Clorazepate (Tranxene) is used adjunctively to treat partial seizures. Children under age 9 should not be given this drug. Clorazepate's antianxiety effects and pharmacokinetic properties are discussed in Chapter 6, Anxiety Disorders. See Table 7-5 for dosage information.

OTHER ANTIEPILEPTICS

Several important antiepileptics do not lend themselves to convenient groupings. The most significant of these are carbamazepine (Tegretol), valproic acid (Depakene), gabapentin (Neurontin), and lamotrigine (Lamictal). In addition, there are a handful of rarely used drugs, such as acetazolamide, lidocaine, magnesium sulfate, and paraldehyde, for which antiepileptic properties are secondary uses. Finally, there are a few antiepileptic medications, namely, phenacemide (Phenurone) and felbamate (Felbatol), that have such adverse or dangerous side effects that they are seldom prescribed. The most significant of these other antiepileptics are carbamazepine and valproic acid. Both of these drugs are now being appreciated for more than their antiepileptic properties. For instance, both are effective in treating refractory bipolar illness (Keltner and Folks, 1991).

CARBAMAZEPINE

Carbamazepine (Tegretol) is a major antiepileptic that is finding considerable use in new and interesting ways. It is related to the TCAs, and some patients taking this antiepileptic testify to improved mood (see Chapter 5, Mood Disorders). Further, carbamazepine is used successfully for patients suffering from bipolar disorder and those with schizophrenia. Both disorders have evidence of ictal or seizure-related phenomena and respond to carbamazepine (Carpenter et al, 1991). Although carbamazepine is an effective antiepileptic, some clinicians are reluctant to prescribe it because of its potential toxic effects.

Pharmacologic Effect

Although its exact mechanism of action is not known, carbamazepine is thought to reduce polysynaptic responses, thus preventing the spread of seizures (Olin, 1995). Carbamazepine is indicated for complex partial, tonic-clonic, or mixed seizures. It is not effective in controlling absence seizures. Other uses for carbamazepine include pain relief in persons with trigeminal neuralgia and restless leg syndrome, posttraumatic stress disorder, and, as just mentioned, schizophrenia and bipolar disorder.

Pharmacokinetics

Carbamazepine is slowly but adequately absorbed from the GI tract. Peak serum levels are reached within 5 hours after oral administration, and steady state is achieved within 2 to 4 days. Carbamazepine is bound to serum proteins (76%). It is metabolized in the liver to an active metabolite. Initially the half-life in drug-naive patients ranges from 25 to 65 hours, but after sustained dosage the half-life is reduced to 12 to 17 hours. Carbamazepine is eliminated through urinary (72%) and fecal (28%) excretions. Table 7-5 contains dosage information.

Side Effects

The most serious side effects of carbamazepine are hematologic reactions. Cases of fatal agranulocytosis have been reported. Although the absolute incidence of this side effect is low (1 in 50,000 persons), it is about 5 to 8 times greater than for the general public (Olin, 1995). Besides agranulocytosis, aplastic anemia, thrombocytopenia, increased prothrombin time, and leukopenia are potential effects of this drug. Patients with a history of bone marrow depression should not receive this drug.

More common yet less severe reactions to carbamazepine than those previously mentioned include drowsiness, dizziness, unsteadiness, nausea, and diplopia. Other adverse reactions include activation of latent psychosis, confusion in elderly patients, hepatic and renal damage, and dermatologic problems.

Implications

Therapeutic versus toxic levels. Therapeutic serum levels are 4 to 12 μg/mL. Levels above 12 μg/mL are potentially toxic. A toxic dose of carbamazepine ranges from 5 g in small children to 30 g in adults. The first signs of overdose appear within 1 to 3 hours of administration and tend to be neuromuscular. Muscle restlessness, twitching, exaggerated reflexes, and, finally, reflex depression are among the initial indications of overdose. Large overdoses lead to respiratory difficulties; cardiovascular symptoms such as arrhythmias, tachycardia, and hypotension or hypertension; and seizures.

Although there is no specific antidote for carbamazepine, supportive care and elimination of the drug from the body can save the patient's life. Supportive care might include elevating the patient's legs when hypotension develops, monitoring blood pressure, continued surveillance of vital signs until full recovery, and intubation for respiratory difficulty.

Gastric lavage, even after several hours have passed, can help the patient recover from overdose. If alcohol is involved, gastric lavage is even more significant. Unless otherwise indicated, vomiting should be induced immediately after discovering an overdose. Activated charcoal given through a nasal gastric tube is warranted as well. Hemodialysis in cases of severe overdose, replacement therapy in small children, and the administration of an osmotic-based diuretic to hasten renal excretion are other interventions for carbamazepine poisoning. Parenteral diazepam or phenobarbital is indicated to control acute seizures brought on by carbamazepine overdose, but they may cause additional respiratory depression.

Use in pregnancy. Carbamazepine is not recommended for use during pregnancy. Breast-feeding is usually discouraged because breast milk can contain a level of the drug as high as 60% of the mother's drug serum level (Vestermark and Vestermark, 1991).

Side effects. Complete blood cell counts, hepatic and renal function tests, and eye examinations should be performed before carbamazepine therapy begins and routinely thereafter. If a significant abnormality in any of the preceding areas should develop, the patient's condition should be carefully monitored or the drug discontinued and a new antiepileptic ordered, to prevent exacerbation of seizure activity. Because fatal agranulocytosis has been reported, when carbamazepine is discontinued based on hematologic grounds, blood levels should be determined regularly, perhaps as often as daily. In the elderly patient, confusion and CNS symptoms necessitate special attention.

Interactions. Carbamazepine interacts with many drugs but can effectively be given concurrently with other antiepileptic agents. When given with drugs such as phenytoin, phenobarbital, or primidone, an increase in the respective doses of these drugs may be necessary because carbamazepine speeds their metabolism.

Drugs that increase serum levels of carbamazepine. Cimetidine, diltiazem, erythromycin, fluoxetine, propoxyphene, and verapamil augment the effect of carbamazepine. Although increased serum carbamazepine levels won't require the clinician to abandon these combinations, careful monitoring of the patient is indicated should any of these drugs be ordered concurrently with carbamazepine.

Drugs that decrease serum levels of carbamazepine. Charcoal, phenobarbital, phenytoin, and primidone decrease the effect of carbamazepine.

Drug serum level increased by carbamazepine. Carbamazepine possibly increases the effect of phenytoin.

Drug serum levels decreased by carbamazepine. Carbamazepine decreases the effect of acetaminophen, haloperidol, oral contraceptives, succinimides, theophylline, and valproic acid.

Additionally, because the interactions of carbamazepine and lithium and carbamazepine and haloperidol can cause a neurotoxic condition, such combinations should be used with caution.

Patient education. As with other antiepileptics, carbamazepine may cause GI tract upset, so the patient is advised to take the drug with food to avoid nausea, vomiting, and the like. Because drowsiness, dizziness, and blurred vision can complicate driving, precautions should also be taken. Because of the seriousness of hematologic reactions, the patient should notify the physician or nurse when any of the signs and symptoms of blood dyscrasia are present, that is, sore throat, bruising, bleeding, fever, chills, and so forth.

VALPROIC ACID AND DERIVATIVES

Valproic acid and its derivatives, sodium valproate and divalproex sodium, are frequently prescribed antiepileptics. Valproic acid is a drug of choice for absence and tonic-clonic seizures and is used to treat myoclonic and complex partial seizures as well (Table 7-2). Valproic acid is gaining acceptance as an effective treatment of bipolar disorder as well (Keltner, Folks, 1991).

Pharmacologic Effects

Valproic acid apparently inhibits the spread of abnormal discharges through the brain. Although the precise nature of this action is not known, it is hypothesized that three mechanisms may be responsible (Olin, 1995): (1) an increase in gamma-aminobutyric acid (GABA), (2) an increased postsynaptic response to GABA, or 3) an increase in the resting membrane potential.

Pharmacokinetics

Valproic acid is rapidly absorbed after oral ingestion, whether taken in capsule or syrup form. Peak serum levels occur in less than 4 hours. Concurrent food intake and use of the enteric-coated form, divalproex sodium, slows absorption. Valproic acid is rapidly distributed in the body and is highly bound to serum proteins. The therapeutic serum level is 50 to 100 μg/mL. Valproic acid is metabolized mostly in the liver and excreted in the urine. The serum half-life is relatively short, 6 to 16 hours. Children with immature livers and older patients with cirrhosis or acute hepatitis have prolonged half-lives (67 hours and 25 hours, respectively). Table 7-5 contains dosage information.

Side Effects

Valproic acid causes relatively few serious side effects. This quality and its broad clinical utility are responsible for its growing acceptance as a major antiepileptic. Some GI tract symptoms are common during early therapy, but these disappear after continued usage. Also, prescription of the enteric-coated form reduces GI tract discomfort. Almost 10% of the patients taking valproic acid gain weight. At therapeutic levels, only phenytoin causes less drowsiness than valproic acid.

Fatal hepatic failure has been associated with valproic acid and is most likely to occur in children under age 2. Valproic acid is often given with other antiepileptics, which confounds efforts to know the true extent of hepatoxicity. Nonetheless, valproic acid and its derivatives are contraindicated in patients with liver disease and in children most at risk, those under 6 months of age.

Other adverse reactions can include emotional upset, some alopecia, and musculoskeletal weakness.

Implications

Therapeutic versus toxic levels. Therapeutic serum levels of valproic acid are 50 to 100 μg/mL. At serum concentrations above this level, CNS depression and coma develop. These events are most likely to result when valproic acid and phenobarbital are given concurrently. Restlessness and visual hallucinations are also symptoms of overdosage. Because valproic acid is absorbed quickly, treatment is supportive unless it begins soon after the drug was ingested. If little time has elapsed, gastric lavage and forced emesis can reduce absorption and should be attempted. If absorption has occurred, support of respiratory and cardiovascular systems is most appropriate. Hemodialysis has been used. Naloxone (Narcan), the narcotic antagonist, may reverse the CNS depressant effects of valproic acid. However, because naloxone could also reverse antiepileptic effects, it should be used cautiously.

Use in pregnancy. Valproic acid is teratogenic and should not be used unless other antiepileptics have been found ineffective. The Centers for Disease Control estimate a risk of 1% to 2% for spina bifida in infants of mothers taking this drug (Olin, 1995). Only when the risk to the mother's health is otherwise so great that withholding valproic acid could be deemed irresponsible practice should this drug be prescribed. Concentrations of valproic acid in breast milk have been found to be 1% to 10% of the mother's serum level of the drug.

Side effects. Again, serious side effects of valproic acid are uncommon. Drowsiness typically disappears after usage. Hepatoxicity, although potentially fatal, can be averted by testing hepatic function before treatment and by screening certain groups of patients, that is, infants and children under age 2 and individuals with liver dysfunction. Gastrointestinal tract problems are alleviated by taking this drug with food.

Interactions. Valproic acid interacts with several drugs. It potentiates the actions of other CNS depressants, such as alcohol and barbiturates, by inhibiting hepatic metabolism of those agents. Some seizure disorders may best be treated with a combination of valproic acid and clonazepam; however, evidence also indicates a potential for decreased efficacy of both drugs.

Drugs that increase serum level of valproic acid. Chlorpromazine *increases* the half-life of valproic acid, as does aspirin. Because valproic acid inhibits platelet aggregation, use with aspirin and warfarin can cause prolonged bleeding and warrants close monitoring.

Drug serum levels increased by valproic acid. Phenytoin serum levels are *increased* by valproic acid (as a result of protein-binding displacement), as are the plasma levels of phenobarbital (inhibition of hepatic metabolism) and ethosuximide. Phenobarbital serum levels are increased by as much as 200% when valproic acid is given concurrently; consequently, when given together, the amount of phenobarbital should be reduced. A similar interaction may occur with the related antiepileptics mephobarbital and primidone.

Patient education. Teach the patient:

To take valproic acid with food, if GI tract upset should occur

To swallow tablets or capsules whole to avoid irritation of mouth and throat

To take the drug at bedtime to minimize effects of drowsiness, and to be cautious when driving

To notify those monitoring for diabetes because valproic acid may give false-positive blood and urine ketone values.

Related Drugs

Valproate (Depakene syrup) is the sodium salt of valproic acid, as is the enteric-coated divalproex sodium (Depakote), a compound that contains equal portions of valproic acid and valproate. Dosages are equivalent. Noticeable differences are the more rapid absorption when the syrup is used and the delayed absorption with the enteric-coated divalproex. Divalproex may reduce GI tract irritation.

GABAPENTIN

Gabapentin (Neurontin), a new antiepileptic approved in early 1994, is an adjunctive treatment for partial seizures in adults and adolescents older than age 12 (Laxer, 1994). This drug is similar to gamma-aminobutyric acid in structure but with molecular alterations to make it more lipophilic and hence better able to penetrate the blood brain barrier (Ramsey et al, 1993).

Absorption of gabapentin is dose-dependent at high dosages (Andrews and Fischer, 1994). Food does not alter absorption. It has a relatively short half-life of 5 to 8 hours. It is not protein bound to any extent ($<3\%$). It is not meaurably metabolized and so is excreted as an unchanged molecule in the urine. Patients with decreased kidney function should be given smaller doses of this drug. Therapeutic serum levels are >2 μg/mL.

Gabapentin is well tolerated and typically produces mild side effects. The most common of these are somnolence, dizziness, ataxia, and nystagmus (Olin, 1995). Gabapentin has no drug interactions with other antiepileptics. Antacids reduce the bioavailability of gabapentin, and cimetidine increases it. Dosage information is found in Table 7-5.

LAMOTRIGINE

Lamotrigine (Lamictal) was approved in late 1994 as an adjunctive treatment for partial seizures and may have implications for more generalized seizures. It is related to the antifolate compound pyrimidine. It blocks sustained repetitive firing of neurons by prolonging the inactivation of sodium channels in animal models (Meldrum, 1994), and it may be by this mechanism that it suppresses seizure activity.

Lamotrigine is rapidly absorbed, reaches peak plasma levels in 1.5 to 4 hours, and is moderately bound to plasma proteins (55%). When patients are prescribed lamotrigine alone, its half-life is 25 hours. When combined with enzyme inducers, that is, carbamazepine, or enzyme inhibitors, that is, valproic acid, the half-life can increase or decrease accordingly (Ramsey, 1993). Therapeutic serum levels are >2 μg/mL.

Side effects are usually mild. Common complaints include diplopia, somnolence, dizziness, ataxia, and blurred vision.

LESS FREQUENTLY USED ANTIEPILEPTICS

Acetazolamide

Acetazolamide (Diamox) is a diuretic that inhibits the enzyme carbonic anhydrase. This mechanism alkalinizes the urine, causing mild systemic acidosis. This reduction in blood pH reduces seizures in some individuals. Acetazolamide is used adjunctively to treat absence, tonic-clonic, and myoclonic seizures. There is convincing evidence that acetazolamide is an effective agent for treating refractory bipolar illness as well (Hayes, 1994).

Lidocaine

Lidocaine (Xylocaine) is a local anesthetic and an antiarrhythmic drug. Its one significant antiepileptic use is as one of the last treatments to be used when attempting to interrupt status epilepticus. The recommended dose is 50 to 100 mg injected IV. High doses of lidocaine can precipitate status epilepticus in otherwise seizure-free patients.

Magnesium sulfate

Patients with lowered levels of magnesium, that is, eclampsia and alcohol withdrawal syndrome, are subject to seizures. Magnesium sulfate given IM (preferred) or IV can prevent these seizures. Because low serum magnesium levels are ongoing in these conditions, it may be necessary to administer magnesium sulfate frequently.

Paraldehyde

Historically paraldehyde has been used to control seizures associated with alcohol withdrawal. New drugs are now being used for this purpose; however, paraldehyde remains a viable agent for treating status epilepticus when other drugs have failed. It is administered IM or IV.

ANTIEPILEPTICS WITH SEVERE OR DANGEROUS SIDE EFFECTS

Phenacemide

Phenacemide (Phenurone), although effective for treating severe forms of mixed complex-partial seizures (psychomotor) refractory to other drugs, is a seldom-used antiepileptic because of the intensity of its side effects. Phenacemide can cause direct toxicity in organs, for example, liver damage.

Phenacemide is well absorbed from the intestine and is metabolized in the liver. Therapeutic serum levels have not been established. To reduce side effects, initial doses are much lower than maintenance doses. Common side effects include anorexia, weight loss, nausea, drowsiness, dizziness, weakness, and ataxia. More serious effects include nephritis and reported fatal blood dyscrasias. A major concern are the psychologic side effects associated with this drug. Aggression, suicidal tendencies, and acute psychosis may necessitate discontinuance of the drug. Table 7-5 provides dosage information.

Felbamate

Felbamate (Felbatol) was approved in 1993 for adjunctive or monotherapy in adults with partial or tonic-clonic seizures and as an adjunctive therapy for children with Lennox-Gastaut syndrome (Laxer, 1994). Because of an unusually high incidence of aplastic anemia associated with felbamate, both the manufacturer and the FDA recommended its immediate withdrawal from the market. As of fall 1995 the suspension remains in place except in those cases in which the physician believes withdrawing felbamate would be a significant setback for the patient.

AGENTS PENDING APPROVAL BY THE FDA

Several new agents may soon be available to the general public. Vigabatrin may be licensed next year and is thought to have a role in managing intractable complex partial seizures when standard antiepileptic therapy has failed (Buchanan, 1994). Other new agents on the horizon include tiagabine, topiramate, and remacemide (Patsalos and Sander, 1994).

REFERENCES

Andrews CO, Fischer JH: Gabapentin: a new agent for the management of epilepsy, *Ann Pharmacother* 28(10):1188, 1994.

Berg AT, Shinnar S: Relapse following discontinuation of antiepileptic drugs: a meta-analysis, *Neurology* 44(4):601-608, 1994.

Borgsdorf LR, Caldwell JW: *Clinical therapeutics: a disease-oriented approach to pharmacology and therapeutics*, Bakersfield, Calif, 1985, Kern Medical Center.

Buchanan N: Vigabatrin use in 72 patients with drug-resistant epilepsy, *Seizure* 3(3):191, 1994.

Carpenter WT et al: Carbamazepine maintenance treatment in outpatient schizophrenics, *Arch Gen Psychiatry* 48(1):69-72, 1991.

Commission on Classification and Terminology of the International League Against Epilepsy, *Epilepsia* 22:489, 1981.

Dalessio JD: Seizure disorders and pregnancy, *New Engl J Med* 312:559, 1985.

Delgado-Escueta AV, Treiman DM, Walsh GO: The treatable epilepsies, *New Engl J Med* 308:1508, 1576, 1983.

Delgado-Escueta AV et al: Management of status epilepticus, *New Engl J Med* 306:1337, 1982.

Engel J, Starkman S: Overview of seizures, *Emerg Med Clin North Am* 12(4):895, 1994.

Hayes SG: Acetazolamide in bipolar affective disorders, *Ann Clin Psychiatry* 6(2):91-98, 1994.

Jallon P: Electroencephalogram and epilepsy, *Eur Neurol* 34(suppl)1:18, 1994.

Jordan KG: Status epilepticus: a perspective from the neuroscience intensive care unit, *Neurosurg Clin N Am* 5 (4):671, 1994.

Keltner NL: Anticonvulsant drugs. In Shlafer M, Marieb EN, editors: *The nurse, pharmacology, and drug therapy,* Redwood City, Calif, 1993, Addison-Wesley.

Keltner NL, Folks, DG: Alternatives to lithium in the treatment of bipolar disorder, *Perspect Psychiatric Care* 27(2):36, 1991.

Keltner NL, Schwecke LH, Bostrom CE, editors: *Psychiatric Nursing,* St Louis, 1995, Mosby.

Laxer KD: Guidelines for treating epilepsy in the age of felbamate, vigabatrin, lamotrigine, and gabapentin, *West J Med* 161(3):309, 1994.

Meldrum BS: Lamotrigine: a novel approach, *Seizure* 3(suppl A):41, 1994.

McKenna PJ, Kane JM, Parrish K: Psychotic syndromes in epilepsy, *Am J Psychiatry* 142:895, 1985.

Norman SE, Browne TR: Seizure disorders, *Am J Nurs* 81:984, 1981.

Olin BR, editor: *Drug facts and comparisons,* St Louis, 1995, Wolters Kluwer.

Parks BR, Dostrow VG, Noble SL: Drug therapy for epilepsy, *Am Fam Physician* 59(3):639, 1994.

Patsalos PN, Sander JW: Newer epileptic drugs: towards an improved risk-benefit ratio, *Drug Safety* 11(1):37, 1994.

Penry JK, Newmark ME: The use of antiepileptic drugs, *Ann Intern Med* 90:207, 1979.

Ramsey RE et al: *Clinical issues in the management of epilepsy,* Miami, 1993, University of Miami Press.

Rogawski MA, Porter RJ: Antiepileptic drugs: pharmacological mechanisms and clinical efficacy with considerations of promising developmental state compounds, *Pharm Rev* 42:223, 1990.

The Medical Letter: Lamotrigine for epilepsy, *The Medical Letter* 37(944):21, 1995.

Trimble MR: *The psychoses of epilespsy,* New York, 1991, Raven.

Vestermark V, Vestermark S: Teratogenic effect of carbamazepine, *Arch Dis Child* 66(5):641, 1991.

Wilder BJ: The treatment of epilepsy: an overview of clinical practices, *Neurology* 45(suppl 3):S7, 1995.

CHAPTER 8

Sleep Disorders

HISTORICAL CONSIDERATIONS

Among the major groups of sleep disorders the dysomnias (insomnia and hypersomnia); the parasomnias; sleep disturbances resulting from narcolepsy, sleep apnea, or periodic leg movements; and psychophysiologic disturbances are most amenable to drug treatment. This chapter focuses primarily on the pharmacologic aspects of disturbed sleep.

Several factors have led to remarkable developments in the basic aspects of sleep disorders. Not until the late 1940s and early 1950s did the pioneering work take place of Nathanial Kleitman and his graduate students, Eugene Aserinsky and William Dement, at the University of Chicago (Aserinsky and Kleitman, 1953). Their work led to technologic advances in the production of reliable electrographic recordings obtained from the human brain and a variety of other organs, which allowed investigation of the neurophysiologic changes that occur on the wakefulness-to-sleep continuum.

The milestone discovery was the realization that sleep, as it progressed through the nocturnal period, was not a unitary phenomenon but indeed was characterized by a sequence of sleep stages. It was noted that physiologic changes occurred as one stage gave way to another. Furthermore, these stages were found to alternate rhythmically throughout the night. Rapid eye movement (REM) sleep was found to be a state distinct from non-REM sleep. The first two decades of sleep research reflected interest in the phenomena of REM and non-REM sleep. This research consisted of a number of studies of REM sleep that resulted in a large body of information about the physiologic, biochemical, and pharmacologic aspects of sleep. A recognition of distinct sleep disorders resulted. The basic tool of sleep research was the simultaneous electrographic recording of multiple physiologic variables, now referred to as *polysomnography* (Holland, Dement, and Raynal, 1974). Valuable to subsequent pharmacologic approaches to insomnia and other sleep disorders were research studies of the effects of hypnotic drugs (Kales et al, 1969).

The study of sleep disturbances has become an interdisciplinary field, perhaps best illustrated in the area of sleep-induced breathing disorders, particularly, obstructive sleep apnea. Half to two thirds of all patients referred to sleep disorder centers in the United States have disorders that reduce sleep. These disorders are a major cause of both social and work disability and contribute to systemic hypertension, cardiac arrhythmia, and other cardiovascular consequences (Coleman et al, 1982; Guilleminault and Dement, 1978). Hence pulmonologists, neurologists, psychiatric professionals, and others, depending on the nature of the patient's problem, work together to assess and diagnose the disorders in patients with disturbed sleep. The ability to help these patients continues to improve. Additionally, the use of questionnaires, sleep diaries, medical history, and physical and laboratory examinations have further improved the basic clinical understanding of sleep disturbances. Together with the polysomnogram, these assessment tools and pharmacologic interventions help guide the management of sleep disorder.

The polysomnogram, a measure of multiple physiologic functions during sleep, involves the patient sleeping one or sometimes two nights at a sleep center. The patient is placed in a sound-controlled private bedroom at a comfortable, controlled temperature. Electroencephalogram (EEG), eye movements, heart rate, and muscle activity from several sources are recorded to determine the physiologic state and the sleep stage. Other values specific to the patient's problems may also be measured, including electrocardiogram (ECG), air flow from the nose and mouth, and blood oxygen saturation. Nighttime recordings are often followed by daytime tests such as multiple sleep latency tests, which are quantitative measures of sleep tendency. A complete review of the physiology of sleep (sleep architecture) and electrophysiology (polysomnography) is beyond the scope of this book; however, for further reading see Mendelson (1987) or Hartmann (1974).

Although the sleep laboratory may not achieve the precise quality and architecture of sleep experienced in the patient's home, surveys indicate that fewer than 1 in 1000 patients sleep so poorly as to invalidate the procedure. Perhaps the most encouraging aspects of the growth of this field have been the high degree of patient satisfaction resulting from the use of current diagnostic and treatment modalities and the many treatment interventions that have been developed to significantly improve the patient's quality of life.

DIAGNOSTIC CONSIDERATIONS

Epidemiologic surveys suggest that 20% to 30% of adults report having sleep difficulties at least occasionally (Kales and Kales, 1984). Approximately 7% of the population use sleeping agents to increase sleep; about 1% use a prescription hypnotic 30 days or more per year (Balter and Bauer, 1975). The incidence of excessive sleepiness has varied from 0.02% to 1% in the general population. Surveys of medical patients suggest that the rate of insomnia is 17% and the rate of hypersomnia is 3% (Bixler, Kales, and Soldatos, 1979). Age and disease tend to increase the prevalence of disturbed sleep.

Quality sleep normally requires good health, comfortable circumstances, and a lengthy daily period that is free of stressful obligations. Also, freedom from the influence of stimulants and other drugs that negatively affect the structure of sleep is required for quality sleep. In short, sleep is easily disrupted. The frenetic demands of an industrial culture may induce a briefer-than-normal average sleeping time. "Ad-lib" sleepers tend to sleep better than those whose obligations compel abbreviated sleep hours; short sleepers (those who require less sleep than normal) tolerate demanding work schedules better than those who require 8 hours or more of sleep (Caraskadon and Dement, 1982).

Insomnia is defined as complaint of sleep insufficient to support good daytime functioning. Epidemiologic surveys suggest that about 15% of adults complain of insomnia, whereas only 2% actually take hypnotic medication (Kales and Kales, 1984). The majority of individuals taking hypnotic drugs use them less than 30 times per year. Thus transient insomnia is relatively common, but persistent insomnia is not. Interestingly, most individuals who come to sleep disorder clinics do so because of hypersomnia rather than insomnia (Coleman et al, 1982).

Common, nonspecific disruptions of sleep may precipitate or aggravate insomnia. Thus many individuals can improve the quality of their sleep by instituting sleep hygiene, as shown in Box 8-1. Instituting a sleep hygiene program requires that the patient's interests and motivations be carefully considered. Some aspects of good

Box 8-1 Measures Used to Improve Sleep Hygiene

1. Arise at the same time each day.
2. Limit daily in-bed time to "normal" amount.
3. Discontinue use of drugs that act on the central nervous system, e.g., caffeine, nicotine, alcohol, and stimulants.
4. Avoid daytime napping except when sleep diary indicates a better night's sleep as a result.
5. Establish physical fitness with a routine of exercise early in the day, followed by other activity.
6. Avoid evening stimulation; substitute either listening to the radio or leisure reading for watching television.
7. Try a warm, 20-minute body bath or soak near bedtime.
8. Eat on a regular schedule; avoid large meals near bedtime.
9. Practice an evening relaxation routine.
10. Maintain comfortable sleeping conditions.
11. Spend no longer than 20 minutes awake in bed.
12. Adjust sleep hours and routine to optimize daily schedule and living situation.

sleep hygiene, such as quitting smoking, are difficult to achieve. Other recommendations shown in the box may be arduous or simply may not be possible.

Persistent insomnia without coexisting medical causes is called *primary insomnia.* Although psychopathologic factors may contribute to the development of primary insomnia, some individuals may not show any comorbid psychiatric condition (Kales and Kales, 1984). Of course, psychologic arousal may result in fears or anxiety. All these psychologic factors may further disrupt sleep. Hypervigilance, anxiety, neuroticism, introversion, and insomnia all theoretically derive from common central nervous system (CNS) profiles of increased internal arousal (Grey, 1982).

Patients and clinicians alike are quick to attribute insomnia to psychologic problems. Specific psychiatric conditions do predispose persons to insomnia, in particular, mood disorders, anxiety, and the dementias. However, insomnia should not be attributed to these conditions unless reasonably good sleep hygiene measures are in place. Many patients have spent fruitless years seeking dependable sleep by means of anxiety reduction and psychotherapy while concomitantly working late, drinking coffee, and sleeping late on weekends.

Patients may complain loudly of insomnia simply because it is debilitating and because it is socially acceptable or quite easy to focus on the symptom. Whether depressed or anxious, patients who complain primarily about insomnia may do so because of a complex mixture of biopsychosocial factors. For example, many patients ascribe their depression to insomnia rather than vice versa. Patients whose moods are dysphoric in concert with insomnia may be promptly helped by sedative hypnotic drugs; however, long-lasting relief of insomnia is sustained only in a minority of patients with depression. In short, the treatment of insomnia caused by a primary psychiatric disturbance necessitates a full understanding of the patient's psychosocial and mental status, and the clinical approach must appreciate any underlying disorder per se. Moreover, drugs, caffeine, nicotine, and alcohol, so ubiquitously disruptive of sleep, must be discontinued or withdrawn in patients with insomnia, if at all possible (Tan et al, 1984).

Additionally, over-the-counter agents with CNS-stimulating actions may disrupt sleep, as may catecholamine reuptake blockers such as stimulating antidepressants (fluoxetine and protriptyline), antiarrhythmic drugs, corticosteroids, thyroid preparations, and methysergide. Diuretics may cause cramps or restless leg syndrome, or both. Sleeping pills paradoxically may worsen sleep. Short-acting agents such as triazolam may cause agitation, amnestic episodes, early-morning awakening, or even next-day anxiety. These may merge together with next-night *rebound insomnia* to compound sleeping difficulties (Kales and Kales, 1984). Thus the chronic administration of hypnotics may actually serve to diminish sleep quality.

A variety of sleep difficulties, including insomnia, may result from suboptimal sleep schedules or from medical problems. In individuals who literally have their days and nights mixed up, a tendency may develop toward later arising times, which results in delayed sleep-phase syndrome. This syndrome is most likely to occur in individuals without regular morning obligations. Disruption of the circadian rhythms may follow. Treatment includes progressively shifting the sleep hours incrementally toward a desirable, fixed schedule.

Many shift workers sleep poorly. Some of those individuals who need little sleep may prefer night work and function well on the few hours of sleep that they are able to obtain. However, other shift workers sleep poorly and feel chronically fatigued. Among those in the country's work force, workers on rotating shifts have perhaps the most difficulty. These rotating-shift workers and their employers should consider the problems associated with disruption of circadian rhythms. A potential partial solution is less frequent changing of shifts, for example, changing shifts monthly rather than weekly. Such a common-sense approach may result in a less significant disturbance of sleep. Individuals who are intolerant of shifting work schedules may have chronic fatigue or may ultimately become disabled or debilitated, in some cases necessitating a career change or a significant change in occupation. Professions that are particularly stressful in this regard include nursing, meteorology, and military service.

Although an individual's work hours may normally vary in relation to sleep hours, those with a tendency toward insomnia may make matters worse by sleeping late on weekends. In fact, rising at a predictable hour, going to bed at a regular time, and the previously discussed normal sequencing of sleep may all be compromised by these disruptions in regular sleep hours. Often patients, after examining a monthly sleep chart, are astounded at what they find, having been unaware of their irregular sleep schedule. In short, what these individuals need is a regular bedtime.

Symptoms of disease, such as itching or pain, may raise the threshold for sleep. Other symptoms, including dyspnea, nocturia, diarrhea, angina, migraine, or other medical problems, may disrupt sleep significantly. Settings in which persons with medical problems are found, such as inpatient hospitals or long-term care settings, may be buzzing with constant activity, have enforced sleeping positions, noises, and periodic crises, which hardly encourage adequate sleep. These clinical settings may sometimes actually exceed the Environmental Protection Agency guidelines for healthy noise levels.

The specifics of a patient's illness and treatment may further worsen the quality of sleep. For example, the patient in the intensive care unit is interrupted an average of five times per hour, even during the calmest of nights (Dlin et al, 1971). Any nonpsychiatric medical condition that potentially disrupts sleep may increase the risk of insomnia. Fear and worry, together with significant symptoms, may indicate the need for an appropriate therapeutic intervention. Direct effects of disease on sleep-regulating mechanisms can cause sleep disruption. Examples of such disease states include alteration of neurotransmitter systems, unpredictable metabolism associated with liver disease, or cortical dysfunction with primary dementia. Individuals with primary sleep problems most often identified with sleep disturbance include those with obstructive sleep apnea (discussed later); those with cardiovascular disorders, especially angina; those predisposed to breathing impairment; and those with an increased metabolic rate in concert with an endocrinopathy such as mild hyperthyroidism or diabetes. Patients with Cushing's disease and individuals with neurologic conditions such as a seizure disorder or Parkinson's disease are at risk for disturbed sleep. Esophageal reflux, chronic renal failure with uremia, other end-organ failure, and urinary frequency, fetal movements, and general discomfort women experience in the third trimester of pregnancy all may cause a diminished quantity and quality of sleep.

DRUGS USED TO TREAT INSOMNIA

Currently sleep disorders are categorized as insomnia, hypersomnia, and a variety of sleep disorders related to a psychiatric disturbance, a secondary sleep disorder, or a substance-induced sleep disorder. Insomnia and hypersomnia are conceptualized as being either primary or secondary. Insomnia and hypersomnia, narcolepsy, the parasomnias, periodic leg movements (nocturnal myoclonus), and sleep apnea are among the disorders most frequently responsive to or affected by pharmacologic intervention (Box 8-2).

Many drugs, including those used to treat insomnia, alter sleep and daytime function. They may mask wakefulness during sleep or diminish alertness during wakefulness. Changes in sleep may remain unnoticed by the individual, and even with daytime sedation, patients may be unaware of their impaired performance. Thus the effects that many drugs may have on the sleep-wakefulness continuum are clinically relevant. Moreover, many drugs modify REM activity. For example, with the tricyclic antidepressants this effect may even correlate with a response to therapy.

The following discussion of psychotropic drugs used to treat sleep disorders addresses the mechanisms of neurotransmission and neuromodulation and outlines implications for the use of sedatives or other psychotropics in specified patients with particular diagnostic sleep-wake problems. This chapter is devoted primarily to the clinical pharmacology of hypnotics and their role in therapeutics, but drugs that, although not used primarily to treat insomnia, may be used to treat other disturbances of sleep or daytime alertness are also identified.

The use of hypnotics to relieve insomnia should be temporary. More prescriptions are written for hypnotic and anxiolytic drugs than for any other class of drugs in the United States. Although the benzodiazepines have almost completely replaced the barbiturates, all known hypnotics promote sleep and inhibit wakefulness. The effects on sleep and wakefulness should not be separated. *All* hypnotic drugs shorten the time that elapses before a person falls asleep (sleep latency), reduce nocturnal wakefulness, increase total sleep time, and decrease body movements during sleep; all also cause difficulty in arousal from sleep. Thus hypnotics are generally viewed as CNS depressants and are specifically viewed as sleep-promoting compounds. This view is supported inasmuch as large doses of long-acting compounds depress and possibly interfere with the wakening function. Thus there are both short- and long-term benefits and risks associated with the use of hypnotics. The benefit-to-risk ratio should be weighed carefully with the knowledge that the aim of

Box 8-2 Sleep Disorders Recognized by the American Sleep Disorders Association

Dyssomnias
Intrinsic sleep disorders
Psychophysiological
Narcolepsy
Hypersomnias
Obstructive sleep
Apnea
Central nervous system sleep apnea
Periodic limb movement disorder
Restless leg syndrome
Extrinsic sleep disorders
Inadequate sleep hygiene
Environmental sleep disorder
Hypnotic-dependent sleep disorder
Stimulant-dependent sleep disorder
Alcohol-dependent sleep disorder
Circadian rhythm sleep disorders
Jet lag
Work, shift-related
Delayed sleep-phase
Advanced sleep-phase

Parasomnias
Arousal disorders
Confusional-arousal disorder
Sleepwalking
Sleep terrors
Sleep-wake transition disorders
Sleep-starts disorder
Sleep-talking disorder
REM sleep-related disorders
Nightmares
Sleep paralysis
REM sleep-related behavior conduct
Hypnotic-dependent sleep disorder

Psychiatric, neurologic, and other medical sleep disorders
Psychiatric
Psychosis
Mood disorders
Anxiety disorders
Panic disorder
Alcoholism
Neurologic
Dementia
Parkinsonism
Epilepsy
Other medical disorders

Proposed sleep disorders
Fragmentary myoclonus
Menstrual-associated sleep disorders
Others

a good night's sleep should be to improve the patient's vigor during the following day. Rarely has this result been demonstrated as a consequence of the use of hypnotic drugs.

Drug treatment for insomnia is all too often casual, and diagnostic features may be incorrect. Long-term use of sedatives usually relieves only sedative-withdrawal insomnia, that is, the insomnia caused by the sedative itself, not the original insomnia. Of the 3% of adults who use prescribed hypnotics, about 20% use drugs more than 120 days per year (Mellinger, Balter, and Uhlenhuth, 1985). Such drugs are disproportionately prescribed for older adults in whom the drugs can aggravate cortical dysfunction and psychologic regression.

As previously noted, the most appropriate and important management approaches to insomnia are removal or treatment of the cause and an alteration of poor sleep habits. Hypnotics, when prescribed, should be administered in short courses and in low doses; alternate or every-other-night therapy is recommended. Treatment should be monitored, and the emergence of nocturnal confusion, agitation, and restlessness, especially in older patients and children, should be carefully considered. As for the patients discussed in Chapters 15, 16, and 17, combining an initial course of pharmacotherapy with a nonpharmacologic approach, such as behavioral techniques, and then optimizing the medical and physiologic status of the patient provide an ideal approach.

A useful initial approach to a patient with insomnia is to consider the duration of the complaint. Long-term insomnia (months or years), short-term insomnia (a week or so), and transient difficulties (periodic bouts of insomnia for 2 to 3 days) should be approached quite differently. The duration of the insomnia not only provides an indication of the origin of insomnia but also may help guide the use of psychotropic agents, specifically, hypnotics. Although hypnotics may be appropriately prescribed for patients with long-term insomnia, in these individuals a diligent evaluation is necessary before hypnotics are prescribed. As shown in Figure 8-1, the drugs are most appropriately prescribed when there is clear evidence of disturbed sleep without an apparent and direct cause. In contrast to long-term insomnia, most other cases involve healthy individuals who wish to carry out their day-to-day activ-

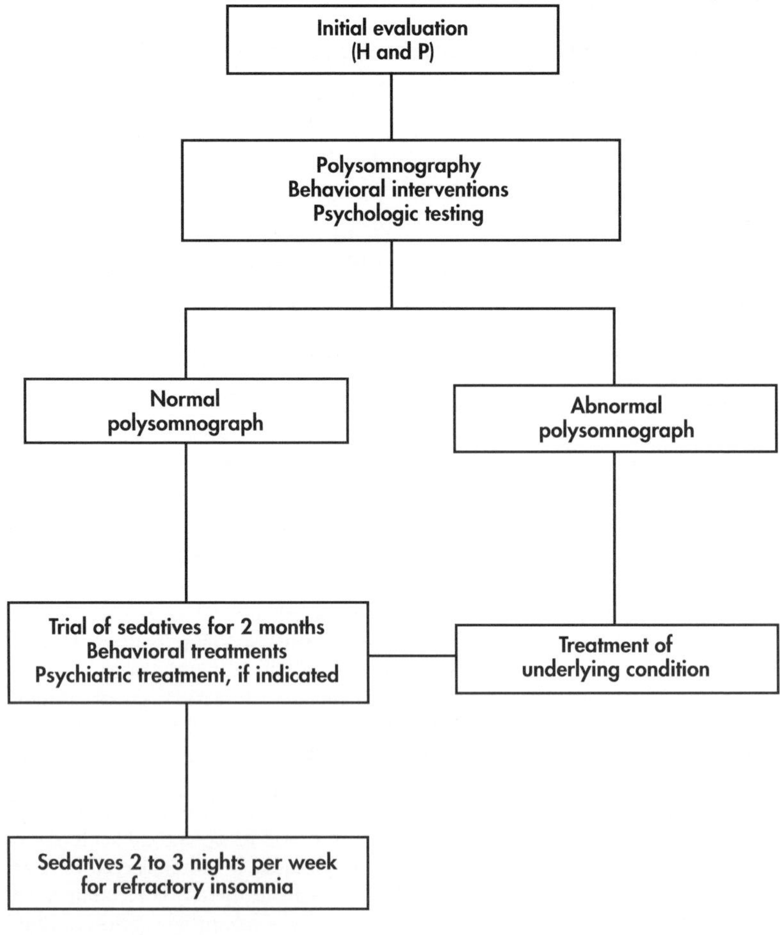

Figure 8-1 Flow chart for the evaluation and treatment of severe insomnia. (From Wooten V: *Psychiatr Ann* 20(8):466, 1990.)

ities free from the residual effects of insomnia. For these individuals benzodiazepines and, to a lesser extent, antidepressant medications are most frequently prescribed. Other drug classes that may be considered useful include phenothiazines, which may improve sleep in psychotic patients; phenytoin to treat the paroxysmal nightmares associated with psychomotor attacks; beta-adrenergic antagonists to treat disturbed sleep in association with hyperthyroidism; and cimetidine or other H_2-receptor blockers for patients with peptic ulcer disease, nonulcer dyspepsia, or reflux. Many patients have "pseudoinsomnia"; they complain of poor sleep, but polysomnograph studies are normal. These patients benefit best from no drug intervention.

Neurochemical Effects of Hypnotics

As with other psychiatric disturbances, changes in sleep and wakefulness are believed to arise from the activity of chemical agents that influence communication between neurons. In particular, monoamines are synthesized as neurotransmitters and are now known to play a particular role in the control of alert states. Other, less well-known neurotransmitter systems (outlined in Chapter 3, Neuropharmacology and Psychotropic Drugs) may also ultimately prove important. These neurochemical processes, of course, can be modulated by drugs. Psychotropics that may have some role in treating sleep disturbances are currently divided into the following categories:

1. Neurotransmitter metabolism modifiers, including precursors such as L-tryptophan or levodopa
2. Enzyme inhibitors that affect the synthesis or catabolism of the neurotransmitter
3. Drugs that alter the distribution or utilization of the transmitter, for example, reserpine, alphamethyldopa, or monoamine oxidase inhibitors (MAOIs).

Psychotropic drug treatment of sleep disturbance is carried out with the recognition that many drugs have distinct or opposite actions on the CNS at different concentrations; that is, complex dose-response relationships exist. For example, some drugs have a stimulatory effect followed by a sedative effect. Feedback mechanisms that operate within the CNS may also be responsible for complex or paradoxic responses to psychotropics.

Considerable attention recently has been devoted to the pharmacology of the benzodiazepines. As discussed in Chapter 6, Anxiety Disorders, these agents modulate gamma-aminobutyric acid (GABA) transmission and interact with specific receptor sites in the brain (Mohler and Okada, 1977). As discussed in Chapter 3, Neuropharmacology and Psychotropic Drugs, GABA is the most abundant inhibitor neurotransmitter in the CNS and about a third of all synapses are GABA-nergic. Most neurons that release this neurotransmitter, however, are interneurons that modulate activity by presynaptic and postsynaptic inhibition. Many intrinsic neurons found within the raphe nuclei and their terminals form inhibitory synapses with serotonergic receptor sites or cells. Terminals are also identified within the locus ceruleus, but the cell bodies of origin are unknown. Although GABA inhibits the activity of the locus ceruleus, the exact mode of action is unclear. A minority of neurons, such as Purkinje's cells in the cerebellum or the GABA-nergic neurons of the striatonigral pathway, project distantly in the brain, probably having complex effects. Moreover, the classic benzodiazepines such as diazepam appear to bind without substantial regional differences. Benzodiazepine-1 receptors located primarily on postsynaptic membranes are distinguished from benzodiazepine-2 receptors, which are presynaptic. The anxiolytic and antiepileptic effects are thought to be related to the agonistic effect on benzodiazepine-1 receptors, whereas sedation may result from activation of the benzodiazepine-2 receptors (Hirsch, Garrett, and Beer, 1985).

BENZODIAZEPINES

Benzodiazepines were first synthesized by Leo Sternback in 1933. In 1956 his colleague Lowell Randell found that chlordiazepoxide (Librium) had tranquilizing effects in animals (Haefely, 1983). Chlordiazepoxide was introduced for clinical use from 1960 to 1961, spawning a series of vastly successful drugs used to treat insomnia. It also is used to treat anxiety, tension, epilepsy, muscle spasm, and neuropsychiatric disturbances. Interestingly, most hypnotic drugs also relieve anxiety (and most CNS stimulant drugs also produce anxiety). As mentioned in Chapter 6, Anxiety Disorders, the effects of benzodiazepines on anxiety and alertness are sometimes difficult to distinguish. Most, if not all, benzodiazepines produce both anxiolytic and hypnotic effects. The selectivity or behavioral effect of benzodiazepines is a product of pharmacokinetic factors. Thus many compounds may have an anxiolytic profile at low doses and a hypnotic profile at high doses. The pattern of metabolism in which many benzodiazepines may be converted to the same metabolite may also account for a specific drug's utility in treatment.

The anxiolytic or hypnotic use of benzodiazepines may have been determined by the pattern of research development or clinical testing. For example, it was found early on that *oxazepam* (Serax) was not an effective sleep inducer but that anxiety was reduced when oxazepam was given in doses that did not cause somnolence (Parkes, 1989). However, two short-acting drugs, *triazolam* (Halcion) 0.5 to 1 mg and *temazepam* (Restoril) 30 mg, were found to cause the least residual impairment (hangover) when used for hypnotic effect (Bond and Lader, 1981). Some studies suggested that the incidence of drowsiness is lower with intermediate half-life benzodiazepines such as *prazepam* (Centrax) and, perhaps, with *lorazepam* (Ativan) and *alprazolam* (Xanax) than with other benzodiazepines of equivalent anxiolytic dose (Cohn, 1981; Dement, Siedel, and Caraskadon, 1982).

The classic benzodiazepines used as hypnotics to treat sleep disturbances are outlined in Table 8-1. These include triazolam, estazolam (ProSom), temazepam, flurazepam (Dalmane), and quazepam (Doral) (Dominguez et al, 1986; Kales, 1990; Greenblatt et al, 1982; Greenblatt et al, 1989). Many conventional antidepressants are also prescribed for enhancing sleep because of their sedating properties. The sedative effect and half-life of antidepressants are profiled in Table 8-2. Antidepressants commonly prescribed to enhance sleep include trazodone (Desyrel), nefazodone (Serzone), amitriptyline (Elavil), trimipramine (Surmontil), doxepin (Sinequan), maprotiline (Ludiomil), imipramine (Tofranil), and nortriptyline (Pamelor). Although these antidepressant compounds are not specifically indicated for treating insomnia, they are often prescribed for that purpose, especially for patients with coexisting depression. The chemical structures for some of the benzodiazepines are presented in Figure 8-2.

Pharmacologic Effects

The classic benzodiazepines generally shorten sleep latency, reduce the number of awakenings and the duration of wakefulness during the night, and increase total sleep time. The latency to REM sleep is prolonged by the benzodiazepines, but this effect may be caused by the suppression of the first episode of REM sleep rather than to a delay in its appearance (Belyavin and Nicholson, 1987). Non-REM sleep

Table 8-1 Clinical Profile of Commonly Prescribed Sedatives

Benzodiazepine sedative	Dosage (mg)	Onset of effect (hr)	Active metabolite	Elimination half-life
Triazolam (Halcion)	0.125-0.5	1-2	None	Rapid
Estazolam (ProSom)	1-2	1-2	None	Intermediate
Temazepam (Restoril)	15-30	2-3	Oxazepam	Intermediate
Flurazepam (Dalmane)	15-30	½-1	1-hydroxyethyl-flurazepam, flurazepam aldehyde, N-desalkylflu-razepam	Slow
Quazepam (Doral)	7.5-15	2	2-oxoquazepam N-desalkyl-2-oxoquapam	Slow
Zolpidem (Ambien)	5-10	½-1	None	Rapid

Table 8-2 Antidepressant Sedative Effect and Elimination Half-Life

Agent	Sedative effect*	Half-life (hr)
Trazodone (Desyrel)	+++	4-9
Amitriptyline (Elavil)	+++	31-46
Doxepin (Adapin, Sinequan)	+++	8-24 (51)†
Maprotiline (Ludiomil)	++	21-25
Imipramine (Tofranil)	++	11-25
Nortriptyline (Aventyl, Pamelor)	++	18-44
Amoxapine (Asendin)	+	8-30
Protriptyline (Vivactil)	+	67-89
Desipramine (Norpramin)	+	12-24
Sertraline (Zoloft)	None to +	26-98‡
Fluoxetine (Prozac)	None	48-216
Fluvoxamine (Luvox)	None to +	15-19
Paroxetine (Paxil)	None to +	21
Venlafaxine (Effexor)	+	5-11‡
Nefazodone (Serzone)	+ to ++	2-4

Modified from Fabre LF: *Trazodone dosing regimen: experience with single daily administration.* Presented at the Eighth World Congress of Psychiatry, Athens, Greece, October 1989.
*+++=marked; ++=moderate; +=mild.
†Active metabolite, desmethyldoxepin, has a longer life than parent compound (51 hours ± 17 hours).
‡Includes active metabolite.

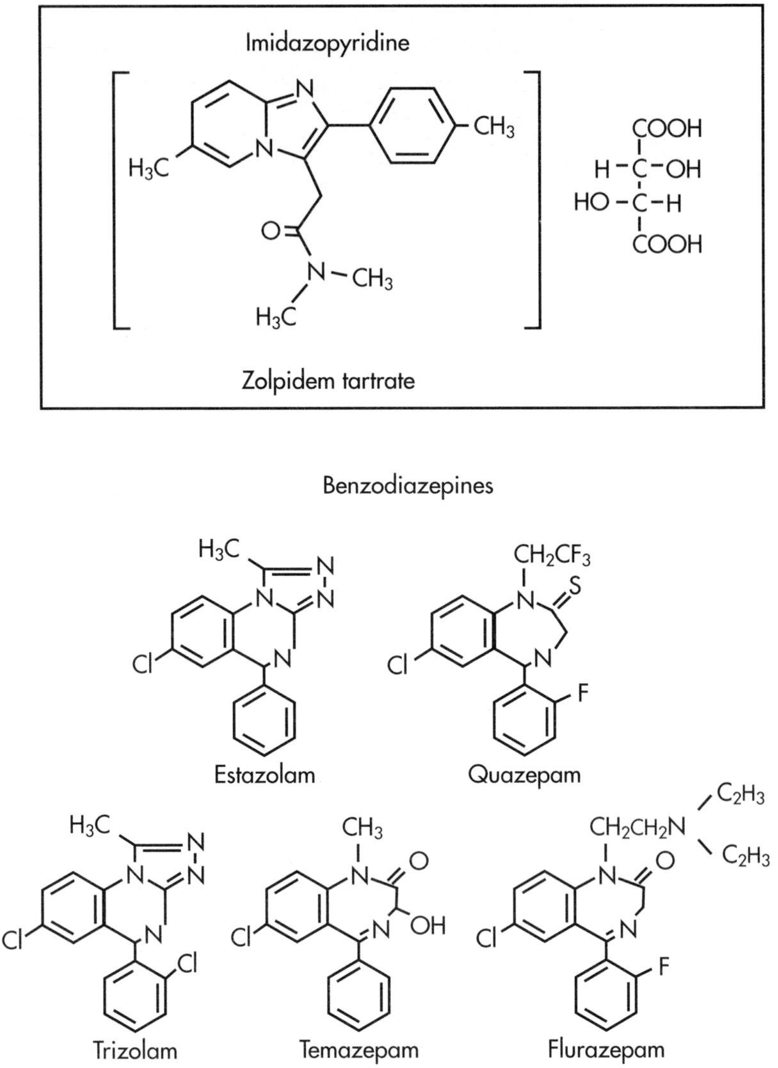

Figure 8-2 Chemical structures for benzodiazepines and zolpidem.

is changed considerably by the classic benzodiazepines. The duration of stage 1 is reduced, and that of stage 2 is increased. Moreover, EEGs show slowing of electrophysiologic activity, in particular, the emergence of delta waves, k-wave potentials, and theta activities that are less abundant. (For a complete discussion of the electroencephalographic changes and physiologic correlates, see Weitzmann and Pollak, 1982.) Perhaps the most significant effects of benzodiazepines are their effects on stage 4 (deep) sleep. Benzodiazepines may diminish release of growth hormone that normally occurs during this stage. This disruption of stage 4 sleep may also decrease REM sleep. Paradoxically some insomniacs may have an increase in REM sleep, because some report having nightmares when taking benzodiazepines. After the withdrawal of benzodiazepines, sleep stages 2 and 4 remain altered much longer than do other sleep stages.

The nonclassic benzodiazepine clonazepam may modify sleep less markedly because it has only a few agonistic effects. Clonazepam is particularly useful as a sleep agent, because it inhibits REM sleep, but stage 4 sleep is actually increased during the night of administration and then decreased during the following night. Clonazepam may be particularly helpful in patients who have a sleep disturbance superimposed on another condition, for example, neurodegenerative disorders such as Alzheimer's or Parkinson's disease or nocturnal myoclonus with periodic leg movement or restless leg syndrome (discussed later in this chapter).

In general all benzodiazepines alter sleep by binding to the benzodiazepine receptor and the GABA receptor–chloride channel molecular complex (see Chapter 3, Neuropharmacology and Psychotropic Drugs). Although barbiturates may affect the chloride channels differently from the benzodiazepines, the activity of both classes of drugs has similar neuropharmacologic effects. For example, pentobarbital and phenobarbital exert a hypnotic effect in patients by shortening sleep latency and reducing intermittent awakenings during the night. In contrast to benzodiazepines, barbiturates, when given for an extended period, may induce a rebound REM sleep when discontinued. This REM sleep is often accompanied by nightmares. Thus benzodiazepines have distinct advantages over their predecessors. Further developments in the pharmacologic study of benzodiazepines may provide compounds that are freer of adverse effects than currently used compounds and may improve our knowledge of the mechanisms involved in the regulation of sleep and wakefulness (Gaillard and Phelippeau, 1976).

Pharmacokinetics

The absorption, metabolism, and elimination of benzodiazepines are nearly identical, but distribution is not. Individual differences are characterized in the latter part of this section. The most important factors governing the choice of benzodiazepines to treat insomnia are the dose, the individual rate of absorption, the distribution (most relevant for single-dose effects), and the elimination half-life (most important in treating chronic insomnia). Sleep induction by means of benzodiazepines depends entirely on the rate of absorption from the gut. Most benzodiazepines are rapidly absorbed, but absorption may be slowed by food and antacids. The absorption rate after intramuscular injection of many benzodiazepines, with the possible exception of lorazepam, is much slower than with oral administration.

The duration of clinical action of benzodiazepines in single doses depends on distribution, whereas accumulation becomes important with multiple doses. This means that absorption rates and distribution to the CNS at the therapeutic level are mostly responsible for a single-dose effect. A long half-life does not necessarily imply a long duration of sedation, nor does a short half-life imply a short duration of action for a hypnotic. Accumulation, of course, is determined by metabolic clearance and elimination half-life. Benzodiazepine metabolism occurs primarily in two ways: conjugation (combining with glucuronic acid and becoming inert) and oxidation (via the hepatic microsomal enzyme system). Some short-acting benzodiazepine derivatives, for example, oxazepam and lorazepam, are almost completely inactivated by one-step conjugation in the liver and therefore have few residual morning-after effects. Indeed, benzodiazepines eliminated as rapidly as these may even result in early-morning insomnia, whereas other benzodiazepines, for example, flurazepam, may produce persistent long-acting metabolites that cause a lingering impairment in alertness, motor performance, and cognitive functioning. Benzodiazepine metabolism is largely age dependent; the elimination half-life of diazepam, for instance, may increase three to fourfold in persons 20 to 80 years of age, thus increasing the bioavailability of the drug (Tables 8-1 and 8-3).

The action of a hypnotic drug depends on its absorption, distribution, and elimination. The rate of absorption determines onset of action because benzodiazepines penetrate the blood-brain barrier easily. The more rapidly absorbed drugs have a faster onset of action, whereas those that are slowly absorbed may not have a desired effect at all. Of the currently marketed hypnotics, flurazepam is the most rapidly absorbed, followed by triazolam, which has an intermediate absorption rate, and temazepam, with a slow absorption rate. Thus the time at which the medication is given to the patient before he or she retires is very important (Greenblatt et al, 1982). Obviously a drug with a slow absorption rate, for instance, oxazepam, may be most appropriate for treating anxiety when a sustained effect with minimal initial drowsiness is sought. Once absorbed, a hypnotic is distributed to the blood and to the highly vascular tissues, that is, the brain, heart, liver, and lungs, and then distributed peripherally to less vascular tissues. This rapid distribution results in an initial drop in the plasma concentration, but the subsequent fall mainly results from elimination by metabolism and excretion.

Because a particular pharmacodynamic effect is related to a specific plasma concentration, knowledge of distribution versus elimination half-life can be of great clinical utility. The duration of activity is short when the plasma level is within the phase that predominantly represents distribution but longer when the plasma level is within the elimination phase. In other words, plasma concentration decay occurs more rapidly during the distribution phase than during the elimination phase. Thus both distribution and elimination influence duration of activity, that is, half-life. In practical terms this means that a relatively short duration of action may be expected when giving a single dose of a hypnotic that is not rapidly eliminated but is rapidly distributed. Thus, although half-life is a familiar concept and often touted as the most important feature of benzodiazepines, it does have limitations in defining the duration of activity of a single dose.

Most benzodiazepines are metabolized in the liver; some produce numerous active metabolites. The pattern of metabolism of various drugs is similar. Benzodiazepines are mainly transformed in the liver by conjugation of attachment of the molecule to glucuronic acid, then excreted in the urine as pharmacologically inactive metabolites. However, some benzodiazepines form active metabolites, which complicates their pharmacologic properties. In addition, if the hepatic-detoxification system is compromised, as in viral hepatitis, benzodiazepine activity is prolonged and potential exists for physical complications.

The influence of distribution on plasma concentration decay is important. Although using the elimination half-life alone to predict duration of action is taught in most pharmacology courses, this guideline is misleading (Nicholson, 1989). However, it is important to note that with repeated ingestion, the elimination half-life again becomes useful as a concept for predicting the rate and extent of metabolic accumulation. Further, the clinician should recognize that slow elimination of a parent compound or an active metabolite is disadvantageous when drugs are being used nightly, particularly because freedom from next-day effects is usually sought.

To show how this information can be translated into clinical usefulness, the compound temazepam is used as an example. Temazepam has a distribution phase similar to that of its parent compound, diazepam, but has an elimination half-life of only 8 hours and insignificant amounts of other metabolites. Thus residual sequelae with temazepam are unlikely unless inappropriately high doses are prescribed.

Table 8-3 Pharmacokinetic Properties of Selected Hypnotic Drugs

Significant pharmacokinetic characteristics	Drug (chemical group)	Recommended dose range (mg)	Tmax (hr)	T½/elim (hr)*	Comments and indications	References
Slow absorption	Oxazepam (benzodiazepine)	15-30 (in elderly patients, 10-20)	2.2 ± 1.9	6.7 ± 1.7	Free of residual effects but rather slowly absorbed; used mainly as an anxiolytic but sustains sleep	Greenblatt DJ et al: *J Pharmacol Exp Ther* 215:86, 1980
Slow elimination of parent compound or metabolite	Flurazepam hydrochloride (benzodiazepine): Active metabolities, 1-hydroxyethylflurazepam, N-desalkylflurazepam	15-30† (in elderly patients, 15)	1.4 ± 0.7 8.0 ± 8.0	0.9 ± 1.1 40 ± 103	Hypnotic effect related to the activity of metabolites; residual efffects likely, and accumulation on continued nightly ingestion inevitable; useful for frequent nocturnal awakenings when some daytime sedation is acceptable; 7.5-mg dose may be useful for elderly patients	Eckert M et al: *Drugs Exp Clin Res* 9:77, 1983

*Half-Life values may vary among different studies.
†Doses exceeding 15 mg may not be appropriate.

Continued

Table 8-3 Pharmacokinetic Properties of Selected Hypnotic Drugs—cont'd

Significant pharmacokinetic characteristics	Drug (chemical group)	Recommended dose range (mg)	Tmax (hr)	$T^{1/2}$/elim (hr)*	Comments and indications	References
Relatively slow elimination, but marked distribution may lead to a short duration of action	Diazepam (benzodiazepine)	5-10 (in elderly patients, 5)	1.1 ± 0.3	32 ± 11	Free of residual effects when given occasionally, because of marked distribution phase; slow elimination of parent compound and active metabolite leads to accumulation and daytime anxiolytic effect with repeated ingestion	Kaplan SA et al: *J Pharm Sci* 62:1789, 1973
Relatively rapid elimination and marked distribution phase in appropriate formulations	Temazepam (benzodiazepine) soft gelatin capsule	10-60† (in elderly patients, 10-20)	0.8 ± 0.3	8.4 ± 0.6	Soft gel cap formulation in the dose range 10-20 mg is free of residual effects and of significant accumulation on daily ingestion; useful for sleep onset	Divoll M et al: *J Pharm Sci* 70:1104, 1981; Fuccella LM: *Br J Clin Pharmacol* 8:315, 1979

Ultrarapid elimination	Triazolam (triazolobenzodiazepine)	0.250‡ (in elderly patients, 0.125)	1.2 ± 0.5	2.6 ± 0.7	Dose range in some countries is 0.25-0.5 mg, but the higher dose leads to residual effects and rebound insomnia; useful for sleep onset	Jochemsen R et al: *Br J Clin Pharmacol* 16:291S, 1983
Rapid absorption and elimination	Zolpidem (imidazopyridine)	5-10	1.8 ± .4	2.5 ± 1	Free of residual effects; no active metabolites. Maintains stage 3 & 4 sleep.§	

*Half-life values may vary among different studies.
†Doses exceeding 20 mg may not be appropriate.
‡A dose of 0.125 mg may also be useful for adults other than the elderly.
§Searle Pharmaceuticals monograph, 1995.

An important clinical consideration (discussed in Chapter 17, Psychopharmacology for Elderly Persons) is the comparison of distribution of hypnotics and other agents in elderly people and young adults. Unless renal function is severely impaired, elimination usually is not significantly affected in an adult. However, metabolism may be different (see Chapter 17, Psychopharmacology for Elderly Persons) and may be slowed in the individual over age 65. Thus the half-lives of compounds may be prolonged in elderly persons and may have a much more profound effect than in young adults.

Clinical decision-making based on pharmacokinetics. Clearly the benzodiazepines and the nonbenzodiazepine agent zolpidem are the sedatives of choice in view of safety and potential for overdose. The more lipid-soluble benzodiazepines readily enter the CNS. For instance, diazepam and flurazepam enter within 10 minutes, whereas oxazepam and clorazepate enter within 18 to 35 minutes, respectively. As shown in Table 8-3, slowly excreted drugs, for example, diazepam and flurazepam, with relatively long half-lives may promote ease of sleep onset the following day and reduce prolonged anxiety throughout the day. Furthermore, long-acting agents are relatively less likely to provoke untoward reactions on abrupt withdrawal. On the other hand, these long-acting benzodiazepines induce next-day levels of subjective sleepiness and may result in hangover. In short, the difference between the slowly and the rapidly excreted benzodiazepines provides a precarious guide for the individual patient, given large differences in tolerance and sensitivity.

The next-day performance and any subjective symptoms of a patient with insomnia are more often influenced by the dose of the drug than by its elimination half-life (Johnson and Cherniak, 1982). Perhaps a choice drug for sleep-onset insomnia is triazolam, and for sleep-maintenance insomnia, temazepam. Early-morning awakening may be best treated with flurazepam, which induces sleep of long duration. That persons with insomnia represent a heterogeneous group is implicit in this discussion. Thus the selection of a drug, the prediction of its effects, and the long-range treatment of most types of insomnia must allow for drug variability among patients. Most patients do not need long-term treatment, and in any case benzodiazepines are best given in short courses. The hazards of well-monitored treatment with hypnotic drugs are small, although true physiologic addiction nonetheless may occur (Clift, 1972; Greenblatt and Shader, 1978). Persons who should not take hypnotic agents include pregnant women, alcoholics, those who must arise and function in the middle of the night, and those with symptomatic sleep apnea (Roth et al, 1982).

Side Effects

Benzodiazepines used as hypnotics are unlikely to have severe adverse effects. As noted in Chapter 6, Anxiety Disorders, unnecessarily high doses and unnecessarily long treatment periods are the main problems associated with benzodiazepine usage. These problems often result in adverse effects, undoubtedly because of misuse. Impaired performance, anterograde amnesia, and other adverse effects of hypnotics may be particularly troublesome (Nicholson and Ward, 1984).

A number of the adverse effects encountered when these compounds are prescribed for a long period are given in Chapter 6, Anxiety Disorders. Also insomnia on cessation of treatment may arise with the misuse of hypnotics when rebound phenomena emerge, in particular, when short-acting drugs are withdrawn

Table 8-4 Other Sedatives (Forerunners of Benzodiazepine Sedatives)

Generic name	Trade name	Comments
Alcohols, aldehydes, and propanediols		
Ethanol	Generic	Not recommended*
Ethchlorvynol	Placidyl	Not recommended*
Chloral hydrate	Generic	1-2 gm to induce sleep
Paraldehyde	Generic	Not recommended*
Meprobamate	Equanil, Miltown, generic	Not recommended*
Tybamate	Tybatran, Solacen, generic	Not recommended*
Barbiturates		
Amobarbital	Amytal, generic	Administer 100-800 mg/hr, intravenously in diagnosis or parenterally for emergency sedation
Methohexital	Brevital	Administer 10 mg/5 sec intravenously (average dose = 70 mg) for electroconvulsive therapy only
Pentobarbital	Nembutal, generic	Can be used for treatment of withdrawal from most sedative addictions†‡
Phenobarbital	Luminal, generic	30-90 mg/day†‡
Secobarbital	Seconal, generic	Not recommended†
Structural relatives of barbiturates (nonbarbiturates)		
Glutethimide	Doriden	Not recommended*
Methyprylon	Noludar	Not recommended*
Methaqualone	Quaalude, generic	Not recommended*
Antihistamines		
Diphenhydramine	Benadryl	25-50 mg parenterally for dystonia§
Hydroxyzine	Atarax, Vistaril	Not recommended*
Promethazine	Phenergan, generic	Not recommended*

Modified from Baldessarini RJ: *Chemotherapy in psychiatry,* Cambridge, Mass, 1985, Harvard University.
*These agents are not recommended for routine use as sedatives.
†Short-acting barbiturates, although not generally recommended, are sometimes used to induce sleep because of their low cost; phenobarbital is an inexpensive sedative and not often abused.
‡Pentobarbital and phenobarbital are often used to treat addiction to sedative-hypnotic drugs.
§Diphenhydramine and other antihistamines are sometimes used as sedatives in pediatric practice. These are not recommended for use in elderly individuals.

suddenly. Rebound insomnia occurs most often when a relatively high dose of a rapidly eliminated drug is prescribed and used nightly. Rebound insomnia is not observed when benzodiazepine sedatives are used in appropriate doses for a limited time (Roehrs et al, 1986). Drug dependence is also a possibility with the use of hypnotics, as with anxiolytics. The potential for dependence can be minimized by the intermittent use of low doses, limited duration of ingestion, and gradual withdrawal when continuous treatment has been given for longer than a month (Ladewig, 1983).

Implications

Therapeutic versus toxic levels. Therapeutic levels of benzodiazepines have a comfortable margin of safety compared with other sedatives. However, overdoses equivalent to approximately two times a monthly supply or less, when taken with alcohol, have led to death. Moreover, the use of long-acting benzodiazepines and intravenous diazepam to control seizures or cardiac arrhythmias is occasionally complicated by respiratory depression, apnea, ventricular arrhythmias, or cardiac arrest. Most deliberate overdoses seem to involve more than one agent; typically alcohol is involved. Thus it is difficult to assess or determine what supply of benzodiazepines would be considered safely dispensed. The continued use of benzodiazepines for more than several weeks should be applied in the context of the critical appraisal of risks and benefits in individual cases.

Use in pregnancy. The safety of benzodiazepines in pregnancy has not been established, and there is no evidence from animal studies to suggest that these drugs are free of hazard. Prolonged administration of benzodiazepines in either low or high dose in the last trimester of pregnancy has been reported to produce arrhythmias, hypertonia, poor sucking, and hypothermia in neonates. Benzodiazepines do cross the placenta and enter breast milk. Thus ingestion during pregnancy and lactation should be avoided.

Side effects. The most common side effects of benzodiazepines are related to mental alertness. The patient should be cautioned about driving or operating hazardous machinery. Tolerance to most side effects quickly develops. Blood pressure of inpatients should be monitored routinely, and a drop in pressure of 20 mm Hg (systolic) on standing warrants withholding the drug and notifying the prescriber.

Interactions. Several of the discussions of drug interactions with benzodiazepines found in Chapter 6, Anxiety Disorders, are relevant to those prescribed primarily as hypnotics. The sedative effect of benzodiazepines is, of course, increased by combination with centrally acting neuroleptics, tranquilizers, sedating antidepressants, other hypnotics, analgesics, anesthetics, and alcohol. In healthy young adults small doses of temazepam and moderate doses of alcohol may produce no significant additive effect and may not necessarily prolong the effects of benzodiazepines, as they clearly do in elderly patients or in those who, indeed, have alcoholism. The elimination half-life of the benzodiazepines is clearly increased by cimetidine; for other interactions see Chapter 6, Anxiety Disorders.

Patient education. Benzodiazepines have a great potential for abuse. Consequently it is important to teach the patient and his or her family about these drugs. The nurse or physician should instruct the patient and the family as follows:

Benzodiazepines prescribed for insomnia should be taken as directed.
Over-the-counter drugs may potentiate the actions of benzodiazepines.
Driving should be avoided until tolerance develops.
Alcohol and other CNS depressants potentiate the effects of benzodiazepines.
Hypersensitivity to one benzodiazepine may indicate hypersensitivity to another.
Benzodiazepine treatment should not be stopped abruptly.

Specific Benzodiazepines

Hypnotics, like anxiolytics, are often characterized based on elimination half-life. Triazolam is the most rapidly excreted hypnotic, with an elimination half-life of 1.5 to 5.5 hours. Oxazepam has an elimination half-life of 5 to 20 hours, and the half-lives of lorazepam, temazepam, alprazolam, and chlordiazepoxide are between 10 and 30 hours and generally longer in elderly individuals. Triazolam may be useful when next-day sedation has occurred, but in some patients its rapid washout may provoke rebound insomnia, next-day anxiety, and anterograde amnesia (Kales and Kales, 1984). Another compound, lorazepam, also has a particular propensity for anterograde amnestic effects. The lack of active metabolites may make oxazepam the preferred drug in patients with liver disease and other conditions in which liver function may be compromised. As mentioned in Chapter 6, Anxiety Disorders, antacids and anticholinergic drugs may decrease the absorption of benzodiazepines, but cimetidine slows their metabolism to a minor degree. Nevertheless, the near-total replacement of the 50 or more previously available barbiturates by the benzodiazepines has resulted in a lower incidence of toxicity and a similar, but not superior, hypnotic effect. These agents cause less respiratory and cardiac depression than do the barbiturates, although overdosage clearly results in respiratory failure. Tolerance of benzodiazepines, in contrast to the barbiturates, is less marked and is never complete.

The choice of an individual hypnotic may depend on the drug's potential to shorten sleep onset when there is difficulty falling asleep, to reduce nocturnal wakefulness, or, when insomnia is accompanied by a marked element of anxiety, to provide an anxiolytic effect the next day. The clinical utility of selected compounds is provided in Table 8-1 (Nicholson, 1980). Three specific compounds, designated short-acting (triazolam), intermediate-acting (temazepam), and long-acting (flurazepam), are discussed in detail in the following sections.

Short-acting benzodiazepines: Prototype drug, triazolam. Triazolam is metabolized principally by hepatic microsomal oxidation. Hepatic clearance occurs at a high rate, depending on blood flow in the liver and activity of hepatic microsomal enzymes. A significant drug interaction (as discussed in Chapter 5, Mood Disorders) occurs with nefazodone (Serzone). Essentially, the dosage of triazolam should be reduced by 50% to 75% when coadministered with nefazodone. This compound is rapidly or very rapidly eliminated after the administration of single doses and does not accumulate. Advantages and disadvantages may occur as a consequence of these properties. The rapid elimination results in no hangover effect, but with the very short-acting compounds early-morning rebound insomnia and anxiety may occur. Furthermore, the complete disappearance of the drug and its metabolites from the blood within a day of discontinuing long-term treatment may result in severe rebound symptoms of drug withdrawal (Kales et al, 1979). Abrupt withdrawal may cause confusion, toxic psychosis, convulsions, or a condition resembling delirium tremor, such as sweating and diarrhea. Long-term treatment should therefore be stopped slowly.

Intermediate-acting benzodiazepines: Prototype drug, temazepam. Among the hypnotics available in alternative formulations with differential rates of absorption is temazepam. This drug is available as a soft gelatin capsule and has a mean peak plasma concentration time of approximately 1 hour. In contrast, the typical hard gelatin capsule is absorbed relatively slowly and has a delay of approximately 2 hours. With temazepam the major metabolite is an inert conjugate. Thus this compound has virtually no active metabolites to prolong its effect.

Because temazepam is metabolized by conjugation rather than by oxidation, its metabolic pathway is less likely to be influenced by factors such as age. Although this knowledge may imply a clinical advantage for temazepam over flurazepam or triazolam among older adults, such an advantage has not been clearly established. The effects of temazepam are thought to be restricted to the night of ingestion as a result of its relatively short half-life. However, with a mean half-life of 13 to 14 hours in some individuals, this drug should be characterized as an intermediate-acting benzodiazepine. Large doses may cause hangover effects.

Long-acting benzodiazepines: Prototype drug, flurazepam. Flurazepam produces a complex mixture of short-acting and long-acting metabolites on repeated dosing. Steady-state levels are reached at 2 to 3 weeks after ingestion. An accumulation may cause impairment of waking performance. Single doses generally cause a full night's sleep, with little residual impairment, and the 30-mg dose may result in an anxiolytic effect throughout the day.

Nonbenzodiazepine Hypnotic: Zolpidem

Zolpidem (Ambien) is a nonbenzodiazepine hypnotic of the imidazopyridine class. Zolpidem is widely prescribed and represents a drug of choice for acute insomnia. This agent has a unique mechanism of action, modulating the GABA A receptor chloride channel complex. This results in sedative, anxiolytic, anticonvulsant, and myorelaxant properties. The major effect occurs on the alpha subunit of the GABA A receptor complex, referred to as the benzodiazepine omega receptor, that is, the benzodiazepine-GABA receptor/complex. Thus this agent shares some properties with the benzodiazepines.

The pharmacologic profile of zolpidem is characterized by rapid absorption and elimination, with an ultra short half-life (Tables 8-1 and 8-3). It has no active metabolites and is unlikely to accumulate with short-term use, that is, several weeks. Daytime drowsiness or residual effects are minimal or lacking, and rebound effects, as described with many benzodiazepine agents, do not occur, including little effect on cognitive functioning. Zolpidem has been shown to have little unfavorable effect on stage 3 or 4 sleep or REM sleep, that is, it maintains the integrity of sleep and sleep architecture (Merlotti et al, 1989).

Zolpidem is viewed by many clinicians to have a very favorable profile, with good tolerability in geriatric and medical patients (Kryger et al, 1991). Common side effects include drowsiness, dizziness, headache, and gastrointestinal upset occurring in a small percentage of cases. Significant drug interactions do not occur except with alcohol, which potentiates the effect of zolpidem. Zolpidem is generally dosed at 10 mg nightly for adults, with an initial dose of 5 mg. Elderly or debilitated patients may respond to the 5-mg dosage, which is recommended for geriatric patients (Scharf et al, 1991). Switching a patient from a benzodiazepine hypnotic to zolpidem may carry risk of rebound or symptoms of abrupt withdrawal, especially if continuous benzodiazepine therapy has occurred at higher dosages. Therefore, the benzodiazepine should be withdrawn gradually, perhaps over 1 to 2 weeks. After a washout of 2 to 3 days, especially for benzodiazepines with longer half-lifes, zolpidem may then be started at 10 mg for adults or 5 mg for older patients or patients with hepatic dysfunction (as noted above).

Treatment Considerations

Hypnotics have sometimes been introduced in unnecessarily high doses because of dose-ranging studies of persons with chronic insomnia. Such studies may provide information relevant to the use of hypnotics to treat chronic insomnia but are not relevant for treating "normal" insomnia. A further trend toward higher dosing is encouraged when an immediate first-night effect is sought and when high doses of ultrarapidly eliminated drugs are prescribed for treating difficulties in sustaining sleep. Such philosophy and approaches initially resulted in significant problems with triazolam, resulting in the 0.5-mg tablet being withdrawn from the market and guidelines for short-term use (up to 21 days) being established.

Dosage strategies. In prescribing any of the hypnotics shown in Figure 8-1, the clinician should strive to use the relatively lowest effective dose by choosing the compound with the most suitable pharmacologic profile. The dose should preserve normal sleep architecture to the extent possible during ingestion and after withdrawal, and the pharmacokinetic profile should meet the clinical requirement to shorten sleep onset, to reduce nocturnal wakefulness, or to provide the anxiolytic effect required during the next day. In every case the goal is to be as free as possible from untoward effects on daytime functioning. The appropriate use of any hypnotic must depend more on whether the profile solves the clinical problems just mentioned and depend less on the particular individual characteristics of the hypnotic.

Effects on electroencephalograms. A significant concern, particularly in patients being evaluated for a primary sleep disorder, may be the effects of benzodiazepines on the EEG. As mentioned earlier, these compounds may cause striking electroencephalographic changes during sleep. There is an overall decrease in the number of sleep-stage shifts throughout the night. Additionally, alterations in normal sleep pattern may change and may be manifested differently in different individuals. Clearly benzodiazepines decrease non-REM sleep stages 1, 3, and 4 and increase sleep stage 2, increasing the latency to REM sleep and diminishing REM sleep for the most part. These effects are similar to but less marked than those of the barbiturates. The effects of zolpidem have been discussed.

REM episodes or bursts in REM latency may have considerable inherent variability in response to benzodiazepines or may be erratic, with either a decrease or an increase in latency during chronic treatment. REM rebound during drug withdrawal tends to be dose related and most obvious after discontinuance of large doses of benzodiazepines.

Benzodiazepine withdrawal. A discussion of withdrawal from regimens of benzodiazepines and other similar sedative hypnotic agents may be found in Chapter 6, Anxiety Disorders. Indeed, withdrawal of hypnotics after long-term use almost always leads to resurfacing of the original symptoms, difficulties in sleeping, and anxiety. Although there is no doubt that rebound insomnia can occur with the benzodiazepines, the frequency and severity vary (Nicholson, 1980). Withdrawal symptoms may be minimized by tapering rather than stopping treatment, and tapering particularly should be considered with drugs that are short acting; also beta-adrenergic blocking drugs and other agents, for example, clonidine, may be useful in difficult cases. Benzodiazepine withdrawal phenomena such as early-morning insomnia and daytime anxiety may occur while the drug is being administered, and on withdrawal symptoms such as rebound insomnia and anxiety may occur (Kales et al, 1983). Moreover, other undesirable side effects such as impaired memory, anxiety, confusion, depersonalization, and hallucinations may be more related to the direct effect of the drug than to withdrawal itself (van der Kroef, 1979).

Tolerance to effects. Benzodiazepine hypnotics and zolpidem remain the most effective agents for sleep disorders, with clinical effects lasting approximately 6 months with continued use (Oswald et al, 1982). These agents do eventually produce adaption and tolerance (Greenblatt and Shader, 1978). Some benzodiazepines lose both their anxiolytic and their hypnotic effects over time.

Dependence. Dependence on the newer benzodiazepine hypnotics and zolpidem has not proven to be a major clinical problem, although frequent review is prudent. Zolpidem has been reported to have lower abuse liability when compared with the benzodiazepine hypnotic triazolam (Evans, Funderburk, and Griffiths, 1990). Dependence and addictions are more likely to occur in patients with a coexisting psychiatric disturbance or a history of an addictive disorder or in patients with personality or somatoform disorders.

Benzodiazepine use in elderly individuals. The metabolism and elimination of CNS depressant drugs (discussed in detail in Chapter 17, Psychopharmacology for Elderly Persons) is decreased in many older adults with low renal glomerular filtration rates, possibly in those with reduced hepatic blood flow, and decreased activity of hepatic drug-metabolizing enzymes. In general, dosages should initially be *cut in half* and daytime alertness should be monitored to detect serious impairment. The elimination half-life of diazepam, for example, is increased significantly in elderly persons, and the apparent volume of distribution of the drug is also increased (Parkes, 1989). In contrast, the elimination half-life of oxazepam does not alter greatly with aging.

Older adults are also known to rely on or to use sleeping pills much more often than do younger adults (Dunnell and Cartwright, 1972). Ideally a short-acting benzodiazepine given in a low dosage should be prescribed for elderly patients. However, some patients may respond poorly to short-acting drugs and prefer longer-acting agents because of their potential to reduce generalized daytime anxiety. As aforementioned, the overall choice for young and old alike depends on the individual clinical characteristics in each case.

OTHER DRUGS USED TO TREAT INSOMNIA

Chloral hydrate, the first hypnotic, was developed in 1868 and is still useful today (Table 8-4). Although it is a potent gastric irritant, chloral hydrate in doses of 0.5 to 1 g is widely used and has a rapid onset of action. Chloral hydrate is cross-tolerant with alcohol, is inexpensive, and is available in syrup form for those who have difficulty swallowing pills. Ethchlorvynol (Placidyl) is another hypnotic; compared with chloral hydrate, ethchlorvynol stimulates dicumarol metabolism, peaks later, and is more slowly excreted. Glutethimide (Doriden) has a rapid onset of action, rapid metabolism, high mortality with overdosage, and great potential for abuse. Among the over-the-counter agents diphenhydramine (Benadryl), a histamine blocker, also possesses a mild sedative effect and is commonly used and prescribed. L-tryptophan, recommended to be withdrawn from the market, has also been shown to exert mild sedative properties in high doses and is an amino acid precursor to CNS serotonin production. L-tryptophan has no side effects and results in maximum benefit at doses of approximately 2 to 3 g.

Discussion

The pharmacotherapy of insomnia often occurs in the context of specific pathophysiologic disturbances of sleep or of psychiatric illness. Thus specific treatments of these conditions may also be indicated. Hypnotics may be quite useful when used in the absence of these conditions or, particularly, when used as an adjunct treatment while patients are receiving behavioral therapy. Daytime residual effects, special problems of elderly patients, interaction with alcohol, dependence, and effects on respiration are just a few of the treatment issues, and a full discussion of these is beyond the scope of this chapter.

Most prescriptions for hypnotics are written for 1 month or less. The vast majority of individuals with insomnia do not take prescribed hypnotic medication; on the other hand, a significant portion of individuals with chronic insomnia self-medicate. Obviously, various disparities exist in the pattern of hypnotic medication prescription, including the disproportionately high rate of prescription among elderly persons. Older sedative hypnotic agents are discussed in Chapter 6, Anxiety Disorders, including barbiturates, chloral hydrate, methylquolone, and meprobamate. Other agents, such as antihistamines and heterocyclic antidepressants commonly prescribed because of their hypnotic effect, are also compared with the benzodiazepines in Chapter 6, Anxiety Disorders. In general there is rarely a good reason to use the older group of sedative hypnotic agents, with the exception of chloral hydrate. Ironically some states require the triplicate form of prescription, which has discouraged the prescription of benzodiazepines, resulting in an increase in the prescription of these older sedative-hypnotic agents, such as meprobamate and barbiturates, for both hypnotic and anxiolytic use in outpatients.

Many so-called natural sleep aids and over-the-counter agents are ultimately quite harmful for patients, whereas the benzodiazepines are remarkably nontoxic and safe when used alone. However, most drug-related suicide attempts involve the combination of several agents, including that of benzodiazepines with alcohol and other agents that are potentially lethal, for example, the tricyclic antidepressants. Despite the overall safety and efficacy of the benzodiazepines, they may produce unwanted effects, particularly in elderly individuals (see Chapter 17, Psychopharmacology for Elderly Persons). Long-acting agents may result in daytime impairment, and ultrashort-acting agents may be associated with rebound insomnia and innocent dose escalating. Recently triazolam has received much attention in the popular press because of its alleged profile of severe side effects. However, data are conflicting and no data exist regarding its ability to produce daytime anxiety or possible disinhibition, resulting in rage, psychosis, or amnesia. For example, a 20% incidence of anterograde amnesia is associated with triazolam, but approximately 45% of untreated patients with insomnia also have memory problems, so it is difficult to determine the clinical significance of triazolam's effect on memory (Mendelson, 1992).

Behavioral approaches to insomnia. The use of behavioral techniques, including progressive relaxation, biofeedback, cognitive approaches, stimulus control instructions, sleep restriction therapy, and other attempts to normalize the sleep-wake cycle, are very important and ideally should be combined with any pharmacologic approach to insomnia. Stimulus control instruction may be especially useful in patients who come to medical attention with a shift in the sleep-wake cycle (Box 8-3).

The judicious use of agents to enhance sleep, particularly the benzodiazepines, should continue. The treatment of persistent insomnia should necessitate an integrated approach, using both pharmacologic and nonpharmacologic strategies. Ac-

Box 8-3 Stimulus Control Therapy*

Retire only when sleepy.
Use bed and bedroom only for sleep (and sexual activity).
Go to another room if unable to sleep and return to bed only when sleepy.
Set alarm at same hour each day, irrespective of amount of sleep attained.
Avoid daytime napping.
Adhere to sleep hygiene guidelines.

Modified from Mendelson WB: *Human sleep,* New York, 1987, Plenum; Wooten V: *Psychiatr Ann* 20(8):466, 1990.
*Method may be repeated as often as needed, and therapy may be continued indefinitely.

curate diagnosis, review of current medications, behavioral changes, cognitive restructuring, or entrainment of the circadian rhythms, together with the potential use of antidepressants, psychotherapy, exercise, biofeedback, progressive muscle relaxation, dietary changes, and phototherapy or other nonpharmacologic approaches, may be appropriate and effective strategies for sleep enhancement.

Stimulus control therapy instructions, which encourage the individual to lie down with the intention of going to sleep only when drowsy, may be more effective than hypnotics. Additionally, individuals should be encouraged not to use the bed for purposes other than sleep or sexual activity. Going to another room and later returning to bed to sleep, if unable to fall asleep, may be a potent intervention. Setting the alarm for the same time each morning, regardless of how much sleep is achieved the night before, and avoiding daytime napping are the crucial factors, among the others listed in Box 8-3, that have led to this nonpharmacologic approach.

Sleep efficiency and sleep hygiene are indeed the key factors in achieving a successful sleep regimen. The sleep laboratory can be useful in refractory cases; unsuspected findings of an organic nature, such as paroxysmal nocturnal dystonias or sleep apnea, may be revealed in as many as 40% of cases. The initial approach outlined in the opening sections of this chapter, combined with accurate history, sleep hygiene instruction, and judicious prescription of appropriate hypnotic agents, generally leads to successful patient outcome.

OTHER SLEEP DISORDERS

Hypersomnia

Hypersomnia is a persistent need for excessive sleep. Any disease or drug state affecting the sleep-wake cycle may be responsible. The sleepiness of neurologic, endocrinologic, or psychiatric problems may be accompanied by other stigmas of disease. Sleepiness is typically provoked by prolonged monotony, for example, watching television or attending meetings. Driving for long distances, particularly on interstate highways, may be a culprit. In this section primarily idiopathic hypersomnia is discussed; the primary goal may simply be to ensure that persistent hypersomnia is assessed and hopefully addressed through a careful evaluation in a sleep physiology laboratory.

Idiopathic hypersomnia involves prolonged nocturnal sleep that is normal on polygraphic study and continuous daytime drowsiness. It commonly develops in young adults who poorly tolerate late-night activities. It may be difficult to identify the onset of hypersomnia, because a change of work requirement or social obligation may precipitate a complaint in an individual who had previously coped with an abnormally increased need for sleep. These individuals often manifest "sleep drunkenness," a period of incapacitating drowsiness on first awakening, sometimes lasting for more than an hour. These individuals often take naps, and the naps are usually prolonged, unlike the shorter naps of narcolepsy. Large sleep requirements often impede fulfilling daytime obligations. Family history of hypersomnia often is present, and hypersomnia may commonly be complicated by depression or impaired daytime concentration in addition to the abnormally prolonged normal night sleep.

The pharmacologic approach to idiopathic hypersomnia involves combining a systematic scheduling of sleep, a prescription of stimulants (discussed in Chapter 13, Drugs Used to Stimulate the Central Nervous System), and the use of a sleep diary with a rigid sleep practice that includes sleep hygiene. Napping is scheduled according to social demands. Stimulants are used primarily as adjuncts in a systematic fashion and are generally prescribed to maintain rather than to restore wakefulness. Two to six 18.75-mg tablets of pemoline, a long-acting stimulant, are prescribed, to be taken in divided doses in the morning. Amphetamines, including dextroamphetamine and methylphenidate, have a short duration of action and are taken in periodic divided doses on arising and for sleep drunkenness, before arising (see Chapter 13, Drugs Used to Stimulate the Central Nervous System, for further discussion of these agents). Occasionally, heterocyclic antidepressants, particularly, protriptyline; activating selective serotonin reuptake inhibitors, for example, fluoxetine; bupropion (Wellbutrin); or MAOIs, especially tranylcypromine (Parnate); are used, with modest clinical response. The outcome of use of these agents often is simply a therapeutic trial in the individual with hypersomnia.

Narcolepsy

Narcolepsy is a sleep disorder with a clear genetic component and occurs in as many as one or two individuals per thousand. Narcolepsy involves features related to REM sleep that suddenly and abnormally intrude on wakefulness during the day. The individual has an irresistible urge to nap for short periods. The paralysis of REM sleep may appear during the daytime, with attacks of cataplexy characterized by brief bilateral paresis, which may be brought on by laughter, anger, or surprise. During these periods of cataplexy, patients are unable to move, talk, or ambulate. However, consciousness and memory for the event are preserved, distinguishing this event from a seizure episode. Sleep paralysis and hypnagogic hallucinations may also occur with narcolepsy. These dreamlike visual experiences may also be accompanied by apprehension that someone else is present in the room.

The clinical features of narcolepsy may be present in a classic case. Paradoxically, wakeful periods may occur during the night. This feature is typically not found in idiopathic hypersomnia. Troublesome dreams and depression are other features seen in association with narcolepsy. Social, familial, and occupational functioning are often impaired. Pharmacologic and clinical approaches to narcolepsy are similar to those for idiopathic hypersomnia. Protriptyline and other conventional antidepressants that suppress REM sleep and therefore narcolepsy symptoms may be especially beneficial. Stimulants, that is, methylphenidate and pemoline, may also be warranted (see Chapter 13, Drugs Used to Stimulate the Central Nervous System). Other cases of narcolepsy may be managed by scheduled naps and small, measured doses of caffeine.

Table 8-5 Sleep Disorders

Disorder	Sleep-laboratory findings	Psychologic evaluation	Management and treatment
Somnambulism	Incidents occur out of stage 4 sleep; critical skills reactivity are impaired during incident	Psychiatric disturbances infrequent in children and frequent in adults	Prophylactic measures; children frequently outgrow disorders, so parents should be reassured; psychiatry evaluation for adults
Enuresis	Occurs during all sleep stages; dreaming is a frequent causal factor	Psychiatric disturbances infrequent with primary enuresis; psychologic evaluation often indicated for secondary enuresis	Parental counseling and reassurance critical so that parental mishandling does not create psychiatric problems; pharmacologic treatment (imipramine) may be indicated in older children
Night terrors	Occur out of stage 4 sleep; characterized by extreme vocalizations, motility, and autonomic response; recall minimal or absent	Psychiatric disturbances infrequent in children and frequent in adults	Parents should be reassured that children frequently outgrow disorder; for adults psychologic evaluation is often indicated; use of stage 4 suppressants is under investigation

Nightmares	Occur out of REM sleep; characterized by less motility and autonomic response than with night terrors; recall is frequent and elaborate	Frequent nightmares in children or adults may indicate psychopathology. Rule out drug withdrawal as a possible cause of nightmares	Parents should be reassured that nightmares in children are often transient; if episodes are frequent in children or adults, psychologic evaluation is indicated
Narcolepsy	Sleep attacks of narcolepsy may be accompanied by three auxiliary symptoms: cataplexy, sleep paralysis, and hypnagogic hallucinations (cataplexy is accompanied by sleep-onset REM periods)	Sleep attacks may be misinterpreted as laziness, irresponsibility, or emotional instability	Establishing diagnosis is critical; stimulants are effective for treatment of sleep attacks; imipramine is effective for treatment of auxiliary symptoms; danger exists in using imipramine and amphetamines simultaneously
Hypersomnia	Sleep-stage patterns normal, but sleep is extended; associated with postdormital confusion and difficulty in awakening; autonomic response variables are increased	Often a symptom of psychologic disorder (e.g., depression)	Stimulant drugs are effective; neurologic and psychologic evaluations are important in establishing diagnosis
Insomnia	Complaints of patients have been verified in sleep laboratory; sleep is more aroused (i.e., heart rate and respiration are increased); most hypnotic drugs lose effecttiveness within 2 weeks	Most often a symptom of psychologic disturbance and not a primary disorder; depression a common feature	When insomnia is secondary to medical conditions, pharmacologic treatment may be useful; if psychologic factors are primary, pharmacologic therapy should be combined with psychotherapy

Sleep Apnea

Sleep apnea is a generic term for breathing disorders that occur during sleep. Commonly the clinical picture is of an obese, middle-aged or older man who smokes, uses large amounts of caffeine, or drinks alcohol frequently, or has a combination of these behaviors. Mild hypertension or cardiac arrhythmias may be present. The cardinal symptom is snoring. This may, however, be absent when CNS sleep apnea or dysregulation of breathing is present, rather than upper airway obstructive mechanisms. Daytime sleepiness may be mild or may be quite noticeable to others or to the patient. It is common for individuals with sleep apnea to be asymptomatic or to have a tendency to deny that their sleep-related problems exist.

Table 8-5 distinguishes some of the other pertinent clinical characteristics of narcolepsy, idiopathic hypersomnia, insomnia, and other disorders that may be characterized by excessive daytime sleepiness. Although antidepressant medications may be useful and indicated in cases of sleep apnea, perhaps the greatest clinical implication is to *withhold benzodiazepines and other sedative hypnotic agents* that may further depress respiratory drive and contribute to the symptoms. Sleep hygiene and surgical intervention to improve the airway are generally the best approaches for treating sleep apnea.

Parasomnias

Parasomnias are unwanted automatisms or automatic behaviors that occur during deep sleep. These often occur when cortical suppression of fixed-action patterns is lessened compared with other sleep stages. Perhaps the most common type of adult parasomnia is adult enuresis, which may be associated with cystitis, diabetes, or other nonpsychiatric medical conditions. Sleepwalking is another relatively rare parasomnia that occurs during adulthood, although a childhood or family history of sleepwalking is frequently found. Sleepwalking movements are usually slow, poorly coordinated, without integrated purpose, and not recalled by the patient, who rarely hurts himself or herself.

Other sleep automatisms that may be considerations for pharmacologic intervention include bruxism and repetitive movements of the head or extremities. Stereotypic behavior such as sitting, standing, stroking the wall, saluting, or punching can also occur. In addition, night terrors, which rarely occur in adults, are distressing. Night terrors arise during deep sleep and, like other parasomnias, the details of the event are not remembered. Unlike nocturnal panic attacks, night terrors are not associated with other symptoms of panic or prolapsed mitral valve syndrome. Night terrors are different from nightmares, which may involve upsetting content, occur during REM sleep, and may not cause the individual to awaken (Table 8-5) (Kales and Kales, 1974).

Periodic Leg Movements (Restless Leg Syndrome)

An organic factor that may require further evaluation and clinical management is periodic leg movements, which may also disrupt sleep and cause an individual to complain of light, broken, or restless sleep. Nocturnal myoclonus entails repetitive, stereotypic leg-muscle jerks. Its incidence increases markedly in individuals over age 45. Although the disorder may be ameliorated by means of benzodiazepines, specifically, clonazepam, it *may worsen with the use of tricyclic antidepressants;* this distinction is crucial, because these agents may be helpful in treating other types of insomnia. Restless leg syndrome is probably a familial disorder. The uncomfortable leg sensations that occur while the patient is at rest are usually relieved by movement.

Thus active patients are asymptomatic during the day but are unable to fall asleep at night; they may also have the sleep-related leg movements that further disrupt sleep. The causes of restless leg syndrome are diverse and include underlying conditions such as amyloidosis and iron-deficiency anemia. Benzodiazepines, as aforementioned, may be useful only to relieve symptoms.

Comorbid Conditions

Using psychotropic drugs to treat sleep disorders has been addressed by largely focusing on insomnia and, to a lesser extent, other disorders. Insomnia and other disturbances often are a harbinger of serious psychiatric illness or are associated with nonpsychiatric medical conditions. Resolution of insomnia may avert subsequent psychiatric morbidity; however, it may be necessary to place the treatment of insomnia in the context of treating associated conditions and comorbid disturbances.

Covert physiologic factors or general medical conditions are the basis for nearly 40% of the cases of insomnia, and if these factors are not identified, the patient's condition may actually worsen, even with effective conventional treatment (Box 8-4). For example, obstructive sleep apnea, as previously characterized, may be asso-

Box 8-4 Nonpsychiatric Causes of Insomnia

Induced by medical conditions
Cardiovascular disorders
Chronic obstructive pulmonary disease
Conditions associated with pruritus
Endocrine and metabolic disorders
Febrile illnesses and infections
Illnesses associated with pain
Inflammatory bowel disease
Neoplastic disorders
Urinary frequency

Induced by drugs
Antihypertensives
Ace inhibitors
Beta-adrenergic blockers
Diuretics
Methyldopa
Reserpine
Autonomic agents
Anticholinergics
Cholinergic agonists
Cimetidine
Central nervous system stimulants
Amphetamines
Caffeine
Methylphenidate
Nicotine
Sympathomimetics
Central nervous system depressants
Alcohol
Anxiolytics
Hypnotics
Narcotics
Opiates
Hormones
Corticotropin
Cortisone
Oral contraceptives
Progesterone
Thyroid hormone preparations
Others
Anticancer medications
Antidepressants
Digoxin
Monoamine oxidase inhibitors
Theophylline

Modified from Erman MK: Insomnia, *Psychiatr Clin North Am* 10:525, 1987.

ciated with cerebral hypoxia and may lead to physical and psychiatric complications. Conventional hypnotic agents may only worsen the condition. Administering antidepressants or improving the airway, for example, by use of continuous positive airway pressure, may be extremely helpful.

Several disorders that affect biologic rhythms may result in problems with initiating or maintaining sleep. As described in the discussion of insomnia, sleep-phase syndromes may occur in which the individual is unable to fall asleep at the desired time and then sleeps substantially longer than desired. These syndromes are particularly common among adolescents, college students, and shift workers. Attempting to compensate by sleeping late on weekends is not particularly effective. Elderly individuals may have an advanced sleep-phase syndrome, retiring quite early and awakening after a normal 7 or 8 hours of sleep, for example, at 3 AM. This sleep pattern creates problems in the home or living situation and leads to inappropriate prescription of medication.

Other cases of insomnia may simply be associated with the use of over-the-counter agents, alcohol, or drugs prescribed for other medical conditions, for example, antibiotics, thyroid preparations, cancer chemotherapeutic agents, and many other medications that can and do affect the sleep-wake cycle (Box 8-4).

REFERENCES

Aserinsky E, Kleitman N: Regularly occurring periods of eye motility and concomitant phenomena during sleep, *Science* 118:273, 1953.

Balter MB, Bauer ML: Patterns of prescribing and use of hypnotic drugs in the United States. In Clift AD, editor: *Sleep disturbances and hypnotic drug dependence,* Amsterdam, 1975, Excerpta Medica.

Belyavin A, Nicholson AN: Rapid eye movement sleep in man: modulation by benzodiazepines, *Neuropharmacology* 26:485, 1987.

Bixler EO, Kales A, Soldatos CR: Sleep disorders encountered in medical practice: a national survey of physicians, *Behav Med* 6:13, 1979.

Bond A, Lader M: After-effects of sleeping drugs. In Weatley D, editor: *Psychopharmacology of sleep,* New York, 1981, Raven.

Caraskadon MA, Dement WC: Nocturnal determinants of daytime sleepiness, *Sleep* 5(suppl 2):73, 1982.

Clift AD: Factors leading to dependence on hypnotic drugs, *Br Med J* 3:4, 1972.

Cohn JB: Multicenter double-blind efficacy and safety study comparing aprazolam, diazepam, and placebo in clinically anxious patients, *J Clin Psychiatry* 42:347, 1981.

Coleman RM et al: Sleep-wake disorders based on a polysomnographic diagnosis, *JAMA* 247:997, 1982.

Dement W, Siedel W, Caraskadon M: Daytime alertness, insomnia and benzodiazepines, *Sleep* 5(suppl 1):S28, 1982.

Dlin BM et al: The problems of sleep and rest in the intensive care unit, *Psychosomatics* 12:155, 1971.

Dominguez RA et al: Comparative efficacy of estazolam, flurazepam, and placebo in outpatients with insomnia, *J Clin Psychiatry* 47:362, 1986.

Dunnell K, Cartwright A: *Medicine takers, prescribers and hoarders,* London, 1972, Routledge & Kegan Paul.

Evans SM, Funderburk FR, Griffiths RR: Zolpidem and triazolam in humans: behavioral and subjective effects and abuse liability, *J Pharmacol Exp Ther* 255(3):1246-55, 1990.

Gaillard JM, Phelippeau M: Benzodiazepine-induced modifications of dream content: the effect of flunitrazepam, *Neuropsychobiology* 2:37, 1976.

Greenblatt DJ, Shader RI: Dependence, tolerance and addiction to benzodiazepines: clinical and pharmacokinetic considerations, *Drug Metab Rev* 8:13, 1978.

Greenblatt DJ et al: Benzodiazepine hypnotics: kinetics and therapeutic options, *Sleep* 5(suppl 1):S18, 1982.

Greenblatt DJ et al: Pharmacokinetic determinants of dynamic differences among three benzodiazepine hypnotics: flurazepam, temazepam, and triazolam, *Arch Gen Psychiatry* 46:326, 1989.

Grey JA: *The neuropsychology of anxiety,* New York, 1982, Oxford University.

Guilleminault C, Dement WC: *Kroc Foundation series. V. Sleep apnea syndromes,* New York, 1978, Alan R Liss.

Haefely W: Alleviation anxiety: the benzodiazepine saga. In Parnaham MJ, Bruinvals J, editors: *Discoveries in pharmacology, vol 1. Psycho- and neuro-pharmacology,* Amsterdam, 1983, Elsevier.

Hartmann EL: *The functions of sleep,* New Haven, Conn, 1974, Yale University.

Hirsch JD, Garrett KM, Beer B: Heterogeneity of benzodiazepine binding sites: a review of recent research, *Pharmacol Biochem Behav* 23(4):681, 1985.

Holland G, Dement WC, Raynal DM: *Polysomnography: a response to a need for improved communication. Fourteenth annual meeting of the Association for the Psychophysiological Study of Sleep,* Jackson Hole, Wyo., June 1974.

Johnson LL, Cherniak DA: Sedative hypnotics and human performance, *Psychopharmacology (Berl)* 76:101, 1982.

Kales A: Quazepam: hypnotic efficacy and side effects, *Pharmacotherapy* 10:1, 1990.

Kales A, Kales JD: Sleep disorders: recent findings in the diagnosis and treatment of disturbed sleep, *N Engl J Med* 290:487, 1974.

Kales A, Kales JD: *Evaluation and treatment of insomnia,* New York, 1984, Oxford University.

Kales A et al: Effects of hypnotics on sleep patterns, dreaming and mood state: laboratory and home studies, *Biol Psychiatry* 1:235, 1969.

Kales A et al: Rebound insomnia: a potential hazard following withdrawal of certain benzodiazepines, *JAMA* 241:1692, 1979.

Kales A et al: Early morning insomnia with rapidly eliminated benzodiazepines, *Science* 220:95, 1983.

Kryger MH et al: Subjective versus objective evaluation of hypnotic efficacy: expeience with zolpidem, *Sleep* 14(5):399-407, 1991.

Kudo Y, Suzuki H, Nakamura Y et al: Tolerance and pharmacokinetics of zolpidem in the healthy volunteers using double-blind manner, *Sleep Research* 96(suppl):353, 1988 (abstract).

Ladewig D: Abuse of benzodiazepines in Western European society: incidence and prevalence of motives in drug acquisition, *Pharmacopsychiatry* 16:103, 1983.

Mellinger GD, Balter MB, Uhlenhuth EH: Insomnia and its treatment, *Arch Gen Psychiatry* 42:225, 1985.

Mendelson WB: *Human sleep,* New York, 1987, Plenum.

Mendelson WB: Pharmacologic treatment of insomnia. In Pies R, editor: *Advances in psychiatric medicine (Psychiatric Times [suppl]),* Santa Ana, Calif., 1992, CME.

Merlotti L et al: The dose effects of zolpidem on the sleep of healthy normals, *J Clin Psychopharmacol* 9(1):9-14, 1989.

Mohler H, Okada T: Benzodiazepine receptor: demonstration in the central nervous system, *Science* 198:849, 1977.

Nicholson AN: Hypnotics: rebound insomnia and residual sequelae, *Br J Clin Pharmacol* 9:223, 1980.

Nicholson AN: Hypnotics: clinical pharmacology and therapeutics. In Kryger MH, Roth T, Dement W, editors: *Principles and practice of sleep medicine,* Philadelphia, 1989, WB Saunders.

Nicholson AN, Ward J, editors: Psychomotor drugs and performance, *Br J Clin Pharmacol* 18(suppl 1), 1984.

Oswald I et al: Benzodiazepine hypnotics remain effective for 24 weeks, *Br Med J* 284:860, 1982.

Parkes JD: Sleep and its disorders. In Kryger MH, Roth T, Dement WC, editors: *Principles and Practice of Sleep Medicine,* Philadelphia, 1989, WB Saunders.

Roehrs TA et al: Dose determinants of rebound insomnia, *Br J Clin Pharmacol* 22:143, 1986.

Roth T et al: Effects of benzodiazepines on sleep and wakefulness, *Br J Clin Pharmacol* 11:315, 1981.

Roth T et al: Pharmacological and medical considerations in hypnotic use, *Sleep* 5(suppl 1):S46, 1982.

Scharf MB et al: Dose response effects of zolipdem in normal geriatric subjects, *J Clin Psychiatry* 52(2):77-83, Feb 1991.

Searle Pharmaceuticals monograph, 1995.

Tan TL et al: Biopsychobehavioral correlates of insomnia. IV. Diagnosis based on DSM-III, *Am J Psychiatry* 141:357, 1984.

van der Kroef C: Reactions to triazolam, *Lancet* 2:526, 1979.

Weitzmann ED, Pollak CP: Effects of flurazepam on sleep and growth hormone release during sleep in healthy subjects, *Sleep* 5(4):343, 1982.

CHAPTER 9

Acute Psychoses and the Violent Patient

SCOPE OF THE PROBLEM

Violence and aggressive behavior are endemic in the mental health treatment setting and constitute a bona fide occupational hazard. Physical assaults on mental health professionals have been reported in all clinical settings, including inpatient wards, outpatient clinics, emergency departments, and institutional facilities (Lion, 1983). Haller and Deluty (1988) and Shah (1993) have reported that the frequency of violence among psychiatric inpatients is rising! However, these patients often can be successfully managed, if the clinical approach is objective, systematic, and appreciative of the underlying dynamics or psychopathologic factors (Dubin, 1981).

Estimates of the incidence of assault on mental health professionals have been drawn from retrospective questionnaires or reviews of incident reports. The reported incidence varies with the profession sampled, the setting, and survey methods. Using a survey questionnaire, Madden, Lion, and Penna (1976) found that 42% of psychiatrists had been assaulted at some point in their careers, generally while working in their younger years with seriously mentally ill patients. Bernstein (1981) surveyed psychiatrists, psychologists, social workers, and counselors working in both inpatient and outpatient settings. These clinicians reported a 14.2% rate of assault. Although the inpatient setting was more often characterized as having great risk for violent behavior and assault (33%), the highest percentage of assaults occurred in an outpatient or a private practice setting (47%). Depp (1976) reported that 12% of 379 documented assaults over an 8-month period in an institutional setting involved the staff. Lion, Snyder, and Merrill (1981) reported 203 incidences of assault against nursing staff over a 1-year period in a Maryland state hospital; as many as 5 times that number were thought to be unreported to the administration.

THE CLINICAL APPROACH

Clinicians' predictions of aggressive behavior or violence have shown some reliability (Lidz, Mulvey, and Gardner, 1993; McNeil and Binder, 1991). Patients with personality disorder, neurologic disorder, psychosis, head trauma, or mental retardation are predisposed (Elliott, 1992; Linaker, 1994; Bjorkly, 1993; Rasmussen and Levander, 1993). Patients tend to become aggressive or violent when they feel helpless or passive. Successful interventions often alleviate these feelings and diminish the chances of loss of behavioral control. Usually a prodromal pattern of behavior precedes overt violence. Sudden, unexpected violence is rare, and most violence is a predictable culmination of a 30- to 60-minute period of escalation.

The patient's posture, speech, and motor activity are key indicators that a violent episode is forthcoming. Most violence is preceded by a period of increasing restlessness and pacing. Hyperactivity may be a sign that immediate intervention is necessary. One study found that confusion, irritability, boisterousness, physical threats, verbal threats, and attacks on objects were common before violence (Linaker and Busch-Iversen, 1995).

POLICIES ON VIOLENCE

Because violent behavior and assault are occupational hazards in all mental health settings, each facility should carefully and thoughtfully develop defined policies and procedures that are appropriate in meeting the problems of its own patient population (Kyser, Diner, and Raulston, 1989). Policies for the care of violent patients who are severely agitated or acutely psychotic should be reviewed, approved, and supported at the highest level of clinical administration. Procedures for the clinical management of a violent patient should be rehearsed regularly by the staff to facilitate safe patient care. Nursing staff and other health care professionals must take the time to learn and practice the steps necessary for the emergency management of a violent patient. This chapter focuses on the emergency pharmacologic management of the aggressive or violent patient, including diagnostic assessment, diagnostic categories, short-term and long-term treatment, and the implications important for successful clinical management.

DIAGNOSTIC CONSIDERATIONS

Assessment and Clinical Approach

The initial clinical approach to the care of the aggressive or violent patient clearly differs from the customary process of clinical diagnosis and treatment as outlined in previous chapters. Rapid assessment and swift symptomatic relief through immediate intervention are often necessary. Treatment is directed against the target symptoms of the agitated or aggressive behavior, often with little time for diagnostic sophistication. The primary goal is to ensure the safety of the patient, the staff, and others who may be innocent bystanders (Hanke, 1984). Once the violence is contained, controlled, or concluded, the staff may begin to work on delineating the origin and pathogenesis of violence (Soreff, 1984).

The clinical approach to aggressive behavior employs a number of strategies as shown in Box 9-1. Initially a variety of nonpharmacologic interventions may be used. Patients who may be on the verge of losing control frequently respond to a well-timed verbal intervention or isolation. Because potentially violent patients are terrified of losing control, they welcome these therapeutic efforts and may actually respond to an empathic response that takes charge of the situation. Of course, the nature of the setting, the staff, and the security resources largely determine whether the patient can be safely managed and will dictate the level of immediate response.

Box 9-1 Clinical Approach to Aggressive Behavior

Talk	Medication—PO
Observation	Medication—IM
Redirection	Seclusion
Isolation	Restraint

Therapeutic practices obviously differ among emergency, outpatient, inpatient, and institutional settings and the locked forensic facility. The sophistication and experience of the staff and the philosophy of care ultimately determine the choice of verbal, pharmacologic, or physical control for the patient. The more secure the setting and the more experienced the staff, the less aggressive and restrictive the preferred intervention is likely to be (Soloff, 1987).

During an interview with a violent or potentially violent patient, the clinician should focus on the patient's underlying feelings. Rationalization and intellectualization are not generally therapeutic and may serve only to increase the patient's sense of frustration. Ventilating anger reduces agitation. By acknowledging the patient's emotional state, the clinician may accomplish some degree of emotional catharsis in the patient, thereby diminishing the need or desire for further aggression (Lion, Levenberg, and Strange, 1972).

During the assessment and interview of an aggressive or violent patient, the interviewer should stay at arm's length. The patient should never be left alone. Police, security personnel, or family should be asked to remain nearby to help control the patient, if necessary. During the verbal intervention, it may be helpful to offer the patient food or drink; hot liquids are avoided, for obvious reasons. Food symbolizes nurturance and caring and may alleviate an angry patient's disruptive behavior. Also the patient's agitated behavior may distinguish the degree of loss of control. For example, the patient who cooperates with the initial verbal intervention and postures himself or herself in a restrained or secure fashion is more likely to comply with treatment.

Box 9-2 Interview Techniques Used with Aggressive or Potentially Violent Patients

1. Secure a private but safe interview environment.
2. Approach the patient respectfully, professionally, and politely.
3. Maintain a nonthreatening, passive clinical approach.
4. Clarify, reassure, and gather data without interpretation or confrontation.
5. Listen uncritically and empathically in an unhurried fashion.
6. Offer food and drink as a symbol of help, assurance, and nurturance.
7. Involve family or friends in the clinical dialogue.
8. Communicate positive expectations for the patient but prepare for the worst.
9. Provide the patient with options and the opportunity for making choices for treatment.
10. Assist the patient in focusing anger and grievances; for example, the staff is not usually a legitimate target.
11. Offer medication to maintain control, as appropriate.
12. Ask security officers to stand by or sit in, as appropriate (show of force).

Modified from Dubin WR. In Stoudemire A, editor: *Psychiatry for medical students,* Philadelphia, 1990, JB Lippincott; Soloff PH. In Hales RE, Frances AJ, editors: *American Psychiatric Association annual review,* vol 6, Washington, DC, 1987, The Association.

The experience and skill of the interviewer is clearly important in defusing the violent threat with directable and responsive patients. Staff may contribute to violent episodes, particularly during inpatient services. Countertransference feelings, racial tensions, treatment structures characterized by authoritarianism, underinvolvement by the staff, or a lack of program clarity may contribute to violent outbursts (Soloff, 1987). Conflicts over issues of power, dependency, or self-esteem constitute the psychodynamic themes that respond to verbal and psychotherapeutic crisis intervention. Thus the agitated paranoid, the borderline, or the mildly psychotic patient, through clarifying his or her grievances and ventilating frustrations, may, in fact, be able to "talk it out."

The ultimate threat is posed by a patient with a weapon. Ideally the mental health professional explores the fear that led the patient to arm himself or herself. A weapon may symbolize a defense against feelings of helplessness and passivity. An immediate request to give up the weapon may heighten these feelings and further exacerbate the threat. Nonthreatening expressions of a desire to help, coupled with an expression of fear, is the response most likely to avert physical harm (Dubin, Wilson, and Mercer, 1988). A similar concern is a threat that may be posed by the staff's potential use of weapons, especially guns carried by police officers and secu-

Box 9-3 Management Approach to Aggressive or Potentially Violent Patients

Do	Do not
Anticipate violence	Ignore gut feelings
Respond to personal fears and feelings	Respond hastily to angry, threatening individuals
Call security at the first sign of violence	Compromise ability to maintain safety and security
Be aware of possible weapons	Antagonize or challenge a patient with a weapon
Offer food, drink, or medication	Touch or startle the individual
Restrain with an organized format	Restrain without a plan or without sufficient personnel
Offer injectable medicines if oral medicines are refused	Neglect "organic" causes of violence
Observe restrained or sedated patient	Bargain about restraint, medication, or need for admission
Hospitalize patients who are violent or uncooperative or patients who are psychotic or cognitively impaired	Forget medical and legal concerns and appropriate documentation
Warn potential victims of threatened violence	Overlook the usefulness of family and friends
Evaluate thoroughly	"Carry the coffin" by yourself: *Do* get help

Modified from Dubin WR. In Stoudemire A, editor: *Clinical psychiatry for medical students*, Philadelphia, 1990, JB Lippincott; Rabin PL, Folks DG, Hollender MH: *Southern Med J* 75:1369, 1982; Weissberg MP: *Am J Psychiatry* 136:787, 1979.

Box 9-4 Diagnostic Features Frequently Associated with Violence

Symptoms of agitation, confusion, or anxiety
Syndromes of mixed anxiety-depression or psychosis
Disorders of mood, thought, cognition, or perception
Disorders of drug and alcohol use
Disorders of personality or interpersonal functioning
Cases involving malingering and noncompliance

rity personnel who may be involved in an intervention. Generally and preferably these employees disarm themselves while in an emergency setting.

Ultimately the agitated or aggressive patient requires symptomatic relief followed by a thorough evaluation as to the origin and pathogenesis of the aggressive behavior. A number of algorithms have appeared in the literature regarding the initial clinical approach to these patients. A standard set of interview techniques with an agitated or aggressive patient is summarized in Box 9-2. Additionally, several management guidelines for the initial assessment are outlined in Box 9-3. Many of these suggested techniques and guidelines are appropriately combined with medication or followed by seclusion or restraint of the patient.

Using drugs to treat aggressive or violent behavior in a patient may occur without clear identification of symptomatic, syndromal, or diagnostic features. The more frequently diagnostic features of these patients are summarized in Box 9-4. The specific drug prescribed varies with the clinical diagnostic problem and involves some consideration of short-term versus long-term treatment, as well as the use of seclusion or physical restraint. Drug treatment is directed toward acute affective or cognitive symptoms responsible for the imminent loss of behavioral control. Thus agitation, hostility, belligerence, suspiciousness, and conceptual disorganization are initially treated, regardless of the underlying process. In some cases drug treatment addresses symptoms of primitive or disruptive forms of personality disorders such as borderline, narcissistic, histrionic, antisocial, schizotypal, or paranoid disorders. In other cases drug treatment relieves symptoms that reflect an acute exacerbation of schizophrenia, bipolar disorder, delusional disorder, or psychotic or agitated depression. Occasionally medication may simply represent the "chemical restraint" for short-term treatment of violence in progress (Monroe, 1970). Thus incidents of violence resulting from psychotic ideation, cognitive impairment or manic excitement, extreme anxiety, or irritability or explosive behavior may all represent cases in which drugs are required to manage the violent behavior.

DRUG TREATMENT

Short-Term Treatment

The acute drug treatment of the agitated or aggressive patient generally involves one of the following classes of agents: (1) the sedative-hypnotic class, usually a benzodiazepine administered orally, (2) the neuroleptic or antipsychotic class, appropriately reserved for patients who are wildly agitated or psychotic, and (3) intravenous sedative-hypnotics, for example, barbiturates or benzodiazepines, or antipsychotics, reserved for cases of extreme agitation or violence in progress in which other medications are not effective. The pharmacologic characteristics of these drugs are described in Chapters 4, Schizophrenia and Other Psychoses, and 6, Anxiety Disorders.

The benzodiazepines are clearly efficacious in treating acute anxiety, but their use in aggressive or agitated patients carries some risk. Anxiolytics may result in disinhibition or further loss of control over feelings and may contribute further to rage, hostility, or aggression. Patients who have a history of outbursts, belligerence, or assaultive or impulsive behavior should probably not be given benzodiazepines except with extreme caution (Salzman, Kochansky, and Shader, 1974). For example, patients with borderline personality disorder have shown marked disinhibition of self-directed and other-directed violence, including suicide attempts and mutilation, when given benzodiazepines (Gardner and Cowdry, 1985). However, widespread acceptance of and familiarity with anxiolytics, as well as the usefulness of a pill "to take the edge off," may well prevent the escalation of anxiety or agitation in a patient who is potentially violent and may facilitate interpersonal interaction (Lion, 1979). Some clinicians recommend the use of low-potency agents, for example, oxazepam or diazepam, in doses of 15 to 30 mg and 5 to 10 mg, respectively.

Neuroleptic or antipsychotic medication is often given in single doses to a potentially violent or agitated patient in the spirit of facilitating an evaluation. For long-term administration, risperidone (Risperdal) has been reported to be especially useful in schizophrenic patients who display hostility. One study showed stabilization over a 2-week period in cases treated with risperidone compared with haloperidol (Czobor, Volavka, and Meibach, 1995). High dosages of 6, 10, and 16 mg per day were all more effective than haloperidol in reducing hostility. However, prompt intervention for the patient who is progressively more agitated is the most common circumstance in which a neuroleptic is prescribed for aggressive behavior. The patient's treatment at this point may no longer be entirely voluntary or lend itself to oral medication. Medication may be initially presented to the patient in a firm but kind manner that indicates to the patient that his or her behavior is slipping out of control and that the medication is now needed to prevent further loss of control. The patient may initially be given a choice of oral or parenteral medication to preserve self-esteem. Therapeutic work or evaluation can then continue after administration of the medication. On the other hand a lack of response on the patient's part may suggest the need for a "show of force," physical restraint, or seclusion. A lack of response may also suggest the need for rapid neuroleptization.

Although verbal intervention is the mainstay, the preferred method of evaluating and treating an acutely agitated or aggressive patient, neuroleptics continue to represent the most effective drug treatment of the acutely violent patient. Rapid neuroleptization is defined as the "careful titrated administration of parenteral high-potency antipsychotic drugs" (Anderson, Kuehnle, and Catanzano, 1976). This therapeutic technique, used during the past 25 years, has been effectively carried out in acutely psychotic, agitated, or violent patients. Rapid neuroleptization has demonstrated both safety and efficacy as an emergency treatment of violent behavior. Rapid tranquilization essentially requires varying doses of medication given at 30- to 60-minute intervals; patients most often begin to respond within 30 to 90 minutes (Dubin, Weiss, and Dorn, 1986).

The technique of rapid neuroleptization is outlined in Box 9-5. Medication and dosages are depicted in Table 9-1. Target symptoms of tension, anxiety, restlessness, hyperactivity, and motor excitement, as well as core psychotic symptoms such as hallucinations, delusions, and disorganized thought, are ultimately addressed. However, rapid tranquilization does not fully relieve psychotic symptoms until appropriate antipsychotic drug treatment has been given for 7 to 10 days. Thus the goal of

Box 9-5 Technique of Rapid Neuroleptization

Use a high-potency neuroleptic.*
Medicate at 4-hour intervals for a low-dose strategy.
Medicate at 30- to 60-minute intervals for a high-dose strategy.
Note response 20 minutes after a dose.
Observe for nontherapeutic effects after each dose.
Document levels of consciousness and vital signs before each dose.
Maintain close observation for patients in seclusion or restraint, as appropriate.

From Dubin WR, Weiss KJ, Dorn JM: *J Clin Psychopharmacol* 6:210, 1986.
*Low-potency neuroleptics and sedative-hypnotics are sometimes employed but are not recommended (see Table 9-1).

rapid neuroleptization is to calm patients so that they may cooperate in the evaluation, treatment, and disposition of their cases. Similarly sedation may not necessarily be an end point, especially because drowsiness may delay evaluation and disposition. Although rapid neuroleptization may indeed obscure the patient's mental status or result in sedation, withholding this effective intervention may serve only to prolong the risk of violence.

Clinical response to rapid neuroleptization is usually amazingly quick. Improvement in symptoms of hostility and belligerence may be noted within 20 minutes of an initial injection of haloperidol 10 mg, with some improvement of core symptoms of psychosis within 6 hours (Donlon et al, 1980). Response rates of 50% to 95% have been reported in acutely psychotic patients within 48 hours of treatment with modest doses of neuroleptic (Anderson and Kuehnle, 1974; Slotnick, 1971). The most important variables in this technique are the choice of agent, the loading dose, the frequency of injection, and the time frame for titration (Box 9-5 and Table 9-1). Although low-potency agents such as chlorpromazine or mesoridazine may be used, they are not preferred because of the potential for nontherapeutic effects (see Chapter 4, Schizophrenia and Other Psychoses). The exception may be when the intent is true chemical restraint such that excessive sedation and parkinsonian slowing, which are usually undesirable in routine treatment, are useful elements of physical control. However, if the goal is continuation of assessment or psychiatric intervention, the preference must be given to high-potency, nonsedating neuroleptics. Thus haloperidol or an equivalent dose of a high-potency antipsychotic in single doses of 2.5 mg to 10 mg every 30 to 60 minutes in total maximum daily doses of 100 mg is standard, as outlined in Box 9-5 and Table 9-1. Studies of low-dose versus high-dose medication indicate that optimal efficacy occurs in the middle range of 15 to 60 mg (Anderson, Kuehnle, and Catanzano, 1976; Donlon et al, 1980).

Baldessarini, Katz, and Cotton (1984) have described the tendency toward using massive doses of high-potency neuroleptics. This phenomenon generally occurs after rapid neuroleptization, when oral doses far in excess of the actual clinical need are given for maintenance. Salzman et al (1986) have recommended the simultaneous use of parenteral lorazepam to reduce the total neuroleptic dosage required in managing violent behavior. A ratio of 5 mg of haloperidol to 1 or 2 mg of lorazepam has been found effective for the acute control of disruptive and violent patients. Thus the patient is spared the long-term use of high doses of neuroleptic medication.

Table 9-1 Rapid Tranquilization: Medications and Doses*

Medication	Parenteral (mg)	Oral (mg)	Range of usual daily dose (mg)	Maximum daily dose (mg)
High-potency neuroleptics				
Haloperidol (Haldol)	5	10	15-100	100
Thiothixene (Navane)	10	20	30-100	100
Trifluoperazine (Stelazine)	10	20	30-100	100
Loxapine (Loxitane)	10	25	30-200	200
Low-potency neuroleptics				
Chlorpromazine (Thorazine)	25	50	100-400	400
Mesoridazine (Serentil)	25	50	50-200	200
Benzodiazepines†				
Diazepam (Valium)	5-10 (IV or IM)	5-10	5-40	40
Chlordiazepoxide (Librium)	25-50	25-50	100-400	400
Lorazepam (Ativan)	0.5-2	1-2	1.5-8	8
Sedative-hypnotic‡				
Sodium amytal	1 mL/min (IV)	—	150-500	—

Modified from Soloff PH. In Hales RE, Frances AJ, editors: *American Psychiatric Association annual review,* vol 6, Washington, DC, 1987, The Association.
*Doses are arbitrary and not recommended for routine use but have been found effective by the authors. Doses for elderly individuals should be half the recommended doses for adults. Adverse effect may occur and should be monitored.
†With the possible exception of lorazepam, benzodiazepines are absorbed erratically or incompletely when given intramuscularly.
‡Use of sodium amytal is reserved for extreme cases of violence-in-progress.

Rapid neuroleptization is an effective approach to the care of the violent patient across all diagnostic categories. Whether the violent or disruptive presentation is secondary to a major psychiatric syndrome such as schizophrenia or mania, a disorder of cognitive impairment, or alcohol or substance abuse, this approach is quite effective (Dubin, Weiss, and Dorn, 1986). In patients with substance abuse or alcohol abuse disorders, rapid neuroleptization serves only to treat loss of behavioral control; cross-tolerant agents such as the benzodiazepines are preferred for the actual treatment of the withdrawal syndrome.

Patients receiving general medical intensive care or critical care sometimes require a different or alternative treatment approach. Patients with burns, debilitated patients, and postsurgical patients may benefit from intravenous administration of medication. Other patients may simply benefit from the rapid intravenous effect (Clinton et al, 1987). Patients receiving intravenous haloperidol may actually possess a lower incidence of extrapyramidal symptoms than patients receiving oral medication (Menza et al, 1987). Goldstein (1987) provides an excellent review of rapid neuroleptization in the intensive care unit and gives guidelines for intravenous use, as summarized in Table 9-2. However, the use of intravenous haloperidol has not been specifically approved by the FDA. Thus documentation of the rationale for this technique must be provided. Coadministration of intravenous lorazepam (Ativan) may also result in a more favorable clinical response. Dosages of 0.5 to 2 mg have been effectively used (Salzman, 1986).

Side effects resulting from rapid neuroleptization are generally uncommon and reversible. Muscle rigidity, drooling, dystonia, akathisia, bradykinesia, and the like

Table 9-2 Guidelines for the Use of Intravenous Haloperidol in Critical Care Settings*

Degree of agitation	Dose (mg)
Mild	0.5-2.0
Moderate	2-10
Severe	Boluses up to 40

Titration and maintenance

Start with a low dose and titrate in increments of 25% to 100%.

Allow 30 minutes before repeating a dose.

If agitation is unchanged, double the initial dose every 30 minutes until patient becomes calm.

If patient calms down, repeat the effective dose at regular dosing intervals, for example, every 2 to 8 hours.

Adjust dose and interval to patient's clinical course. Gradually increase the interval between doses until the interval is every 8 hours.

Once the patient's condition is stable for 24 hours, administer doses on a regular schedule, with supplemental doses as needed.

Once the patient's condition is stable for 36 to 48 hours, attempt to gradually taper dosage.

If agitation is severe, high boluses (up to 40 mg) may be required.

Modified from Dubin WR. In Stoudemire A, editor: *Clinical psychiatry for medical students,* Philadelphia, 1990, JB Lippincott; Tesar GE, Murray GB, Cassem NH: *J Clin Psychopharmacol* 5:344, 1985.

*Haloperidol is not specifically approved by the Food and Drug Administration for the intravenous route; careful documentation of the necessity and rationale must be achieved.

may occur in the first 24 hours after treatment. Extrapyramidal side effects that are not dose related may occur early, as may dystonic reactions. The most serious form of dystonia is laryngospasm, which compromises the airway by contracting the muscles of the larynx and leads to severe respiratory distress.

The sedative or anticholinergic effects of neuroleptics may mask or aggravate certain delirious or toxic metabolic confusional states. In general these effects are more common with low-potency neuroleptics, whereas the extrapyramidal symptoms are more typical of high-potency agents. Akathisia is a sometimes subtle or unrecognized side effect that is too frequently misdiagnosed in a patient who is agitated or is having psychotic decompensation. The inability to sit still, restlessness, or an inner feeling of anxiety induced by akathisia is relieved only by pacing. The patient is literally wound up like a spring; he or she is irritable and feels like "jumping out of his or her skin" (Van Putten and Marder, 1987). This drug-induced phenomenon can literally worsen the patient's clinical outcome and has been reported to lead to acts of suicide, violence, or homicide. Thus the patient who has received rapid tranquilization and appears to be worsening, the patient who responds initially but becomes agitated subsequently, or the patient who complies with drug treatment but has an apparent relapse should be considered a likely prospect for akathisia. See Chapter 14, Drugs Used to Treat Extrapyramidal Side Effects, for a discussion of treatment of this side effect.

Less common problems that may emerge with rapid neuroleptization are discussed in Chapter 4, Schizophrenia and Other Psychoses. Neuroleptic malignant syndrome, the potential for tardive dyskinesia (not well defined in these patients) or other serious side effects, and, the possibility of sudden death generally develop with long-term neuroleptic use. A final concern with rapid neuroleptization arises when low-potency drugs are used, for example, chlorpromazine, requiring large volumes of injectable medication. As much as 25 mg/mL, when resulting in local tissue irritation, requires adequate nursing techniques and prohibits the administration of individual volumes any larger than 3 mL per site. Of course, a high-concentration, high-potency neuroleptic is preferred for this practical reason alone.

Sedative-hypnotic agents may be useful in situations involving violence in progress. Acutely violent patients under temporary physical control or restraint may benefit greatly from sedatives, if the goal is immediate sedation. Sodium amytal in doses of 200 to 500 mg may be given by slow intravenous push as a 2.5% or 5% solution at the rate of 1 mL per minute until sleep is induced. The advantage of this technique is rapid and total control of behavior through sedation. Complications include potentiation of excitement when insufficient doses are given, laryngeal spasm, or respiratory depression. Barbiturates may potentiate the effects of other central nervous system depressants, including alcohol or other sedative hypnotic agents, as discussed in Chapter 6, Anxiety Disorders. Another alternative is the use of intravenous diazepam in 5- to 10-mg doses (Tupin, 1975).

Other sedative-hypnotic agents that may be used to treat alcohol or sedative-hypnotic withdrawal in less profoundly ill patients or when neuroleptics are ineffective include diazepam, chlordiazepoxide, and lorazepam (Table 9-1). The intramuscular use of lorazepam in 1- to 2-mg doses is discussed in Chapter 6, Anxiety Disorders, and is given in Table 9-1. Side effects may include ataxia, nausea, vomiting, amnesia, and confusion. Aggression is usually well controlled by means of a regimen of 10 mg or less of lorazepam in a 24-hour period, but sedative-hypnotics are not particularly effective in psychotic patients. Lorazepam or an equivalent dose of clonazepam may be especially useful in managing acute mania (Lenox et al, 1992), as discussed in Chapter 5, Mood Disorders.

A discussion of the use of restraints and seclusion is beyond the scope of this text. However, some general guidelines for the use of restraints with or without seclusion are provided in Table 9-3. When verbal intervention and voluntary medication are refused or fail to benefit the violent patient, seclusion and restraint may be necessary to ensure safety and facilitate treatment. Seclusion or restraint may be needed the following instances: (1) to prevent imminent harm to the patient or other persons when other means of control are ineffective or inappropriate, (2) to prevent serious disruption of the treatment program or significant damage to the physical environment, (3) for treatment as part of an ongoing plan of behavior therapy, (4) to decrease the stimulation that a patient is receiving, and (5) at the request of the patient (American Psychiatric Association, 1985). Thus "the containment of the violent impulse, the isolation from frightening or confusing external stimuli, and the definition of disrupted ego boundaries may result in a therapeutic response" (Soloff, 1987). An emergency setting may include patients brought by the police in handcuffs; in such cases restraint is necessary so that a further measure of security and control is provided while assessment is carried out or treatment begun.

Physical control such as seclusion and restraint are used when the patient's behavior exceeds the tolerance of the setting, a tolerance which may be defined by staffing patterns, patient population, or philosophy of care (Gerlock and Solomons, 1983). With rare exceptions mechanical restraint or seclusion is, indeed, an involuntary treatment requiring the use of force and suspension of the patient's right to refuse (Outlaw and Lowery, 1992; Keltner and Folks, in press). The choice of either seclusion or restraint as a means of control is all too often made based on legal,

Table 9-3 Intensive Care of the Violent Patient: Guidelines for Restraint With or Without Seclusion

Guideline	Comment
Personnel and approach	A team of four or five personnel approach the patient confidently and calmly, with a firm but kind "show of force"; an explanation is provided for the seclusion and restraint; reassurance and clarification are provided throughout the process.
Technique	Restraint is achieved by use of leather straps, with patient's legs "spread eagle," one arm to one side, and one arm above the head with the head slightly raised.
Monitoring	Restraints are checked every 5 to 15 minutes as appropriate; toileting occurs at least every 4 hours, and requests for food and beverage are promptly met; the attending physician is notified of the restraint within 1 to 3 hours and attends the patient, in keeping with established policies.
Treatment	Verbal or drug intervention ensues immediately, and rapid tranquilization is carried out, if appropriate, per protocol; restraint and then seclusion are discontinued only after the patient is calm, communicative, and cooperative.
Removal	Restraints are removed one at a time, except for the last two, which are removed simultaneously; the patient is debriefed, that is, given a clear explanation for the seclusion and restraint.

Modified from Binder, RL, McCoy SM: *Hosp Community Psychiatry* 34:1052, 1983; Dubin WR. In Stoudemire A, editor: *Clinical psychiatry for medical students,* Philadelphia, 1990, JB Lippincott; Dubin WR, Weiss KJ. In Michels R et al: *Psychiatry,* vol 2, Philadelphia, 1985, JB Lippincott.

rather than clinical, wisdom (Phillips and Nast, 1983). The mental health professional should be familiar with the legal aspects of seclusion and restraint, as well as the clinical advantages and disadvantages of both (Soloff, Gutheil, and Wexler, 1985).

Long-Term Treatment

Long-term treatment of the aggressive or violent patient is often carried out in more restrictive settings. However, shorter hospital stays have resulted in the need to effectively intervene in crisis units and outpatient settings in some cases. Management of aggressive behavior or violence in patients may also be carried out within the community or in a long-term care setting. Patients with mental retardation or psychosis or who are cognitively impaired may represent the majority of these cases.

The long-term drug treatment of aggressive or violent behavior ideally combines medication with psychosocial interventions. Psychotherapy for patients with personality disorders, as well as medication and social intervention for those who may be cognitively impaired, has proven beneficial. Compliance with a medical regimen may also be a significant problem in such cases. The motivation of the patient, the patient's ability to achieve self-control, issues regarding transference and countertransference, the development of affective awareness and insight, and the appreciation of the consequences of violence all represent psychotherapeutic tasks that are imperative in these cases.

Generally there is no one drug treatment for long-term management of the violent patient, who may be potentially disruptive or aggressive. A variety of drugs have been suggested, depending on the underlying cause. Neuroleptics, lithium, sodium valproate, carbamazepine, antidepressants, beta blockers, and the anxiolytics have been used effectively, as depicted in Table 9-4. Most recently buspirone, valproate, and perhaps the SSRIs have emerged as potentially beneficial long-term medications. Also, the novel antidepressant trazodone has been suggested as possibly useful in a variety of patients, either in single doses of 25 to 50 mg or larger doses given primarily at bedtime (Folks, 1990; Folks and Fuller, in press).

As outlined in Table 9-4, neuroleptics are mostly useful for treating schizophrenia, mania, and other syndromes in which delusional thinking, significant agitation, or psychotic symptoms are present. Haloperidol and loxapine are particularly popular because they can be administered rapidly in high doses and are safe for use in patients with epilepsy (Donlon, Hopkin, and Tupin, 1979). Haloperidol or fluphenazine may be reasonable choices for the patient in whom depot administration is desirable in aftercare, for example, the patient with paranoid schizophrenia. Of course, long-term treatment patients are subject to the long-term side effects of neuroleptics including tardive dyskinesia, as outlined in Chapter 4, Schizophrenia and Other Psychoses.

Lithium is an effective treatment for aggression or hypersexuality, or both, in patients with mania and for the prophylaxis of manic depressive disorder. Lithium is also useful in decreasing agitation, aggression, and the potential for violence in many patients. However, no study has shown that lithium has been effective in treating aggression associated with epilepsy (Lion and Tardiff, 1987). Lithium has been successfully applied to treating children and adolescents with chronic aggressive behavior and conduct disorders (Campbell et al, 1982). Although no significant difference is evident between lithium and haloperidol, the advantages of lithium with respect to short-term and long-term side effects are obvious in these cases. Generally lithium produces the best results in children or adolescents with a strong mood component related to the aggressive or violent behavior. Lithium is not currently approved for uses other than to treat manic depressive illness and is not generally recommended for use in children under age 12, as noted in Chapters 15, Psychopharmacology for Children, and 16, Psychopharmacology for Adolescents.

Valproate has received recent attention as a useful agent for aggressive behavior and for acute agitation. It is commonly used as an alternative to lithium. This agent may be uniquely effective in rapid mood cycling (Pope et al, 1991) and in geriatric patients (Mazure, Druss, and Cellar, 1992; Lott, McElroy, and Keys 1995; Mellow, Solano-Lopex, and Davis, 1993). Posttraumatic stress syndrome, behavioral dyscontrol, agitated dementia, and "organic" psychotic patients have been reported to respond to treatment with valproate at concentrations of 50 to 150 μg/mL (Wilcox, 1994).

Carbamazepine continues to be useful for treating aggression in psychiatric patients without epilepsy. This drug is discussed in detail in relation to bipolar disorder (see Chapter 5, Mood Disorders) and epilepsy (see Chapter 7, Seizure Disorders). Psychotic patients, predominantly patients with schizophrenia or cognitive impairment associated with aggression and excitability, benefit greatly from carbamazepine with or without haloperidol as an adjunct (Luchins 1983; Klein et al, 1980). Carbamazepine may be particularly useful in patients with temporal lobe abnormalities on electroencephalogram (Folks et al, 1982; Luchins, 1984). Carbamazepine may also be useful in decreasing agitation, aggressiveness, and emotional

Table 9-4 Long-Term Psychopharmacologic Treatment of Aggression

Agent	Indications	Approximate dose*(mg)	Special clinical considerations†
Neuroleptic	Aggression directly related to psychotic symptoms; management of violence or aggression by use of single dose or rapid neuroleptization	Standard antipsychotic doses	Oversedation; multiple side effects, including risk of tardive dyskinesia when used long-term
Carbamazepine or valproate	Aggression related to mood cycling or seizures; aggression possibly related to general medical condition	Maintain serum levels at 6-12 μg/mL of carbamazepine and 50-120 μg/mL of valproate	Monitor for evidence of toxic effects; watch for microsomal induction and drop in serum level of carbamazepine
Lithium	Aggression and irritability related to manic excitement or cyclic mood	Maintain serum levels at 0.6-1.2 mEq/L	May augment effects of antidepressants, antipsychotics, or carbamazepine
Benzodiazepines	Acute management of agitation by use of sedative-hypnotic properties	Standard anxiolytic doses	Possible induction of paradoxic rage; problems with over-sedation
Buspirone	Long-term management by use of antianxiety and serotonergic properties	15-60 mg in divided doses	Onset of action up to 30 days at sufficient dose; may be used secondarily as an adjunct to another agent
Beta blockers	Recurrent aggression in patients with cognitive impairment or irritability when aggression is not directly related to psychosis	50-400 mg/day of propranolol in divided doses	Latency period before onset of action may be 4-6 weeks; metaprolol, atenolol, and nadolol are alternative agents
SSRIs	Aggression associated with dysphoric mood or personality disorder or cognitive impairment	Low doses	Onset of action at 3-4 weeks

Modified from Maletta GJ: *Psychiatr Ann* 20:454-1990.
*Doses for geriatric patients should be started at lower levels and individually titrated over time.
†Trazodone in 25- to 50-mg doses may also be useful alone or as an adjunct to another agent.

lability in patients with episodic dyscontrol syndrome (Monroe, 1970; Stone et al, 1986).

Buspirone (BuSpar) has shown promise in patients with agitated dementia or other aggressive syndromes associated with cognitive impairment. Aggressive or agitated patients with brain injury and mental retardation or developmental disorder also appear to respond to buspirone alone or when coadministered with another agent. Standard therapeutic doses of 15 to 60 mg have been effective (Stanislav et al, 1994; Ratey et al, 1992). The serotonergic affect is thought to be responsible for buspirone's beneficial effect, which can take up to 6 weeks to occur. Similarly, a number of clinicians have noted positive effect from the SSRIs, generally at low doses, for example, sertraline 25 to 50 mg or fluoxetine 10 to 20 mg (Burke et al, 1994). Further studies are needed to confirm their usefulness.

Propranolol is useful in treating chronic or recurrent aggression, especially in patients with brain injury or psychiatric syndromes secondary to general medical conditions. Chronic or recurrent aggression or irritability in patients whose aggression is not directly related to psychotic ideation may also benefit particularly from this class of drug. Silver and Yudofsky (1985) have reviewed the beta blockers, noting their successful application for treating aggression in patients with head trauma, seizures, Wilson's disease, mental retardation, minimal brain dysfunction, Korsakoff's psychosis, and other neuropsychiatric disorders. Doses lower than 640 mg per day and a response time of 2 days to 6 weeks are typical. Side effects include lowered blood pressure, decreased pulse rate, and, rarely, respiratory difficulties, nightmares, ataxia, and lethargy. Most patients receive concomitant treatment with haloperidol or other neuroleptic medication. Some adverse effects, including central nervous system intoxication, severe sedation, and cardiovascular reactions, have been reported (Alexander, McCarty, and Giffen, 1984). Thus a careful medical examination should be performed to identify patients with cardiopulmonary distress, asthma, insulin-dependent diabetes mellitus, cardiac disease, severe renal disease, or hyperthyroidism.

The initial dosages of propranolol are 20 mg 3 times a day; dosages may be increased by 60 mg every 3 to 4 days, usually to a maximum of 640 mg per day. Dizziness, wheezing, and ataxia are all indications for decreasing the dosage. The highest tolerated dose should be given for at least 1 month before concluding that the patient is nonresponsive. Plasma levels of neuroleptics and antiepileptics should also be monitored in concert with beta-blocker treatment. Prospective studies and further use of propranolol and other, similar agents are needed. Recently Ratey et al (1992) showed a significant decline in the frequency of nadolol-treated aggression when compared with controls. Thus nadolol and other beta blockers, for example, metaprolol or pindolol, may prove to be of significant benefit in treating aggression in psychiatric patients with chronic conditions.

IMPLICATIONS AND TREATMENT ISSUES

There are many special concerns about the treatment of aggression and violence in patients with psychiatric disorders, particularly in an outpatient setting. Lion and Tardiff (1987) have noted that countertransference issues, inappropriate response, safety concerns for staff and bystanders, the duty to protect potential victims, and other ongoing issues must be addressed. As patients become less violent, a risk of despondency ensues. Aggressive patients presumably value being aggressive. To relinquish such behaviors is to be confronted with passivity, dependence, and the helplessness inherent in being weak. Thus the therapeutic task in treating violence, both short-term and long-term, includes consideration of these aspects of management of patient care. These considerations, together with drug treatment, supportive interventions, and seclusion, restraint, and maintenance medication, are intended to culminate in improved therapeutic outcome and to reduce the potential for harm.

REFERENCES

Alexander HE, McCarty K, Giffen MD: Hypotension and cardiopulmonary arrest associated with concurrent haloperidol and propranolol therapy, *JAMA* 252:87, 1984.

American Psychiatric Association: *Report of the task force on psychiatric uses of seclusion and restraint of the council on governmental policy and the law of the American Psychiatric Association,* Task Force Report No. 22, Washington, DC, 1985, The Association.

Anderson WH, Kuehnle JC: Strategies for the treatment of acute psychosis, *JAMA* 229:1884, 1974.

Anderson WH, Kuehnle JC, Catanzano DM: Rapid treatment of acute psychosis, *Am J Psychiatry* 133:1086, 1976.

Baldessarini RJ, Katz B, Cotton P: Dissimilar dosing with high-potency and low-potency neuroleptics, *Am J Psychiatry* 141:748, 1984.

Bernstein HA: Survey of threats and assaults directed toward psychotherapists, *Am J Psychother* 35:542, 1981.

Bjorkly S: Scale for the prediction of aggression and dangerousness in psychotic patients: an introduction, *Psychol Rep* 73:1363-1377, 1993.

Burke WJ et al: Serotonin reuptake inhibitors for the treatment of coexisting depression and psychosis in dementia of the Alzheimer type, *Am J Geriatr Psychiatry,* 2(4):352-3, 1994.

Campbell M et al: Lithium and haloperidol in hospitalized aggressive children, *Psychopharmacol Bull* 18:126, 1982.

Clinton JE et al: Haloperidol for sedation of disruptive emergency patients, *Ann Emerg Med* 16:319, 1987.

Czobor P, Volavka J, Meibach RC: Effect of risperidone on hostility in schizophrenia, *J Clin Psychopharmcol* 15:4:243-9, 1995.

Depp FC: Violent behavior patterns on psychiatric wards, *Aggressive Behavior* 2:295, 1976.

Donlon PT, Hopkin J, Tupin JP: Overview: efficacy and safety of the rapid neuroleptization method with injectable haloperidol, *Am J Psychiatry* 136:273, 1979.

Donlon PT et al: Haloperidol for acute schizophrenic patients: an evaluation of three oral regimes, *Arch Gen Psychiatry* 37:691, 1980.

Dubin WR: The evaluation and management of the violent patient, *Ann Emerg Med* 10:481, 1981.

Dubin WR, Weiss KJ, Dorn JM: Pharmacotherapy of psychiatric emergencies, *J Clin Psychopharmacol* 6:210, 1986.

Dubin WR, Wilson S, Mercer C: Assaults against psychiatrists in outpatient settings, *J Clin Psychiatry* 49:338, 1988.

Elliott FA: Violence. The neurologic contribution: an overview, *Arch Neurol* 49:595-603, 1992.

Folks DG: Clinical approaches to anxiety in the medically ill elderly, *Drug Ther Suppl,* August 1990, p 72-80.

Folks DG, Fuller WC: Uses of anxiolytics and sedatives in geriatric practice: clinical selection and treatment considerations, *Psychiatr Clin North Am,* New York, (in press).

Folks DG et al: Carbamazepine treatment of selected affectively disordered inpatients, *Am J Psychiatry* 139:115, 1982.

Gardner DL, Cowdry RW: Alprazolam-induced dyscontrol in borderline personality disorder, *Am J Psychiatry* 142:98, 1985.

Gerlock A, Solomons HC: Factors associated with the seclusion of psychiatric patients, *Perspect Psychiatr Care* 21:47, 1983.

Goldstein MG: Intensive care unit syndromes. In Stoudemire A, Fogel BS, editors: *Principles of medical psychiatry,* Orlando, Fla, 1987, Grune & Stratton.

Haller RM, Deluty RH: Assaults on staff by psychiatric inpatients: a critical review, *Br J Psychiatry* 152:174-9, 1988.

Hanke N: *Handbook of emergency psychiatry,* Lexington, Mass, 1984, DC Health.

Keltner NL, Folks DG: Legal considerations in the administration of psychotropic drugs, *Perspect Psychiatr Care* (in press).

Klein DF et al: *Diagnosis and drug treatment of psychiatric disorders: adults and children,* ed 2, Baltimore, 1980, Williams & Wilkins.

Kyser JG, Diner BC, Raulston GW: A practical approach to the assessment and management of psychiatric emergencies, *Jefferson Psychiatry* 7:81, 1989.

Lenox RH et al: Adjunctive treatment of manic agitation with lorazepam versus haloperidol: a double-blind study, *J Clin Psychiatry* 53:47, 1992.

Lidz CW, Mulvey EP, Gardner W: The accuracy in prediction of violence to others, *JAMA* 269:1007-11, 1993.

Linaker OM: Assaultiveness among institutionalised adults with mental retardation, *Br J Psychiatry* 164:62-8, 1994.

Linaker OM, Busch-Iversen H: Predictors of imminent violence in psychiatric inpatients, *Acta Psychiatr Scand* 92:250-4, 1995.

Lion JR: Benzodiazepines in the treatment of aggressive patients, *J Clin Psychiatry* 40:70, 1979.

Lion JR: Special aspects of psychopharmacology. In Lion JR, Reid WC, editors: *Assaults within psychiatric facilities,* New York, 1983, Grune & Stratton.

Lion JR, Levenberg LB, Strange RE: Restraining the violent patient, *J Psychosoc Nurs Ment Health Serv* 10:9, 1972.

Lion JR, Snyder W, Merrill GL: Underreporting of assaults on staff in state hospitals, *Hosp Community Psychiatry* 32:497, 1981.

Lion JR, Tardiff K: The long-term treatment of the violent patient. In Hales RE, Frances AJ, editors: *Psychiatry update: American Psychiatric Association annual review,* vol 6, Washington, DC, 1987, The Association.

Lott AD, McElroy SL, Keys MA: Valproate in the treatment of behavioral agitation in elderly patients with dementia, *J Neuropsychiatry Clin Neurosci* 7:314-9, 1995.

Luchins DJ: Carbamazepine for the violent psychiatric patient, *Lancet* 1:766, 1983.

Luchins DJ: Carbamazepine in psychiatric syndromes: clinical and neuropharmacological properties, *Psychopharmacol Bull* 20:569, 1984.

Madden DJ, Lion JR, Penna MW: Assaults on psychiatrists by patients, *Am J Psychiatry* 133:422, 1976.

Mazure CM, Druss BG, Cellar JS: Valproate treatment of older psychotic patients with organic mental syndromes and behavioral dyscontrol, *J Am Geriatr Soc* 40:9:914-6, 1992.

McNeil DE, Binder RL: Clinical assessment of the risk of violence among psychiatric inpatients, *Am J Psychiatry* 128:1317-21, 1991.

Mellow AM, Solano-Lopex C, Davis S: Sodium valproate in the treatment of behavioral disturbance in dementia, *J Geriatr Psychiatry Neurol* 6:205-9, Oct-Dec 1993.

Menza MA et al: Decreased extrapyramidal symptoms with intravenous haloperidol, *J Clin Psychiatry* 48:278, 1987.

Monroe RR: *Episodic behavioral disorders,* Cambridge, Mass, 1970, Harvard University.

Outlaw FH, Lowery BJ: Seclusion: the nursing challenge, *J Psychosoc Nurs Ment Health Serv* 30:13, 1992.

Phillips MA, Nast SJ: Seclusion and restraint and prediction of violence, *Am J Psychiatry* 140:229, 1983.

Pope HG et al: Valproate in the treatment of acute mania: a placebo-controlled study, *Arch Gen Psychiatry* 48:62-8, 1991.

Rasmussen K, Levander S: Lack of self-monitoring competency in aggressive schizophrenics, *Pers Individual Differences* 15:397-402, 1993.

Ratey JJ et al: Nadolol to treat aggression and psychiatric symptomology in chronic psychiatric inpatients: a double-blind, placebo-controlled study, *J Clin Psychiatry* 53:41, 1992.

Ratey J et al: Low-dose buspirone to treat agitation and maladaptive behavior in brain-injured patients: two case reports, *J Clin Psychopharmacol* 12:362-4, 1992 (letter).

Salzman C, Kochansky GE, Shader RI: Chlordiazepoxide-induced hostility in a small group setting, *Arch Gen Psychiatry* 31(3):401, 1974.

Salzman C et al: Benzodiazepines combined with neuroleptics for management of severe disruptive behavior, *Psychosomatics* 27(suppl 1):17, 1986.

Shah AK: An increase in violence among psychiatric patients: real or apparent? *Med Sci Law* 33:227-30, 1993.

Silver JM, Yudofsky S: Propranolol for aggression: literature review and clinical guidelines, *Int Drug Ther Newsletter* 20:9, 1985.

Slotnick VB: *Management of the acutely agitated psychotic patient with parenteral neuroleptics: a comparative symptoms effectiveness profile of haloperidol and chlorpromazine.* Paper presented at the Fifth World Congress of Psychiatry, Mexico City, Nov 1971.

Soloff PH: Emergency management of violent patients. In Hales RE, Frances AJ, editors: *American Psychiatric Association annual review,* vol 6, Washington, DC, 1987, The Association.

Soloff PH, Gutheil TG, Wexler DB: Seclusion and restraint in 1985: a review and update, *Hosp Community Psychiatry* 36:318, 1985.

Soreff SM: Violence in the emergency room. In BS Comstock et al, editors: *Phenomenology and treatment of psychiatric emergencies,* New York, 1984, Spectrum.

Stanislav SW et al: Buspirone's efficacy in organic-induced aggression, *J Clin Psychopharmacol* 14(2):126-30, 1994.

Stone JL et al: Episodic dyscontrol disorder and paroxysmal EEG abnormalities: successful treatment with carbamazepine, *Biol Psychiatry* 21:208, 1986.

Tesar GE, Murray GB, Cassem NH: Use of high-dose intravenous haloperidol in the treatment of agitated cardiac patients, *J Clin Psychopharmacol* 5:344, 1985.

Tupin JP: Management of the violent patients. In Shader RI, editor: *Manual of psychiatric therapeutics,* Boston, 1975, Little, Brown.

Van Putten T, Marder SR: Behavioral toxicity of antipsychotic drugs, *J Clin Psychiatry* 48(suppl 9):13, 1987.

Wilcox J: Divalproex sodium in the treatment of aggressive behavior, *Ann Clin Psychiatry* 6:1:17-20, 1994.

CHAPTER 10

Alcoholism and Other Substance Abuse Disorders

SCOPE OF THE PROBLEM

Abuse of drugs and alcohol in American society is widespread, despite concerted efforts to educate the public and curb their use. Substance-related health care costs are staggering, accounting for an estimated $140 billion of the total U.S. health care budget of more than $900 billion. Substance abuse is embedded in most of our other social problems. Dependence on alcohol and drugs has moved to the forefront of issues in psychiatric medicine and nursing. Many new developments have taken place in the field. Studies of genetic and environmental influences, neurobiologic contributors, and the clinical approach have provided important insights about treatment. Moreover, a greater understanding of individuals with dual diagnoses and sequelae resulting from alcohol or drug use has further improved the ability to develop effective treatment strategies. This chapter focuses on pharmacologic agents used to ameliorate withdrawal syndromes, modify drug-seeking behavior, and treat psychiatric disorders in drug-dependent individuals. Chapter 12, Drugs of Abuse, examines drugs of abuse without reference to treatment considerations. Although there is some overlap in the content of these two chapters, there is little redundancy.

EPIDEMIOLOGY

Accurate assessment of the extent and character of substance abuse and dependence patterns is difficult because of several significant measurement problems. Because the use of most drugs is illicit or unacceptable, most surveys are likely to provide conservative estimates of prevalence as a result of underreporting by respondents. Because drug-taking patterns change rapidly, national survey data may also be outdated by the time they are reported. Also, marked variation exists in patterns among persons from various cultural groups and different geographic regions. Further, data from emergency departments and other treatment facilities, as well as data from arrest records or reports of overdose deaths, measure only those individuals who are largely unsuccessful in their drug use patterns. Despite these limitations, it is possible to outline some of the trends in substance abuse that are pertinent to pharmacologic interventions.

Historical Perspective

Before the 1960s the abuse of all psychoactive drugs except alcohol was relatively rare and confined primarily to certain underprivileged inner-city populations, individuals within the entertainment world, or criminals. Marijuana use began to increase in the 1960s, particularly among urban men. This use increased with the emergence of a counterculture that rejected traditional values and sought to find meaning, truth, or escape in pharmacologically induced altered states of consciousness. Subsequently the civil rights movement, the Vietnam war, birth control pills, and the development of a range of legitimate psychotropic medicines were contributing factors in a sharp rise in nonmedical psychoactive drug taking. For example, during the 1960s and 1970s marijuana use spread to rural areas, increasing the incidence of use at least once in a lifetime (lifetime experience incidence) in 1979 to 31% in 12- to 17-year-olds and 68% in young adults (Fishburne, Abelson, and Cisin, 1980). During the 1980s the use of marijuana and other hallucinogens declined. Also, the nonmedical use of sedative-hypnotic agents, in particular, barbiturates, appeared to level off. Cocaine became a more frequently employed drug of abuse, its use rising in 1982 to a lifetime experience rate of 28.3% among young adults. Since the mid-1980s cocaine use has remained stable or even decreased slightly. Heroin use has remained stable, although it has moved from predominantly inner-city, impoverished groups to more affluent populations (Johnston, Bachman, and O'Malley, 1984; Miller, et al, 1983). Also during the 1980s and 1990s a major shift in the gender pattern of substance abuse took place. Traditionally men were more likely to smoke, drink alcoholic beverages, or use drugs, but in recent years more women have been noted to be drug users than in the past (Clayton, 1984).

National Surveys

The National Institute on Drug Abuse sponsors two key national surveys: the National Survey of High School Seniors and the National Household Survey on Drug Abuse. The National Survey of High School Seniors has noted a steadily declining annual prevalence of substance abuse since 1987, to an annual incidence of 5.3% in 1990 (Johnston, Bachman, and O'Malley, 1991). The use of crack cocaine, an inexpensive freebase form of the drug, has steadily decreased from a lifetime experience incidence of 5.4% in 1987 to 4.7% in 1989 and 3.5% in 1990. Despite the general overall decreases and the decline in the use of crack cocaine, 48% of high school seniors in 1990 had tried one illicit drug and almost a third had tried an illicit drug other than marijuana (Johnston, Bachman, and O'Malley, 1991). One problem with such surveys is that they do not include high school dropouts, among whom there is a higher incidence of drug abuse.

Data from the National Household Survey on Drug Abuse (1991) indicated that in general, substantial declines in the prevalence of drug use had occurred, beginning in 1985. Marijuana appears to be the most widely abused illegal drug in the United States, with an estimated 67.7 million Americans having used marijuana at least once in their lifetimes (National Household Survey on Drug Abuse, 1991). Some critics challenge the validity of the National Household Survey on Drug Abuse because homeless individuals, prison inmates, and others living in institutions or treatment centers are not counted. The segment of the population that is not counted by the survey is, perhaps, the one most affected by drug addiction. Many scientists, educators, and politicians have expressed the fear that the numbers reported by the National Institute on Drug Abuse will be used to underestimate the amount of resources needed to combat the drug problem (Kaufman and McNaul, 1992).

The most current estimates for the United States concerning substance dependence are depicted in Table 10-1. These estimates from the National Comorbidity Study represent a large-scale epidemiologic project completed between 1990 and 1992 (Anthony et al, 1994; Kessler et al, 1994). Comparing alcohol with tobacco, more 15- to 54-year-olds consumed alcohol (91.5%) than tobacco, but fewer alco-

Table 10-1 Estimated Prevalence (± SE) of Extramedical Use and Dependence in Total Study Population and Lifetime Dependence Among Users

Drugs	Proportion with a history of dependence	Proportion with a history of extramedical use	Dependence among extramedical users
Tobacco*	24.1 ± 1.0	75.6 ± 0.6	31.9†
Alcohol	14.1 ± 0.7	91.5 ± 0.5	15.4 ± 0.7
Other drugs	7.5 ± 0.4	51.0 ± 1.0	14.7 ± 0.7
Cannabis	4.2 ± 0.3	46.3 ± 1.1	9.1 ± 0.7
Cocaine	2.7 ± 0.2	16.2 ± 0.6	16.7 ± 1.5
Stimulants	1.7 ± 0.3	15.3 ± 0.7	11.2 ± 1.6
Anxiolytics‡	1.2 ± 0.2	12.7 ± 0.5	9.2 ± 1.1
Analgesics	0.7 ± 0.1	9.7 ± 0.5	7.5 ± 1.0
Psychedelics	0.5 ± 0.1	10.6 ± 0.6	4.9 ± 0.7
Heroin	0.4 ± 0.1	1.5 ± 0.2	23.1 ± 5.6
Inhalants	0.3 ± 0.1	6.8 ± 0.4	3.7 ± 1.4

From Anthony JC, Arria AM, Johnson EO: Epidemiological and public health issues for tobacco, alcohol, and other drugs. In Oldham JM and Riba MB, editors: *Review of psychiatry,* vol 14, Washington, DC, 1995, American Psychiatric Press.
Note: Weighted estimates from National Comorbidity Survey data gathered in 1990–1992; N = 8098 persons ages 15-54. Extramedical use refers to the use of the drug listed without a physician prescription and supervision or in ways not intended by such a prescription if one was given.
*N = 4414.
†Not estimated.
‡Anxiolytics, sedatives, and hypnotic drugs, grouped.

hol users became dependent (15.4%). Thus the lifetime prevalence of alcohol dependence is 14.1%, compared with 24.1% for tobacco dependence. Psychoactive drug use other than tobacco and alcohol is at 12.4% for males compared with 7.1% for females.

The comorbidity of psychoactive substance dependence with psychiatric disorders is significant. Substance abusers are at risk to develop psychiatric disturbance and anxiety; depression and other psychiatric disorders are often associated with self-medication, including alcohol use. Substance-dependent patients with a comorbid psychiatric condition are much more likely to relapse and have a poorer prognosis (Anthony et al, 1995).

Pregnancy Considerations

Drug abuse, particularly, cocaine use, in pregnant women and its effects on the fetus and infant is also an epidemiologic concern. The consequences of cocaine use during pregnancy include complications both prenatally and during delivery, as well as other toxic effects that can result in congenital malformations and drug withdrawal symptoms in infants. These withdrawal symptoms may last for several weeks beyond birth (Dixon, 1989; Neerhof et al, 1989; Little et al, 1988; Giacoia, 1990).

Psychologic Considerations

Psychologic alterations induced by drug abuse may have significant influences on the personalities of those exposed persistently to drugs. Drug-related nonfatal emergencies, deaths, and emergency room visits for the treatment of alcohol abuse are well-known phenomena. Thus there is the need to continue studying determinants of drug and alcohol abuse and to further develop pharmacologic agents that may be useful in treatment.

GENETIC, ENVIRONMENTAL, AND OTHER INFLUENCES

Genetic Influences

The study of genetic contributors to alcohol and substance abuse is just beginning. The lack of knowledge about the genetic aspects of drug addiction is marked, in contrast to the wealth of knowledge about the genetic aspects of alcoholism, for which a hereditary relationship has been well established for years. Adoption studies and twin studies focusing on drug abuse have begun to improve our understanding of genetic and environmental factors that contribute to drug abuse (Cadoret et al, 1986; Grove et al, 1990; Pickens and Svikis, 1989). Generally drug abuse is highly correlated with antisocial personality disorder, and antisocial personality disorder, in turn, is often predicted by the presence of antisocial personality behavior in a first-degree relative. Alcohol problems among biologic relatives often predict increased drug or alcohol abuse, or both, in those without antisocial personality disorder who are adopted but not in adoptees with the disorder (Cadoret et al, 1986). Offspring of tobacco smokers are more likely to become tobacco smokers and to become tobacco dependent than is the general population (Krasnagor, 1979). A higher rate of opiate dependence is found among the siblings and relatives of opiate addicts than among the general population (Kaufman, 1981). Interestingly one study measured a euphoric response to a single 1-mg oral dose of alprazolam in a sample of 12 nonalcoholic sons of alcoholics (Ciraulo et al, 1989). Nine of the men with a family history of alcoholism experienced euphoria, whereas only two of the 12 control subjects without a family history of alcoholism had a euphoric response.

Other studies of risk or possible genetic contributors to substance abuse include the longitudinal study of Kandel, Simcha-Fagan, and Davis (1986), who found that delinquency was highly predictive of drug abuse in adolescents and young adults. Wallace (1990) has found that 61% of a sample of individuals referred for crack cocaine detoxification were adult children of alcoholics and that another 36% had dysfunctional family characteristics other than alcoholism. Another recent study identified the influence of older brothers, peers, and parents on younger brothers' drug use (Brook et al, 1990). The results showed that older brothers who did not use drugs could offset the effects of parental drug use on younger brothers. Also, younger brothers were least likely to use drugs if both older brothers and peers abstained.

Environmental Influences

Drug-taking patterns are apparently influenced by factors relating to the family constellation and psychosocial environment. Possibly the lack of realistic, rewarding alternatives and the paucity of legitimate role models may render drug-taking behaviors more attractive (Millman and Khuri, 1981). Peer influence plays a central role in the initiation, development, and maintenance of drug abuse patterns (Sadava, 1973). The media may also have a profound effect on substance abuse patterns. Alcohol, marijuana, and tobacco have been romanticized such that engaging in these behaviors sometimes may confer on the user a variety of attributes perceived to be positive. Although the dangers of cocaine, alcohol, and tobacco use are receiving a great deal of attention in newspapers and magazines and on television, these drugs also are portrayed as an exciting province of the rich, the famous, and the popular.

Moreover, young individuals growing up in families with parents or older siblings who are substance abusers tend to become substance abusers themselves. Parental attitudes or perceived parental attitudes influence the adolescent's decision to start drinking alcoholic beverages or taking drugs. Other familial factors possibly related to drug abuse include family instability, parental rejection, and divorce (Maloff et al, 1982; Millman, 1986).

Psychiatric Influences

Whether drug abuse or dependence results from specific personality factors or psychodynamics and whether particular drug-use patterns are associated with certain personality types remain controversial (Millman, 1986). Youthful drug abusers have been characterized as having external locus of control (Williams, 1973), and lowered self-esteem and increased anxiety and depression have been noted among these abusers (Braucht et al, 1973; Weider and Kaplan, 1969). Psychodynamic conceptualizations have suggested that abuse of alcohol and drugs is an attempt to self-medicate a variety of dysphoric states. In addition, the muting and antiaggression properties of the opiates and other compounds may diminish painful psychic states, at least temporarily, and allow the narcotic-dependent individual to cope (Khantzian, 1974; Wurmser, 1974).

Sometimes it is difficult to tell whether the psychopathologic features associated with alcohol or substance abuse are secondary or primary to the pharmacologic effect of the chronic use of the particular drug. Also, the adaptation to the experience of becoming and being a drug-dependent person in a society that stigmatizes and punishes such behavior must be appreciated (Zinberg, 1975). Most likely, substance abusers vary markedly in premorbid personality patterns and in psychopathologic features. Systematic studies of narcotic addicts in methadone treatment have demonstrated the heterogeneity of psychiatric diagnoses in these populations (Rounsaville, Gawin, and Kleber, 1985; McLellan, Woody, and O'Brien, 1979). Perhaps the choice of drug may reflect personality patterns or psychopathology, thus whether stimulants, narcotics, opiates, alcohol, or other sedative-hypnotic depressants are used may depend on the specific individual's makeup and may account for great heterogeneity among substance-abuse populations. As noted in Chapters 6, Anxiety Disorders, and 8, Sleep Disorders, alcohol or other depressants may be used to suppress or treat symptoms of anxiety or, by contrast, to allow expression of long-suppressed anger (Millman, 1986). Some individuals may avoid the use of marijuana, hallucinogens, or stimulants that weaken the connection to reality and amplify paranoid, psychotic, or anxiety states. Generally a careful drug-use history, with particular emphasis on which drugs are perceived as pleasant and beneficial and which have led to adverse reactions, may facilitate the clinical approach.

Drug-Related Influences

All too often the sense of control that derives from drug abuse is related to the effect of a rapid rate of change of consciousness or perception in almost any direction (Millman, 1985). For example, cocaine is perceived to be more desirable than an oral amphetamine; a rapidly acting benzodiazepine may be more subject to abuse than are drugs that are slower in onset. Moreover, the conditioned learning important in maintaining drug abuse patterns and in initiating relapse may also be an important environmental influence. For example, the dysphoric symptoms that the drug-taking behavior allayed or controlled or certain situations that have come to be associated with drug-taking behaviors become in time the conditioned stimulus for the experience of drug craving and drug-seeking behavior. Learning may be an important determinant of the subjective perception of the drug experience; for example, marijuana is used in some cultures as a work enhancer and an appetite suppressant, in contrast to its publicized effects in America as a drug that decreases motivation and stimulates the appetite for sweet food.

Neurobiologic Influences

The most recent neurochemical research has focused on opioids and cocaine. Cocaine and other abusable stimulants have varied actions on multiple neurotransmitter systems. Essentially these compounds exert their primary effect on dopaminergic systems, but they also affect noradrenergic, serotonergic, and cholinergic systems (Gawin, 1988). Cocaine increases dopamine concentration in the synaptic cleft, resulting in increased neurotransmission in brain reward systems. Chronic use of cocaine or other stimulants causes catecholamine receptor supersensitivity. Autoreceptor feedback systems may ultimately decrease dopaminergic transmission. This action may explain the anhedonia seen in chronic cocaine users. Cocaine may also impair the ability of neurons to use dopa (Baxter et al, 1988; Volkow et al, 1990). Also, the benzodiazepine receptor may be affected by cocaine through complex interactions. Studies of these receptors and their interactions with the gamma-aminobutyric acid (GABA) neurotransmitter systems may further explain some of the phenomena seen in both cocaine and benzodiazepine withdrawal (Kolata, 1982). In addition to the opiates, a receptor specific for tetrahydrocannabinol (THC), the active ingredient in marijuana, has recently been identified in the human brain (Culhane, 1990). This discovery may lead to a better understanding of the effects of marijuana, both positive, for example, appetite stimulation and nausea prevention, and negative, such as perceptual and memory disturbance. The toxic effects of marijuana may be caused by its effect on the cells of the hippocampus, which are known to be important in learning and memory (Schuster, 1990).

The availability of animal models that simulate drug addiction in humans has enabled identification of specific regions in the brain that are important in addictive disorders. The locus ceruleus plays an important role in physical dependence to opiates. The mesolimbic dopamine system is involved in clinically evident drug-seeking behavior. Molecular and cellular changes or adaptions occur in various brain regions responsible for behavioral features of addiction and dependence. Intracellular messengers, especially G proteins and cyclic AMP systems, are involved. As pathophysiologic mechanisms are understood, pharmacologic interventions can be developed (Nestler et al, 1995).

DIAGNOSTIC CONSIDERATIONS

The appropriate treatment of an individual with substance abuse or dependence relies not only on the characterization of the specific drug and pattern of use but also on an understanding of the psychologic set and social situations attendant to the behavioral patterns. The nature and degree of drug-induced psychoactive effects, as well as the presence of abstinence phenomena, should be evaluated, which requires careful history and physical assessment, including a complete history of drug use.

The recognition and treatment of alcoholism and other types of substance abuse and dependence require knowledge of the pharmacokinetics and pharmacodynamics of specific psychoactive substances. The presence of substance abuse or dependence must be considered with respect to known therapies for the acute management of intoxication and withdrawal and options for long-term rehabilitation. Several aspects of substances that are often abused have been reviewed in a previous chapter. However, some consideration of the diagnostic approach is necessary in examining those pharmacologic agents that are used to treat alcohol and drug abuse and dependence.

Frequently no clear delineation distinguishes the appropriate use of a psychoactive substance from misuse, abuse, or dependence. Although the scope of this problem has been considered with respect to epidemiologic, genetic, environmental, and neurobiologic contributors, most of the factors determining an individual's susceptibility to substance abuse are not well understood. Studies of populations at risk for developing substance abuse have identified factors that foster the development and continuance of substance abuse. However, the relative contribution of these factors varies among individuals, and no single factor appears to account entirely for the risk. Diagnosis and classification of substance abuse disorders reflect prevailing cultural attitudes and theoretic biases. In recent years it has become recognized that these disorders may exist independent of other psychiatric conditions. Thus the current nomenclature permits the independent diagnosis of substance use and dependence apart from other psychiatric disorders.

American Psychiatric Association Considerations

The American Psychiatric Association has considered the problem of psychiatric substances to be a medical disorder when the use of psychoactive substances constitutes or meets certain criteria. From a pharmacologic perspective *dependence* is a state in which a syndrome of specific withdrawal signs and symptoms follows reduction or cessation of the drug use. *Tolerance* refers to a state in which the physiologic or behavioral effects of repeated doses of a psychoactive substance decrease over time or a greater dose of drug is necessary to achieve the same effect. *Withdrawal* is a physiologic state that follows cessation or reduction in the amount of the drug used. *Abuse* is a residual category for patterns of drug use that do not meet the criteria for dependence. Psychoactive substance abuse is therefore defined as a pattern of substance use of at least 1 month's duration that impairs social or occupational functioning and the presence of psychologic or physical problems or situations in which use of the substance is physically hazardous, for example, driving while intoxicated. "Addiction" is often used as a synonym of "dependence" but carries a more negative and pejorative connotation. Specific criteria for substance abuse are shown in Box 10-1. Box 10-2 lists the *DSM-IV* categories of psychoactive substances.

Comorbidity

Much of the current treatment approach to alcoholism and other substance use disorders has focused on the association with other psychopathologic features (Meyer, 1986; Butcher, 1988; Kosten and Kleber, 1988). Dually diagnosed patients constitute 30% to 50% of psychiatric patients and up to 80% of substance abusers. The comorbid pathologic characteristics found consist of both axis I and axis II disorders within the nomenclature (American Psychiatric Association, 1994). The most prevalent disorders include mood disorders, disorders within the affective spectrum, psychotic disorders, attention deficit and conduct disorders, and personality disorders, particularly those that fall within the cluster characterized as antisocial, histrionic, borderline, and narcissistic (Kaufman and McNaul, 1992; Woody et al, 1995). Several personality characteristics measured by the Minnesota Multiphasic

Box 10-1 Criteria for Substance Dependence

At least *three* of the following persist for at least 1 month or have occurred repeatedly over a significant period of time:

Substance taken in larger amounts or over a longer period than originally intended

Substance use to relieve or avoid stress (may not apply to cannabis, hallucinogens, or PCP)

One or more unsuccessful attempt to cut down or to control substance use or a persistent desire to do so

Considerable time spent in activities necessary to obtain the substance, using the substance, or recovering from its effects

Symptoms of intoxication or withdrawal occur when expected to fulfill major obligations at work, school, or home

Important activities or obligations are reduced or unmet due to the substance use

Continued substance use despite knowledge that a persistent or recurrent social, psychological, or physical problem is related to use of the substance

Marked tolerance with increased amount of the substance (at least 50%) to achieve intoxication or a desired effect: markedly diminished effect with use of the same amount of substance

Characteristic withdrawal symptoms

Modified from *Diagnostic and Statistical Manual of Mental Disorders,* ed 4, American Psychiatric Association, 1994, Washington, DC, The Association.

Box 10-2 Psychoactive Substance Categories According to the DSM-IV

Alcohol
Amphetamines (sympathomimetics)
Caffeine
Cannabis
Cocaine
Hallucinogens
Inhalants
Nicotine
Opioids
Phencyclidine (arylcyclohexylamines)
Sedative-hypnotics* or anxiolytics

*These drugs may precipitate drug-drug interactions.
From *Diagnostic and Statistical Manual of Mental Disorders,* ed 4, American Psychiatric Association, 1994, Washington, DC, The Association.

Personality Inventory (MMPI) have been shown to be associated with substance abuse.

Dually diagnosed individuals are prevalent among all treatment settings for substance abuse. Covert diagnosis is important; substance use disorders will follow their course, and independent disorders will follow their own course. Most substances of abuse will magnify psychiatric symptoms. Nicotine and opiates are the exception. Opiates may even suppress comorbid conditions. Whether symptoms are drug-induced or not, they must be treated. Treatment involves a combination of drug-focused and psychiatric approaches, usually involving a multidisciplinary team approach. Progress is usually shown with dual diagnosis cases, and prognosis is improved when both conditions are treated. Additional psychotherapy or counseling is often necessary in such cases.

DRUG TREATMENT

The pharmacologic approach to the treatment of alcohol and drug use or dependence ideally includes a combination of psychotherapy, behavioral techniques, and adjunctive interventions that may also serve to improve compliance with the medical regimen. To provide appropriate treatment, it is necessary to consider the psychosocial characteristics of the patient, as well as the pharmacology and pattern of abuse of the particular psychoactive substance. Treatment should be conceptualized as including initial and long-term phases.

Short-Term Treatment Objectives

During the initial phase, terminating drug use and establishing a stable, drug-free state must be the primary therapeutic goal. Identifying the substance use problem and helping the patient accept the proposed intervention may require some degree of confrontation in a family, work, social, or school setting (Blume, 1984). During the initial treatment phase, provisions must be made for long-term interventions. Whereas the therapeutic relationship and trust are essential to the treatment process, patients often resume abuse without informing the therapist. Thus intermittent or routine screens may be performed, and objective data on drug abuse status may actually facilitate an open and trusting therapeutic alliance. In the context of this relationship the following objectives of short-term treatment have been outlined by Swift (1990):

1. Relieving subjective symptoms of distress and discomfort resulting from intoxication or withdrawal
2. Preventing and treating serious complications of intoxication, withdrawal, or dependence
3. Establishing a drug- or alcohol-free state
4. Preparing for and referral to longer-term treatment or rehabilitation
5. Engaging the family in the treatment process

Long-Term Treatment Objectives

The objective of long-term treatment or rehabilitation is to maintain the alcohol- or drug-free state through ongoing psychologic, family, and vocational interventions. Long-term treatment involves behavioral and psychologic interventions to maintain abstinence. Changes in lifestyle, work, or friendships may be necessary. Halfway houses, therapeutic communities, and other residential treatment situations may also be useful. Treatment of underlying psychiatric or medical illnesses may reduce the impetus for self-medication. Self-help groups such as Alcoholics Anonymous (AA) and Narcotics Anonymous (NA) provide education, emotional support, and hope to substance abusers and their families. Many patients who come to medical attention for treatment do so in the context of a dysfunctional family structure. For these individuals, involving the family, particularly spouses and children, may provide great benefit.

Drugs Used in the Treatment of Alcoholism

An estimated 5% to 7% of Americans have alcoholism in a given year; 13% have alcoholism at some time during their lives. Simply defined, alcoholism is a repetitive but inconsistent and sometimes unpredictable loss of control of drinking that produces symptoms of serious dysfunction or disability (Clark, 1981). There are marked sex differences in alcohol dependence and abuse; the prevalence is about 5% to 6% for men and 1% to 2% for women. The prevalence is highest among men ages 18 to 64 and women ages 18 to 24, with a gradual drop afterward (Regier et al, 1988). Alcoholism is believed to account for 20% to 50% of all hospital admissions but is diagnosed in less than 5% (Lewis and Gordon, 1983; Holden, 1985). Alcohol use is also highly correlated with suicide, homicide, and accidents (Goodwin, 1967).

Drug treatment of alcohol intoxication or withdrawal (short-term). Patients who come to medical attention for treatment of alcohol intoxication or withdrawal may show various types of impairment. Many alcoholics have profound social and financial problems that our health care system is ill equipped to handle. Particularly frustrating is the alcoholic with profound social needs who does not require medical treatment or who refuses medical treatment. The acute alcohol withdrawal syndrome varies greatly in severity. Although severity of withdrawal is generally proportional to the level and duration of alcohol intake, many other factors such as previous episodes of dependence and concurrent medical illness influence the syndrome's severity. Most episodes are mild and require neither hospitalization nor pharmacologic intervention (Whitfield, 1980).

Although prescribing sedative-hypnotic agents to manage withdrawal on an ambulatory basis may seem taboo, these drugs are useful among hospitalized alcoholics (Jaffe and Ciraulo, 1985). Generally, comprehensive nursing care, the routine use of nutritional supplements, and prompt attention to complicating illnesses are responsible for the present low rates of delirium tremens and mortality resulting from alcohol withdrawal. Although the benzodiazepines, paraldehyde, chloral hydrate, barbiturates, and other sedative-hypnotic agents are effective in suppressing the alcohol withdrawal syndrome, the benzodiazepines are superior when given in adequate dosage for sufficient periods of time (Sellers and Kalant, 1982). Available benzodiazepines vary greatly in complexity, as outlined in Chapters 6, Anxiety Disorders, and 8, Sleep Disorders.

Use of benzodiazepines. The basic principle in using benzodiazepines to treat alcohol withdrawal is rapid substitution of a sufficient amount to suppress withdrawal, followed by a gradual tapering of the drug level over several days. Drugs with long-acting properties, such as chlordiazepoxide (Librium), diazepam (Valium), and clonazepam (Klonopin), are useful in that they self-taper. These long-acting agents enable once-daily dosing for alcohol withdrawal. They may also be used for single high-dose loading to facilitate detoxification without any subsequent benzodiazepine dosing (Sellers, Naranjo, and Peachey, 1981). Parenteral administration must be considered for patients who cannot take drugs by mouth. Lorazepam (Ativan), which is promptly and reliably absorbed from intramuscular sites, may be preferred. If suppression of withdrawal is delayed and hallucinosis develops, dopaminergic blockers such as haloperidol may be required in addition to benzodiazepines (Sellers and Kalant, 1982).

Symptoms of acute withdrawal may benefit from beta blockers such as atenolol to decrease autonomic arousal (Kraus et al, 1985). Coadministration with benzodiazepines facilitates detoxification. For milder withdrawal, clonidine may be as effective as chlordiazepoxide (Baumgartner and Rowen, 1987), and lofexidine can have similar efficacy, with less hypotension and sedation (Brunning et al, 1986).

Other agents. Barbiturates may be preferred for treating alcohol withdrawal. Chloral hydrate and paraldehyde, however, should be considered obsolete because of toxic effects. Phenytoin is sometimes used as part of the treatment for alcohol withdrawal, but there is no evidence that it should be used routinely except in patients who have a history of seizures unrelated to alcohol withdrawal. Unlike phenytoin, valproic acid does suppress alcohol withdrawal seizures in animals and may be useful in treating alcohol withdrawal in humans. Carbamazepine and buspirone may be of future interest in the management of acute alcohol withdrawal syndrome (Jaffe, 1987).

Thiamine should be administered to all alcohol users as soon as possible (and before the administration of glucose) to prevent the development of Wernicke's encephalopathy, which is characterized by ataxia, nystagmus, ophthalmoplegia, and changes in mental status. The encephalopathic symptoms tend to improve with thiamine repletion. Levels of magnesium and other electrolytes should be determined and deficits replaced. Other details of detoxification management are beyond the scope of this chapter.

Maintenance treatment of alcoholism (abstinence). The goal of long-term treatment of alcoholism is to maintain abstinence through a comprehensive treatment program that includes psychologic, family, and social interventions. Pharmacologic agents can deter alcohol consumption by making the ingesting of alcohol aversive (sensitizing agents) or by producing unpleasant effects that deliberately lengthen the metabolism of alcohol to create an aversion to alcohol (conditioning agents). *Disulfiram (Antabuse)* has been widely used to treat alcoholism. This agent inhibits the enzyme aldehyde dehydrogenase, which metabolizes acetaldehyde to acetic acid. When this enzyme is inhibited, ingestion of alcohol causes a rise in the acetaldehyde level and brings on an unpleasant syndrome characterized by facial flushing, tachycardia, pounding in the chest, decreased blood pressure, nausea, vomiting, shortness of breath, sweating, dizziness, and confusion (Sellers, Naranjo, and Peachey, 1981). Recently the toxic effects of disulfiram have raised the question whether it should be used therapeutically under any circumstances. Patients taking disulfiram must be informed about the danger of the drug's combination with even small amounts of alcohol. Alcohol present in foods, shaving lotion, mouthwashes, or over-the-counter medications may produce a reaction. The usual dose of disulfiram is 250 to 500 mg daily. Disulfiram may interact with other medications, notably, anticoagulants and phenytoin. It should not be used in patients with liver disease. Other contraindications may include myocardial disease, severe pulmonary insufficiency, renal failure, disorders of cognitive impairment, neuropathy, psychosis, difficulty with impulse control, or suicidal ideation. Certain medications such as vasodilators, beta-adrenergic agonists, monoamine oxidase inhibitors (MAOIs), or antipsychotic agents may also represent relative contraindications.

More recently two classes of agents have demonstrated efficacy: opioid antagonists and serotonergic agents such as SSRIs and buspirone. Two carefully controlled trials have examined the opioid antagonist naltrexone (ReVia) in reducing relapse among chronic alcoholics (O'Malley et al, 1992; Volpicelli et al, 1992). Both trials showed that 50 mg per day significantly reduced relapse and placebo. Naltrexone is well tolerated and reduces consumption rates. Patients treated with naltrexone show increased ability to participate in therapy or counseling.

Serotonergic agents have also shown good efficacy in reducing alcohol relapse (Sellers et al, 1992). Recent studies with selective serotonin reuptake inhibitors, for example, fluoxetine and sertraline, have been effective in reducing alcohol use in nondepressed heavy drinkers (Swift, 1990; Schuckit, 1986). Most beneficial are citalopram and viqualine, which are unavailable in the United States. Other agents that reduce consumption include buspirone ($5HT_{1A}$), ritanserin ($5HT_2$), and ondansetron ($5HT_3$) (Kosten and McCance-Katz, 1995).

A number of drugs that have been useful in treating postwithdrawal anxiety and depression associated with reduction of alcohol consumption include TCAs, MAOIs, benzodiazepines, dopaminergic antagonists such as haloperidol, and other dopaminergic blockers. The TCAs are frequently prescribed, but there is little firm evidence for their efficacy, even in alcoholics with primary depression. However, it is now clear that alcoholics metabolize imipramine much more rapidly than do controls, and in all probability, in most previous studies, insufficient dosages were used. Thus using TCAs to treat postwithdrawal syndrome may be useful (Jaffe and Ciraulo, 1985).

Drugs Used to Treat Narcotic (Opioid) Dependence and Abuse

Estimates of the incidence and prevalence of narcotic or opioid use and dependence have been relatively stable over the past several years. Generally the term *addict* has been used to mean someone with severe dependence on opiate drugs. The term *opioid* generally refers to a large number of chemically diverse substances that have in common the capacity to bind specifically and to produce actions at several distinct types of opioid receptors. The term *narcotic analgesic* has also been used to describe this class of drugs.

The physiologic effects of opiates are caused by stimulation of receptors that modulate endogenous hormones, enkephalins, endorphins, and dynorphins. Mu, kappa, sigma, delta, and epsilon opioid receptors have been identified (Jaffe and Martin, 1985). Morphine, heroin, and methadone act primarily through mu receptors and produce analgesia, euphoria, and respiratory depression. Drugs that appear to be mediated through the kappa receptors include the so-called mixed agonist-antagonists butorphanol and pentazocine, which produce analgesia but less respiratory depression. The sigma receptor appears to imitate the receptor for the hallucinogen phencyclidine (PCP). The delta receptor binds endogenous opioid peptides. At high doses opioid drugs lose their receptor specificity and have agonist or antagonist properties at multiple receptor subtypes.

The treatment of acute opiate withdrawal became of interest with the use of clonidine in 1978 (Gold et al, 1979). Administering naloxone and naltrexone to precipitate withdrawal is generally combined simultaneously with giving high doses of clonidine (Kleber and Gawin, 1986). This technique can speed withdrawal and lessen withdrawal symptoms. For example, a dose of naltrexone, 12.5 mg, can be followed by clonidine, up to 6 mg, with an average daily dose of approximately 3 mg (Charney et al, 1982).

A more recent technique has been opioid detoxification with buprenorphine (Buprenex), a partial opioid agonist (Kosten and Kleber, 1988). Daily sublingual doses of 2 to 8 mg of buprenorphine have enabled the switch from methadone and detoxification of heroin. The coadministration technique with naltrexone, as with clonidine, has also been successful (Shi et al, 1993).

Maintenance therapy: Methadone. Methadone (Dolophine) maintenance continues to be a major modality for treating opioid dependence. The maintenance approach alleviates drug hunger with high doses of methadone, blocking the dependency by means of cross-tolerance. Decreases in criminal activity and increases in legitimate productive work have been shown to be outcomes of this type of treatment. Methadone is typically administered orally. Because of its reliable absorption and delay in peak plasma levels of 2 to 6 hours after ingestion, patients are protected against sharp peaks in serum levels and continuation of tolerance. Methadone can ultimately be administered once daily, and opioid maintenance programs using methadone can be undertaken with confidence. Patient progress is monitored by means of interviews and urine testing.

The objective in managing withdrawal is to suppress severe withdrawal symptoms. However, some discomfort is almost always experienced; the discomfort and associated craving can sometimes be reduced by gradual reduction in opioid dosage. Hospitalized patients are generally more able than outpatients to tolerate rapid dosage reductions, often starting with 15 to 20 mg of methadone repeated after 2 to 4 hours when withdrawal symptoms are not suppressed or if they reappear. The dosage is generally not more than 40 mg per day, and dosage reductions of approximately 10% to 20% per day can be started and the entire process completed within 1 to 2 weeks (Fultz and Senay, 1975). Some low-level withdrawal symptoms, including sleep and mood disturbance, may persist for weeks after the last dose. Constipation and sweating are side effects of methadone and may persist.

Patients who have been on a maintenance regimen of high doses of methadone or professionals with access to pure opioids may have more severe degrees of physical dependence. They may require higher stabilization doses and may be unable to tolerate a rapid withdrawal protocol. Successful detoxification is more difficult to achieve with outpatients. Some clinicians recommend a slow dose reduction of 10% per week, then 3% per week when the dosage drops below 20 mg per week (Senay et al, 1977; Jaffe, 1986).

An alternative to methadone is LAAM, a long-acting methadone cogener with a half-life of 96 hours. A fixed dose of 80 mg every other day is achieved through titrations during a 1-month period of stabilization in which methadone may be coadministered.

Buprenorphine is the most recent opioid maintenance treatment. It is widely used in other countries and is gaining in popularity in the United States (Bickel et al, 1988). Administering daily 8-mg doses (as with detoxification) is equivalent to administering 65 mg of methadone. Unfortunately, this agent has been abused intravenously, and precautions are required (Quigley et al, 1984). Common side effects are similar to methadone. Overall, this drug shows promise as an alternative to methadone for heroin-addicted individuals.

Narcotic antagonists. The use of opioid antagonists in treating opioid dependence was originally based on the high relapse rate after detoxification. Naltrexone is a long-acting, orally effective agent that, when given either as 50 mg per day or 3 times weekly in doses of 100 mg, produces substantial blockade of the effects of large doses of injected opioid drugs (Resnick, Schuyten-Resnick, and Washton, 1980). Naltrexone is contraindicated in patients with acute hepatitis or liver failure. Patients must be free of opioid dependence for 1 week before naltrexone can be used.

Opioid overdose, a life-threatening emergency, should be suspected in any patient who comes to medical attention with coma and respiratory suppression. Treatment of suspected overdose includes emergency support of respiration and cardiovascular functions. Parenteral administration of the opioid antagonist, naloxone (Narcan), 0.4 to 0.8 mg, rapidly reverses the coma and respiratory suppression but does not result in the depression caused by other sedatives such as alcohol or barbiturates. Naloxone can precipitate opioid withdrawal, causing the patient whose life has just been saved to be extremely ungrateful.

Drugs Used to Treat Effects of Central Nervous System Stimulants

Drugs used to treat cocaine abuse and dependence. The use of cocaine and crack cocaine has undergone an epidemic increase. Cocaine has emerged as a major drug of abuse after a relatively long quiescent period during which its use was limited to a small subgroup of the population. The pure drug has been available for only approximately 100 years, but chewing coca leaves has been a practice for 2000 years. Cocaine is an alkaloid extracted from the leaves of the native South American plant. Cocaine is a local anesthetic that blocks the initiation and propagation of nerve impulses and is a potent sympathomimetic agent that potentiates the actions of catecholamines in the autonomic nervous system, causing tachycardia, hypertension, and vasoconstriction. Cocaine is also a central nervous system stimulant, increasing arousal and producing mood elevation and psychomotor activation.

There has been a major shift from snorting cocaine to intravenous injection and smoking freebase cocaine. Freebase cocaine, known as *crack,* is inexpensive and widely available. Thus the dramatic increases in hospital admissions for treatment, emergency care, and deaths reflect not only the increased number of users but also new ways of ingesting this drug.

Cocaine intoxication is characterized by elation, euphoria, excitement, pressured speech, restlessness, stereotypic movements, and bruxism. Sympathetic nervous system stimulation occurs, including tachycardia, mydriasis, and sweating. Paranoia, suspiciousness, and psychosis may occur with prolonged use. Overdosage produces hyperpyrexia, hyperreflexia, seizures, coma, and respiratory arrest (Swift, 1990).

Cocaine produces effects in multiple neurotransmitter systems, including reuptake block of dopamine, norepinephrine, and serotonin (Koe, 1976). Dopamine reuptake inhibition results in increased extracellular dopamine concentration in the mesolimbic and mesocortical reward pathways (Kosten and McCance-Katz, 1995).

Cocaine has a short plasma half-life of 1 to 2 hours, which correlates with its behavioral effects (Van Dyke et al, 1978). Along with the decline in plasma levels, most users experience a period of dysphoria, which often leads to additional cocaine use within a short period. The dysphoria of the "crash" is intensified and prolonged after repeated usage. Abusers uniformly report control over early stimulant usage. As use continues, however, the individual binges until immediate supplies are exhausted (Gawin and Kleber, 1985). This compulsive use pattern and impairment of self-control are the best indicators of stimulant abuse and of the severity of abuse.

Clinical presentations involving cocaine abuse and dependence include a mixture of acute and chronic symptoms with different intensities. Cocaine intoxication, delirium, delusions, post-use dysphoria, and withdrawal may be present. Cocaine may cause severe drug intoxication or death through an extension of its sympathomimetic properties. Chronic medical complications may include malnutrition, anorexia, nutritional deficiencies, dehydration, endocrine abnormalities, and complications linked to the route of administration (Cohen, 1981).

The major new developments in pharmacologic treatment of substance abuse involve cocaine abuse and dependence. New agents and strategies are based on the premise that altered neurochemical substrate underlies the chronic high intensity use (binge) and "crash" that follows (Kuhar et al, 1991). Before the 1980s the scientific evaluation of the treatment of cocaine abuse was sparse, and no consensus existed regarding optimal treatment strategies. Clearly, accurate psychiatric characterization of the cocaine abuser is important because symptoms appearing during abstinence might provide guides to when and what pharmacologic adjuncts are indicated. Treatment generally focuses on one of three areas: acute sequelae, craving, and withdrawal. Psychologic supports and behavioral therapy are generally applied when treating these patients. Hospitalization may be required for individuals who are chronic freebase or intravenous cocaine users or concurrent alcohol users, or for individuals who have significant psychiatric or medical comorbidity, psychosocial impairment, or lack of motivation or who were not successfully treated as outpatients (Kleber and Gawin, 1986; Rounsaville, Gawin, and Kleber, 1985).

Although no panacea exists for treating cocaine dependence, a wide range of psychotropic medications have been used, including stimulants, antidepressants, precursors to neurotransmitters, neuroleptics, and other agents that have multiple effects on brain neurotransmission. Pharmacologic agents that aid the recovering addict may be divided into those that are useful as anticraving agents and those that may be more useful for maintaining abstinence and preventing relapse. Agents that have a relatively rapid onset of action, including amantadine, bromocriptine, levodopa (L-dopa), carbidopa, methylphenidate, and carbamazepine, may be useful; in addition, the TCAs may be useful against craving. Although no long-term, placebo-controlled, double-blind studies have been made of any of these agents, their efficacy has been touted in case reports and in some single-dose placebo cross-over trials (Gawin and Ellinwood, 1988; Giannini and Baumgartel, 1987; Tennant and Segherian, 1987).

Dopaminergic drugs. Amantadine (Symmetrel) may exert its therapeutic effect by releasing neuronal stores and delaying uptake of dopamine and norepinephrine, thereby increasing availability to the postsynaptic receptor sites. This drug theoretically could be given with L-dopa, carbidopa, or tyrosine to enhance the clinical effect. Doses of 200 to 300 mg per day reduce cocaine craving for several days to a month. Although amantadine initially is effective without significant side effects, its usefulness appears to be limited to the acute withdrawal phase (Gawin et al, 1989; Morgan et al, 1988).

Bromocriptine, a dopamine agonist, also appears to reduce the density of the inhibitory receptors or autoreceptors on dopamine neurons that exert a rapid anticraving effect (Giannini et al, 1989). Doses of 0.5 to 1.5 mg per day may be useful. Abstinent cocaine users report an antagonist effect of bromocriptine when using cocaine. Higher doses are poorly tolerated because of the side effects. Oral craving is reduced in many cases (Dackis and Gold, 1985). Thus bromocriptine may be useful in abstinent cocaine abusers as an antagonist, similar to the way disulfiram or naltrexone is used with alcoholics or opiate addicts, respectively.

Methylphenidate (Ritalin) has been studied for treatment of cocaine abuse. Treated subjects report tolerance, diminished craving, and a mild sense of stimulation. Disadvantages include tolerance, abuse potential, and poor patient acceptance (Gawin, Riordan, and Kleber, 1985).

Masinidol, a catecholamine reuptake blocker, has been useful in Parkinson's disease and may significantly reduce craving. Tolerance and abuse do not occur nor does rebound depression. (Diakogiannis et al, 1990). Bupropion (Wellbutrin) has also been reported to be useful in doses of 100 mg three times a day (Margolin et al, 1991).

Carbamazepine. Carbamazepine (Tegretol) has been used in treatment-resistant addicts. Theoretically carbamazepine, through its ability to reverse cocaine-induced kindling, reverses cocaine receptor supersensitivity that results from chronic cocaine use (Halikas et al, 1989). Patients receiving treatment in an open trial have shown significant reductions in cocaine craving with use of this drug.

Tricyclic antidepressants. Tricyclic antidepressants have had success in the treatment of cocaine users, but because of the delayed onset of action of TCAs, their use may be better suited for the later phases of maintaining abstinence and preventing relapse (Kosten, 1989; Gawin et al, 1989b). The rationale for their effectiveness is that they reduce dopaminergic receptor sensitivity and thereby reduce cocaine-induced supersensitivity. Most of the better-controlled studies of drug treatment of cocaine dependence have used the TCAs. Several trials have used desipramine, resulting in significant decreases in cocaine use and craving. However, desipramine was found useful only when given in adequate doses for sufficient duration. Daily doses of 2.5 mg per kg body weight for up to 6 weeks may result in the full therapeutic effect. The efficacy of lower doses such as 75 to 100 mg daily may not be much better than that of a placebo (Kaufman and McNaul, 1992).

The anhedonia, anergia, and consequences of chronic cocaine abuse can result in a syndrome known as *intracranial self-stimulation.* Desipramine, imipramine, and amitriptyline treatment have been employed, and use in an animal model seems to reverse the changes that occur at catecholamine receptors as a result of repeated stimulant use. In essence the TCAs restore hedonic capacity and decrease cocaine craving. Whether desipramine and, possibly, other antidepressants, for example, trazodone or nefazodone or the SSRIs, have some ability to block the physiologic effects of cocaine has been the subject of speculation (Rowbotham et al, 1984; Ritz and Kuhar, 1989). However, to determine conclusively whether antidepressants block cocaine's effects or have anticraving effects, or both, remains a subject of further study.

Other agents. The central role of depression in cocaine abuse is demonstrated not only by the striking resemblance of the cocaine withdrawal syndrome to depression but also by findings that depressive disorders predict increased cocaine use in follow-up. Because depression predicts subsequent cocaine abuse, pharmacologic treatment of depression may, indeed, be an important preventive strategy. Methylphenidate (Ritalin) may be a useful agent for treating the abstinent cocaine abuser but is not recommended because it stimulates cocaine craving (Khantzian, 1983). Lithium or valproate may also diminish craving, particularly in persons who meet diagnostic criteria for cyclothymia or who have a family history of bipolar disorder. However, these agents are not generally considered blocking agents for cocaine euphoria and have not been established as particularly useful for these patients.

Cocaine has no specific antagonist for the treatment of acute sequelae. Management of overdose is largely symptomatic and is aimed at reversing epileptogenic, cardiorespiratory, and metabolic effects (Gay, 1982). Diazepam for transient agitation, together with propranolol, may be useful for persistent symptoms. Suicidal ideation and depressive symptoms that often occur during the postcocaine "crash" are transient and require no acute treatment other than close observation. Neuroleptics may be used briefly for severe psychotic symptoms; chlorpromazine, because of its sedative effects and potential to antagonize the lethal effects of cocaine, may be particularly useful (Kleber and Gawin, 1986). Haloperidol may also be used effectively to treat cocaine-induced psychosis (Smith, 1984). However, psychotic symptoms seem to be short-lived and usually remit after sleep normalization. Symptoms of depression or psychosis that do not remit within approximately 3 days may necessitate conventional treatment.

In summary, several pharmacologic agents have shown promise as adjuncts in the treatment of cocaine abuse, both for craving and for withdrawal. Imipramine, desipramine, trazodone, fluoxetine, and lithium may reduce craving or usage, or both. The dopamine antagonists, bromocriptine and amantadine may block craving as well. Many treatment facilities provide short-term intensive psychologic treatment and drug education in a drug-free environment. Ideally this approach, followed by a long-term residential drug-free program for those with more severe difficulties, may be most efficacious. Self-help groups such as Narcotics Anonymous may also be useful as a primary treatment modality or as an adjunct to another treatment. Certain psychiatric disorders such as depression, cyclothymia, and attention deficit disorder may be common in cocaine users and should be treated. In addition, many cocaine users also use alcohol or other drugs, particularly sedatives and heroin, and may require treatment for abuse of these substances as well.

Drugs used to treat amphetamine dependence. Although the subjective effects of amphetamines are similar to those of cocaine, there are important differences in their mechanisms of action. It is not clear why cocaine epidemics have stimulated so many more attempts at pharmacologic intervention than did the amphetamine epidemic that occurred in the 1960s. Nevertheless, remarkably little is known about the pharmacologic treatment of amphetamine dependence or its complications (Jaffe, 1987).

As a group amphetamines are structurally related to the catecholamine neurotransmitters norepinephrine, epinephrine, and dopamine. These drugs release endogenous catecholamines from nerve endings and are catecholamine agonists at receptors in the peripheral, autonomic, and central nervous systems. Thus intoxication with stimulants such as amphetamines, methylphenidate, or other sympathomimetics produces a clinical picture similar to that of cocaine intoxication. Agitation, paranoia, delusions, and hallucinosis may follow the chronic use of these drugs (Ellinwood, 1969; Swift, 1990). Chronic users engage in a pattern similar to that of chronic cocaine abusers, escalating doses for several days, then abstaining. Paranoid psychosis similar on diagnosis to schizophrenia may result (amphetamine psychosis). Underlying psychiatric illnesses such as affective disorder may also be present, as in cocaine dependence.

Over-the-counter sympathomimetic amines may be abused. Use of these medications, sold as appetite suppressants, decongestants, or bronchodilators, may become evident with signs of intoxication similar to those present with amphetamine intoxication. However, a greater tendency for autonomic effects is present with use of these over-the-counter sympathomimetic amines and may result in a hypertensive crisis.

Dopaminergic blockers such as haloperidol are generally preferred for treating amphetamine-induced paranoid and psychotic states that do not subside spontaneously within a few days. Lithium may be useful to blunt or block the euphoric effects of amphetamines. However, this agent tends to be useful in patients with affective symptoms or alcoholism. The use of TCAs has been recommended to reduce postamphetamine depression and drug craving. However, there are no definitive reports of success with the use of TCAs, not even in cases in which depression was a significant motivating factor for the use of the amphetamines (Jaffe, 1987).

Drugs used to treat caffeine dependence. The use of caffeine and related compounds such as theophylline is ubiquitous in the United States. Caffeine is present in chocolate and a variety of prescription and over-the-counter agents that are used as stimulants, appetite suppressants, analgesics, and cold and sinus preparations (Dews, 1982). The physiologic effects of these agents include cardiac stimulation, diuresis, bronchodilation, and CNS stimulation. These compounds may augment the actions of neurotransmitters, such as norepinephrine, and may have a direct stimulatory effect on nerve endings. Central nervous system effects of caffeine include psychomotor stimulation, increased attention and concentration, and suppression of the need for sleep. Caffeine may exacerbate the symptoms of anxiety disorders and increase requirements for neuroleptic or sedative medications (Charney, Henninger, and Jatlow, 1985). In moderate to heavy users a withdrawal syndrome characterized by lethargy, hypersomnia, irritability, and severe headache may ensue. Treatment of caffeine dependence consists of limiting consumption and substituting decaffeinated forms of beverages such as coffee or cola. No other definitive treatments are available.

Drugs Used to Treat Nicotine Dependence

Heavy or persistent smokers who abruptly stop smoking typically experience tobacco withdrawal syndrome, consisting of craving, irritability, impatience, hostility, restlessness, anxiety, depression, difficulty in concentrating, confusion, disturbed sleep patterns, increased appetite, decreased heart rate, and increased slow waves on the electroencephalogram (EEG). As with individuals dependent on alcohol and opioids, pharmacologic treatments for tobacco dependence are divided into the following groups: (1) agents that produce some of the effects produced by nicotine, (2) agents that deliver nicotine but with reduced toxicity, and (3) agents intended to block the reinforcing effects of smoking or to make smoking aversive.

Nicotine is an alkaloid drug present in the leaves of the tobacco plant. Nicotine addiction and tobacco use are legally sanctioned forms of substance abuse. Tobacco is clearly the most lethal substance in our society. The percentage of Americans who smoke has declined (Swift, 1990); however, the number of young women who smoke tobacco products has increased, because tobacco companies continue to market tobacco as a chic product.

Nicotine has several effects on the peripheral, autonomic, and central nervous systems. It agonizes the nicotinic cholinergic receptor sites and stimulates autonomic ganglia in the parasympathetic and sympathetic nervous systems, producing salivation, increased gastric motility and acid secretion, and increased catecholamine release. Thus tobacco is a mild psychostimulant, producing increased alertness, increased attention and concentration, and appetite suppression. Tobacco can be used to prevent weight gain, which makes this drug attractive, particularly to some individuals concerned about weight control. Repeated use of nicotine produces tolerance and dependence. The degree of dependence is considerable: 70% of those who quit using tobacco relapse within 1 year.

The treatment of nicotine-dependent patients follows the general principles common to treatment of dependence on all psychoactive substances. Short-term goals consist of reducing or stopping the tobacco use, followed by treatment designed to support and encourage abstinence. Few patients can reduce tobacco use on their own; most require a smoking cessation program (Greene, Goldberg, and Ockene, 1988). The most successful treatment combines pharmacologic and behavioral therapies.

Generally attempts to produce stimulation, appetite suppression, or other amphetamine-like effects in smokers do not reduce tobacco use. Employing sedatives, tranquilizers, or propranolol has not been of substantial aid in smoking cessation. Lobeline, an alkaloid that is structurally similar to nicotine, has been proposed as a treatment for tobacco dependence and withdrawal. Although this compound has some cross-tolerance with nicotine and is marketed as an over-the-counter preparation, it is not significantly superior to placebo in helping smokers stop smoking (Jaffe, 1987).

There is evidence that nicotine in the form of chewing gum can suppress important components of tobacco withdrawal and be particularly useful in achieving long-term success. Symptoms that are relieved include irritability and impatience, with some reduction in restlessness, anxiety, hunger, insomnia, and changes in heart rate. The gum is a sweet-flavored resin containing 2 mg of nicotine, which is released slowly when the gum is chewed. Proper use of the gum can somewhat reduce the craving for tobacco and decrease the discomfort during the withdrawal period (Jarvik and Schneider, 1984; Schneider, Jarvik, and Forsythe, 1984). It is not clear whether the failure to relieve all symptoms of tobacco withdrawal is related to the dose or to the route of administration. However, nicotine gum does *not* substantially alleviate craving and generally must be combined with both careful instruction on its use and a smoking cessation program.

In addition to nicotine gum, other means of delivery of nicotine itself have been developed, such as nicotine nasal sprays or skin patches (Jaffe, 1987). Currently three types of nicotine patches are available, as depicted in Table 10-2. Use of these patches significantly increases abstinence rates when combined with a behavioral or a smoking cessation program. Their use significantly reduces craving for cigarettes or other tobacco products. They maintain a steady blood level of nicotine by means of a simple, convenient, once-daily therapy. Nicotine patches are generally prescribed beginning with the highest dosing system, except for individuals weighing less than 100 pounds. Regardless of the product choice, Prostep, Habitrol, or Nicoderm, each is prescribed for 4 to 6 weeks, with subsequent weaning to the next lower dose for 2 to 4 weeks. Generally the weaning process takes from a minimum of 6 weeks to a maximum of 12 weeks. Again, these treatments are best combined with a behavioral or a smoking cessation program, because psychologic factors such as stress and negative emotions can trigger the urge for tobacco, as do social and behavioral factors of dependence (Bonowitz, 1988; Stitzer and Gross, 1988). Box 10-3 presents guidelines for nicotine patch use.

Table 10-2 Nicotine Transdermal Systems

Agents (trade name)	Dosages (delivery rate in vivo)	Comments (apply to all three systems)
Nicoderm	21 mg/day 14 mg/day 7 mg/day	Rotate skin sites; consider nontherapeutic effects, i.e., nicotine excess versus withdrawal symptoms; topical reactions are most common side effect; other side effects, in descending order of frequency, are diarrhea, dyspepsia, muscle ache, abnormal dreams, and insomnia.
Habitrol	21 mg/day	
Prostep	14 mg/day 7 mg/day 22 mg/day 11 mg/day	

Box 10-3 Guidelines for Use of the Nicotine Patch (Nicotine Transdermal Systems)

The goal of the program is complete abstinence.
Patients must read instructions and have questions answered for appropriate use.
Quality, frequency, and intensity of support and a formal smoking cessation program are recommended.
Patients who fail to quit using nicotine should be given a "therapy holiday" before another attempt.
Symptoms of withdrawal and excess overlap and should be considered assiduously.*
Nicotine transdermal systems should not be used for longer than 3 months.
Patches should be applied to a nonhairy, clean, dry site.
Skin sites should be alternated and should not be reused for 1 week.

*Excess nicotine causes abnormal dreams, insomnia, and gastrointestinal symptoms. Withdrawal from nicotine causes anxiety, somnolence, and depression, including somatic symptoms.

The use of nicotine patches requires absolute motivation and abstinence during the treatment phase. Adjustments in the dosages of concomitant medications may be necessary, for example, decreases in benzodiazepines, TCAs, beta blockers, theophylline, insulin, or beta-adrenergic antagonists. In contrast, an increase in the dose of adrenergic agonists such as phenylephrine may be necessary when the patient ceases to smoke.

Nontherapeutic effects such as allergic reactions and topical effects may occur as a result of the patch itself. The regimen for patients with cardiovascular and peripheral vascular diseases should be started carefully, and the benefits of nicotine replacement should be considered in the context of the cardiovascular disease. Patients with ischemic heart disease, severe cardiac arrhythmia, and vasospastic diseases should be carefully screened and evaluated before nicotine replacement is prescribed. Nicotine patches should be used with caution in patients with hyperthyroidism, pheochromocytoma, or insulin-dependent diabetes, because nicotine causes the release of catecholamines by the adrenal medulla. Nicotine may delay the healing of peptic ulcers and accelerate hypertension. Data regarding the teratogenic effects of nicotine in humans are inconclusive. Nicotine has been shown to produce skeletal abnormalities in the offspring of mice and therefore is not recommended for use during pregnancy. Because dependence on nicotine chewing gum has been reported, the use of a patch system beyond 3 months should be discouraged. To minimize the risk of dependence, the patient should also be encouraged to gradually withdraw from the treatment after 4 to 6 weeks, progressively decreasing the dosage every 2 to 4 weeks, as previously noted. Recently the alpha-2 receptor agonist clonidine has been reported as partially efficacious in reducing nicotine withdrawal symptoms (Glassman et al, 1988). Nonetheless, the most successful treatment of nicotine dependence combines both pharmacologic and behavioral approaches.

Many former smokers have adopted the use of oral tobacco in the form of snuff or chewing tobacco. This practice may reduce the hazards associated with smoke inhalation but does not qualify as a pharmacologic treatment of tobacco dependence.

Drugs Used to Treat Cannabis (Marijuana) Dependence

Some individuals use cannabis daily or almost daily. In many of these persons the capacity to function normally is seriously impaired. A withdrawal syndrome that is not life threatening but resembles mild sedative withdrawal has been reported. The relationship of this syndrome to marijuana-seeking behavior remains unclear (Jaffe, 1987). There are no specific therapeutic agents for cannabis withdrawal or dependence.

Drugs Used to Treat Abuse of Phencyclidine and Similar Agents

Phencyclidine (PCP) is used as an anesthetic in veterinary medicine. The mechanism of action is not well understood, although recently this drug has been shown to bind the so-called sigma opioid receptor in the brain.

PCP intoxication has several definitive features based on empirical data. PCP and other similar agents produce amnestic, euphoric hallucinatory states, and their effects may be unpredictable, resulting in a prolonged agitated psychosis with impulsive violence directed at self and others (Peterson and Stillman, 1979; Walker, Yesavage, and Tinklenberg, 1981). The general approach to detoxification also includes isolation in a quiet environment, supportive measures to prevent patients from harming themselves, maintenance of cardiorespiratory functions, and drug treatment that ameliorates psychotic symptoms. The removal of PCP, which is sequestered in acidic gastric fluids, can be aided by judicious use of gastric drainage. Acidification of urine accelerates excretion but is no longer routinely used. Dopamine blockers such as haloperidol appear to be of value in treating PCP-induced acute psychotic states. Opioids such as meperidine and morphine may be valuable in certain cases but are not conventionally prescribed. In addition to haloperidol, benzodiazepines have been described as useful in decreasing agitation and psychosis. Psychiatric hospitalization may be necessary in those individuals with prolonged psychosis.

Drugs Used to Treat Sedative-Hypnotic and Anxiolytic Abuse and Dependence

Sedatives, unlike heroin, cocaine, amphetamines, marijuana, and other abusable substances, are produced almost entirely by pharmaceutical companies. Thus the diversion of these substances originates primarily from pharmaceutical and medical sources. Many adverse effects of sedative abuse may result, including acute drug effects and bodily damage resulting from accidents or overdoses. Discussion of the chronic effects of sedative-hypnotics is beyond the scope of this chapter. The treatment of sedative abuse or dependence usually occurs in two stages: detoxification and long-term treatment. The primary goal of treatment is abstinence.

The type of detoxification recommended is determined by evaluation of the patient's medical condition and social and personal circumstances. If no physical dependence exists, individuals may be treated as outpatients. However, hospitalization is usually necessary for successful detoxification. Abrupt withdrawal from sedatives can lead to seizures or to toxic psychosis; deaths have been reported as a consequence (O'Brien and Woody, 1986). Several detoxification techniques are used; each method involves substituting a prescribed sedative for one that has been abused. Once the patient's condition has been stabilized on a substitute drug regimen, the drug is reduced by approximately 10% per day, a generally acceptable rate of detoxification. The pentobarbital challenge test, as presented in Table 10-3, involves the oral administration of 200 mg of pentobarbital followed by close observa-

Table 10-3 Pentobarbital Challenge Test: Initial Response to 200 mg of Pentobarbital

Patient's condition	Degree of tolerance	24-hour pentobarbital requirement* (mg)
Asleep and sedate	None	None
Drowsy; marked intoxication	Mild	400-600
Comfortable; minimal intoxication	Marked	600-1000
No effect	Extreme	1000

*Phenobarbital may be preferred and substituted at a dose of 30 mg for pentobarbital, 100 mg.

tion to assess the degree of tolerance. Based on the patient's condition after the test dose, an estimated 24-hour pentobarbital requirement is determined; similarly a phenobarbital substitution technique may be carried out, with the oral substitution of 30 mg of phenobarbital for each 100 mg of the estimated pentobarbital requirement. Medication is administered every 6 hours for approximately 24 hours. If a stabilization dose is reached, the substituted agent may then be reduced as previously described. Phenobarbital is generally preferred because it is longer acting and has better anticonvulsant activity than does pentobarbital.

The condition of patients who are addicted to both sedatives and narcotics must be stabilized on a regimen of both types of drugs before detoxification can occur. It is important to remember that patients are restless and anxious and often have insomnia during and after detoxification. Given the significant heterogeneity of sedative abusers, it is essential to attempt to categorize the social and psychologic correlates of drug use in each patient so that a long-term treatment plan can be formulated (Wesson and Smith, 1975; Wikler, 1968).

Long-term treatment of sedative abuse is customized and may include residential drug-free programs or self-help groups such as AA and NA, or a combination of these. Some patients may be found to have an underlying psychiatric disorder. If pharmacologic treatment is deemed necessary, the use of antidepressant medication or a nondependence-producing anxiolytic such as buspirone should be considered.

REFERENCES

American Psychiatric Association: *Diagnostic and Statistical Manual of Mental Disorders,* ed 4, revised, Washington, DC, 1994, The Association.

Anthony JC, Warner LA, Kessler RC: Comparative epidemiology of dependence on tobacco, alcohol, controlled substances and inhalants: basic findings from the National Comorbidity Survey, *Clin Exp Psychopharmacol* 2:244, 1994.

Anthony JC, Arria AM, Johnson EO: Epidemiological and public health issues for tobacco, alcohol, and other drugs. In Oldham JM and Riba MB, editors: *Review of Psychiatry,* vol 14, Washington, DC, 1995, American Psychiatric Press.

Baumgartner GR, Rowen RC: Clonidine versus chlordiazepoxide in the management of acute alcohol withdrawl syndrome, *Arch Intern Med* 107:880, 1987.

Baxter LR et al: Localization of neurochemical effects of cocaine and other stimulants in the human brain, *J Clin Psychiatry* 49(suppl):23, 1988.

Bickel WK et al: A clinical trial of buprenorphine comparison with methadone in the detoxification of heroin addicts, *Clin Pharmacol Ther* 43:72, 1988.

Blume SB: Psychotherapy in the treatment of alcoholism: psychiatry update. In Grinspoon L, editor: *The American Psychiatric Association annual review,* vol 3, Washington, DC, 1984, The Association.

Bonowitz NI: Pharmacologic aspects of cigarette smoking and nicotine addiction, *New Engl J Med* 319:1318, 1988.

Braucht G et al: Deviant drug use in adolescence: a review of psychosocial correlates, *Psychol Bull* 79:92, 1973.

Brook JS et al: The role of older brothers in younger brothers' drug use viewed in context of parent and peer influences, *J Genet Psychol* 151:59, 1990.

Brunning J, Mumford JP, Keaney FP: Lofexidine in alcohol withdrawal states, *Alcohol* 21:167-172, 1986.

Butcher JN: *Personality factors in drug addiction,* NIDA Research Monograph Series, No. 89, Rockville, Md, 1988, National Institute on Drug Abuse.

Cadoret RJ et al: An adoption study of genetic and environmental factors in drug abuse, *Arch Gen Psychiatry* 43:1131, 1986.

Charney DS, Henninger GR, Jatlow PI: Increased anxiogenic effects of caffeine in panic disorders, *Arch Gen Psychiatry* 42:233, 1985.

Charney DS et al: Clonidine and naltrexone: a safe, effective, and rapid treatment of abrupt withdrawal from methadone therapy, *Arch Gen Psychiatry* 39:1327, 1982.

Ciraulo DA et al: Parental alcoholism as a risk factor in benzodiazepine abuse: a pilot study, *Am J Psychiatry* 146:1333, 1989.

Clark WD: Alcoholism: blocks to diagnosis and treatment, *Am J Med* 71:275, 1981.

Clayton R: Extent and consequences of drug abuse. In *Drug abuse and drug abuse research,* Rockville, Md, 1984, National Institute on Drug Abuse.

Cohen S: *Cocaine today,* New York, 1981, American Council on Drug Education.

Culhane C: Marijuana's brain receptor found, *US Journal,* Dec. 11, 1990, p 11.

Dews PB: Caffeine, *Annu Rev Nutr* 2:323, 1982.

Dackis CA, Gold MS: Bromocriptine as a treatment of cocaine abuse, *Lancet* 1:1151, 1985.

Diakogiannis IA, Steinberg M, Kosten TR: Mazindol treatment of cocaine abuse: a double-blind investigation, *NIDA Res Monogr Ser* 105:514, 1990.

Dixon SD: Effects of transplacental exposure to cocaine and methamphetamine on the neonate, *West J Med* 150:436, 1989.

Ellinwood EH: Amphetamine psychosis: a multidimensional process, *Semin Psychol* 1:208, 1969.

Fishburne PM, Abelson HI, Cisin I: *National survey on drug abuse. Main finding: 1979,* Department of Health and Human Services Pub No. ADM-80-976, Washington, DC, 1980, US Government Printing Office.

Fultz JM Jr, Senay EC: Guidelines for the management of hospitalized narcotic addicts, *Ann Intern Med* 82:815, 1975.

Gawin FH: Chronic neuropharmacology of cocaine: progress in pharmacotherapy, *J Clin Psychiatry* 49(suppl):11, 1988.

Gawin FH, Ellinwood EH: Cocaine and other stimulants: actions, abuse, and treatment, *New Engl J Med* 318:1173, 1988.

Gawin FH, Kleber HD: Cocaine abuse in a treatment population: patterns and diagnostic distinctions. In Kozell NJ, Adams EH, editors: *Cocaine use in America: epidemiologic and clinical perspectives,* NIDA Research Monograph Series, No. 61, Rockville, Md, 1985, National Institute on Drug Abuse.

Gawin FH, Riordan CA, Kleber HD: Methylphenidate use in non-ADD cocaine abusers: a negative study, *AM J Drug Alcohol Abuse* 11:193-197, 1985.

Gawin FH et al: Double-blind evaluation of the effect of acute amantadine on cocaine craving, *Psychopharmacology* 97:402, 1989.

Gay GR: Clinical management of acute and chronic cocaine poisoning, *Ann Emerg Med* 11:562, 1982.

Giacoia GP: Cocaine in the cradle: a hidden epidemic, *Southern Med J* 83:947, 1990.

Giannini AJ, Baumgartel PD: Bromocriptine therapy in cocaine withdrawal, *J Clin Pharmacology* 27:267, 1987.

Giannini AJ et al: Bromocriptine and amantadine in cocaine detoxification, *Psychiatr Res* 29:11, 1989.

Glassman AH et al: Heavy smokers, smoking cessation and clonodine: results of a double-blind, randomized trial, *JAMA* 259:2863, 1988.

Gold MS et al: Opiate withdrawal using clonidine: a safe, effective and rapid non-opiate treatment, *JAMA* 234:343, 1979.

Goodwin DW: Alcohol in homicide and suicide, *Q J Stud Alcohol* 28:517, 1967.

Greene HL, Goldberg R, Ockene JK: Cigarette smoking: the physician's role in cessation and maintenance, *J Gen Intern Med* 3:75, 1988.

Grove WM et al: Heritability of substance abuse and antisocial behavior: a study of monozygotic twins reared apart, *Biol Psychiatry* 27:1293, 1990.

Halikas J et al: Carbamazepine for cocaine addiction? *Lancet* 1:623, 1989 (letter).

Holden C: The neglected disease in medical education, *Science* 229:741, 1985.

Jaffe JH. Opioids. In Frances AJ, Hales RE, editors: *American Psychiatric Association annual review,* vol 5, Washington, DC, 1986, The Association.

Jaffe JH: Pharmacological agents in treatment of drug dependence. In Meltzer HY, editor: *The third generation of progress,* New York, 1987, Raven.

Jaffe JH, Ciraulo D: Drugs used in the treatment of alcoholism. In Mendelson JH, Mello NK: *The diagnosis and treatment of alcoholism,* New York, 1985, McGraw-Hill.

Jaffe JH, Martin WR: Opioid analgesics and antagonists. In Gilman AG et al: *The pharmacological basis of therapeutics,* ed 7, New York, 1985, Macmillan.

Jarvik ME, Schneider NG: Degree of addiction and the effectiveness of nicotine gum therapy for smoking, *Am J Psychiatry* 141:790, 1984.

Johnston LD, Bachman JG, O'Malley PM: *Drug use, drinking, and smoking: national survey results from high school, college, and young adult populations, 1975-1990,* Rockville, Md, 1991, National Institute of Mental Health.

Johnston LD, Bachman JG, O'Malley PM: *1983 highlights: drugs and the nation's high school students,* Washington, DC, 1984, US Government Printing Office.

Kandel D, Simcha-Fagan O, Davis M: Risk factors for delinquency and illicit drug use from adolescence to young adulthood, *J Drug Issues* 16:67, 1986.

Kaufman E: Family structures of narcotic addicts, *Int J Addict* 16:273, 1981.

Kaufman E, McNaul JP: Recent developments in understanding and treating drug abuse and dependence, *Hosp Community Psychiatry* 43:223, 1992.

Kessler RC et al: Lifetime and 12 month prevalence of DSM-IIIR psychiatric disorders in the United States: results from the National Comorbidity Survey, *Arch Gen Psychiatry* 51:8-19, 1994.

Khantzian EJ: A critique of therapy and some implications for treatment, *Am J Psychother* 28:59, 1974.

Khantzian EJ: Extreme case of cocaine dependence and marked improvement with Ritalin, *Am J Psychiatry* 140:784, 1983.

Kleber HD, Gawin FH: Cocaine. In Frances AJ, Hales RE, editors: *American Psychiatric Association annual review,* vol 5, Washington, DC, 1986, The Association.

Koe BK: Molecular geometry of inhibitors of the uptake of catecholamines and serotonin in synaptosomal preparations of rat brain, *J Pharmacol Exp Ther* 199:649, 1976.

Kolata G: New valiums and anti-valiums on the horizon, *Science* 216:604, 1982.

Kosten TR: Pharmacotherapeutic interventions for cocaine abuse: matching patient to treatments, *J Nerv Ment Dis* 177:379, 1989.

Kosten TR, Gawin F, Shumann B: *Treating cocaine-abusing methadone patients with desipramine,* NIDA Research Monograph Series, No. 81, Rockville, Md, 1988, National Institute on Drug Abuse.

Kosten TR, Kleber HD: Differential diagnosis of psychiatric comorbidity in substance abusers, *J Subst Abuse Treat* 5:201, 1988.

Kosten TR, McCance-Katz E: New pharmacotherapies. In Oldham JM and Riba MB, editors: *Review of Psychiatry,* vol 14, Washington, DC, 1995, American Psychiatric Press.

Krasnagor NA, editor: *The behavioral aspects of smoking,* NIDA Research Monograph Series, No. 26, Rockville, Md, 1979, National Institute on Drug Abuse.

Kraus ML et al: Randomized clinical trial of atenolol in patients with alcohol withdrawal, *N Engl J Med* 313:905, 1985.

Kuhar MJ, Ritz MC, Boja JW: The dopamine hypothesis of the reinforcing properties of cocaine, *Trends Neurosci* 14:299-302, 1991.

Lewis D, Gordon A: Alcoholism and the general hospital: the Roger Williams intervention program, *Bull NY Acad Med* 59:181, 1983.

Little BB et al: Cocaine use in 46 pregnant women in a large public hospital, *Am J Perinatol* 5:206, 1988.

Maloff D et al: Informal social controls and their influence on substance use. In Zinberg N, Hardin WM, editors: *Control over intoxicant use,* New York, 1982, Human Sciences.

Margolin CH et al: Bupropion reduces cocaine abuse in methadone-maintained patients, *Arch Gen Psychiatry* 48:87, 1991.

McLellan AT, Woody GE, O'Brien CP: Development of psychiatric illness in drug abusers, *New Engl J Med* 201:1310, 1979.

Meyer RE: *Psychopathology and addictive disorders: how to understand the relationship between psychopathology and addictive disorders,* New York, 1986, Guilford.

Miller JD et al: *National survey of drug abuse. Main findings: 1982,* Department of Health and Human Services Pub No. ADM-83-1263, Washington, DC, 1983, US Government Printing Office.

Millman R: Drug abuse and dependence. In Wyngaarde JB, Smith LH, editors: *Textbook of medicine,* ed 17, Philadelphia, 1985, WB Saunders.

Millman RB: General principles of diagnosis and treatment. In Frances AJ, Hales RE, editors: *American Psychiatric Association annual review,* vol 5, Washington, DC, 1986, The Association.

Millman RB, Khuri ET: Adolescence and substance abuse. In Lowinson JH, Ruiz P, editors: *Substance abuse: clinical problems and perspectives,* Baltimore, 1981, Williams & Wilkins.

Morgan CH et al: A pilot trial of amantadine for cocaine abuse, *NIDA Res Monogr Ser* 81:81, 1988.

National Household Survey on Drug Abuse, Rockville, Md, 1991, National Institute of Mental Health.

Neerhof MG et al: Cocaine abuse during pregnancy: peripartum prevalence and perinatal outcome, *Am J Obstet Gynecol* 161:633, 1989.

Nestler EJ, Fitzgerald LW, Self DW: Neurobiology. In Oldham JM and Riba MB, editors: *Review of Psychiatry,* vol 14, Wahington, DC, 1995, American Psychiatric Press.

O'Brien CP, Woody GE: Sedative-hypnotics and antianxiety agents. In Frances AJ, Hales RE, editors: *American Psychiatric Association annual review,* vol 5, Washington, DC, 1986, The Association.

O'Malley SS et al: Naltrexone and coping skills therapy for alcohol dependence: a controlled study, *Arch Gen Psychiatry* 49:894, 1992.

Peterson RC, Stillman RC, editors: *PCP (phencyclidine) abuse: an appraisal,* NIDA Research Monograph Series, No. 21, Department of Health, Education, and Welfare, Washington, DC, 1979, US Government Printing Office.

Pickens RW, Svikis DS: *The twin method in study of vulnerability to drug abuse,* NIDA Research Monograph Series No. 89, Rockville, Md, 1989, National Institute on Drug Abuse.

Quigley AJ, Bredemeyer DE, Seow SS: A case of buprenorphine abuse, *Med J Aust* 142:425, 1984.

Regier DA et al: One-month prevalence of mental disorders in the United States, *Arch Gen Psychiatry* 45:977, 1988.

Resnick RB, Schuyten-Resnick E, Washton AM: Assessment of narcotic antagonists in the treatment of opioid dependence, *Annu Rev Pharmacol Toxicol* 20:463, 1980.

Ritz MC, Kuhar MJ: Relationship between self-administration of amphetamine and monoamine receptors in brain: comparison with cocaine, *J Pharmacol Exp Ther* 248:1010, 1989.

Rounsaville BJ, Gawin FH, Kleber HD: Interpersonal psychotherapy adapted for ambulatory cocaine users, *Am J Drug Alcohol Abuse* 11:171, 1985.

Rowbotham MC et al: Trazodone–oral cocaine interactions, *Arch Gen Psychiatry* 41:895, 1984.

Sachs DPL: Advances in smoking cessation treatment, *Curr Pulmonol* 12:139, 1991.

Sadava SW: Initiation to cannabis use: a longitudinal social psychological study of college freshmen, *Can J Behav Sci* 5:371, 1973.

Schneider NG, Jarvik ME, Forsythe AB: Nicotine vs placebo gum in the alleviation of withdrawal during smoking cessation, *Addict Behav* 9:149, 1984.

Schuckit MA: Genetic and clinical implications of alcoholism and affective disorder, *Am J Psychiatry* 143:140, 1986.

Schuster CR: The National Institute on Drug Abuse in the decade of the brain, *Neuropsychopharmacol* 3:315, 1990.

Sellers EM, Higgins GA, Sobell MB: 5-HT and alcohol abuse, *Trends Pharmacol Sci* 13:69, 1992.

Sellers EM, Kalant H. In Kaufman E, Pattison EM, editors: *Encyclopedic handbook of alcoholism,* New York, 1982, Gardner.

Sellers EM, Naranjo CA, Peachey JE: Drug therapy: drugs to decrease alcohol consumption, *New Engl J Med* 305:1255, 1981.

Senay EC et al: Withdrawal from methadone maintenance: rate of withdrawal and expectation, *Arch Gen Psychiatry* 34:361, 1977.

Shi JM et al: Three methods of ambulatory opiate detoxification, *NIDA Res Monogr Ser* No. 132, NIH Publ No. 93-3505, Washington, DC, 1993, US Government Printing Office.

Smith DE: *Treatment and aftercare for cocaine dependency.* Presented at the Institute of Alcoholism and Drug Abuse Studies Conference on Cocaine: Problems and Solutions, Baltimore, Jan. 1984.

Stitzer ML, Gross J: Smoking relapse: the role of pharmacological and behavioral factors, *Prog Clin Biol Res* 261:163, 1988.

Swift RM: Alcoholism and substance abuse. In Stoudemire A, editor: *Clinical psychiatry for medical students,* Philadelphia, 1990, JB Lippincott.

Tennant FS, Segherian AA: Double-blind comparison of amantadine and bromocriptine for ambulatory withdrawal from cocaine dependence, *Arch Intern Med* 147:109, 1987.

Van Dyke C et al: Oral cocaine: plasma concentration and central effects, *Science* 200:211, 1978.

Volkow ND et al: Effects of chronic cocaine abuse on postsynaptic dopamine receptors, *Am J Psychiatry* 147:719, 1990.

Volpicelli J et al: Naltrexone in the treatment of alcohol dependence, *Arch Gen Psychiatry* 49:867, 1992.

Walker S, Yesavage JA, Tinklenberg JR: Acute phencyclidine (PCP) intoxication: quantitative urine levels and clinical management, *Am J Psychiatry* 138:674, 1981.

Wallace BC: Crack cocaine smokers as adult children of alcoholics: the dysfunctional family link, *J Subst Abuse Treat* 7:89, 1990.

Weider H, Kaplan E: Drug use in adolescents, *Psychoanal Study Child* 24:339, 1969.

Wesson DR, Smith DE: A new method for the treatment of barbiturate dependence, *JAMA* 231:294, 1975.

Whitfield C. In Fann WE et al, editors: Nondrug detoxification. *Phenomenology and treatment of alcoholism,* New York, 1980, Spectrum.

Wikler A: Diagnosis and treatment of drug dependence of the barbiturate type, *Am J Psychiatry* 125:758, 1968.

Woody GE, McLellan AT, Bedrick J: Dual diagnosis. In Oldham JM and Riba MB, editors: *Review of psychiatry,* vol 14, Wahington, DC, 1995.

Williams AF: Personality and other characteristics associated with cigarette smoking among young teenagers, *J Health Soc Behav* 14:374, 1973.

Wurmser L: Psychoanalytic considerations of the etiology of compulsive drug use, *J Am Psychoanal Assoc* 22:820, 1974.

Zinberg NE: Addiction and ego function. In Fissler BS et al, editors: *The psychoanalytic study of the child,* New Haven, 1975, Yale University.

UNIT III

Drug Issues Related to Psychopharmacology

CHAPTER 11

Drugs Used for Electroconvulsive Therapy

Sallie Jones, a 71-year-old African-American woman with major depression was admitted on March 6, 1995, to the geropsychiatric unit of a large Southeastern medical center. She had been experiencing psychiatric symptoms since the summer of 1994 but had no history of psychiatric illness before that date. Her symptoms on admission were lack of interest in anything, lying in bed all day, sadness, decreased appetite, lack of energy, crying spells, and insomnia. Ms. Jones denied having experienced hallucinations or delusions. Previous outpatient treatment had involved antidepressant medication, but Ms. Jones' condition continued to deteriorate. Her outpatient physician arranged for her admission to the geropsychiatric unit, with the expressed intent of providing electroconvulsive therapy (ECT) for Ms. Jones. After appropriate assessments were made, Ms. Jones received a series of six ECT treatments. Within 3 weeks of her admission she was much improved, and discharge plans were finalized. Although unresponsive to antidepressants, Ms. Jones responded dramatically to ECT.

Electroconvulsive therapy (ECT) is an effective and predictable treatment option (90% efficacy) for individuals with severe or refractory depression (Murugesan, 1994; Potter and Rudorfer, 1993). Although this treatment form has undergone considerable negative scrutiny, it has emerged in the past decade as a major psychiatric intervention. In 1995 approximately 60,000 people in the United States underwent ECT, with a total of about 1 million individual treatments being given (Shulins, 1995). This once reviled and supposedly barbaric treatment has recaptured a strong endorsement from clinicians (American Psychiatric Association, 1990) and the interest of the media. A new book, titled "Undercurrents: A Therapist's Reckoning With Her Own Depression," tells the story of Dr. Martha Manning, a clinical psychologist, whose depression became so debilitating that she agreed to ECT. In a television appearance, Dr. Manning convincingly advocated ECT for those who are not helped by antidepressants. Like most patients who benefit from ECT, her attitude toward this treatment is favorable (Pettinati et al, 1994).

A SUMMATIVE HISTORY OF ECT

Electroconvulsive therapy has now been used for more than half a century (Hay, 1991) and has proved to be a remarkably safe treatment (American Psychiatric Association, 1990). During those 50 years a number of critics emerged and affected public and professional perceptions of this treatment form. Because of its efficacy, however, and for no other reason, ECT has weathered these misperceptions and continues to be used effectively today.

Electroconvulsive therapy, also referred to as *electroshock therapy* (EST) or "shock therapy," emerged as a treatment form in 1938. It was introduced by Ugo Cerletti and Luciano Bini, two Italian psychiatrists. ECT had been preceded by other forms of convulsive therapy. Convulsants included camphor oil, metrozol, and insulin. Each were rejected for reasons ranging from lack of predictability to instillation of doom.

Although ECT has proved to be effective, paradoxically the theoretical premise on which it was built was faulty. Early twentieth-century psychiatrists believed schizophrenia and epilepsy were incompatible. Although we now know that this is not true, the conceptual extension of this false belief led to the development of an effective treatment form.

The early advocates of ECT envisioned a dramatic relief from the curse of mental illness. Over time, inappropriate use and disappointing results, coupled with growing distrust of psychiatric hospitals, created a climate of hostility toward ECT. The emergence of antipsychotics and other psychopharmacologic agents in the 1950s foreshadowed the decline of ECT. By the 1960s and early 1970s, ECT came under harsh criticism, and legislation was passed to limit its use. By 1980 the use of ECT had come to a virtual standstill (Thompson and Blaine, 1987).

During the 1980s ECT once again emerged as a viable alternative when more conventional treatment approaches failed. With the application of rigid treatment criteria and careful pretreatment evaluation, many psychiatric patients, particularly those with depression, have responded to ECT. Currently ECT is recognized as an effective treatment for a variety of affective disorders.

Historical Perspective on the Negative View

To appreciate the safety and effectiveness of modern ECT, it is important to understand why the "old" ECT procedure caused such great distress (Box 11-1). The "old" ECT was literally applied as an electrical current that passed through the brain, causing an epileptic, or grand mal, seizure. The convulsion was accompanied by various complications, including muscle soreness, fractures, dislocations, sprains, and tongue lacerations. In its heyday ECT was given to almost every patient who did not respond to other treatment forms. In large state hospitals ECT was given on Mondays, Wednesdays, and Fridays to as many as 20 or more patients on a psychiatric ward. One patient after another—some under their own power, others literally overpowered and held—would take his or her place on the bed to be given ECT. Nursing staff would hold the patient in place (to decrease fractures, dislocations, and the like), insert the mouth guard (to prevent tongue bites), put paste on the electrodes and hold them in place on each side of the head (usually in the temple area), and hold the chin and jaw in proper alignment (similar to cardiopulmonary resuscitation [CPR] positioning to prevent dislocation and maintain the airway); the physician, stationed in the background, would deliver the shock. A full grand mal

Box 11-1 Consequences of "old" ECT

- Full grand mal seizure
- Problems associated with full seizure
  - Muscle soreness
  - Fractures
  - Dislocations
  - Sprains
  - Tongue lacerations
  - 1 in 1000 patients died
  - 40% of patients were injured

seizure would occur. After convulsion activity stopped, the patient would be turned on his or her side and tied in place (to prevent aspiration) while a staff member or "helper patient" would stay at the bedside until consciousness returned. The ECT team would then move on to the next patient.

This unforgettable scene, the media (including novels and films), and reports from former patients contributed to the stigma and public fear of ECT. Despite this historically negative view of ECT, the addition of several important drugs and refinements in the delivery of the stimulus have revitalized the technique. Many psychiatric professionals view ECT as the treatment of choice for major depression, finding it safe and economical (Markowitz et al, 1987).

MODERN ELECTROCONVULSIVE THERAPY

During ECT an electrical current is passed through the brain for 0.5 to 2 seconds. The seizure resulting from ECT should be between 20 and 120 seconds in duration (more typically 30 to 60 seconds) to be of therapeutic value. Collectively, between 220 to 250 seconds is usually required for a therapeutic series of ECT. As the treatment series progresses, the seizure threshold can increase as much as 200%, necessitating a stronger stimulus. (This seizure suppression appears to have implications for treating epilepsy [Swartz, 1993a].)

The events performed before, during, and after the treatment, including primarily nursing, medical, or shared responsibilities, follow in roughly sequential order and are outlined in Box 11-2. Electrodes are typically placed bilaterally, but unilateral placement is also common.

Seizure activity is monitored by an electroencephalograph (EEG). Blood pressure and heart rate are also monitored. Oxygen is administered immediately before and after the treatment because of the interruption of breathing caused by succinylcholine (Anectine) and the electrically induced seizure. Typically patients are given ECT two to three times per week up to a total of six to twelve treatments (or until the patient improves or is obviously not going to improve).

Indications

Electroconvulsive therapy is most useful in treating major depression (typically 6 to 12 treatments are prescribed). Patients with major depression respond better (Bowden, 1985) and faster (Coffey and Weiner, 1990) to ECT than to other treatments. Approximately 85% to 90% of ECT patients suffer from severe depression (Potter and Rudorfer, 1993; Tancer et al, 1989). Patients with refractory depression, suicidal tendencies, acute mania (80% efficacy), catatonia (1 to 4 treatments), and some catatonic or prominently affective schizophrenia (up to 15 treatments required) are significantly helped by ECT (American Psychiatric Association, 1978, 1990; Hay, 1991; Mukherjee, Sackeim, and Schnur, 1994). Box 11-3 lists the disorders, depressive symptoms, and conditions that respond to ECT. The clinical example in Box 11-4 details the use of ECT for symptoms of parkinsonism.

Electroconvulsive therapy seems to be particularly suited to the elderly patient because there are no drug side effects, and it is safe and effective (Alexopoulos, Young, and Abrams, 1989; Fogel, 1988; Hay, 1989; Hay, 1991; Greenberg and Fink, 1992; Zwil and Pelchat, 1994; Rice et al, 1994). Administering ECT to children is more controversial, but a number of clinicians advocate its use in this population (Chatterjee, 1995; Fink, 1995; Kellett, 1995). Electroconvulsive therapy is *not* useful for treating mild depressions, behavior disorders, phobias, anxiety, somatoform disorders, or personality disturbances (Box 11-5).

Box 11-2 Electroconvulsive Therapy Administration

Preparation

Medical

The patient must have a pretreatment evaluation, including physical examination, electrocardiogram, laboratory work (blood cell count, blood chemistry studies, and urinalysis), and baseline mental status examination that includes a formal assessment of cognition. A computed tomography scan or magnetic resonance imaging of the head may also be indicated and performed.

Nursing

A consent form must be signed. Because ECT is often given as a treatment of last resort, some patients are so profoundly depressed by the time ECT is ordered that obtaining their "informed consent" is not possible. In such cases, involving family members and requesting assistance form the facility's legal staff may be necessary.

Medical

1. Eliminate the routine use of benzodiazepines or barbiturates for nighttime sedation because of their ability to raise the seizure threshold and cause shorter seizures (less than 25 to 30 seconds in duration).* Chloral hydrate may be used as an alternative drug regimen. A subconvulsive stimulus may be harmful to the patient.† Discontinue antidepressant and lithium regimens to avoid adverse effects or the potential for neurotoxicity.‡
2. Obtain the services of a trained electrotherapist and an anesthesiologist. Whether an anesthesiologist provides care significantly different from that of a psychiatrist is a subject of debate. The new American Psychiatric Association guidelines on ECT§ carefully skirt this issue. Pearlman, Loper, and Tillery† found no deaths attributable to ECT in surveying 9 years of psychiatrist-administered anesthesia ($N = 8161$).
3. Obtain an ECT treatment device (e.g., MECTA SA-1 (MECTA, Inc., Portland, Oregon).

Before treatment

Nursing

1. The patient should receive nothing by mouth from the midnight preceding treatment until after the treatment.
2. Give atropine as ordered. Atropine can be given 1 hour before treatment or given by intravenous (IV) administration immediately before treatment. Atropine reduces secretions and subsequent risk of aspiration. Metoclopramide (Reglan) or glycopyrrolate (Robinul) may also be given in concert with atropine or as an alternative agent.
3. Ask the patient to urinate before treatment. (Seizure-induced incontinence is common.)
4. Remove the patient's hairpins and dentures.

*Fink M: *Am J Psychiatry* 144:1995, 1987.
†Pearlman T, Loper M, Tillery L: *Am J Psychiatry* 147:1553, 1990.
‡Coffey CE, Weiner RD: *Hosp Community Psychiatry* 41:515, 1990.
§American Psychiatric Association: *APA Task Force on Electroconvulsive Therapy,* task force No. 14, Washington, DC, 1990, The Association.

Continued.

Box 11-2 Electroconvulsive Therapy Administration—cont'd

Before treatment
***Nursing*—cont'd**
5. Take the patient's vital signs.
6. Be positive about the treatment and attempt to reduce the patient's pretreatment anxiety.

During treatment
Medical or nursing
1. Insert an intravenous line.
2. Attach electrodes to the proper place on the head. Electrodes are typically held in place with a rubber strap.

Nursing
Insert bite-block.
Medical
1. Give methohexital (Brevital), 1.5 mg/kg body weight, or another short-acting barbiturate (occasionally, thiopental sodium, 3.5 mg/kg body weight) by the intravenous route for anesthesia. The barbiturate causes immediate anesthesia, pre-empting the anxiety associated with waiting for the "jolt to hit" and the anxiety caused by succinylcholine (Anectine). (Succinylcholine causes paralysis but not sedation, thereby leaving the patient conscious but unable to breath.)
2. Place blood pressure cuff on one arm. Inflate cuff before giving/administering succinylcholine.
3. Give succinylcholine IV. Fasciculations should occur in all muscles except those below the blood pressure cuff. Stimulate with nerve stimulator to ascertain paralysis.* Succinylcholine prevents the external manifestations of a grand mal seizure, thus minimizing the risk of fractures, dislocations, and the like while not affecting the "brain seizure."
4. The anesthesiologist mechanically ventilates the patient with 100% oxygen immediately before the treatment.
5. Give the electrical impulse: up to 150 volts for 0.5 to 2 seconds.
6. Observe the length of the seizure. The seizure must be greater than 20 to 30 seconds in duration to be of therapeutic value. If the seizure is less than 30 seconds long, a decision must be made whether to stimulate another seizure. Up to four attempts may be made. Coffey et al† augmented ECT with the administration of caffeine, 242 mg IV push pretreatment to maintain or increase seizure duration.

Medical or nursing
1. Monitor the patient's heart rate, heart rhythm, and blood pressure; electroencephalography is also used.
2. Ventilation and monitoring should continue until the patient recovers.

*Henneman, EA, Bellamy P, Togashi C: Peripheral nerve stimulators in the critical care setting, *Critical Care Nurse* (6):82, 1995.
†Coffey CE et al: *Am J Psychiatry* 147:579, 1990.

Box 11-2 Electroconvulsive Therapy Administration—cont'd

After treatment

Medical

The anesthesiologist mechanically ventilates the patient with 100% oxygen until the patient can breathe on his or her own.

Nursing

1. Monitor for respiratory problems.
2. Because ECT causes confusion and disorientation, it is important to help reorient the patient to time, place, and person as he or she emerges from this groggy state.
3. Observe the patient until he or she is oriented and is steady on his or her feet.

Medical and nursing

Carefully document all aspects of the treatment for the patient record.

Box 11-3 Disorders, Depressive Symptoms, and Conditions that Respond to ECT

Disorders	Depressive Symptoms	Conditions
Severe depression	Anhedonia	Tardive dystonia
Treatment-refractory depression	Anorexia	Tardive dyskinesia
Catatonia	Delusions	Akathisia
Mania	Insomnia	Parkinsonian symptoms
Some types of schizophrenia	Muteness	Neuroleptic malignant syndrome
	Psychomotor retardation	
	Suicidal ideations	

From Swartz CM: Seizure benefit: grand mal or grand bene? *Neurol Clin* 11(1):151, 1993b.

Although ECT is most often prescribed after another treatment option has failed, for example, psychotropic medications, there are several situations in which it can be considered a first-line treatment (Beale, Pritchett, and Kellner, 1995). They are:

1. When immediate intervention is warranted, for example, where there is catatonia, suicidality, or malnutrition
2. When the risks of other treatments are greater than the risk of ECT
3. When a history of successful response from ECT exists
4. When the patient prefers ECT

Contraindications

Although there are no absolute contraindications for ECT, it is relatively contraindicated for patients with recent myocardial infarctions or cerebrovascular accidents and when intracranial tumors are present. Ziring (1993) likens ECT to life-

Box 11-4 Clinical Example of ECT: Patient with Parkinsonism

Mr. X is an approximately 62-year-old retired veteran with parkinsonism and depression. Mr. X had experienced a complicated course with his illness over the past 5 years. Having tried all medications for the treatment of parkinsonism and the accompanying depression, Mr. X, along with his wife, decided to contact a psychiatrist in a large teaching hospital in the South to discuss the option of ECT. Mr. X was severely depressed; on admission to the facility, he was unable to walk, had difficulty speaking, and was unable to tend to activities of daily living (ADLs). The patient and his wife drove across two states to find a psychiatrist who was willing to administer ECT as a specific treatment for parkinsonism. ECT was administered in the normal fashion for a total of eight treatments. Following completion of the ECT, Mr. X was able to converse with others with relative ease. He began walking and attended his own ADLs with minimal assistance from the staff. Mr. X even demonstrated a sense of humor with the staff and his wife, which was a very dramatic change from his pretreatment restricted affect, cognitive deficits, and virtual muteness. These effects lasted approximately 4 months before another exacerbation of his symptoms occurred. Needless to say, Mr. X, his family, and the staff were pleased with this treatment modality for parkinsonism.

(Courtesy Jan Findlay, MSN.)

Box 11-5 Conditions That Do Not Respond to ECT

Anxiety disorders
Behavioral disorders
Mild depressions
Personality disorders
Phobic disorders
Somatoform disorders

saving surgery; if a patient's life is in jeopardy, using of life-saving procedures outweighs almost all potential risk. Box 11-6 presents conditions known to be high risk for ECT. Physiologic effects associated with ECT are presented in Box 11-7.

Advantages

"Even with the host of psychotropic agents now available, ECT still represents for some patients the safest, most rapid, and most effective form of treatment . . ." (Frances, Weiner, and Coffey, 1989).

Electroconvulsive therapy is a safe procedure. Death as a result of ECT is rare (Sackeim et al, 1993). The morbidity rate for an individual treatment is about 1 per 50,000, with approximately 1 death per 10,000 patients occurring. This mortality

Box 11-6 Conditions Resulting in Increased Risk for ECT

Very high risk:	Recent myocardial infarction Recent cerebrovascular accident Intracranial mass lesion
High risk:	Angina pectoris Congestive heart failure Severe pulmonary disease Severe osteoporosis Major bone fractures Glaucoma Retinal detachment Thrombophlebitis Pregnancy

Modified from Ziring B: Issues in the perioperative care of the patient with psychiatric illness, *Med Clin North Am* 77(2):443, 1993.

Box 11-7 Physiologic Effects of ECT

Cardiac effects
- hypertension
- arrhythmias
- alteration of cardiac output
- changes in cerebrovascular dynamic

Increased oxygen consumption*
Hyponatremia†
Migraine headaches‡

*Ziring B: Issues in the perioperative care of the patient with psychiatric illness, *Med Clin North Am* 77(2):443, 1993.
†Greer R, Stewart R: Hyponatremia and ECT, *Am J Psychiatry* 150(8):1272, 1993.
‡Weinstein MD: Migraine occurring as sequela of electroconvulsive therapy, *Headache* 33(1):45, 1993.

rate approximates that for uncomplicated anesthesia (Gitlin et al, 1993). Mortality rates for ECT (0.002% to 0.004% per treatment) are lower than mortality rates for childbirth (0.01%) (Coffey and Weiner, 1990). Mortality is most often associated with cardiovascular complications; however, even these complications are less problematic with ECT than with tricyclic antidepressants (TCAs). Regardless, when contrasted to the death by suicide of those diagnosed with major depression (15 per 100), the use of ECT is easily justified. Electroconvulsive therapy is not only safe but also appears to be equieffective with antidepressants (Potter and Rudorfer, 1993), and because ECT works faster than TCAs, it provides an economic advantage (Markowitz et al, 1987).

Disadvantages

The major disadvantage of ECT is that it provides only temporary relief; it does not provide a permanent cure. Certainly many patients are able to remain depression free for long periods, and still others may never need treatment again. However, about 20% of those treated relapse within 6 months and will need another series of treatments. Some psychiatrists order maintenance or continuation ECT (once per month for 6 to 12 months). Maintenance ECT has been found safe, efficacious, and well tolerated, with minimal adverse effects (Stiebel, 1995).

Memory impairment, both retrograde (memory before treatment) and anterograde (ability to learn new things and memory after treatment), has been frequently cited as a side effect of ECT. Anterograde amnesia is typically transient and may be related to reversible inhibition of protein synthesis in the hippocampus (Chatterjee, 1995). Retrograde memory loss is more problematic but also returns in time (Chatterjee, 1995).

Memory of events closest in time to ECT is most frequently affected. Although it is true that memory is impaired for events that occur before and after each treatment and that confusion occurs immediately after each treatment, there seems to be no substantial loss of mental function once the treatment series is completed. By 6 months, all patients have recovered their full memory. Furthermore, because depression, too, can cause memory loss, it is not always clear whether memory impairment is related to ECT or to depression. Confusion, no matter how severe, clears within days to weeks (Sackeim, 1993).

Although bilateral electrode placement is thought to be more effective, unilateral electrode placement appears to reduce anterograde memory loss and disorientation after treatment (Beale, 1995). Frances, Weiner, and Coffey (1989) reported memory may actually have improved after unilateral nondominant-hemisphere stimulation ECT was begun. When the unilateral approach is used, both electrodes are placed on the nondominant hemisphere (usually the right hemisphere) instead of one being placed on each side of the head. This approach is now a recommended method of delivering ECT; however, some patients only respond to bilateral ECT (Murugesan, 1994).

HOW ELECTROCONVULSIVE THERAPY WORKS

More than 100 theories have been proposed to explain the efficacy of ECT (Sackeim, 1994). Although ECT's efficacy is established, the mechanism of that effectiveness is not well understood. However, most likely ECT's efficacy is associated with the many changes in the various neurotransmitter systems that are affected, including changes in second-messenger systems and down regulation of beta receptors postsynaptically.

DRUGS USED IN ELECTROCONVULSIVE THERAPY

Three major drugs are used to enhance ECT: atropine, methohexital (Brevital), and succinylcholine (Anectine). Before treatment atropine is given to reduce secretions and to minimize aspiration. Atropine can be given 1 hour before treatment by mouth or may be given intravenously immediately before the treatment. Once the patient is ready for the treatment, methohexital is given intravenously. Methohexital induces anesthesia, which reduces pretreatment anxiety. One can easily imagine the fear associated with waiting for the "jolt" to hit that patients in the premodern ECT era experienced. A second, and perhaps more important, rationale for the use of methohexital is that it induces anesthesia before succinylcholine is given. Succinylcholine is a muscle relaxant that prevents the external manifestations of seizure activity long associated with ECT. Although brain seizures continue to occur and can be measured by EEG, tonic and clonic seizures do not occur, sparing the patient from the physical consequences associated with convulsions. However, succinylcholine does not affect consciousness or cerebration (Olin, 1995). Without the addition of methohexital, the suffocating effect of succinylcholine would terrify the patient.

SUCCINYLCHOLINE

Succinylcholine is an ultrashort-acting (30 to 60 seconds), noncompetitive neuromuscular blocker used for several short-duration procedures, including ECT. Succinylcholine is a depolarizing blocker as opposed to most neuromuscular blockers, which are nondepolarizing. Nondepolarizing agents block the nicotinic receptors on the muscle cell, thus preventing muscle activation by acetylcholine (ACh). Depolarizing agents such as succinylcholine are ACh agonists that mimic ACh but are longer acting. Initially the muscle is highly stimulated, but because succinylcholine is longer acting, the depolarized muscle becomes insensitive to further stimulation by the ACh. The resulting paralysis prevents the external manifestations of grand mal seizures. The initial stimulation caused by succinylcholine lasts about 30 seconds and produces strong muscle contractions (fasiculations) in a rostrocaudal (head to toe) direction. Recovery of muscle tone occurs in reverse order (Olin, 1995). Succinylcholine has been reported to cause bone fractures in a few weakened individuals.

Pharmacokinetics and Interactions

Succinylcholine is given intravenously about 1 minute after methohexital administration and is metabolized rapidly by plasma and liver pseudocholinesterases; however, because succinylcholine is noncompetitive, the paralysis it induces cannot be reversed by pharmacologic treatment. Complete paralysis occurs within 30 to 60 seconds. Succinylcholine has the shortest duration—about 5 minutes—of all neuromuscular blockers. For ECT an intravenous dose of succinylcholine, 0.6 mg per kg body weight, is given. Propranolol, quinidine, and other drugs, including phenelzine, promazine, oxytocin, procainamide, lithium carbonate, and furosemide, can prolong paralysis, leading to hypotension; digoxin increases the risk of cardiac arrhythmias, and lidocaine enhances respiratory depression when combined with succinylcholine. An important interaction is the one succinylcholine has with neostigmine, a drug that inhibits the destruction of ACh and is used as an antidote for nondepolarizing neuromuscular blockers. When combined with succinylcholine, neostigmine inhibits succinylcholine metabolism and intensifies the initial depolarization of muscles. Neostigmine should not be used with succinylcholine in most situations. An exception to this rule occurs when the neuromuscular block evolves to a phase II block. Discussion of phase I versus phase II blockade is beyond the scope of this text.

METHOHEXITAL

Methohexital is an ultrashort-acting barbiturate used to induce anesthesia and is the preferred agent for inducing a light coma preceding delivery of ECT. Less often, thiopental sodium (Pentothal) is used for this purpose, but it causes more postictal confusion. Although the primary efforts in modern ECT have been directed at eliminating the overt manifestations of seizure activity, induction of anesthesia is the first step in that process. Succinylcholine provides the sought-after muscle relaxation needed to reduce observable convulsions, but it does not induce anesthesia. Consequently, as noted above, if succinylcholine alone were to be given to the patient, the patient would experience muscle paralysis, including respiratory paralysis, while conscious. The emotional reaction to suffocation would be panic; therefore, anesthesia induction with methohexital is required.

Pharmacokinetics

Methohexital is given intravenously just before the intravenous administration of succinylcholine. Methohexital rapidly crosses the blood-brain barrier and quickly depresses the central nervous system, causing unconsciousness within 10 to 15 seconds. The duration of effect is relatively short (5 to 7 minutes) as a result of a natural redistribution to adipose tissue and other less vascular sites. Methohexital is metabolized by the liver, excreted in the urine, and has a half-life of 3 to 8 hours.

The amount of methohexital employed for ECT is typically 50 to 120 mg given intravenously (or 1.5 mg per kg body weight) for adults. Pettinati et al (1990) recommended a dose of 0.9 mg per kg for their ECT patients.

Side Effects

The major side effects of methohexital are respiratory depression, hypotension, myocardial depression, and decreased cardiac output. Consequently, methohexital is used cautiously in persons with asthma, hypotension, and severe cardiovascular disease. Other potentially life-threatening reactions include anaphylactic reactions, cardiac arrhythmias, peripheral vascular disease, apnea, laryngospasm, and bronchospasm. Bothersome and occasionally serious side effects include prolonged unconsciousness, headache, restlessness and anxiety, nausea and vomiting, dyspnea, hiccups, and a variety of skin rashes.

Interactions

Methohexital has several potentially serious drug interactions. Most notably, other CNS depressants increase CNS and respiratory depression. Furosemide (Lasix), a commonly prescribed drug in older patients, interacts with methohexital to cause substantial orthostatic hypotension. In addition, a number of drugs have decreased effectiveness when given concurrently with methohexital.

ATROPINE

Atropine is the prototypical anticholingeric agent. Anticholingeric drugs inhibit the effects of ACh on the parasympathetic system. Atropine is derived from a common plant, *Atropa belladonna.* Atropine and all anticholinergics have a wide effect in the body; however, atropine is given before ECT for several specific responses, including inhibition of salivation and respiratory tract secretions (thereby decreasing potential for aspiration respiratory problems) and vagal stimulation (thereby decreasing the potential for cardiovascular depression resulting from ECT, succinylcholine, and/or methohexital).

Pharmacokinetics

Atropine is well absorbed when given orally (onset 30 minutes) or intramuscularly/subcutaneously (onset 15 minutes) 1 hour before ECT and can be given intravenously (onset 1 minute) just before delivery of ECT. Atropine readily crosses the blood-brain barrier, is metabolized in the liver, and is excreted primarily in the urine. It has a duration of action of 4 hours and a half-life of 2 to 3 hours. A typical dose ranges from 0.4 to 0.6 mg.

Side Effects

The most common side effects associated with atropine are dry mouth, blurred vision, constipation, urinary hesitancy, and, possibly, urinary retention. More serious reactions include paralytic ileus, mydriasis, and anaphylactic reactions. Occasional adverse responses include nervousness, flushing, confusion, fever, restlessness, tremor, bradycardia, palpitations, nausea and vomiting, photophobia, and skin rashes.

Atropine is used cautiously when a patient is known to have a history of glaucoma, prostatic hypertrophy, cardiac arrhythmias, current fever, or obstructive uropathy. Interventions for anticholinergic side effects are found in Chapters 4, Schizophrenia and Other Psychosis, and 5, Mood Disorders.

Interactions

When atropine is given concurrently with other anticholinergic drugs, an additive effect occurs. Particularly common drug-drug interactions are found between atropine and the following drugs with anticholinergic properties: antihistamines, antipyschotics, antiparkinson agents, TCAs, amantadine, benzodiazepines, and MAOIs. Caution should also be used when atropine is given concurrently with sympathomimetics (an increased sympathomimetic response), cholinesterase inhibitors (decreased cholinesterase effect), digitalis, slow-release digoxin, and neostigmine (an increased potential for side effects).

Patients with hypertension or cardiovascular disease or those who are frail or medically ill can usually be safely treated with ECT. However, additional drugs to reduce the autonomic changes (sympathetic rush) protect the patient. Esmolol, 1.3 or 4.4 mg per kg, or labetalol, 0.13 or 0.44 mg per kg, has been shown effective in reducing cardiovascular response to ECT (Castelli et al, 1995). Other agents used to maintain cardiac integrity include nitroglycerin and lidocaine. Several other drugs routinely employed by anesthesiologists to maintain homeostasis may also be used in complicated cases but are beyond the scope of this chapter.

REFERENCES

Alexopoulos G, Young R, Abrams RC: ECT in the high-risk geriatric patient, *J Am Geriatr Soc* 32:651, 1989.

American Psychiatric Association: *APA task force on electroconvulsive therapy,* Task Force No. 14, Washington, DC, 1978, The Association.

American Psychiatric Association: *The practice of electroconvulsive therapy, recommendations for treatment, training, and privileging: a task force report of the American Psychiatric Association,* Washington, DC, 1990, The Association.

Beale MD, Pritchett JT, Kellner CH: Recent developments in electroconvulsive therapy, *J S C Med Assoc* 91(3):93, 1995.

Bowden CL: Current treatment of depression, *Hosp Community Psychiatry* 36:1192, 1985.

Castelli I et al: Comparative effects of esmolol and labetalol to attenuate hyperdynamic states after electroconvulsive therapy. *Anesth Analg* 80(3):557, 1995.

Chatterjee A: Electroconvulsive therapy, *Lancet* 345(8948):518, 1995 (letter).

Coffey CE et al: Caffeine augmentation of ECT, *Am J Psychiatry* 147:579, 1990.

Coffey CE, Weiner RD: Electroconvulsive therapy: an update, *Hosp Community Psychiatry* 41:515, 1990.

Fink M: Electroconvulsive therapy, *Lancet* 345(8948):519, 1995 (letter).

Fogel B: Electroconvulsive therapy in the elderly: a clinical research agenda, *Int J Geriatr Psychiatry* 3:181, 1988.

Frances A, Weiner RD, Coffey CE: ECT for an elderly man with psychotic depression and concurrent dementia, *Hosp Community Psychiatry* 40:237, 1989.

Gitlin MC et al: Splenic rupture after electroconvulsive therapy, *Anesth Analg* 76:1363, 1993.

Greenberg L, Fink M: Use of electroconvulsive therapy in geriatric patients, *Clin Geriatr Med* 8(2):349-354, 1992.

Greer R, Stewart R: Hyponatremia and ECT, *Am J Psychiatry* 150(8):1272, 1993.

Hay DP: Electroconvulsive therapy in the medically ill elderly, *Convuls Ther* 5(1):8, 1989.

Hay DP: Electroconvulsive therapy. In Sadavoy J, Lazarus LW, Jarvik LF, editors: *Comprehensive review of geriatric psychiatry,* Washington, DC, 1991, American Psychiatric Association.

Henneman EA, Bellamy P, Togashi C: Peripheral nerve stimulators in the critical care setting, *Crit Care Nurs* 15(6):82, 1995.

Kellett JM: Electroconvulsive therapy, *Lancet* 345(8948):518, 1995 (letter).

Markowitz J et al: Reduced length and cost of hospital stay for major depression in patients treated with ECT, *Am J Psychiatry* 144:1025, 1987.

Mukherjee S, Sackeim HA, Schur DB: Electroconvulsive therapy of acute manic episodes: a review of 50 years' experience, *Am J Psychiatry* 151(2):169, 1994.

Murugesan G: Electrode placement, stimulus dosing and seizure monitoring during ECT, *Aust N Z J Psychiatry* 28(4):675, 1994.

Olin, BR: *Drug facts and comparisons.* St. Louis, 1995, Wolters Kluwer.

Pearlman T, Loper M, Tillery L: Should psychiatrists administer anesthesia for ECT? *Am J Psychiatry* 147:1553, 1990.

Pettinati HM et al: Evidence of less improvement in depression in patients taking benzodiazepines during unilateral ECT, *Am J Psychiatry* 147(8):1029, 1990.

Pettinati HM et al: Patient attitudes toward electroconvulsive therapy, *Psychopharmacol Bull* 30(3):471, 1994.

Potter W, Rudorfer M: Electroconvulsive therapy: a modern medical procedure, *N Engl J Med* 328(12):882, 1993.

Rice EH et al: Cardiovascular morbidity in high-risk patients during ECT, *Am J Psychiatry* 151(11), 1637-1641, 1994.

Sackeim HA et al: Effects of stimulus intensity and electrode placement on the efficacy and cognitive effects of electroconvulsive therapy, *N Engl J Med* 328(12):839, 1993.

Sackeim HA: Central issues regarding the mechanisms of action of electroconvulsive therapy: directions for future research, *Psychopharmacol Bull* 30(3):281, 1994.

Shulins N: Reviled electroshock therapy improved and effective, *Las Vegas Sun,* March 19, 1995, p 11b.

Stiebel VG: Maintenance electroconvulsive therapy for chronic mentally ill patients: a case series, *Hosp Community Psychiatry,* 46(3):265, 1995.

Swartz CM: ECT or programmed seizures? *Am J Psychiatry* 150(8):1274, 1993a.

Swartz CM: Seizure benefit: grand mal or grand bene? *Neurol Clin* 11(1):151, 1993b.

Tancer ME et al: Use of electroconvulsive therapy at a university hospital: 1970 and 1980-1981, *Hosp Community Psychiatry* 40(1):64, 1989.

Thompson JW, Blaine JD: Use of ECT in the United States in 1975 and 1980, *Am J Psychiatry* 144:557, 1987.

Weinstein MD: Migraine occurring as sequela of electroconvulsive therapy, *Headache* 33(1):45, 1993.

Ziring B: Issues in the perioperative care of the patient with psychiatric illness, *Med Clin North Am* 77(2):443, 1993.

Zwil AS, Pelchat RJ: ECT in the treatment of patients with neurological and somatic disease, *Int J Psychiatry Med* 24(1):1-29, 1994.

CHAPTER 12

Drugs of Abuse

LELAND N. ALLEN III

This chapter represents a departure from the intervention model used in this book. The scope of alcohol and substance abuse and diagnostic guidelines relevant to the pharmacologic interventions for drug abuse are discussed in Chapter 10, Alcoholism and Other Substance Abuse Disorders. For nonpharmacologic interventions the reader is referred to other sources.

Once associated (in about the mid-nineteenth century) with genteel women addicted to prescribed opiates, drug abuse is now the province of a social underclass that traffics in theft and violence to support drug acquisition (Jonnes, 1995). Drug abuse has become what some believe to be the single most significant issue of our day. Unfortunately, it is underrecognized and undertreated. The broad net of substance abuse ranges from the 10% of the adult general population who suffer from some type of substance disorder (7+% with alcoholism and 3+% with drug disorders) (Regier et al, 1993) to the "addiction" of nearly 50% of people with mental illness who crowd our city streets (Federal Task Force on Homelessness and Severe Mental Illness, 1992). The cost to the United States associated with treatment, reduced productivity, mortality, criminal justice expenditures, and other related factors is thought to exceed $161 billion (National Foundation for Brain Research, 1992). Drugs of abuse are also prominently involved in other disorders. For example, in 1991 27% of the men and 48% of the women with acquired immunodeficiency syndrome (AIDS) were intravenous (IV) drug users, and the rate of new HIV infections is highest among IV drug abusers (Kaufman and McNaul, 1992). Tables 12-1 to 12-3 capture the categories of drugs of abuse and provide information on key variables.

Smith et al (1986) defined dependence as a pathologic process involving a compulsion to use a psychoactive drug, loss of control over use of the drug, and continued use of the drug despite adverse consequences. The term *dependency* has replaced *addiction* for describing compulsive drug use because it more precisely defines the condition. The *Diagnostic and Statistical Manual of Mental Disorders, Fourth Edition (DSM-IV)* (American Psychiatric Association, 1994) differentiates between substance dependence and substance abuse. Substance dependence "is a cluster of cognitive, behavioral, and physiological symptoms indicating that the individual continues use of the substance despite significant substance-related problems." (*DSM-IV*, p. 176) The *DSM-IV* then lists the 7 criteria listed in Box 12-1 and requires that 3 or more be present in a 12-month period for the diagnosis of dependence. Abuse is defined by the *DSM-IV* as "a maladaptive pattern of substance use manifested by recurrent and significant adverse consequences related to the repeated use of substances." (*DSM-IV*, p. 182) Essential features of substance abuse are listed in Box 12-1. In 1987 the American Medical Association declared all drug dependencies to be diseases. Such a view seeks to reduce the guilt and blame traditionally associated with chemical dependency, thereby facilitating treatment.

Table 12-1 Drugs of Abuse: Trade or Other Names

Drugs, controlled substances	Trade or other names	Medical uses
DEA schedules		
Narcotics		
Opium: II, III, V	Dover's powder, Paregoric, Parapectolin	Analgesic, antidiarrheal
Morphine: II, III	Morphine, MS-Contin, MS-IR, Roxanol, Roxanol-SR	Analgesic, antitussive
Codeine: II, III, V	Codeine, Tylenol with codeine	Analgesic, antitussive
Heroin: I	Diacetylmorphine, horse, smack	none
Hydromorphone: II	Dilaudid	Analgesic
Meperidine: II	Demerol, Mepergan	Analgesic
Methadone: II	Methadone, Methadose, Dolophine	Analgesic, narcotic withdrawal
Other narcotics: I, II, III, IV, V	Lortab, Lorcet, Tylox, Talwin, Lomotil, Fentanyl	Analgesic, antidiarrheal, antitussive
Depressants		
Chloral hydrate: IV	Noctec, "knockout drops"	Hypnotic
Barbiturates: II, III, IV	Amytal, Butisol, Fiorinal, Lotusate, Phenobarbital, Seconal, Tuinal	Anesthetic, anti-convulsant, sedative, hypnotic
Benzodiazepines: IV	Ativan, Dalmane, Diazepam/Valium, Librium, Xanax, Serax, Tranxene, Vestran, Versed, Halcion, Restoril	Anxiolytic, anticonvulsant, sedative, hypnotic
Methaqualone: I	Quaalude	Sedative, hypnotic
Glutethimide: III	Doriden	Sedative, hypnotic
Other depressants: III, IV	Equanil, Miltown, Noludar, Placidyl, Valmid	Anxiolytic sedative, hypnotic, anticonvulsant
Stimulants		
Cocaine: II	Coke, flake, snow, crack, rock	Local anesthetic, vasoconstrictor
Amphetamines: II	Biphetamine, Delcobase, Desoxyn, Dexedrine, Obetrol	Attention deficit hyper-activitiy disorder, narcolepsy, obesity
Phenmetrazine: II	Preludin	Obesity control
Methylphenidate: II	Ritalin	Attention deficit hyper-activity disorder, narcolepsy, failure to thrive

Continued

Table 12-1 Drugs of Abuse: Trade or Other Names—cont'd

Drugs, controlled substances	Trade or other names	Medical uses
Stimulants—cont'd		
Other stimulants: III, IV	Adipex, Cylert, Didrex, Ionamin, Melfiat, Plegine, Sanorex, Tenuate, Tepanil, Prelu-2	Obesity control
Hallucinogens		
LSD: I	Acid, microdot	none
Mescaline and peyote: I	Mesc, buttons, cactus	none
Amphetamine variants: I	STP, MDA, MDMA, DOM, DOB	none
Phencyclidine: I	PCP, angel dust, hog	none
Phencyclidine analogues: I	PCE, TCP	none
Other hallucinogens: I	DMT, psilocybin, psilocin	none
Cannabinoids		
Marijuana: I	Pot, Acapulco gold, grass, reefer, sinsemilla, weed, Thai sticks	none
Tetrahydrocannabinol: I, II	THC	Antinauseant for cancer chemotherapy
Hashish: I	Hash	none
Hashish oil: I	Hash oil	none

Modified from *Federal Register* 55(159):33590, Washington, DC, Aug. 16, 1990.
DMT, N, N-dimethyltriptamine; *DOB,* 4-bromo-2, 5-dimethoxyamphetamine; *DOM,* 4-methyl-2, 5-dimethoxyamphetamine; *LSD,* lysergic acid diethylamide; *MDA,* 3, 4-methylenedioxyamphetamine (methylene dioxyamphetamine); *MDMA,* 3, 4-methylenedioxymethamphetamine; *PCE,* N-ethyl-l-phenylcyclohexylamine; *PCP,* phencyclidine; *STP,* 2, 5-dimethoxy-4-methyl; *TCP,* l-[1-phenylcyclohexyl]-pyrrolidine; *THC,* tetrahydrocannabinol.

Although not all psychiatrists and psychiatric nurses embrace the disease concept of drug dependencies, there are convincing arguments for accepting the disease hypothesis. Using alcoholism as an example, Ohlms (1988) points out that alcoholism (1) causes the person to function abnormally, (2) has a characteristic chain of symptoms reflecting specific stages of the disease that are both reliable and predictable, and (3) has the inevitable outcome of death, if continued. These characteristics satisfy the definition of a disease model.

ALCOHOL

Alcohol abuse is the number one problem in North America and is addressed separately because of its enormity. The cost to the United States in health problems, lost work hours, family disruption and disintegration, and criminal activity is cur-

Table 12-2 Drugs of Abuse: Effects, Overdose, and Withdrawal

Drugs	Effects	Overdose	Withdrawal
Narcotics	Euphoria, respiratory depression, constricted pupils, nausea, constipation	Slow, shallow breaths; clammy skin; coma; convulsions; respiratory arrest; death	Watery eyes, runny nose, yawning, loss of appetite, irritability, tremors, panic, cramps, nausea, chills, sweating
Depressants	Slurred speech, disorientation, drunken behavior without evidence of alcohol	Shallow respirations, clammy skin, dilated pupils, weak & rapid pulse, coma, death	Anxiety, insomnia, tremor, delerium, convulsions, death
Stimulants	Increased alertness, excitation, euphoria, rapid pulse, hypertension, insomnia, anorexia	Agitation, hyperthermia, hallucinations, convulsions, death	Apathy, sleep, irritability, depression, disorientation
Hallucinogens	Illusions and hallucinations, poor time and distance perception	Longer and more intense "trips," psychosis, death	No withdrawal syndrome reported
Cannabinoids	Euphoria, disorientation, relaxed inhibitions, increased appetite	Fatigue, paranoia, psychosis	Insomnia, hyperactivity, anorexia

From *Federal Register* 55(159):33590, Washington, DC, Aug. 16, 1990.

rently estimated at more than $90 billion. An estimated 12.1 million Americans have one or more symptoms of alcoholism (Noble, 1985); after cardiovascular disease and cancer, alcoholism ranks third among the causes of death and disability in the United States (Whitfield, Davis, and Barker, 1986). Alcoholics have a death rate two to four times higher than that of nonalcoholics and die, on average, 20 years earlier than their nondrinking counterparts (Poldrugo et al, 1993). Approximately 100,000 deaths each year are directly related to alcohol (Institute of Medicine, 1992). At least 50% of all traffic fatalities involve a drunken driver. Other causes of alcohol-related mortality are suicide, liver disease, heart disease, homicide, and cancer. Low to moderate alcohol intake produces in some drinkers a pleasant, uninhibited feeling; however, even moderate amounts of alcohol can

Table 12-3 Diagnoses Associated with Class of Substances

	Dependence	Abuse	Intoxication	Withdrawal	Intoxication delirium	Withdrawal delirium	Dementia	Amnestic disorder	Psychotic disorders	Mood disorders	Anxiety disorders	Sexual dysfunctions	Sleep disorders
Alcohol	X	X	X	X	I	W	P	P	I/W	I/W	I/W	I	I/W
Amphetamines	X	X	X	X	I				I	I/W	I	I	I/W
Caffeine			X								I		I
Cannabis	X	X	X		I				I		I		
Cocaine	X	X	X	X	I				I	I/W	I/W	I	I/W
Hallucinogens	X	X	X		I				I*	I	I		
Inhalants	X	X	X		I		P		I	I	I		
Nicotine	X			X									
Opioids	X	X	X	X	I				I	I		I	I/W
Phencyclidine	X	X	X		I				I	I	I		
Sedatives, hypnotics, or anxiolytics	X	X	X	X	I	W	P	P	I/W	I/W	W	I	I/W
Polysubstance	X												
Other	X	X	X	X	I	W	P	P	I/W	I/W	I/W	I	I/W

From American Psychiatric Association: *Diagnostic and statistical manual of mental disorders*, ed 4, Washington, DC, 1994, The Association.

*Also Hallucinogen persisting perception disorder (flashbacks).

Note: The letters X, I, W, I/W, or P indicate that the category is recognized in DSM-IV. In addition, *I* indicates that the specifier With Onset During Intoxication may be noted for the category (except for Intoxication Delirium); *W* indicates that the specifier With Onset During Withdrawal may be noted for the category (except for Withdrawal Delirium); and *I/W* indicates that either With Onset During Intoxication or With Onset During Withdrawal may be noted for the category. *P* indicates that the disorder is Persisting.

Box 12-1 DSM-IV Criteria for Substance Dependence and Substance Abuse

Substance dependence

Maladaptive use of a substance that leads to impairment or distress as manifested by any three of the following occurring in a single year:

1. Tolerance to the effect of the substance
2. Withdrawal symptoms when use is stopped
3. Increasing frequency or quantity of use
4. Efforts to cut down or quit are unsuccessful
5. Time is devoted to getting or using the substance
6. Ordinary activities are curtailed in favor of the substance
7. Substance use is continued despite knowledge of adverse effects

Substance abuse

Maladaptive use of a substance leading to impairment or distress as manifested by one of the following occurring in a single year, but not having met the criteria for dependence:

1. Major role obligations at work, school, or home are curtailed in favor of or because of substance use
2. Use of a substance when it is hazardous
3. Substance-related legal problems
4. Continued use despite adverse social/interpersonal effects

Modified from American Psychiatric Association: *Diagnostic and statistical manual of mental disorders,* ed 4, Washington, DC, 1994, The Association.

cause significant impairment. The legal blood alcohol level for drunkenness is 0.1% in some states. Many states have lowered the legal blood alcohol level to 0.08% in the hope of reducing highway deaths caused by drunken drivers. Table 12-4 summarizes the clinical effects of alcohol that are associated with different blood alcohol levels.

The effects of alcoholism are commonly found among medical and psychiatric patients. It is estimated that among general hospital inpatients, 25% of the men (Wallerstedt et al, 1995) and 4% to 35% of the women are alcoholics (Lewis and Gordon, 1983). Regans (1985) reported that one third of American adults (56 million persons) have been adversely affected by alcohol.

Etiologic Theories

Psychodynamic theories. A number of psychologic theories have attempted to explain how people become alcoholics. Traditionally people with alcoholism have been viewed as psychologically weak-willed, irresponsible, selfish, self-destructive, and morally bankrupt individuals who easily succumb to the escape provided by alcohol. Over time the search for an "alcoholic personality" has given way to a multivariate model that incorporates the biopsychosocial components of the disease (Hough, 1989). Current researchers think that many of the stereotypic characteris-

Table 12-4 Clinical Effects of Alcohol

Blood alcohol level	Clinical signs and symptoms
0.05 to 0.15 g/dL	Euphoria, labile mood, cognitive disturbances (decreased concentration, impaired judgment, loss of sexual inhibitions)
0.15 to 0.25 g/dL	Slurred speech, staggering gait, diplopia, drowsiness, labile mood with wild outbursts
0.3 g/dL	Stupor, aggressive behavior, incoherent speech, labored breathing, vomiting
0.4 g/dL	Coma
0.5 g/dL	Severe respiratory depression, death

From Antai-Otong D: Helping the alcoholic patient recover, *Am J Nurs* 95(8):22-30, 1995.

tics found among alcoholics, such as dependency, low self-esteem, passivity, and introversion, are the result of, not the cause of, alcoholism.

Biologic theories. Heredity as an etiologic factor has been studied for many years and continues to provide insight into understanding the genesis of alcoholism. Genetic predisposition is considered to be the single most significant piece of information in identifying alcoholism (Hill, 1995; Ohlms, 1988). Children of alcoholic parents, even if raised in an alcohol-free environment, are more likely to develop alcoholism than are the children of nonalcoholic parents (Goodwin et al, 1973). Mueller and Ketcham (1987) found that even when the child of a person with alcoholism does not drink, an inherited susceptibility to alcoholism is passed on to his or her children. Hereditary explanations provide a good basis for understanding the vulnerability to alcohol apparent in people with alcoholism.

Pharmacokinetics

The chemical name for beverage alcohol is ethanol (CH_3CH_2OH). It is primarily metabolized in the liver. The oxidation process can be described chemically as follows:

$$\underset{\text{(ethanol)}}{CH_3CH_2OH} \rightarrow \underset{\text{(acetaldehyde)}}{CH_3CHO} + H_2 \rightarrow \underset{\text{(acetic acid)}}{CH_3 - C - OH - O} \rightarrow \underset{\text{(carbon dioxide [water])}}{CO_2 - H_2O}$$

At each step of the metabolizing process, an enzyme breaks down the chemical. Ethanol is broken down by alcohol dehydrogenase to acetaldehyde and hydrogen. The hydrogen molecule causes the liver to bypass normal energy sources, that is, the hydrogen from glucose metabolism, and to use the hydrogen from ethanol. This excess of hydrogen production erroneously signals the liver that the body is in a "fed" state, causing the liver to cease producing glucose. This can lead to profound, life-threatening hypoglycemia. Aldehyde dehydrogenase breaks down acetaldehyde to acetic acid, which is an innocuous substance. When enzymatic action on acetaldehyde is blocked by the aldehyde dehydrogenase blocker disulfiram (Antabuse) or by loss of normal hepatic function, acetaldehyde can accumulate, causing an unpleasant illness consisting of malaise, nausea, and flushing. Large concentrations of acetaldehyde in the liver can cause hepatocyte (liver cell) necrosis, leading to cirrhosis and ultimately death. Acetaldehyde also interferes with vitamin activation. The alcohol dehydrogenase in the gastrointestinal tissue of nonalcoholic men oxidizes a significant amount of the alcohol in the gut before it enters the bloodstream. However, Frezza et al (1990) have discovered that the gastrointestinal tissue of women and of alcoholic men contains little alcohol dehydrogenase. The inability of women's bodies to make this "first-pass metabolism" accounts for their enhanced vulnerability to the effects of alcohol and confirms an age-old suspicion that women become intoxicated more easily than men, even when studies are controlled for size differences.

Some researchers postulate that some of the excess acetaldehyde travels to the brain and reacts chemically with neurotransmitters to make tetrahydroisoquinolines (TIQs) and beta-carbolines (Figure 12-1). Tetrahydroisoquinolines are similar to the addictive substance found in heroin and morphine (Mueller and Ketcham, 1987). When TIQs are infused into the brains of monkeys, the monkeys develop an irreversible preference for alcohol over water. Beta-carbolines have been shown to cause severe anxiety, and it is hypothesized that people with alcoholism use alcohol to reduce the anxiety caused by previous ingestion of alcohol (Wallace, 1985).

Alcohol is absorbed partially from the stomach but mostly from the small intestine. If alcohol is ingested by a person with an *empty stomach,* it is in the bloodstream within *20 minutes.* The rate of absorption is affected by the type of alcohol consumed. Beer contains 4% to 6% ethanol; wine, 12% ethanol; and whiskey, 40% to 50% ethanol. Alcohol in beer and wine is absorbed more slowly than that in liquor, but the alcohol content does not account completely for its absorption rate. Food also slows alcohol absorption.

Ethanol is distributed equally in all body tissue according to water content. Large persons or persons with great amounts of body water can ingest more alcohol than small persons or persons with less body water. Alcohol affects the cerebrum and

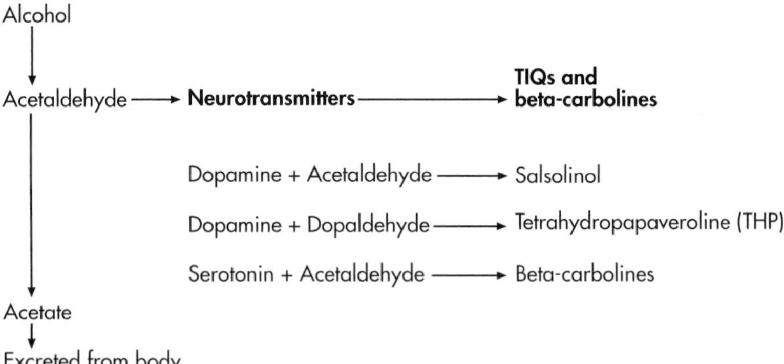

Figure 12-1 How addictive products, tetrahydroisoquinolines (TIQs), and beta-carbolines are formed in the body. Alcohol is metabolized to acetaldehyde. Acetaldehyde and other aldehydes condense with neurotransmitters to produce TIQs and beta-carbolines. These compounds, formed when we drink alcohol, appear to be highly addictive brain substances similar to morphine precursors. Infused into animal brains, they produce what seems to be irreversible addictive drinking. (From Wallace J: *Alcoholism: new light on the disease,* Newport, RI, 1985, Edgehill.)

cerebellum before it affects the spinal cord and the vital centers because the former areas contain more water.

The rate of absorption largely determines how quickly a person will become intoxicated, but the metabolic rate largely determines how long alcohol will affect the body. The metabolic rate is constant. The body can metabolize 10 mL of alcohol (1 ounce of whiskey or 1 glass of beer) every 60 minutes. In persons who drink alcohol frequently for years, hepatic drug-metabolizing levels are increased to hasten alcohol metabolism. Hot coffee, "sweating it out," and other home remedies do not increase alcohol metabolism nor do they speed the "sobering-up" process. Scientists have attempted unsuccessfully to develop a drug to prevent or decrease intoxication. In late-stage alcoholism the metabolism rate decreases because the damaged liver can no longer adequately metabolize the alcohol.

Tolerance to alcohol occurs and is probably related to elevated hepatic enzyme levels and to cellular adaptations. The naive drinker may be noticeably intoxicated after two to three drinks, whereas the long-term drinker may walk around almost unaffected by drinking five times that amount. This is an example of tolerance. "Drinking someone under the table" is a function of practice rather than of manhood (Scavnicky-Mylant and Keltner, 1991).

Physiologic Effects

The initial neurophysiologic and neuropsychologic responses to alcohol consumption are disinhibition, impaired judgment, and impaired cognition. These signs represent cerebrum intoxication. In many situations this mental relaxation is pleasant. Alcohol also depresses psychomotor activity. Alcohol has been described as a social lubricant because it relaxes self-imposed barriers that tether sociability. Anxiety and tension are relieved, usually for a couple of hours after a drink is taken. Unfortunately, once the anxiety-reducing effect wears off, more tension and anxiety remain, so the drinker must consume more alcohol to regain the anxiety-free state again. Eventually, at least for people with alcoholism, drinking becomes defensive; that is, the individual often drinks to avoid the effects of years of drinking. Many persons with alcoholism, even after drinking all they can hold, are not able to quell the psychomotor rebound upheaval caused by years of alcohol-related central nervous system (CNS) irritation.

Alcohol adversely affects both the central nervous system and the peripheral nervous system (PNS). CNS effects are related to sedation and toxicity. As the vital centers become depressed, a slower, stuporous-to-unconscious mental state develops. Large amounts of alcohol can cause progressive depression of brainstem functions to the point that reflexes such as the gag reflex or automatic functions such as respiratory drive are impaired. Other common symptoms of intoxication include slurred speech, a short attention span, loud talk, and memory deficits. *Blackout* is a period during which a person with alcoholism functions socially but for which he or she has no memory.

Historically the brain damage associated with alcoholism was thought to be caused by alcohol-related nutritional deficiencies. Persons with alcoholism eat poorly, which leads to pathologic change. It is now known, however, that brain damage occurs when drinking, even when a nutritious diet is maintained. In fact, all persons with alcoholism have some brain cell loss, and atrophy of the brain can be seen on computed tomograms (CT) of the brain (Ibañez et al, 1995; Sullivan et al, 1995).

Wernicke-Korsakoff syndrome is caused by thiamine deficiency in the diet. Patients for whom alcohol comprises a significant percentage of their caloric intake are likely to be thiamine-deficient. Additionally, thiamine absorption is blocked directly by alcohol, further exacerbating the deficiency. The syndrome is probably associated with a genetic predisposition and is characterized by gait disturbances, confusion, memory loss, and ophthalmoplegia (loss of control of eye movements) (Manzo et al, 1994). Recovery is usually complete if thiamine is administered parenterally.

Alcohol effects the PNS primarily through nutritional deficiencies. Peripheral neuropathy may be either motor or sensory. Sensory neuropathy is usually the initial manifestation, with patients complaining of vague pain, burning, or numbness in the extremities. Untreated, this can predispose the patient to pressure sores identical to those found in people with diabetes. Sensory neuropathy can be objectively demonstrated by a loss of deep-tendon reflexes or loss of pinprick sensation or of heat-cold discrimination in the legs or arms. Motor neuropathy presents as weakness, typically affecting distal muscle groups more than proximal. Treatment involving abstinence from alcohol and nutritional replacement often fails to fully resolve neuropathy.

Cirrhosis and other diseases of the liver are the physical health problems most commonly associated with alcohol abuse. Cirrhosis is the fifth-leading cause of death in the United States. In cirrhosis normal hepatocytes are replaced with fibrous, nonfunctioning scar tissue, which obstructs blood flow, leading to portal hypertension, ascites, and esophageal varices. As the functioning liver is replaced by scar tissue, symptoms and signs of liver failure become evident. The patient with liver dysfunction has low serum protein levels, high serum ammonia and bilirubin levels, and clotting problems. The reduction in normal hepatocytes decreases the liver's ability to metabolize drugs and toxins, leading to an increased sensitivity of the patient to the side effects or toxic effects of common medications. Alcohol metabolism is also reduced in the cirrhotic liver, leading to a loss of tolerance to the effects of alcohol. Alcohol may also cause an acute hepatitis, or inflamation of the liver. This is clinically characterized by abdominal pain, fever, nausea, vomiting, malaise, jaundice, and occasionally, overt liver failure and death.

Alcohol is a chemical irritant. It burns the mouth and throat and prompts the stomach to secrete more hydrochloric acid. Gastric ulcers and gastritis are caused and then worsened by alcohol. People with alcoholism experience ulcers, gastritis, bleeding, and hemorrhage in the stomach. Ulcers can eventually perforate, creating a life-threatening situation.

The pancreas is both directly and indirectly affected by alcohol. Acute and chronic pancreatitis are common in chronic drinkers and may lead to diabetes (Gupta, al-Kawas, 1995). A malabsorption syndrome is caused by irritation of the intestinal lining. This seems to affect B vitamins generally and to lead to a deficiency of vitamin B1 (thiamine) in particular. Thiamine deficiency contributes to peripheral neuropathy. Alcohol also directly affects muscle tissue, a condition known as *alcohol myopathy.* Other organs affected by alcohol include the eyes (loss of peripheral and night vision), the heart (hypertension, enlarged left ventricle, disturbances in the normal cardiac rhythm, and a reduction in systolic function), and reproductive organs (as a depressant, alcohol can cause impotence).

Related Issues

Overdose. People who overdose on alcohol can die as a result of CNS depression. Vital centers become anesthetized, compromising both respiration and heart rate and leading to coma or death. Gastrointestinal bleeding or hemorrhage can occur because of ulcers or gastritis. Alcohol also impairs the body's thermoregulatory system, which leads to heat loss. Many people have succumbed to hypothermia in cold climates. People consistently underestimate the potency of alcohol, and deaths have occurred simply because individuals drank too much. Yearly, newspapers report the death of a college student coerced into drinking too much alcohol. Although alcohol used alone can kill, most alcohol-related deaths result from combining alcohol with CNS depressants or use of an automobile.

Disulfiram. Disulfiram (Antabuse) inhibits the breakdown of acetaldehyde by the enzyme aldehyde dehydrogenase (see Chapter 10, Alcoholism and Other Substance Abuse Disorders). Because acetaldehyde is toxic, the person who drinks alcohol while taking disulfiram becomes ill (sweating, flushing of the neck and face, a throbbing headache, nausea and vomiting, palpitations, dyspnea, tremor, and weakness). This combination can also cause arrhythmias, myocardial infarction, cardiac failure, seizures, coma, and death. The unpleasant response to alcohol reinforces the efforts of the person with alcoholism to stop drinking.

Naltrexone. Naltrexone (ReVia), an opiate receptor antagonist, reduces the urge to drink while also diminishing the alcoholic high and has recently been approved for treating alcoholism (Miller, 1995; O'Brien, 1994; Volpicelli et al, 1995).

Interactions. Alcohol taken with other CNS depressants causes profound CNS depression, often leading to death. For instance, diazepam, which is seldom lethal when taken alone (even in large doses), can lead to death when it is combined with alcohol. Individuals taking barbiturates, antipsychotic drugs, antidepressants, benzodiazepines, and other CNS depressants should avoid alcohol. Chloral hydrate and lorazepam (Ativan) have been associated with intentional sedating of unsuspecting persons in bars. A combination of chloral hydrate and alcohol (the legendary "knock-out drops") was used years ago to "recruit" men for ship duty or for robbery. Lorazepam and alcohol have been used recently by prostitutes to debilitate their clients so they can rob them.

Use in elderly persons. Individuals with impaired liver function or lower lean body mass do not metabolize alcohol as efficiently and therefore can tolerate less of the drug than can young, heavier people. Decreased liver function is a product of aging; consequently many older persons cannot drink much alcohol without becoming inebriated, confused, and sedated. The nurse or physician should be particularly watchful for combinations of alcohol with other CNS depressants in members of this age group.

Fetal alcohol syndrome. Pregnant women who drink alcohol risk seriously harming their unborn children. Fetal alcohol syndrome (FAS) is the result of alcohol's inhibition of fetal development during the first trimester. It is the third most commonly recognized cause of mental retardation and has been particularly devastating among some Native American tribes. Characteristic signs of FAS include microcephaly, cleft palate, altered palmar creases, cardiac defects, anomalous genitalia, severe mental retardation, and a depressed sucking reflex. The risk of FAS is directly related to the amount of alcohol the mother drinks.

Withdrawal and detoxification. Withdrawal from alcohol can be painful, scary, and even lethal. As the person abstains from alcohol, he or she begins to reap the consequences of the CNS irritation caused by alcohol: tremulousness, nervousness, anxiety, anorexia, nausea and vomiting, insomnia and other sleep disturbances, rapid pulse rate, high blood pressure, profuse perspiration, diarrhea, fever, unsteady gait, difficulty concentrating, exaggerated startle reflex, and a craving for alcohol and other drugs. As the withdrawal symptoms become more pronounced, hallucinations can occur. Table 12-2 provides an overview of the withdrawal courses for addictive drugs (Mueller and Ketcham, 1987). Treatment for alcoholism is further discussed in Chapter 10, Alcoholism and Other Substance Abuse Disorders.

Increased psychomotor activity as a consequence of alcohol is called the *alcohol-withdrawal syndrome*. Sedation is the predominant effect of alcohol, but as sedation wears off, psychomotor activity increases. This is referred to as a *rebound phenomenon*. As the CNS becomes more irritated, the normal drinker feels sick and irritable (a hangover) but lives through it. People who drink heavily or who have alcoholism have to drink again to resedate the psychomotor system. Eventually people with alcoholism have to drink large amounts of alcohol just to feel normal. Some reach the point at which they cannot drink enough and CNS irritability is not sedatable. Alcoholic tremors, sweating, palpitations, and agitation then occur. Most often these symptoms occur after alcohol ingestion has stopped, but in some cases they occur while the person with alcoholism is drinking.

Alcoholic hallucinosis, a state of auditory hallucinations, is a phenomenon that alcoholics sometimes experience. The brain begins to invent sensory input. Alcoholic hallucinations typically begin 48 hours or so after drinking has stopped. Frightening voices or sounds are heard, usually within the context of a clear sensorium.

The ultimate level of CNS irritability is delirium tremens (DTs). In DTs the body not only invents sensory input but also has extreme motor agitation. Hallucinations become visual, for example, the proverbial pink elephants, and the sufferer is tremulous and terrified. Tonic-clonic (grand mal) seizures can occur.

OTHER CENTRAL NERVOUS SYSTEM DEPRESSANTS

Central nervous system depressants are relatively new pharmacologic agents. Barbiturates were first used medicinally as sedatives in the last half of the nineteenth century. It was not until 1950 that researchers confirmed the ability of CNS depressants to produce physical dependence. CNS depressants decrease the awareness of and response to sensory stimuli. Two classes of CNS depressants discussed in this chapter are barbiturates and inhalants. Antipsychotic drugs and antianxiety agents, which also depress the CNS, were discussed in previous chapters.

BARBITURATES

Barbiturates are used to relieve anxiety or to produce sleep (see Chapter 8, Sleep Disorders). They have a narrow therapeutic index, the lethal dose being only slightly higher than the therapeutic dose. These drugs produce both physical and psychologic dependence.

Barbiturates are classified according to the duration of action as follows: ultrashort (30 minutes to 3 hours), short (3 to 4 hours), intermediate (6 to 8 hours), and long (10 to 12 hours). Uses range from anesthesia (ultrashort-acting barbiturates such as thiopental) to long-term use in epilepsy (long-acting barbiturates such as phenobarbital).

Pharmacokinetics

Barbiturates, when abused, are usually taken orally. They are metabolized by the liver and excreted by the kidneys. When barbiturates are combined with alcohol, dangerous levels of CNS depression can occur.

Physiologic Effects

Barbiturates depress the CNS, thus decreasing awareness of external stimuli, shortening the attention span, and decreasing intellectual ability. Regular sleep patterns are changed, with loss of rapid eye movement sleep. Barbiturates are used to treat insomnia, to soften withdrawal from heroin, and as anticonvulsants. People who abuse drugs take barbiturates to maintain a state of relatively anxiety-free living. These drugs are also taken to counteract the effects of amphetamines, to "come down," or to replace heroin when it is not available. The acutely intoxicated person has an unsteady gait, slurred speech, and sustained nystagmus. Chronic users have mental symptoms that include confusion, irritability, and insomnia. Persons who regularly use barbiturates develop tolerance to them.

Related Issues

Overdose. The toxic dose of barbiturates varies; in general, an oral dose of 1 g results in serious poisoning, and doses of 2 to 10 g can be fatal. Acute overdose is manifested by CNS and respiratory depression. Coma and death are possible. Treatment is supportive.

Interactions. Barbiturates interact with many drugs, but the most significant are those that increase CNS depression. Alcohol, sedatives, tranquilizers, and antihistamines can cause serious CNS depression. Barbiturates also induce hepatic microsomal enzymes and by doing so can increase the metabolism and shorten the half-life of important drugs such as oral anticoagulants, steroids, and some antibiotics.

Use in elderly persons. Barbiturates frequently cause excitement in elderly individuals. Elderly persons are also prone to confusion caused by barbiturates.

Use during pregnancy. Barbiturates can cause fetal abnormalities. These drugs cross the placental barrier, and fetal serum levels approach maternal blood levels. Infants born to mothers who take barbiturates during the last trimester of pregnancy have withdrawal symptoms and may be intoxicated at birth.

Withdrawal and detoxification. Symptoms of withdrawal from barbiturates are severe and can cause death. Symptoms usually begin 8 to 12 hours after the last dose is taken. Minor withdrawal symptoms include anxiety, muscle twitching, tremor, progressive weakness, dizziness, distorted visual perception, nausea and vomiting, insomnia, and orthostatic hypotension. More serious withdrawal symptoms include convulsions and delirium beginning approximately 16 hours after the last dose and lasting up to 5 days. Untreated, withdrawal symptoms may not decline in intensity for some time. Detoxification requires a cautious and gradual reduction of these drugs. One approach is to reduce the patient's regular dose by 10% each day. Barbiturates can be detected in the urine for up to 3 weeks (Table 12-5).

INHALANTS

Three basic forms of inhalants are hydrocarbon solvents (gasoline), aerosol propellants (found in spray cans), and anesthetics (chloroform and nitrous oxide). Inhalants usually depress the CNS and increase hilarity. They are particularly dangerous because the amount inhaled cannot be controlled. Deaths resulting from asphyxiation have been reported. Inhalants cross the blood-brain barrier quickly. Common side effects include mouth ulcers, gastrointestinal problems, anorexia, confusion, headache, and ataxia.

NARCOTICS (OPIOIDS)

Narcotics or opioids are widely abused and include heroin, morphine, codeine, meperidine (Demerol), methadone, and fentanyl. Until the relatively recent cocaine crisis the public viewed heroin as the most significant drug of abuse. However, heroin abuse has again become the focus of attention, because users find the drug less expensive than cocaine. Illicit drugs can be swallowed, smoked, snorted, injected into soft tissue (skin popping), and mainlined (injected intravenously). Parenteral use of heroin, for example, involves (1) "cooking" the substance in a spoon or bottlecap, (2) filtering it with a cotton ball, (3) "sterilizing" a needle with a match, and (4) injecting the drug into a vein. Initially veins in the antecubital space are used, but as veins scar and sclerosis ("tracks") develops other veins are used, requiring the abuser to inject less accessible vascular structures such as the subclavian vein, the dorsal vein of the penis, or even directly into the heart. The needle is frequently passed from one user to another. Infections, including AIDS and hepatitis, are commonly spread by shared needles and have prompted the controversial needle exchange programs.

Table 12-5 Period of Time After Ingestion That Drugs Can Be Detected in Urine

Drug	Detection period
Narcotics	
Heroin	2-4 days
Morphine	2-4 days
Meperidine (Demerol)	2-4 days
Methadone	2-4 days
Fentanyl	Can be <1 h
Depressants	
Barbiturates	12 h-3 wk
Benzodiazepines	Up to 1 wk
Stimulants	
Amphetamines	2-4 days
Cocaine	2-4 days
Hallucinogens	
Marijuana	3 days to >1 mo
Phencyclidine (PCP)	1 day-1 mo

Modified from Sullivan E, Bissell L, Williams E: *Chemical dependency in nursing,* Redwood City, Calif, 1988, Addison-Wesley.

Pharmacokinetics

Opioids are metabolized in the liver and excreted by the kidneys. They are not absorbed well in the gut but are readily metabolized there and in the liver. Opioids can be given orally but are usually given parenterally. Drugs that compete for liver metabolism increase the effect of opioids.

Physiologic Effects

Opioids relieve pain by increasing the pain threshold and by reducing anxiety and fear. They do this by stimulating specific neurotransmitter receptor sites in the brain. These naturally occurring neurotransmitters, the endorphins, mediate pain and regulate mood. The opioids are endorphin agonists. It is their effect on mood (a feeling of euphoria) that attracts people who abuse drugs. Such individuals frequently refer to the euphoric mood created by heroin as "better than sex." In addition to the euphoria, an overall CNS depression occurs. Drowsiness, or "nodding," and sleep are common effects.

Heroin has a higher abuse potential than morphine because it more readily passes the blood-brain barrier. Once heroin enters the brain, it is metabolized to morphine, so it becomes trapped in the brain (Goldstein and Betz, 1986). This property of heroin causes a more sustained high than that of morphine.

CNS effects of opioids include respiratory depression related to decreased sensitivity to hypercarbia as a stimulus for respiration at the medullary center. Respiratory depression is the primary cause of death among people who abuse opioids. Peripheral effects include reduced gastrointestinal mobility, causing nausea and vomiting, and constipation; decreased gastric, biliary, and pancreatic secretions; urinary retention; hypotension; and reduced pupil size. Pinpoint pupils are a sign of opioid overdose.

Related Issues

Overdose. At therapeutic doses prescribed and administered by professionals, narcotics are helpful and safe analgesics. People who abuse drugs, however, are never sure of how much drug they are taking. Street purchases are not standardized, and occasionally users obtain more pure drug than they anticipated. Inadvertent overdose occurs. The primary effect of overdose is respiratory depression. A respiratory rate below 12 breaths per minute is cause for concern. The following recognizable symptom pattern for overdose is documented:

The person becomes stuporous and then sleeps.
The skin is wet and warm.
Coma develops, accompanied by respiratory depression and hypoxia.
The skin becomes cold and clammy.
The pupils dilate.
Death quickly ensues.

Provision of adequate airway and assisted ventilation, if needed, are treatment priorities. A narcotic antagonist (see Chapter 10, Alcoholism and Other Substance Abuse Disorders) is administered to reverse the effects of opioids.

Narcotic antagonists. Opioids are the only class of commonly abused drugs that have a specific antidote. Naloxone (Narcan), a narcotic antagonist, is the drug of choice when opioid overdose is suspected. Naloxone blocks the neuroreceptors affected by opioids, so the patient responds in a few minutes to an intravenous injection of naloxone. Respirations improve, and the patient consciously responds. However, because most opioids have a longer-lasting effect than naloxone has, the antagonist must often be repeated to maintain adequate respirations. The nurse administering naloxone must carefully observe the patient to determine whether additional antagonist will be needed. Naltrexone (ReVia) is also a narcotic antagonist used to treat alcohol dependence. Narcotic antagonists do not interrupt the effects of nonnarcotics. The treatment strategy with these agents is further discussed in Chapter 10, Alcoholism and Other Substance Abuse Disorders.

Interactions. The effects of opioids are increased when they are combined with other CNS depressants. Because substance abusers commonly use multiple drugs, the potential for deadly combinations is real. If it is known that heroin has been taken and naloxone does not reverse CNS depression, it can be safely assumed that other depressants were also taken. In such cases supportive care is indicated.

Use in elderly persons. Elderly persons are particularly at risk for decreased pulmonary ventilation associated with opioids.

Use during pregnancy. Pregnant women who abuse opioids give birth to babies who have withdrawal symptoms. These drugs can cross the placental barrier and produce respiratory depression in neonates.

Withdrawal and detoxification. The unassisted withdrawal from alcohol or barbiturates can be fatal, but the unassisted withdrawal from opioids is rarely fatal. Withdrawal symptoms are related to the degree of dependence and to the abruptness of discontinuance. Maximum intensity is reached within 36 to 72 hours and subsides in 5 to 10 days. Withdrawal symptoms can be categorized as early, intermediate, and late appearing. Early symptoms of withdrawal include yawning, tearing, rhinorrhea, and sweating. Intermediate symptoms include flushing, piloerection, tachycardia, tremor, restlessness, and irritability. Symptoms that are late appearing include muscle spasm, fever, nausea, diarrhea, vomiting, repetitive sneezing, abdominal cramps, and backache. Treatment is primarily symptomatic and supportive.

Specific Drugs

Drugs related to morphine include hydromorphone (Dilaudid), a derivative of morphine and more potent; levorphanol (Levo-Dromoran), a drug whose action is identical to that of morphine but that is used for less severe pain; meperidine, a synthetic narcotic analgesic; pentazocine (Talwin), which has weaker analgesic effects than other narcotic drugs, is less addicting, and has partial opioid antagonist activity and therefore does not cause euphoria; and several related drugs such as oxymorphone (Numorphan), alphaprodine (Nisentil), anileridine (Leritine), butorphanol (Stadol), and nalbuphine (Nubain). Fentanyl (Sublimaze), an anesthetic, is similar to but 100 times stronger than morphine and 20 to 40 times stronger than heroin. It is said to produce an "unbelievable" high.

Morphine. Morphine is the prototype opioid and is useful in alleviating pain. Oral administration has a variable onset, but intravenous morphine provides almost immediate effect. It is metabolized in the liver, excreted in the urine, and has a half-life of 2.5 to 3 hours.

Methadone. Methadone (Dolophine), although an opioid similar to morphine, is used to prevent withdrawal symptoms. Methadone is given orally and is poorly metabolized in the liver. Accordingly, it has a much longer half-life (15 to 30 hours) than does morphine. Because of the long half-life, once-a-day dosage is effective and conducive to outpatient care and has led to the founding of methadone clinics where people who abuse opioids may recieve a tapering dose of methadone so they may be gradually weaned from narcotics.

Heroin. Heroin is derived from morphine and is referred to as a *semisynthetic* drug. It was originally thought to be a cure for morphine addiction but proved to be far more addictive than morphine. A super-pure heroin known as "People's Choice" has been linked to many deaths. The bodies of users have been found adjacent to where they injected their last dose. Accustomed to heroin cut by B vitamins or lactose, their systems could not tolerate such pure doses.

Codeine. Codeine is used primarily as a cough suppressant. Its abuse preceded the general drug abuse of the mid- to late 1960s because codeine was easily available in over-the-counter cough syrups. Ease of access was eliminated at about the same time that drug abuse became recognized as an emerging national problem. Codeine is not a drug choice for many substance abusers today because it causes a significant degree of nausea in many who use it, even at therapeutic doses for legitimate purposes.

STIMULANTS

Use of stimulants by Americans is widespread, for instance, in caffeine-containing drinks. If they do not start their day with a cup of coffee, many people say they feel sluggish. Should they remain caffeine-free all day, they have the withdrawal symptoms associated with stimulant withdrawal, including headache, nausea, and vomiting. Nicotine is also a common stimulant abused by much of the population.

COCAINE

Coca leaves have been used as stimulants for thousands of years. Coca plants grow high in the Andes, and the Inca Indians chewed coca leaves long before the Spanish explorers arrived. Cocaine is extracted from the coca plant and is a fine, white, odorless substance with a bitter taste. It was introduced to Western medicine as an anesthetic in 1858. Freud was known to use cocaine and believed it to be a remedy for morphine addiction. It was once used in Coca-Cola, and advertisements extolled Coke's ability to refresh. After the Pure Food and Drug Law was passed in 1906, cocaine was eliminated from Coca-Cola. Cocaine and its offspring *crack* are the most costly illicit drugs to society with respect to crime, morbidity, and mortaliy. The number of persons who have tried cocaine at least once increased from 5.4 million in 1974 to 30 million in 1989 (DiGregorio, 1990). The list is long of famous and not-so-famous persons struck down in their youth by these stimulants. The problems associated with these drugs extend to every level of society. The United States Senate Judiciary Committee has said that the rising murder rate in America can be blamed on rising stockpiles of assault weapons and shrinking supplies of cocaine. In a 1-year study of suicides in New York City, fully 20% of suicide victims under age 61 had taken cocaine within days of their deaths (Marzuk et al, 1992). Among those killed by others, a full 31% had medical evidence of cocaine in their system at the time of death (Tardiff et al, 1995). If viewed as a separate category, cocaine-caused deaths would rank as the fifth-leading cause of death among young men in New York City (Marzuk et al, 1995).

Pharmacokinetics

Cocaine passes the blood-brain barrier quickly, causing an instantaneous high. When administered intravenously, cocaine is rapidly metabolized by the liver, so the "rush," although exhilarating, does not last long. Cocaine affects both the CNS and PNS because it blocks norepinephrine and dopamine reuptake into neurons. It depletes these neurotransmitters. Cocaine can also be swallowed or snorted. Snorting, in which cocaine is absorbed through the nasal mucous membranes, is the preferred route for people who abuse cocaine. Freebasing is another way of using cocaine.

Freebasing is used to rid "street cocaine" of its adulterants and reduce it to a pure cocaine base. The cocaine base is volatile, and explosions have occurred. Freebase cocaine is smoked and produces incredibly powerful feelings of euphoria instantaneously. Euphoria is quickly followed by discomfort, so more smoking is required to relieve the discomfort. A vicious cycle ensues.

Crack, or "rock," a form of cocaine, may be the most addictive drug on the streets today. It is produced in a relatively uncomplicated procedure (mixed with baking soda and water, heated, and hardened) and then smoked. It produces an instantaneous high and a "crash" almost as instantaneous. An intense desire to smoke again is produced. Crack is cheap and easy to find.

Tolerance to CNS and PNS effects develops quickly with crack use because neuronal norepinephrine stores are depleted (and decreased norepinephrine levels is one explanation for depression), causing a need to increase drug amounts to achieve the desired effect. Tolerance develops to otherwise lethal amounts.

Physiologic Effects

Cocaine and its derivatives are addictive stimulants. Although physical dependence is less severe than with opiate abuse, psychologic dependence is intense. Abusers become tongue-tied when attempting to describe the sensations of cocaine. Euphoria, increased mental alertness, increased strength, anorexia, and supposed increased sexual stimulation are major desired effects of cocaine and its derivatives. The primary effect is a dopaminergic stimulation of mesolimbic and mesocortical reward pathways (Kaufman and McNaul, 1992). Chronic cocaine use leads to catecholamine receptor supersensitivity and probably the eventual destruction of dopaminergic neurons. This result may account for the anhedonia found in some chronic cocaine users (Kaufman and McNaul, 1992).

Increased motor activity, tachycardia, and high blood pressure are PNS-mediated effects. Cocaine can also provoke cardiac arrest. Two primary mechanisms for cardiotoxic actions are cocaine's anesthetic potential and its powerful sympathomimetic response, (for example, tachycardia, vasospasm, increased contractile force, and cardiac arrhythmias) (Billman, 1995). In a survey of unexpected, nontraumatic deaths of men between ages 20 and 40, Shen et al (1995) found a full third between 1980 and 1989 were cocaine related. Sensory and motor nerve endings are numbed, causing blood vessels to contract. Other complications of cocaine use include headache and chronic cough (Warner, 1995).

CNS effects include stimulation of the medulla, resulting in deeper respirations, euphoria, increased mental alertness, dilated pupils, anorexia, and increased strength. The person who uses cocaine also talks a lot and is stimulated sexually. Less common reactions are specific hallucinations and delusions. Persons taking cocaine report "bugs" crawling beneath the skin (formication) and foul smells. Nasal septum perforation is associated with snorting cocaine and is caused by extreme vasoconstriction, which impedes blood supply to this area and thus causes nasal necrosis.

Cocaine use during pregnancy leads to prematurity, stillbirth, small gestational size, and CNS damage (Buehler, 1995).

AMPHETAMINES

"Call it crank, speed, ice, or poor man's coke—methamphetamine, already the illegal drug of choice in the West, is now spreading across the country."

Birmingham Post-Herald, July 31, 1995, p. A6.

Amphetamines were developed in 1887. They have medicinal uses, such as in the short-term treatment of obesity, attention deficit hyperactivity disorder in childhood (see Chapters 15, Psychopharmacology for Children, and 16, Psychopharmacology in Adolescents), and narcolespy (see Chapter 8, Sleep Disorders). Amphetamine and amphetamine variants are known as speed, crank, ice, and MDMA (3,4-methylenedioxymethamphetamine).

Pharmacokinetics

Amphetamines (speed or crank) are indirect-acting sympathomimetics that cause the release of norepinephrine from nerve endings. Amphetamines also block norepinephrine reuptake in presynaptic nerve endings. Amphetamines are well absorbed from the gastrointestinal tract. They are given orally. Therapeutic parenteral administration is illegal in the United States, but many "speed freaks" self-administer amphetamines intravenously. "Ice," a smokable form of methamphetamine, is known to be twice as toxic as amphetamine and to be a strong CNS stimulant (Beebe and Walley, 1995).

Physiologic Effects

As with cocaine, individuals take amphetamines because they make them feel good. CNS effects include wakefulness, alertness, heightened concentration, energy, improved mood to euphoria, insomnia (sometimes desired, sometimes not), and amnesia.

The most common side effects of amphetamine use are restlessness, dizziness, agitation, and insomnia. PNS effects are palpitations, tachycardia, and hypertension. Respirations also increase because, like cocaine, the amphetamines stimulate the medulla. A psychiatric side effect of amphetamine use is amphetamine-induced psychosis. In the emergency room this psychotic presentation can be almost indistinguishable from paranoid schizophrenia.

Related Issues

Overdose. Cocaine overdose has resulted in a number of deaths, primarily brought about by arrhythmias and respiratory collapse. Freebasing adds to the problem because large amounts reach the system quickly. Toxic levels of amphetamines cause severe hypertension, cerebral hemorrhage, seizures, and coma. Treatment includes induction of vomiting, acidification of the urine, and forced diuresis. In patients with amphetamine psychosis related to toxic levels of these drugs, chlorpromazine or haloperidol given intramuscularly antagonizes the amphetamine effect.

Interactions. The effects of cocaine and amphetamines are augmented when they are combined with other CNS stimulants. Many over-the-counter products such as hay fever medications and decongestants contain stimulants. Urinary alkalinizing agents such as sodium bicarbonate decrease the elimination of stimulants, whereas urinary acidifying agents increase the elimination of stimulants.

Use during pregnancy. Amphetamines should be used during pregnancy only when clearly needed because harm to the fetus has been demonstrated. Cocaine-addicted mothers give birth to addicted babies with multiple problems. Use of cocaine and crack among pregnant women in New York City is responsible for a dramatic decrease in the birth weight of infants in that city (Joyce, 1990). Other obstetric consequences of cocaine use include abruptio placentae, preterm delivery, premature rupture of membranes, microcephaly, and increased neonatal morbidity (Kaufman and McNaul, 1992).

Withdrawal and detoxification. Although cocaine and amphetamines are highly addictive, physical withdrawal is relatively mild. Psychologic withdrawal is severe, however, because the drugs are so pleasurable. The process is gradual and safe for persons withdrawing from amphetamines under medical supervision. "Cold turkey" withdrawal without medical supervision causes agitation, irritability, and severe depression. As a rule of thumb, the low of withdrawal will be inversely proportional to the high experienced. Withdrawal from cocaine causes intense craving for the drug. A number of approaches are used, all aiming to restore depleted neurotransmitters. Amino acid precursors such as tyrosine and phenylalanine, TCAs, and the dopamine agonist bromocriptine are three approaches for increasing the availability of neurotransmitters.

HALLUCINOGENS

Hallucinogens, also referred to as *psychotomimetics* or *psychedelics,* alter perception. There are two basic groups of hallucinogens: natural and manufactured, or synthetic. Natural hallucinogenic substances include mescaline (peyote [from cactus]), psilocybin (psilocin [from mushrooms]), and marijuana *(Cannabis sativa).* Synthetic or semisynthetic substances include lysergic acid diethylamine-25 (LSD), 2,5-dimethoxy-4-methyl amphetamine (STP), phencyclidine (PCP), N,N-dimethyltryptamine (DMT), and methylenedioxyamphetamine (MDA).

Hallucinogens can heighten awareness of reality or can cause a terrifying psychosis-like reaction. Users report distortions in body image and a sense of depersonalization. Particularly frightful is a loss of the sense of reality. Hallucinations depicting grotesque creatures such as a "dog with a snake for a tongue" can be extremely frightening. Emotional consequences of such effects are panic, anxiety, confusion, and paranoid reactions. Some people have had frank psychotic reactions after minimal use. In the jargon of the hallucinogens, such an experience is a "bad trip."

MESCALINE AND RELATED SYNTHETIC SUBSTANCES

Mescaline (peyote) is derived from cactus plants found in America. Native Americans harvested peyote "buttons" from cacti and used them in their religious ceremonies. This practice is still protected by law and is part of their worship. Manufactured forms of mescaline are STP, DMT, and MDA.

Pharmacokinetics

Mescaline, whether naturally occurring or synthetically produced, is taken orally and is quickly absorbed. Its site of action is probably the norepinephrine synapses. Mescaline passes the blood-brain barrier within 2 hours and usually takes effect within 30 to 40 minutes. Its effects last up to 12 hours. It is excreted in the urine.

Physiologic Effects

With mescaline use, colors are vivid, music is more beautiful, and sounds are more intense. When the user closes his or her eyes, colors and images can be seen. A distorted sense of space and time occurs. A young man who drove his car after taking peyote stated that it seemed to take an eternity to reach a stop sign no more than 50 feet away. The experience is directly related to preingestion expectations. "Good" experiences include hilarity and joy. The user may feel especially insightful. The answers to questions such as those involving the "meaning of life" may seem quite clear. Such insights can easily add to a sense of religious experience.

So-called bad trips are the side effects of concern. Although less potent than LSD, peyote nonetheless can cause panic, paranoid thinking, and anxiety when the trip is too intense. Dependence does not occur in the strict sense, yet users enjoy the experience and seek to repeat it. Pupil dilation and tremors sometimes occur.

PSILOCYBIN, PSILOCIN

Psilocybin is derived from the mushroom *Psilocybe mexicana.*

Pharmacokinetics

Psilocybin is taken orally. Once in the stomach, it is converted to psilocin by enzymatic action. Psilocybin decreases the reuptake of serotonin in the brain. Onset of action is experienced in 25 to 40 minutes. Effects last up to 8 hours.

Physiologic Effects

Hallucinations and time, space, and perceptual alterations are experienced and are the sensations that cause Native Americans to continue to use psilocybin. It dilates the pupils and increases heart rate, blood pressure, and body temperature. Tingling of the skin and involuntary movements can occur. As with other hallucinogens, a sense of unreality can occur. An inability to concentrate may add to feelings of anxiety and lead to panic and paranoia. Hallucinations and illusions may occur. Although no deaths resulting from psilocybin intoxication have been reported, deaths related to perceptual distortions have occurred.

MARIJUANA

Marijuana is the drug most widely used illegally in the United States; typically it is used by teenagers and young adults, often as the first illicit substance used. Marijuana *(Cannabis sativa)* and other related drugs (hashish and tetrahydrocannabinol [THC]) come from hemp plants. Marijuana is difficult to categorize. Placement with the hallucinogens seems appropriate, but other categorizations are defensible.

Pharmacokinetics

The active ingredient in marijuana is Δ−6−3,4−THC. Tetrahydrocannabinol is changed to metabolites in the body and is stored in fatty tissues. It remains in the body for up to 6 weeks after it is smoked and can be detected in blood and urine for 40 days. The effects of smoked marijuana last between 2 and 4 hours. If marijuana is ingested, effects may last up to 12 hours.

Physiologic Effects

Marijuana produces a sense of well-being, is relaxing, and alters perceptions. Euphoria results and is the cause of drug-seeking behaviors. It can cause increased hunger ("munchies"), making it useful for anorexic persons such as cancer patients. Marijuana's antiemetic properties make it attractive to some patients for treating nausea and vomiting associated with chemotherapy, although much more effective antinauseants are available. It also has been used to lower intraocular pressure in patients with glaucoma.

Balance and stability are impaired for up to 8 hours after marijuana use. Short-term memory, decision making, and concentration are also impaired. Research has found that marijuana is toxic to hippocampal cells, which are important to these cognitive functions (Schuster, 1990).

Dry mouth, sore throat, increased heart rate, dilated pupils, conjunctival irritation, and perceived keener sight and hearing are physical responses to marijuana. It has been thought to be amotivational, but not all research supports this thinking.

Other effects associated with marijuana use include harmful pulmonary effects (bronchitis), weakening of heart contractions, immunosuppression, and reduction of serum testosterone and sperm count. Anxiety, impaired judgment, paranoia, and panic are not uncommon reactions to marijuana. These terrifying experiences may culminate in some health-compromising behavior.

Flashbacks, more commonly associated with LSD, have also been reported with marijuana use. A flashback is a spontaneous reliving of feelings experienced during a high.

LYSERGIC ACID DIETHYLAMIDE

Lysergic acid diethylamide (LSD) use is increasing among young people while rates for other abused substances are declining (Abraham and Aldridge, 1993).

Pharmacokinetics

LSD stimulates the sympathetic nervous system by inhibiting the reuptake of serotonin. It is taken orally, and onset of action occurs within 30 to 40 minutes. Effects are experienced for up to 12 hours. Extremely small amounts of LSD, usually only 50 to 300 μg, produce these effects.

Physiologic Effects

Lysergic acid diethylamide causes a phenomenon known as *synesthesia.* Synesthesia is the blending of senses (for example, smelling a color or tasting a sound). Expectations and environment govern the "quality" of the LSD trip.

LSD causes an increase in blood pressure, tachycardia, trembling, and dilated pupils. CNS effects include a sense of unreality, perceptual alterations and distortion, and impaired judgment. Another problem associated with LSD is flashbacks. Flashbacks, or hallucinogen persisting perception disorder, are frightening and can heighten a sense of "going crazy." These post-hallucinogen perceputal disorders can persist for up to 5 years after the last exposure to LSD (Abraham and Aldridge, 1993). Bad trips from LSD use cause anxiety, paranoia, and acute panic. Some persons have had psychotic "breaks" as a result of LSD use and have never fully recovered. A number of persons have killed themselves while under the influence of LSD.

PHENCYCLIDINE

Phencyclidine (PCP), a synthetic drug, traditionally has been used as an animal tranquilizer. Many emergency room nurses are familiar with this drug because PCP-intoxicated persons are often brought to the emergency room: their unpredictable outbursts of violent behavior are legendary. They literally change from coma to violent behavior and back. Caution must be exercised when caring for these patients because of their unpredictable behavior.

Pharmacokinetics

Phencyclidine is taken orally or intravenously and is smoked and snorted. Oral PCP takes effect in 5 minutes. Injected or snorted PCP takes hold immediately; effects from smoking PCP take longer. Phencyclidine is well absorbed by all routes. Effects last for 6 to 8 hours. Phencyclidine can be found in the blood and urine for up to 10 days after intake.

Physiologic Effects

The user experiences a high. Euphoria and a peaceful, easy feeling can occur and are sought. Perceptual distortions are common.

Undesired effects of PCP are many and serious. Blood pressure and heart rate are elevated. Other PNS effects include ataxia, salivation, and vomiting. Psychologic symptoms include hostile, bizarre behavior, a blank stare, and agitation. A catatonic type of muscular rigidity alternating with violent outbursts is particularly frightening to bystanders. PCP is toxic to neurons in both the cortex and cerebellum (Nakki et al, 1995).

Related Issues

Overdose. High doses of mescaline are not generally toxic, but high doses of STP and MDA can cause hyperexcitability. Deaths have occurred because of these drugs. Psilocybin overdose has not been associated with any deaths, and usually a calm environment is all that is needed to assist withdrawal. LSD- and PCP-related deaths are not uncommon. Deaths can be caused by overdose but are more likely to be associated with perceptual disorientation and unresponsiveness to environmental stimuli. Confusion and acute panic can result from an overdose of marijuana. Diazepam (Valium) can be administered for psilocybin, LSD, and mescaline overdoses. Phencyclidine presents greater problems. Diazepam may be given for seizures and agitation, and haloperidol (Haldol) for psychotic behavior. Acidifying the urine to a pH of 5.5 accelerates excretion of PCP. Urine screening is the best means of identifying abused substances.

Interactions. Mescaline, psilocybin, and LSD can potentiate sympathomimetics. Marijuana should not be used with alcohol, because marijuana masks the nausea and vomiting associated with excessive alcohol consumption. Respiratory depression, coma, and death can occur.

Use during pregnancy. Birth defects have been associated with these drugs.

Withdrawal and detoxification. Hallucinogens do not commonly produce physical dependence, so there are no withdrawal symptoms. Symptoms of withdrawal from marijuana are insomnia, restlessness, and hyperactivity. One of the clinician's biggest concerns is developing an approach for dealing with the intoxicated person. Basically, one should provide a calm, reassuring environment. Patients acutely intoxicated with hallucinogens rarely need any other treatment than "talking down," but sedatives such as haloperidol or a benzodiazepine may be used in extreme circumstances.

Remarks

The goal of treatment for the chemically dependent person is abstinence from alcohol and drugs. The person who is dependent on one substance can easily become cross-dependent on another. Because patients are rarely cured, most clinicians view treatment as a lifelong process in which the persons are continually recovering or in remission of their dependence. The *DSM-IV* contains as modifiers of its definition of dependence six "course specifiers" that indicate the degree and duration of remission. The term *recovering* indicates an ongoing and dynamic process but also indicates the ever-present possibility of slipping.

In the psychiatric hospital every patient should be assessed for chemical dependency. It is estimated that one third to half of all psychiatric patients abuse alcohol or drugs, including homeless people who are mentally ill (Ananth et al, 1989; Carey, 1989). Always ask whether the patient drinks or uses other drugs, whether he or she has had problems associated with alcohol and drugs, and whether any relative has had alcohol- or drug-related problems. If the patient's responses indicate that he or she is at risk, a more definitive screening tool should be used.

Estes and Heinemann (1986) recommended avoiding the terms *alcoholic* or *addict* early in the assessment process and instead suggested using phrases such as "problem with drinking" or "difficulties with drug use." It may also be helpful initially to focus on legal drugs or more culturally accepted drugs such as caffeine and nicotine.

The best known intervention programs are Alcoholics Anonymous (AA) and Narcotics Anonymous (NA). These programs use self-help, a support group model comprising fellow users in various stages of recovery. Philosophically AA and NA view psychosocial problems as stemming from substance abuse and reject the idea that an underlying psychopathologic disease or disorder is responsible for drinking or drug abuse. AA has established the 12-step system in which people begin by admitting their powerlessness over alcohol and end by making themselves available, night or day, to another alcoholic person in need. The popular bumper sticker slogan "Easy does it" reflects a philosophy of taking life one day at a time and avoiding a frenetic lifestyle. Both AA and NA believe that only total abstinence can free the chemically dependent person from the bondage of alcohol and drugs.

Screening Tests

Several screening questionnaires have been developed to assist the health care professional in diagnosing chemical dependency. The Michigan Alcoholism Screening Test (MAST) is reliable and can be given without extensive training (Powers and Spickard, 1984). It can be modified to identify other drug problems.

The acronym *CAGE,* a questionnaire, is an effective, efficient, and easy-to-use instrument (Liskow et al, 1995). It is less discriminating than the MAST. The following questions make up the *CAGE* questionnaire:

1. Have you ever felt you should *Cut* down on your drinking?
2. Have people *Annoyed* you by criticizing your drinking?
3. Have you ever felt bad or *Guilty* about your drinking?
4. Have you ever had a drink first thing in the morning *(Eye-opener)* to steady your nerves or get rid of a hangover?

Two positive responses are suggestive of alcoholism, and three or four positive responses are diagnostic (Whitfield, Davis, and Barker, 1986). Schofield (1988) pointed out that questions 1 and 3 assess introspection and reflection on personal drinking, and question 2 provides reinforcement of this introspection by external cues. Question 4 reflects a change in behavior.

Another tool that distinguishes severity of alcoholism is the Drinking and You self-report instrument (Harrell and Wirtz, 1988). It was specifically developed for use with adolescents and taps four areas: loss of control and social, psychologic, and physical symptoms.

The problem with most screening tests has been their susceptibility to faking and denial on the part of the patient (Creager, 1989). The MacAndrew Scale (MacAndrew, 1965), made up of appropriate items from the Minnesota Multiphasic Personality Inventory (MMPI) scale (Allen, Eckardt, and Wallen, 1988), and the Substance Abuse Scale have been developed to overcome denial and lying. The Substance Abuse Scale requires only 10 minutes to complete and claims 90% accuracy of diagnosis (Creager, 1989).

REFERENCES

Abraham HD, Aldridge AM: Adverse consequences of lysergic acid diethylamide, *Addiction* 88(10):1327, 1993.

Allen JP, Eckardt MJ, Wallen J: Screening for alcoholism: techniques and issues, *Public Health Rep* 103:6, 1988.

American Psychiatric Association: *The diagnostic and statistical manual of mental disorders,* ed 4, Washington, DC, 1994, The Association.

Ananth J et al: Missed diagnosis of substance abuse in psychiatric patients, *Hosp Community Psychiatry* 40:297, 1989.

Antai-Otong D: Helping the alcoholic patient recover, *Am J Nurs* 95(8):22-30, 1995.

Beebe DK, Walley E: Smokable methamphetamine ("ice"): an old drug in a different form, *Am Fam Physician* 51(2):449,1995.

Billman GE: Cocaine: a review of its toxic actions on cardiac function, *Crit Rev Toxicol* 25(2):113, 1995.

Buehler BA: Cocaine: how dangerous is it during pregnancy? *Nebr Med J* 80(5):116, 1995.

Carey KB: Emerging treatment guidelines for mentally ill chemical abusers, *Hosp Community Psychiatry* 40:341, 1989.

Creager C: SASSI test breaks through denial, *Professional Counselor* July-August, 1989, p 65.

DiGregorio GJ: Cocaine update: abuse and therapy, *Am Fam Physician* 41:247, 1990.

Estes N, Heinemann ME: Issues in identification of alcoholism. In *Alcoholism: development, consequences, and interventions,* ed 3, St. Louis, 1986, Mosby.

Federal Task Force on Homelessness and Severe Mental Illness: *Outcasts on Main Street,* Washington, DC, 1992, DHHS.

Frezza M et al: High blood alcohol levels in women: the role of decreased gastric alcohol dehydrogenase activity and first-pass metabolism, *N Engl J Med* 322(2):95, 1990.

Goldstein GW, Betz AL: The blood-brain barrier, *Sci Am* 255:74, 1986.

Goodwin DW et al: Screening adolescents in adoptees raised apart from alcoholic biological parents, *Arch Gen Psychiatry* 28:238, 1973.

Gupta PK, al-Kawas FH: Acute pancreatitis: diagnosis and management, *Am Fam Physician* 52(2):435, 1995.

Harrell AV, Wirtz PW: *Screening adolescents for drinking problems.* Paper presented at 1988 National Alcoholism Forum, Arlington, Va, April 1988.

Hill, SY: Vulnerability to alcoholism in women: genetic and cultural factors, *Recent Dev Alcohol,* 12:9, 1995.

Hough ESE: Alcoholism: prevention and treatment, *J Psychosoc Nurs Ment Health Serv* 27(1):15, 1989.

Ibañez J et al: Chronic alcoholism decreases neuronal nuclear size in the human entorhinal cortex, *Neurosci Lett* 183(1-2):71, 1995.

Institute of Medicine: Prevention and treatment of alcohol-related problems: research opportunities, *J Stud Alcohol* 53(1):5, 1992.

Jonnes J: The rise of the modern addict, *Am J Public Health* 8598 (Pt 1):1157, 1995.

Joyce T: The dramatic increase in the rate of low birthweight in New York City: an aggregate time-series analysis, *Am J Public Health* 80:682, 1990.

Kaufman E, McNaul JP: Recent developments in understanding and treating drug abuse and dependence, *Hosp Community Psychiatry* 43(3):223, 1992.

Lewis DC, Gordon AJ: Alcoholism and the general hospital: the Roger Williams Intervention Program, *Bull NY Acad Med* 59:181, 1983.

Liskow B et al: Validity of the CAGE questionnaire in screening for alcohol dependence in a walk-in (triage) clinic, *J Stud Alcohol* 56(3):277, 1995.

MacAndrew C: The differentiation of male alcoholic outpatients from non-alcoholic psychiatric outpatients by means of the MMPI, *Q J Stud Alcoholism* 26:238, 1965.

Manzo L et al: Nutrition and alcohol neurotoxicity, *Neurotoxicology* 15(3):555, 1994.

Marzuk PM et al: Prevalence of cocaine use among residents of New York City who committed suicide during a one-year period, *Am J Psychiatry* 149(3):371, 1992.

Marzuk PM et al: Fatal injuries after cocaine use as a leading cause of death among young adults in New York City, *N Engl J Med* 332(26):1753, 1995.

Miller NS: Pharmacotherapy in alcoholism, *J Addict Dis* 14(1):23, 1995.

Mueller LA, Ketcham K: *Recovering: how to get and stay sober,* New York, 1987, Bantam.

Nakki R et al: Cerebellar toxicity of phencyclidine, *J Neurosci* 15(3 Pt 2):2097, 1995.

National Foundation for Brain Research: *The cost of disorders of the brain,* Washington, DC, 1992, The Foundation.

Noble J: *Working paper: projections of alcohol abusers, 1980, 1985, 1990,* Washington, DC, 1985, NIAAA, Department of Biometry and Epidemiology, National Association of Private Psychiatric Hospitals.

O'Brien CP: Treatment of alcoholism as a chronic disorder, *Alcohol* 11(6):433, 1994.

Ohlms D: *The disease of alcoholism,* Millstadt, Ill, 1988, Gary Whitaker (videotape).

Poldrugo F et al: Mortality studies in the long-term evaluation of treatment of alcoholics, *Alcohol Alcohol* 2(suppl):1551, 1993.

Powers JS, Spickard A: Michigan alcoholism screening test to diagnose early alcoholism in a general practice, *South Med J* 77:852, 1984.

Regans P: *ABC News and Washington Post poll,* Survey No. 0190, Washington, DC, 1985, Washington Post.

Regier DA et al: The de facto US mental and addictive disorders service system, *Arch Gen Psychiatry* 50(2):85, 1993.

Scavnicky-Mylant M, Keltner NL: Chemical dependency. In Keltner NL, Schwecke LH, Bostrom C, editors: *Psychiatric nursing: a psychotherapeutic management approach,* St Louis, 1991, Mosby.

Schofield A: The CAGE questionnaire and psychological health, *Br J Addict* 83:761, 1988.

Schuster CR: The National Institute on Drug Abuse in the decade of the brain, *Neuropharmacology* 3:315, 1990.

Shen WK et al: Sudden unexpected nontraumatic death in 54 young adults: a 30-year population-based study, *Am J Cardiol* 76(3):148, 1995.

Smith AR et al: Trends in psychotropic prescribing in general practice and general medical patients, *Postgrad Med J* 62:637, 1986.

Sullivan EV et al: Anterior hippocampal volume deficits in nonamnesic, aging chronic alcoholics, *Alcohol Clin Exp Res* 19(1):110, 1995.

Tardiff K et al: Cocaine, opiates, and ethanol in homicides in New York City: 1990 and 1991, *J Forensic Sci* 40(3):387, 1995.

Volpicelli JR et al: Effect of naltrexone on alcohol "high" in alcoholics, *Am J Psychiatry* 152(4):613, 1995.

Wallace J: *Alcoholism: new light on the disease,* Newport, RI, 1985, Edgehill.

Wallerstedt S et al: The prevalence of alcoholism and its relation to cause of hospitalization and long-term mortality in male somatic inpatients, *J Intern Med* 237(3):339, 1995.

Warner EA: Is your patient using cocaine? Clinical signs that should raise suspicion, *Postgrad Med* 98(2):173, 1995.

Whitfield C, Davis J, Barker L: Alcoholism. In Barker LR, Burton JR, Zieve PD, editors: *Principles of ambulatory medicine,* Baltimore, 1986, Williams & Wilkins.

CHAPTER 13

Drugs Used to Stimulate the Central Nervous System

"Through the ages, humanity's diligent search for stimulants has been rewarded by the discovery of the coffee bean (Coffea arabica) *in Arabia, the tea leaf (*Thea *[or* Camellia*]* sinensis*) in China, the kola nut* (Cola nitida *and* Cola aluminata) *in West Africa, the cocoa bean* (Theobroma cacao) *in Mexico, and other plant sources of caffeine."*

Tony Chou, 1992, p. 544.

Two basic categories of drugs that stimulate the central nervous system (CNS) are cerebral stimulants, which mainly affect the cerebral cortex, and analeptics, which primarily stimulate the brain stem. Analeptics are used to increase respirations in patients who are having difficulty with breathing. Analeptics do this by stimulating the medullary respiratory control center in the brain stem and by actions on the peripheral carotid chemoreceptors that regulate respiration by sensing blood carbon dioxide levels. A discussion of analeptics is not consistent with the objectives of this book. More information on these drugs can be found in a basic pharmacology text.

The drugs discussed in this chapter are the cerebral stimulants, commonly referred to as *psychostimulants.* These agents affect the cerebral cortex and have beneficial psychopharmacologic effects. The potential therapeutic use of cerebral stimulants is compromised by their great potential for abuse. Specific therapeutic uses of cerebral stimulants are also presented in Chapters 8, Sleep Disorders; 15, Psychopharmacology for Children; 16, Psychopharmacology for Adolescents; and 17, Psychopharmacology for Elderly Persons. Specific abuses are discussed in Chapters 10, Alcoholism and Other Substance Abuse Disorders, and 12, Drugs of Abuse.

CEREBRAL STIMULANTS

The amphetamines and amphetamine congeners (chemical derivatives of amphetamines) represent the major classes of cerebral stimulants, but other drugs are used in a similar manner. Caffeine in beverages; drugs, such as methylphenidate (Ritalin) and pemoline (Cylert), for attention deficit hyperactivity disorder (ADHD); and phenylpropanolamine and other related compounds found in many over-the-counter cold, hay fever, stimulant, and anorectic preparations are examples of other cerebral stimulants. Amphetamines are addressed most thoroughly in this chapter, because understanding these drugs enables understanding of other CNS stimulants.

AMPHETAMINES

The amphetamines were first synthesized in 1887, but not until 40 years later were their stimulant effects discovered (Lovgren, 1985; Pickering and Stimson, 1994).

They were first marketed in the United States in 1932 as nasal inhalers, were later used as respiratory stimulants (indicating a broader range of effect than just the cerebral cortex), and in 1937 gained acceptance as a treatment for narcolepsy (Roccaforte and Burke, 1990; Lovgren, 1985).

Amphetamines gained popularity during World War II because they were helpful in overcoming battle fatigue. Close to 200 million amphetamine tablets were issued to American soldiers stationed in Britain during the war (Warneke, 1990). Psychostimulants were used in the 1950s to treat depression (Arana and Hyman, 1991). By 1970, 10 billion stimulants were being legally manufactured in the United States (Warneke, 1990). These drugs came to be used by certain groups of individuals, for example, long-distance truck drivers, students, and night-shift workers, who valued the alertness stimulants provided (Pickering and Stimson, 1994).

Today stimulants are the only drugs approved by the FDA to treat ADHD (see Chapters 15, Psychopharmacology for Children, and 16, Psychopharmacology for Adolescents), narcolepsy (see Chapter 8, Sleep Disorders), and refractory obesity. Although amphetamines formerly were a preferred treatment for obesity, the aforementioned propensity to abuse these drugs, coupled with pronounced tolerance and tachyphylaxis (unusually rapid tolerance), have made their prescription for obesity all but unheard of.

Three amphetamines are used clinically: dextroamphetamine, or d-amphetamine (Dexedrine); racemic amphetamine, or amphetamine sulfate; and methamphetamine (Desoxyn). The two forms of amphetamine that are molecular "mirror images" are designated as *d* (dextro) form and *l* (levo) form. These forms are more correctly referred to as *isomers* and differ pharmacologically. To explain the mirror-image metaphor, visualize pointing your hand directly into a mirror. Your actual thumb is farthest away from the mirror, and the mirror image of your thumb is set most deeply into the mirror image. This identical yet opposite molecular configuration accounts for a difference in effect. Thus the d-isomer amphetamine, that is, dextroamphetamine and methamphetamine, is three to four times more potent than the l-isomer amphetamine (Roccaforte and Burke, 1990) and is a more potent CNS stimulant. The *l* form is a more effective cardiovascular system stimulator. Racemic amphetamine is a mixture of *d* and *l* forms.

Pharmacologic Effect

Amphetamine is a potent catecholamine agonist that causes the release of biogenic amines and blocks their reuptake (Goldberg et al, 1991; Kuczenski, 1983). Amphetamines have both a CNS and a peripheral nervous system (PNS) effect. These effects are caused indirectly through the release of norepinephrine, dopamine, and serotonin from the nerve endings. The concept of indirect action is important, simply meaning that amphetamines stimulate the body by causing the release of these neurotransmitters, which, in turn, trigger neuronal firing. Examples of direct-acting sympathomimetics include norepinephrine bitartrate (Levophed), epinephrine (Adrenalin), and phenylephrine hydrochloride (Neo-Synephrine). Amphetamines increase catecholamine bioavailability by blocking the reuptake of norepinephrine and dopamine back into the presynaptic nerve ending.

Central nervous system effects. Amphetamines stimulate the cerebral cortex, the brain stem, and the reticular activating system (RAS). The RAS is a group of ill-defined, interconnected nuclei located in the medulla, pons, and midbrain. These nuclei receive sensory input from the major sensory pathways and relay it to the cerebral cortex via the thalamus, the sensory relay center for the nervous system

(Liebman, 1991). When the RAS is not stimulated, sleep can occur. When the RAS is stimulated, one awakens. Individuals already awake experience greater alertness when the RAS is stimulated (Liebman, 1991). Amphetamines and other CNS stimulants stimulate the RAS. Amphetamine's cortical effects that account for its abuse potential include wakefulness, alertness, increased concentration, increased motor activity, improved physical performance, decreased fatigue, improved mood, inhibited sleep, and an anorexigenic effect. As noted in the section on side effects, an exaggeration of these pharmacologic effects is precisely the element of amphetamine usage associated with adverse outcomes.

Amphetamines appear to stimulate the reward center of the brain; this stimulation accounts for the great appeal of these drugs. The nucleus accumbens, a small subdivision of the basal ganglia, appears to be a major component of the reward center (Fischbach, 1992; Graybiel, 1995). By stimulating the reward center, amphetamines produce a sense of well-being usually reserved for accomplishment, love, or some other rewarding external source of gratification. Amphetamines and other stimulants essentially enhance or perpetuate this sense of well being. This enhancement is followed by rebound depression. This rebound phenomenon is linked to a dopaminergic stimulation of the autoreceptor (which sends a signal to *not release* more dopamine) (Grace, 1995). Obviously abuse of stimulants can result, as discussed in Chapters 10, Alcoholism and Other Substance Abuse Disorders, and 12, Drugs of Abuse.

Research indicates that the euphoric properties of amphetamines may be more closely related to their effects on dopaminergic systems than on norepinephrine or serotonin systems, as formerly thought. This hypothesis stems from the ability of haloperidol (a dopamine antagonist) to block euphoria, which noradrenergic blockers do not do. Amphetamine's anorectic effect probably results from the stimulation of the lateral hypothalamic satiety center.

Because they stimulate the medulla, psychostimulants increase respirations. Such an effect serves to illustrate the well-known fact that drugs have many intersystem and intrasystem effects and that, although amphetamines produce primarily a cortical effect, they also stimulate subcortical areas.

Paradoxically, amphetamines in low doses may depress the CNS. Occasionally, individuals report a sedative effect after taking a low dose. Nonetheless, CNS activity is really a balancing of opposing actions between excitatory and inhibitory neurons, and low doses of amphetamines show a preference for inhibitory neurons, consequently causing a shift in the "norm" toward an overall inhibitory response, that is, CNS depression. This "paradox" is particularly beneficial in normalizing hyperkinetic motor activity and behavior.

Low doses of amphetamines and related drugs such as methylphenidate apparently stimulate the immature RAS in children with ADHD; thus improved functioning results. Normalization of this system presumably enables the ADHD patient to sit and listen, to tune out extraneous stimuli, and to control bothersome motor activity. The precise mechanism of amphetamines and other stimulants used to treat ADHD is not clear.

The sought-after effects of amphetamines begin to reverse themselves as the drugs wear off. A sense of well being gives way to despair, concentration turns to irritation and distractibility, and improved physical performance and alertness become fatigue. Some have viewed this reversal of emotions as a roller-coaster ride, with the "downs" roughly paralleling the "ups." For many beginning users such swings in emotion discourage further experimentation, but others find the highs irresistible and endure the lows, as discussed in Chapter 12, Drugs of Abuse.

Peripheral nervous system effect. The PNS effects of psychostimulants with the greatest potential for harm involve the cardiovascular system. Amphetamines may increase blood pressure and heart rate. Tachycardia and tachyarrhythmias can also have serious implications in individuals with pre-existing conditions. Paradoxically amphetamines can decrease heart rate through activation of the baroreceptor reflex as a result of increased blood pressure. This baroreceptor reflex increases parasympathetic input to the heart, thus causing bradycardia. Amphetamines also dilate the pupils and cause decongestion of the mucous membranes. Other effects related to abuse are outlined in Chapter 12, Drugs of Abuse, and treatment of abuse is discussed in Chapter 10, Alcoholism and Other Substance Abuse Disorders.

Pharmacokinetics

Amphetamines given orally are well absorbed from the gut, are distributed throughout the body, and are highly lipophilic, crossing the blood-brain barrier readily (Chiarello and Cole, 1987). When given orally (the only legally approved route in the United States), they exert both CNS and PNS effects within 30 to 60 minutes. Amphetamines are available in several oral forms, including timed-release capsules, immediate-acting tablets, and an elixir. Other amphetamines come in a chewable, slow-release form.

Amphetamines are not metabolized per se and continue to produce an effect until excreted in the urine. Renal excretion of dextroamphetamine and other amphetamines is altered by urine pH; acidic urine expedites excretion (a pH of less than 5.6 equals a half-life of 7 hours), whereas urine alkalinization slows elimination (a half-life of up to 30 hours) (Olin, 1995). The average half-life of an amphetamine is 12 hours (Roccaforte and Burke, 1990). Urinary alkalinization extends half-life because molecules are unchanged and hence diffuse quickly back into the bloodstream. An average 7-hour increase in amphetamine half-life results from every 1-unit increase in pH (Olin, 1995). Thus the clinician should avoid using dietary and pharmacologic substances that alkalinize the urine.

Side Effects

Amphetamine side effects are largely extensions of effects previously mentioned (Box 13-1). Through the CNS these drugs cause anorexia and consequent weight loss (sometimes desired), insomnia (sometimes desired), overly anxious behavior and moodiness, euphoric feelings that can lead to inappropriate or overly ambitious decisions, and irritability or dysphoria. Growth retardation is a concern in children who are given these drugs for ADHD (see Chapters 15, Psychopharmacology for Children, and 16, Psychopharmacology for Adolescents). Other CNS effects include restlessness, irritability, dizziness, tremor, talkativeness, aggressive behavior, confusion, panic, and increased libido.

A toxic paranoid psychosis or toxic delirium, or both, can develop in some individuals. Traditionally the toxic psychosis caused by amphetamines has been viewed as a schizophrenia-like manifestation, in keeping with amphetamine's dopamine-potentiating properties. Some clinicians think that such an analysis, although tempting in light of the dopamine hypothesis of schizophrenia, is oversimplified and argue that this phenomenon closely parallels a dysphoric manic episode. Because amphetamines increase norepinephrine, psychotic symptoms arising from amphetamine intoxication could be attributable to increased norepinephrine bioavailability as well (Breier et al, 1990).

Box 13-1 Side Effects of Central Nervous System Stimulants

Central nervous system
Restlessness, dizziness, insomnia, overstimulation, euphoria, anorexia, weight loss

Eye
Mydriasis, photophobia

Metabolic
Hyperglycemia, worsening of diabetic symptoms

Cardiovascular
Palpitations, tachycardia, hypertension, angina, arrhythmias

Gastrointestinal
GI upset, diarrhea, constipation, dry mouth, anorexia

PNS effects, as mentioned previously, include cardiovascular effects (more pronounced with racemic amphetamine), with elevated blood pressure, chilling, palpitations and, less frequently, tachycardia and tachyarrhythmias. Some patients have died of circulatory collapse (Clark, Queener, and Karb, 1993). Headaches, pallor, facial flushing, mucous membrane decongestion, mydriasis and photophobia, diarrhea, cramps, vomiting, dry mouth, and abdominal pain are also potential side effects of amphetamines.

Implications

Therapeutic versus toxic levels. Toxic effects generally reflect autonomic overstimulation and cause an extreme exaggeration of side effects previously mentioned. Therapeutic blood levels of amphetamines range from 5 to 10 μg/dL (Olin, 1995). Some individuals can ingest much more than the recommended levels of amphetamines without serious effects, because of tolerance and tachyphylaxis.

Tolerance, as defined in Chapter 10, Alcoholism and Other Substance Abuse Disorders, is an important dimension of treatment with amphetamines. Tolerance to amphetamines occurs in two ways, one more significant than the other. The more significant mechanism is the depletion of norepinephrine from the nerve endings. As norepinephrine is depleted, more and more amphetamine is required to maintain a consistent response. Tolerance to amphetamine can occur after only one or two doses. The second mechanism of amphetamine tolerance is ketosis, a byproduct of amphetamine-caused anorexia. As the individual stops eating, an alteration in metabolism occurs, resulting in ketosis that, in turn, leads to acidic urine. As noted previously, acidic urine hastens the excretion of amphetamine.

Although tolerance to almost all of the CNS and PNS effects can occur, no tolerance is observed for the psychotic effects of amphetamines. What this means is that abusers can take doses of amphetamines hundreds of times greater than therapeutic doses without harmful physical effects but remain vulnerable to amphetamine psychosis. High levels of amphetamine ingestion would kill someone who has not developed amphetamine tolerance (Keltner, 1989).

Overdose results in sympathetic hyperactivity, that is, hypertension, tachycardia, and hyperthermia accompanied by the delirium and toxic psychosis previously mentioned (Arana and Hyman, 1991). Grand mal seizures can occur as a physiologic response to an overdose of amphetamine. Deaths have been reported when tachycardias, tachyarrhythmias, hyperthermia, and seizures have converged to compromise body systems (Arana and Hyman, 1991).

Acute overdose treatment includes emptying the stomach of its contents, the administration of activated charcoal 1 g per kg body weight, and urine acidification. Strategies to treat overdose of amphetamines should also include using adrenergic blockers such as phentalomine to reduce blood pressure and lower pulse rate. Other measures for overdose are supportive. Airway support is critical for patients who are unconscious, and external cooling approaches, including the use of cooling blankets, are required for hyperthermia. Seizures can be controlled with intravenous (IV) benzodiazepine, for example, lorazepam (Ativan), 1 to 2 mg, or diazepam (Valium), 5 to 10 mg (Arana and Hyman, 1991). Fluids should be administered until urine flow reaches 3 to 6 mL per kg per hour (Olin, 1995).

Use in pregnancy. Amphetamines are highly lipophilic and cross the placental barrier. Although the d-amphetamines have a federal pregnancy category C rating (potential risk to the fetus), racemic amphetamine is in category X, which is an absolute prohibition against use during pregnancy.

Side effects. Side effects can be minimized somewhat by the following sensible yet conventional supportive measures:

Mydriasis and photophobia: Wearing protective eyewear out of doors

Weight loss: Taking medication after meals to minimize anorectic effect

Insomnia: Taking the last dose at least 6 hours before bedtime; insomnia and restlessness associated with overdose can be treated with lorazepam at 1 to 2 mg or diazepam at 5 to 10 mg every 1 to 2 hours as needed (Arana and Hyman, 1991)

Cardiovascular effects: Monitor blood pressure and vital signs frequently; guard against other subtle sympathomimetic substances such as coffee and colas that could add to existing system stimulation; severe hypertension and tachyarrhythmias can be treated with IV propranolol at 1 mg every 5 to 10 minutes as needed, to a total of 8 mg (Arana and Hyman, 1991) or with an IV vasopressor (Olin, 1995)

Gastrointestinal (GI) upset: Taking amphetamines with meals reduces GI upset

Central nervous system effects: When patients become too restless, euphoric, or agitated, reduce the dosage until therapeutic effects are experienced but these side effects are minimized

Toxic psychosis or delirium: Chlorpromazine (Thorazine) at 50 mg 4 times a day IM or haloperidol (Haldol) at 5 mg 2 times a day IM is an effective intervention (Arana and Hyman, 1991); because chlorpromazine also has antiadrenergic properties, it reduces blood pressure and pulse rate as well.

Interactions. The major concern with drug interactions is the additive effect of other CNS stimulants (Table 13-1). Prescription, nonprescription, and common

Table 13-1 Major Interactions Between Central Nervous System Stimulants and Other Drugs

Interactant	Result of interaction
Acidifying agents (urinary) (ascorbic acid, fruit juices, etc.)	Decreased CNS and PNS effects of cerebral stimulants
Alkalinizing agents (urinary) (sodium bicarbonate)	Increased CNS and PNS effects of stimulants
Antidepressants	Increased antidepressant blood levels
Antihypertensives	Decreased antihypertensive effect with most CNS stimulants
Antipsychotic drugs	Decreased cerebral stimulant effect, decreased peripheral sympathomimetic effect
Central nervous system depressants, including alcohol	Antagonism of desired stimulant effect
Hypoglycemic drugs (insulin, oral hypoglycemics)	Increased or decreased blood glucose levels; poor diabetes control
Lithium	Decreased effect of one or both interactants, poor control of psychiatric disorder
Monoamine oxidase inhibitors	Risk of severe hypertensive episode, stroke
Sympathomimetics	Increased and potentially serious cardiac effects; CNS stimulation; hypertension

dietary substances can potentiate the stimulating effects of amphetamines. Some of the more common interactions include the following:

Common dietary substances: Coffee, tea, and colas can potentiate the effects of amphetamines

Over-the-counter sympathomimetics such as cold, cough suppressant, allergy, and appetite suppressant medications: These agents enhance the effects of amphetamines

Monoamine oxidase inhibitors: Monoamine oxidase inhibitors generally should not be given with amphetamines because this combination floods the peripheral synapses with norepinephrine, causing a potential hypertensive crisis

Tricyclic antidepressants: Tricyclic antidepressants in combination with amphetamines may cause increased anticholinergic effects and increased cardiac stimulation

Guanethidine: Amphetamines decrease the antihypertensive effect of guanethidine

Urinary acidifiers: These agents *decrease* the half-life, hence the effect of amphetamines; higher doses of amphetamine might be needed; ascorbic acid and fruit juices acidify the urine

Urinary alkalinizers: These agents *increase* the half-life, hence the effect of amphetamines; lower doses of amphetamine might be indicated; sodium bicarbonate (used for heartburn, particularly in elderly persons) and acetazolamide are examples of urinary alkalinizers

Antipsychotic drugs: These drugs antagonize the effects of amphetamines

Patient education. The patient and family should be taught:

To take these drugs early in the day to avoid insomnia

To decrease caffeine consumption

To avoid over-the-counter preparations, as previously described
To avoid alcohol consumption
To observe for rest deficits, because these agents tend to cause patients to avoid rest behaviors
To avoid chewing sustained-released forms of the drug
To increase dosage only on the advice of the prescriber
That amphetamines can mask extreme fatigue, so care should be observed when undertaking potentially hazardous tasks
That these agents can cause nervousness, restlessness, insomnia, dizziness, anorexia, and GI disturbances but that by notifying the prescriber, measures may be developed that can modify these effects

OTHER PRESCRIPTION CENTRAL NERVOUS SYSTEM STIMULANTS

Two other prescription CNS stimulants are available for clinical use. Methylphenidate (Ritalin) and pemoline (Cylert) are two drugs frequently prescribed for both ADHD (see Chapters 15, Psychopharmacology for Children, and 16, Psychopharmacology for Adolescents) and narcolepsy (see Chapter 8, Sleep Disorders).

METHYLPHENIDATE

Methylphenidate is the most commonly prescribed drug for ADHD and is structurally related to amphetamine (Figure 13-1). It is a milder cortical stimulant than amphetamine (Chiarello and Cole, 1987), being about half as potent, and appears to have a greater effect on mental activities than on motor activities. Its mechanism of action is not fully understood; however, tolerance to the effects of this drug does occur to some extent.

Pharmacokinetics

Methylphenidate is well absorbed from the GI tract and reaches peak blood levels within 1 to 3 hours. Its half-life ranges from 1 to 3 hours, but its effects last up to 6 hours. Methylphenidate is metabolized in the liver to inactive products (unlike the amphetamines), so urinary acidification or alkalinization does not affect its stimulatory abilities. It is excreted in the urine. Methylphenidate is also available in a slow-release form (Ritalin SR).

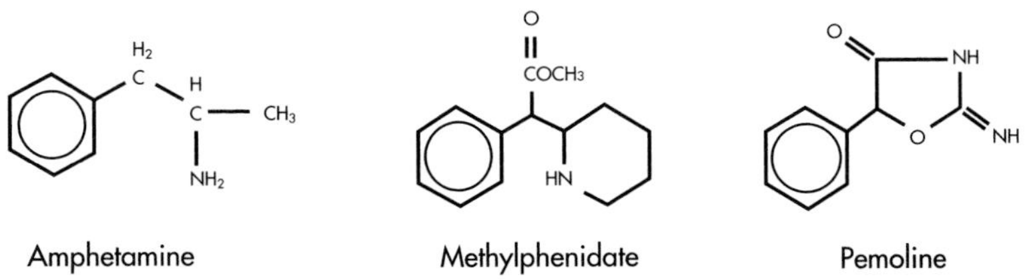

Figure 13-1 Chemical structures of amphetamine, methylphenidate, and pemoline.

Side Effects

The side effects of methylphenidate are similar to those of the amphetamines already discussed. Insomnia, restlessness, and nervousness are the most common effects. Anorexia and consequent weight loss are of particular concern to parents of children with ADHD. This concern is addressed in Chapters 15, Psychopharmacology for Children, and 16, Psychopharmacology for Adolescents. In a few individuals anemia and other blood dyscrasias have been linked to methylphenidate treatment. Periodic complete blood cell counts can help the clinician monitor for an untoward hematologic effect.

Implications

Therapeutic versus toxic levels. An overdose of methylphenidate manifests as CNS overstimulation, that is, agitation, tremors, muscle twitching, euphoria, confusion, hallucinations, delirium, headache, facial flushing, fever, and cardiovascular stimulation such as palpitations, tachycardia, tachyarrhythmias, and hypertension. Treatment is supportive. The patient's environment should be controlled to guard against excessive stimulation that would aggravate physiologic stimulation. If the patient is conscious and if not too much time has elapsed since ingestion, gastric lavage or forced emesis would be appropriate. Maintaining adequate circulation and airway are important. External cooling would be appropriate should hyperpyrexia occur.

Use in pregnancy. Although no evidence of fetal malformation has been documented, methylphenidate should not be given to a pregnant woman unless the benefits outweigh the risk to the fetus.

Side effects. The side effects of methylphenidate are similar to those of amphetamines, and interventions discussed for amphetamines are appropriate for methylphenidate. One notable exception is that because methylphenidate is metabolized, acidifying the urine does not hasten its excretion.

Interactions. Most of the interactions associated with amphetamines are also of concern with methylphenidate (see Table 13-1). However, methylphenidate also inhibits the metabolism of several antiepileptics, for example, phenobarbital and phenytoin. Essentially the half-lives of these drugs are prolonged, leading to increased effects such as sedation.

Patient education. Patients and families should be taught:

To take the last dose of methylphenidate in the afternoon, to avoid methylphenidate-induced insomnia

To take methylphenidate with meals to reduce anorectic effects

To use caution when driving and the like because methylphenidate can mask fatigue

To notify the prescriber when nervousness, insomnia, palpitations, vomiting, and fever occur

To refrain from chewing timed-release capsules

PEMOLINE

Pemoline is an FDA-approved drug for treating ADHD. It is only remotely similar to amphetamine and has minimal sympathomimetic activity (Warneke, 1990). Pemoline is well absorbed from the stomach, and peak serum levels occur within 2 to 4 hours. The half-life is 12 hours, which facilitates once-per-day dosage. About half of each dose is excreted unchanged in the urine; the rest is metabolized before excretion (Keltner, 1989).

Pemoline apparently acts by increasing storage or synthesis of dopamine. A beneficial effect does not occur for 3 to 4 weeks. Pemoline causes less cerebral stimulation than do the amphetamines and methylphenidate; it also has fewer peripheral sympathomimetic effects. Side effects, adverse responses, toxic effects, and appropriate interventions are similar to those for amphetamines (Keltner, 1989). The abuse potential for pemoline is less than that for amphetamines and methylphenidate.

OTHER STIMULANTS: CAFFEINE AND AMPHETAMINE-LIKE ANORECTICS

Many other drugs with stimulant qualities are available. Most of these drugs are sold as anorectics (also referred to as *anorexigenics* or *anorexiants*), which are used for weight loss. Other stimulants can be found in foodstuff (caffeine), headache tablets, hay fever and cold remedies, and decongestants. Although some anorectics require a prescription, many other stimulants can be purchased over the counter.

Caffeine

"Hail, hail, hail to thee coffee
Hail, hail best of blisses
Ah coffee, ah sweet coffee
Coffee, if my Pa would please me
Only coffee will appease me."

Cantata No. 211 (Coffee Cantata, 1732)
Quoted by Glass, 1994, p. 1065.

Caffeine is the most widely used stimulant in the world (Chou, 1992). Caffeine is found in coffee, tea, and colas. It is an ingredient in more than 1000 over-the-counter medications (Lecos, 1984). More than half of the people in the United States could not start their day without their eye-opening cup of coffee. In fact, 80% of Americans ingest some form of caffeine daily, with an average adult consumption of 200 to 280 mg per day (about 2 cups of coffee) (Schreiber et al, 1988; Strain et al, 1994). It is coffee's CNS-stimulating potential, with the accompanying "mini-euphoria," that makes it so popular (Greden, 1974; Greden et al, 1978). Caffeine users often have the characteristics associated wtih substance abusers: tolerance, withdrawal, persistent desire, and unsuccessful attempts to reduce or stop consumption despite physical and psychologic consequences (Glass, 1994; Pickworth, 1995).

The psychiatric significance of caffeine is related to its ability to produce a sustained anxiety-like syndrome in individuals hypersensitive to its sympathomimetic effects. The *Diagnostic and Statistical Manual of Mental Disorders, Fourth Edition (DSM-IV)* identifies this disorder as caffeine intoxication (305.90). Essential symptoms of this disorder include restlessness, nervousness, excitement, insomnia, flushed face, diuresis, and GI disturbance (American Psychiatric Association, 1994). These symptoms can occur with doses less than 250 mg per day (in caffeine-sensitive individuals), but in individuals diagnosed with caffeinism, higher doses are usually required (Nehlig, Daval, and Debry, 1992). When doses have exceeded 10 g per day, deaths have been reported (Olin, 1995). Table 13-2 lists sources of caffeine. Because 10 g of caffeine are equivalent to 89 to 100 cups of coffee, overdose occurs most often with tablets.

Coffee was discovered around AD 850 by Khaldi, a goatherder in northern Eygpt. Technically it was Khaldi's wayward goats that first sampled berries from the coffee bush and, noting their euphoric state, Khaldi partook and was stimulated as well (Chou, 1992). Coffee ingestion accounts for about 75% of all caffeine consumed (Chou, 1992). The *DSM-IV* (American Psychiatric Association, 1994) notes that coffee contains 100 to 150 mg of caffeine per cup, tea about half that amount, and colas about one third. Caffeine-containing headache powders have one third to half the amount of caffeine found in a cup of coffee. Chocolate and cocoa contain significantly less caffeine. Between 20% and 30% of persons in the United States ingest between 500 and 600 mg of caffeine per day (Pilette, 1983), and about 10% consume more than 1000 mg per day, the defining point for overuse (Hughes et al, 1992). As many as 10% of persons in the United States could be described as having caffeinism. However, caffeine "abuse" is significantly different from what is popularly called "drug abuse" (Glass, 1995). Caffeine users do not need incrementally larger doses, and antisocial behaviors are not associated with caffeine use (Adamson and Roberts, 1995).

Excessive caffeine intake is prevalent among psychiatric patients (Hughes et al, 1992). A number of inpatient units across the country have become caffeine free in an attempt to reduce the synergistic effect of too much caffeine on other diagnostic conditions. Anecdotal summaries indicate improvement in patient interactions, a decrease in aggressive outbursts, and facilitation of treatment strategies.

Caffeine stimulates the CNS and heart and relaxes smooth muscle in blood vessels and the bronchi. A faster heart rate coupled with vasodilation leads to increased urine output. Gastric acid and other secretions are also increased, leading to a variety of GI tract ailments. Not all the GI tract disorders associated with coffee are caffeine related. Oils found in coffee, for example, are irritating to the stomach; however, such a discussion lies outside the objectives for this text. The basal metabolic rate of regular coffee drinkers is increased by about 10% (Greden, 1974).

Caffeine apparently inhibits the breakdown of cyclic adenosine monophosphate (cAMP), a second messenger in norepinephrine and dopamine neurotransmitter systems. The increase in cAMP bioavailability intensifies other CNS and PNS sympathomimetic effects (Olin, 1995).

Caffeine withdrawal. Caffeine withdrawal is accompanied by headache (and occasionally, vomiting), decreased arousal, and fatigue. Withdrawal effects are reversible with readministration of caffeine.

Phenylpropanolamine

Phenylpropanolamine is an ingredient in more than 100 prescription and over-the-counter anorectics, nasal decongestants, psychostimulants, and treatments for premenstrual syndrome (Dilsaver, Votolato, and Alessi, 1989). Table 13-3 lists several well-known compounds that are sold as anorectics. Phenylpropanolamine is often combined with caffeine but can be the only stimulant in the product. The amount of phenylpropanolamine ranges from 25 to 75 mg per tablet and should be used only by adults. At somewhat lower doses, that is, 12.5 mg, it is used in allergy, cough suppressant, and cold medications.

Psychiatrically, phenylpropanolamine is important because it intensifies stimulant properties of other sympathomimetics or antagonizes the effects of other

Table 13-2 Sources of Caffeine

Source	Caffeine content (approximate)
Beverages	
Coffee, brewed (drip)	60-180 mg/5 oz
Coffee, brewed (percolator)	40-170 mg/5 oz
Coffee, instant	30-120 mg/5 oz
Coffee, decaffeinated, brewed	2-5 mg/5 oz
Tea, brewed, major US brands	20-90 mg/5 oz
Tea, instant	25-50 mg/5 oz
Tea, iced	67-76 mg/12 oz
Cocoa	2-20 mg/5 oz
Soft drinks*	
Jolt	100 mg/12 oz
Sugar-free Mr. Pibb	59 mg/12 oz
Mountain Dew	54 mg/12 oz
Tab	47 mg/12 oz
Coca-Cola	46 mg/12 oz
Diet Coke	46 mg/12 oz
Mr. Pibb	41 mg/12 oz
Dr. Pepper	40 mg/12 oz
Big Red	38 mg/12 oz
Pepsi-Cola	38 mg/12 oz
Diet Pepsi	36 mg/12 oz
RC Cola	36 mg/12 oz
7-Up, ginger ale, most root beers	0 mg/12 oz
Over-the-counter analgesics*	
Anacin, Midol, Vanquish	32 mg/tablet
Excedrin Extra Strength	65 mg/tablet or capsule
Over-the-counter cold preparations*	
Dristan	16 mg/tablet
Triaminicin†	32 mg/tablet
Over-the-counter stimulants*	
No Doz	100 mg/tablet
Vivarin	200 mg/tablet
Prescription medications*	
Darvon compound	32 mg/capsule
Fiorinal	40 mg/tablet or capsule
Cafergot	100 mg/tablet

From Keltner NL. In Schlafer M, editor: *The nurse, pharmacology, and drug therapy,* Redwood City, Calif, 1989, Addison-Wesley.

*A representative sampling of the caffeine-containing preparations in these categories.

†These products also contain phenylpropanolamine.

Data for beverages; over-the-counter analgesics, cold preparations, and stimulants; and prescription medications adapted from Lecos C: *FDA Consumer* 18:14, 1984; Chou, T: *West J Med* 957:544, 1992.

Box 13-2 Clinical Signs and Symptoms Associated with Phenylpropanolamine Use*

Hypertension
Throbbing bilateral headache
Nausea and emesis
Anxiety
Palpitations
Seizures
Paresthesias
Stroke
Tremor
Hallucinations
Tachycardia
Ventricular ectopy or tachycardia
Myalgias
Reversible renal failure
Increased intracerebral pressure verified by lumbar puncture
Disorientation to person, place, or time
Paranoid psychosis
"Bizarre" behavior (e.g., disrobing in public)
Suicidal behavior

From Dilsaver SC et al: Complications of phenylpropanolamine, *Am Fam Physician* 39(4):201, 1989.
*Listed in order of decreasing frequency.

Table 13-3 Representative Over-the-Counter Weight-Loss Products Containing Phenylpropanolamine

Product	Phenylpropanolamine content (mg)
Acutrim	75 (tablet)
Appedrine*	25 (tablet)
Dexatrim capsules*	25, 75 (capsule)
Grapefruit diet plan with Diadax	12.5, 30, 75 (capsule)
Phenoxine	25 (tablet)
Unitrol	75 (capsule)

*Also contains caffeine.

psychotropic agents. Phenylpropanolamine is molecularly similar to amphetamine; however, it is a direct-acting sympathomimetic. It acts as a pressor agent because of a strong alpha-1 effect and a relatively weak beta effect. Subsequent hypertension associated with phenylpropanolamine is often accompanied by a reflex bradycardia (Dilsaver, Votolato, and Alessi, 1989). Box 13-2 lists signs and symptoms associated with phenylpropanolamine use in descending order, from most common to least common.

Other anorectics include drugs containing phentermine, phenmetrazine, benzphetamine, phendimetrazine, diethylpropion, mazindol, and fenfluramine (Olin, 1995). These prescription drugs have effects and precautions similar to amphetamines.

TREATMENT CONSIDERATIONS

Amphetamines, methylphenidate, and pemoline are used primarily to treat ADHD and narcolepsy (Table 13-4). Of children with ADHD, 60% to 70% remain symptomatic as adults (Garfinkel and Amrami, 1992), and drug dosages given in Chapter 16, Psychopharmacology for Adolescents, may be applicable. Information on the pharmacologic treatment of ADHD is found in Chapters 15, Psychopharmacology for Children, and 16, Psychopharmacology for Adolescents. Information on the treatment of narcolepsy is found in Chapter 8, Sleep Disorders.

Treatment of Depression

Psychostimulants have been prescribed for treating depression (Levin, 1991; Masand, Pickett, and Murray, 1991). Although anecdotal reports are encouraging, research does not support using psychostimulants over more conventional antidepressant approaches (Arana and Hyman, 1991). After an extensive review of the literature beginning with the first article by Myerson (1936), Chiarello and Cole (1987) concluded that treating depression with stimulants ". . . is intriguing but clearly insufficient to warrant consideration for FDA approval." In a case study ($N = 1$) Gupta, Ghaly, and Dewan (1992) reported that a combination of dextroamphetamine and fluoxetine resulted in a "robust response" in only 6 days in a woman previously considered refractory to treatment. A number of other studies support the augmentation role for stimulants in depression (Metz and Shader, 1991; Warneke, 1990).

Treatment of Depressed Medically Ill Patients

Myers and Stewart (1989) reported that methylphenidate has shown promising results with or without TCAs to treat depressed medically ill patients. As an example

Table 13-4 Adult Dosages of Major Central Nervous System Stimulants

Drug	Indications	Usual adult dose (mg/day)
Dextroamphetamine (Dexedrine), schedule II	ADHD Narcolepsy	10-30* 5-60 in divided doses
Racemic amphetamine, schedule II	ADHD Narcolepsy	10-30* 5-60 in divided doses
Methamphetamine (Desoxyn, Gradument SR), schedule II	ADHD	10-30*
Methylphenidate (Ritalin), schedule II	ADHD Narcolepsy	20-40* 20-60 in divided doses
Pemoline (Cylert), schedule IV	ADHD	56.25-75.0*

*Modified from Arana GW, Hyman SE: *Handbook of psychiatric drug therapy,* Boston, 1991, Little, Brown.

of a dosing strategy, they reported that 25 mg of desipramine twice a day coupled with 10 mg of methylphenidate every morning successfully launched a depressed cancer patient on an appropriate antidepressant regimen. Stimulants may have fewer and less powerful cardiovascular side effects than do traditional antidepressants.

Use as a Challenge Test for Predicting a Response to Antidepressants

Goff and Jenike (1986) suggested that a positive response (a euphoric response) to a dose of amphetamine may be an indication that a particular patient will respond positively to noradrenergic TCAs. Patients who have a dysphoric response may respond more favorably to serotonergic antidepressants. However, research on this topic is not conclusive.

Use in Elderly Persons

Roccaforte and Burke (1990) in a review of the literature have found evidence to support the notion that psychostimulants can be particularly helpful in elderly persons who have an amotivational syndrome and depression. Effects on cognition were less remarkable. Kaplitz (1975) and Pickett, Masand, and Murray (1990) found that methylphenidate and dextroamphetamine, respectively, were helpful in treating apathetic and withdrawn elderly patients. This topic is further discussed in Chapter 17, Psychopharmacology for Elderly Persons.

Caffeine Augmentation of Electroconvulsive Therapy

Giving pretreatment caffeine can help lengthen ECT-induced seizure time without increasing the electrical stimulus (Ancill and Carlyle, 1992; Coffey et al, 1990; Nehlig, Daval, and Derby, 1992). Clinical efficacy does not appear to be compromised; furthermore, Coffey et al (1990) reported a higher response rate in the pretreatment caffeine group (95%) than in the control group (80%).

Treatment of Schizophrenia

Goldberg et al (1991) sought to improve mood and cognition by coadministering dextroamphetamine and haloperidol. Although the theoretic underpinning of their effort seems reasonable (that amphetamine would selectively stimulate D-1 receptors in the frontal cortex), patients in the study did not improve. Chiarello and Cole (1987) reviewed 10 studies of stimulant-treated schizophrenia ($N = 430$). Ninety-six patients improved, and 162 patients were either unaffected or worsened. The authors remained hopeful that a role exists for stimulants in treating schizophrenia. A more recent study (Carpenter, Winsberg, and Camus, 1992) found no benefit when methylphenidate augmentation therapy was used for patients with schizophrenia.

Miscellaneous Uses

Central nervous system stimulants have been used to treat mania, neurasthenia, pathologic fatigue, and obsessive-compulsive disorder. Further studies may reveal a more important role for this group of psychotropic drugs than now realized.

REFERENCES

Adamson RH, Roberts HR: Caffeine dependence syndrome, *JAMA* 27(18):1418, 1995.

American Psychiatric Association: *Diagnostic and statistical manual of mental disorders,* ed 4, Washington, DC, 1994, The Association.

Ancill MB, Carlyle W: Oral caffeine augmentation of ECT, *Am J Psychiatry* 149(1):137, 1992.

Arana GW, Hyman SE: *Handbook of psychiatric drug therapy,* Boston, 1991, Little, Brown.

Breier A et al: Plasma norepinephrine in chronic schizophrenia, *Am J Psychiatry* 147(11):1467, 1990.

Carpenter MD, Winsberg BG, Camus LA: Methylphenidate augmentation therapy in schizophrenia, *J Clin Psychopharmacol* 12(4):273, 1992.

Chiarello RJ, Cole JO: The use of psychostimulants in general psychiatry, *Arch Gen Psychiatry,* 44:286, 1987.

Chou T: Wake up and smell the coffee: caffeine, coffee, and the medical consequences, *West J Med,* 157:544, 1992.

Clark JB, Queener SF, Karb VB: *Pharmacological basis of nursing practice,* ed 4, St Louis, 1993, Mosby.

Coffey CE et al: Caffeine augmentation of ECT, *Am J Psychiatry* 147(5):579, 1990.

Dilsaver SC, Votolato NA, Alessi NE: Complications of phenylpropanolamine, *Am Fam Physician* 39(4):201, 1989.

Fischbach GD: Mind and brain, *Sci Am* 267(3):48, 1992.

Garfinkel BD, Amrami KK: A perspective on the attention-deficit disorders, *Hosp Community Psychiatry* 43(5):445, 448, 1992.

Glass RM: Caffeine dependence: what are the implications? *JAMA,* 272:1065, 1994.

Glass RM: Caffeine dependence syndrome, *JAMA,* 273:1419, 1995.

Goff DC, Jenike MA: Treatment-resistant depression in the elderly, *J Am Geriatr Soc* 34:63, 1986.

Goldberg TE et al: Cognitive and behavioral effects of coadministration of dextroamphetamine and haloperidol in schizophrenia, *Am J Psychiatry* 148(1):78, 1991.

Grace AA: The tonic/phasic model of dopamine system regulation: its relevance for understanding how stimulant abuse can alter basal ganglia function, *Drug Alcohol Depend* 37(2):111, 1995.

Graybiel AM: The basal ganglia, *Trends Pharmacol Sci,* 18:60, 1995.

Greden JF: Anxiety or caffeinism, *Am J Psychiatry* 131(10):1089, 1974.

Greden JF et al: Anxiety and depression associated with caffeinism among psychiatric inpatients, *Am J Psychiatry* 135(8):963, 1978.

Gupta S, Ghaly N, Dewan M: Augmenting fluoxetine with dextroamphetamine to treat refractory depression, *Hosp Community Psychiatry* 43(3):281, 1992.

Hughes JR et al: Should caffeine abuse, dependence, or withdrawal be added to DSM-IV and ICD-10? *Am J Psychiatry* 149(1):3340, 1992.

Kaplitz SE: Withdrawn apathetic geriatric patients responsive to methylphenidate, *J Am Geriatr Soc* 23:271-276, 1975.

Keltner NL: Central nervous system stimulants. In Shlafer M, Marieb E, editors: *The nurse, pharmacology, and drug therapy,* Redwood City, Calif, 1989, Addison-Wesley.

Kuczenski R: Biochemical actions of amphetamines and other stimulants. In Creese I, editor: *Stimulants: neurochemical, behavioral, and clinical perspectives,* New York, 1983, Raven.

Lecos C: The latest caffeine scorecard, *FDA Consumer* 18:14, 1984.

Levin R: Psychostimulants for depression, *Am Fam Physician* 44(3):758, 763, 1991 (letter).

Liebman M: *Neuroanatomy made easy and understandable,* ed 4, Gaithersburg, MD, 1991, Aspen Publishers, Inc.

Lovgren K: Amphetamines, *Emergency* 17(6):10, 1985.

Masand P, Pickett P, Murray GB: Psychostimulants for secondary depression in medical illness, *Psychosomatics* 32(2):203, 1991.

Metz A, Shader RI: Combination of fluoxetine with pemoline in the treatment of major depressive disorder, *Int Clin Psychopharmacol* 6(2):93, 1991.

Myers WC, Stewart JT: Use of methylphenidate, *Hosp Community Psychiatry* 40(7):754, 1989.

Myerson A: The effect of benzedrine sulfate on mood and fatigue in normal and neurotic persons, *Arch Neurol Psychiatry* 36:816-822, 1936.

Nehlig A, Daval J-L, Derby, G: Caffeine and the central nervous system: mechanisms of action, biochemical, metabolic and psychostimulant effects, *Brain Res Rev* 17:139, 1992.

Olin BR: *Facts and comparisons,* St. Louis, 1995, Wolters Kluwer.

Pickering H, Stimson GV: Prevalence and demographic factors of stimulant use, *Addiction,* 89:1385, 1994.

Pickett P, Masand P, Murray GB: Psychostimulant treatment of geriatric depressive disorders secondary to medical illness, *J Geriatr Psychiatry Neurol* 3(3):146, 1990.

Pickworth WB: Caffeine dependence, *Lancet,* 345:1066, 1995.

Pilette WL: Caffeine: psychiatric grounds for concern, *J Psychosoc Nurs Ment Health Serv* 21:19, 1983.

Roccaforte WH, Burke WJ: Use of psychostimulants for the elderly, *Hosp Community Psychiatry* 41(12):1330, 1990.

Schreiber GB et al: Measurement of coffee and caffeine intake: implications for epidemiologic research, *Prev Med* 17:280, 1988.

Strain EC et al: Caffeine dependence syndrome: evidence from case histories and experimental evaluations, *JAMA* 272(13):1043, 1994.

Warneke L: Psychostimulants in psychiatry, *Can J Psychiatry* 35:3, 1990.

CHAPTER 14

Drugs Used to Treat Extrapyramidal Side Effects

Most patients on neuroleptic therapy experience some form of extrapyramidal side effect (EPSE) (Bezchlibnyk-Butler and Remington, 1994). Accordingly this chapter should, perhaps, precede the chapter on antipsychotic drugs. Generally understanding the primary group of drugs presented here, that is, anticholinergic antiparkinson drugs, can better delineate and characterize the pharmacologic effects of neuroleptic agents. The mention of antipsychotic drugs is deliberate because that class of drug is most often responsible for side effects that are routinely treated with other drugs.

Antipsychotic drugs cause side effects ostensibly created by a reduction in central nervous system (CNS) dopamine in the basal ganglia portion of the brain. These undesired effects are referred to as *extrapyramidal side effects* (EPSEs) and include akathisia, dystonia, akinesia, drug-induced parkinsonism, dyskinesia and tardive dyskinesia, and neuroleptic malignant syndrome. A narrative review of these reactions is given in Chapter 4, Schizophrenia and Other Psychoses. Box 14-1 summarizes the information found in Chapter 4 and provides a ready reference in this chapter. We think the best approach to understanding EPSEs is, first, to review the biochemical mechanisms associated with parkinsonism and then, based on that discussion, to trace the concept of EPSEs.

REVIEW OF PARKINSONISM

Parkinsonism is a chronic and progressive neurodegenerative disorder. Degeneration is known to occur in pigmented brain-stem nuclei, particularly in the substantia nigra, a major dopamine-generating portion of the brain. About 1% of these neurons are lost per year (Scherman et al, 1989), and total cell loss can approach 90% in severely impaired patients with parkinsonism (Agid, 1991). A certain cell-depletion threshold of about 50% to 60% in the substantia nigra and perhaps 70% to 80% of the dopaminergic neurons that project to the basal ganglia must occur before symptoms become evident (Agid, 1991). Increased activity by remaining healthy cells and hypersensitivity of dopaminergic receptors account for the lack of symptoms in individuals with dopaminergic cell loss below this threshold. Figure 14-1 compares a normal substantia nigra with one from a patient with parkinsonism.

The substantia nigra is part of a larger system, the extrapyramidal system. The extrapyramidal system differs from the pyramidal system both functionally and anatomically. The extrapyramidal system coordinates involuntary movement, which supports voluntary movement. For example, when a person walks, a host of involuntary muscle activities support and facilitate those voluntary movements associated with walking. The extrapyramidal system coordinates or fine-tunes those involuntary actions. Another example is the simple act of sitting in a chair. Muscle tone

Box 14-1 Extrapyramidal Side Effects (EPSEs)

Akathisia	Subjective feeling of restlessness, restless legs, jittery feeling, "nervous energy." It is the most common EPSE and responds poorly to treatment. Approximately 50% of patients on long-term, high-potency neuroleptics have akathisia. If treatment with anticholinergics does not help, noncholinergics such as clonidine or a benzodiazepine may help. Dosage reduction from the neuroleptic typically works.
Akinesia	Weakness (hypotonia), fatigue, painful muscles, anergy, absence of movement. Typically a bradykinesia occurs more often. Akinesia is treated effectively with most anticholinegics.
Dystonias	These EPSEs manifest as abnormal postures that are caused by involuntary muscle spasms. Dystonias tend to appear early in neuroleptic treatment. They include oculogyric crises, tongue protrusion, torticollis, laryngeal-pharyngeal constriction, which can be life threatening. Younger males are more likely to develop dystonias. These EPSEs are relatively rare among elderly individuals.
Drug-induced parkinsonism	Loss of associated movements, tremor, dysphagia, dysarthria, loss of facial expression, sialorrhea, festinating gait, increased muscle tone, rigidity. Its incidence increases with age.
Tardive dyskinesia	Tardive means "late appearing." This disorder seldom occurs before 6 months of neuroleptic usage. It is not related to dopamine-ACh imbalance but is probably caused by hypersensitivity of dopamine receptors. About 15% to 25% of patients receiving chronic neuroleptic therapy develop this EPSE. It affects muscles of the mouth and face, causes lipsmacking, grinding of teeth, rolling or protrusion of tongue, tics, and diaphragmatic movements that may impair breathing. Its severity fluctuates, and it disappears with sleep. There are no drugs that "cure" tardive dyskinesia; anticholinergics worsen the condition.
Neuroleptic malignant syndrome (NMS)	Cardinal symptoms are hyperthermia (103°F or higher), muscular rigidity, impaired ventilations, muteness, altered consciousness, and autonomic hyperactivity. It occurs in up to 1% of patients receiving neuroleptics. NMS can be fatal. See Box 14-2 for more information.

Modified from Malhotra and Pickar, 1993; Schwartz and Brotman, 1993.

A

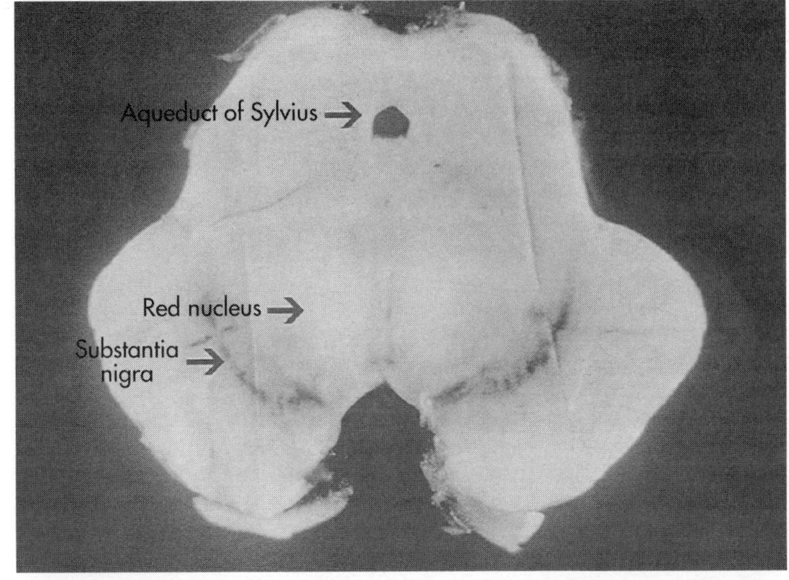

B

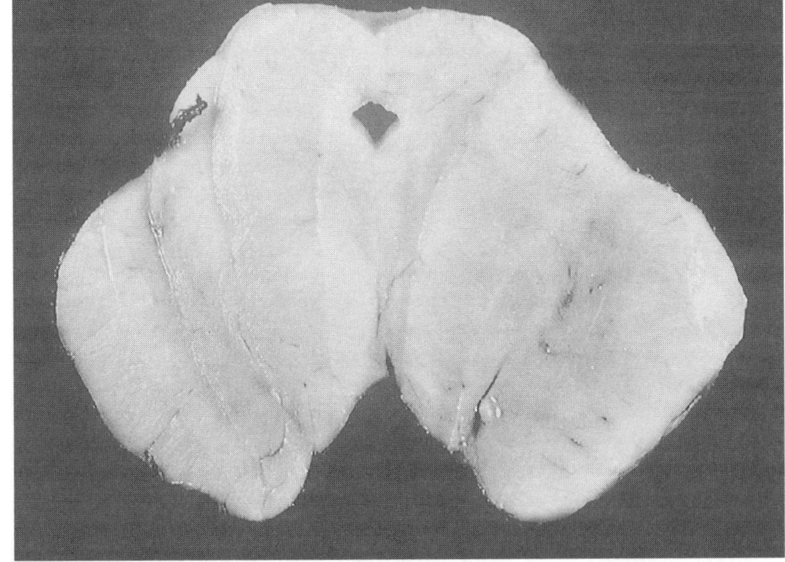

Figure 14-1 **A,** Brain slice illustrating a normal substantia nigra with adequate pigmentation. The substantia nigra is located in the zona compacta area of the midbrain. **B,** This midbrain is from a patient who suffered from parkinsonism. Note the loss of pigmentation. (Courtesy Dr. Cheryl Palmer, Department of Neuropathology, University of Alabama at Birmingham Brain Resource Program.)

and support, though involuntary, is required to successfully sit in a chair without falling over, slipping down, or slumping.

The pyramidal system is responsible for voluntary movement, for example, walking. Anatomically the pyramidal system begins in the motor strip, extends down through the brain to the brain stem, crosses over (decussates), and continues down the spinal cord, emerging at various points along the way to synapse with neurons innervating voluntary muscle throughout the body. Several terms are used to describe this system anatomically *(motor strip, precentral gyrus, corticospinal tract)* and/or functionally *(the voluntary system, the motor system)*. The motor strip of a normal brain, an intact motor strip in the brain of a patient with Alzheimer's disease, and the abnormal motor strip of a patient with amyotrophic lateral sclerosis are shown in Figures 14-2 to 14-4.

Anatomically the extrapyramidal system lies rostral to (in front of) the motor strip in the premotor area and projects to the basal ganglia. Some authorities treat the extrapyramidal system and the basal ganglia synonymously. This only underscores the frontier nature of brain function study.

The major cause of involuntary motor system disruption is a decrease in the availability of dopamine and a subsequent decrease in dopamine transmission. Reductions in dopamine cause a profound effect on posture, walking, balance, and

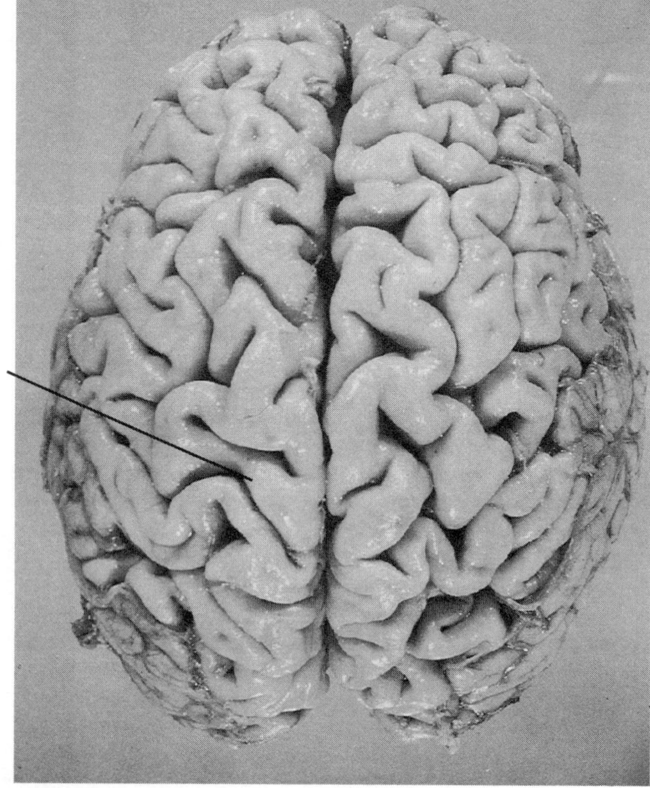

Figure 14-2 Normal brain and precentral gyrus (motor strip). (Courtesy Dr. Richard Powers, Director, University of Alabama at Birmingham Brain Resource Program.)

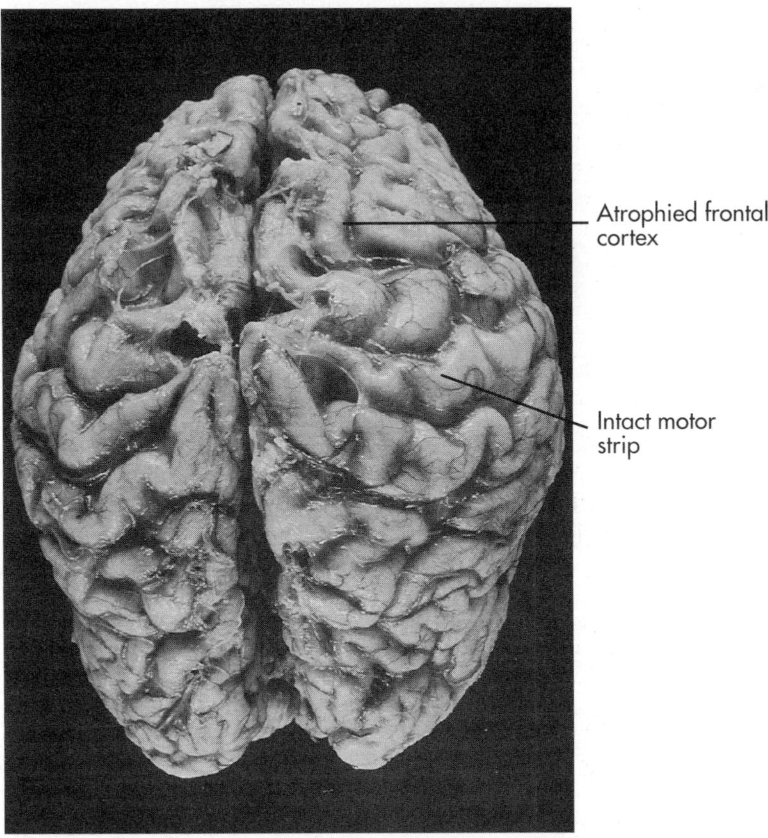

Figure 14-3 Brain of a patient with Alzheimer's disease. Note the atrophied frontal gyri, with the relative sparing of the motor strip. This pattern of pathology is consistent with the clinical observation that patients with Alzheimer's disease have cognitive impairment but adequate motor function. (Courtesy Dr. Richard Powers, Director, University of Alabama at Birmingham Brain Resource Program.)

other muscle-dependent activities. For an individual to successfully negotiate everyday movement, two neurotransmitter systems, dopamine and acetylcholine (ACh), must be in balance. In parkinsonism there is too little dopamine and a relative excess of ACh. Dopamine is an inhibitory neurotransmitter in the basal ganglia, and ACh is an excitory neurotransmitter. However, the role of acetylcholine seems to be secondary. That is, though drugs that deplete dopamine, for example, antipsychotics, will cause parkinsonism, drugs tht enhance acetylcholine, for example, choline and physotigmine, do not cause parkinsonism (Borison and Diamond, 1987).

Dopamine deficiency can occur in the following three ways (Keltner, Schwecke, and Bostrom, 1995):

1. The brain produces less dopamine because of loss of dopamine-generating cells and dopaminergic tracts, that is, parkinsonism.
2. Neuronal dopamine is depleted chemically such as occurs with reserpine.

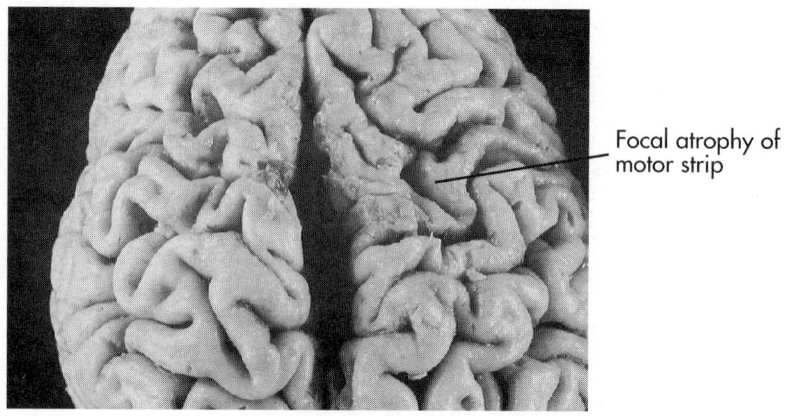

Figure 14-4 Brain of a patient with amyotrophic lateral sclerosis. Note the obvious focal atrophy of the motor strip (and to a lesser extent the sensory postcentral gyrus), with sparing of frontal areas. These patients suffer from severe motor impairment. (Courtesy Dr. Richard Powers, Director, University of Alabama at Birmingham Brain Resource Program.)

3. Dopamine is blocked at the postsynaptic receptor such as occurs with antipsychotic drugs.

The primary symptoms of parkinsonism—resting tremor, bradykinesia, rigidity, and loss of postural reflexes—are caused by massive destruction of nigrostriatal dopaminergic neurons in the zona compacta of the substantia nigra (Agid, 1991; Liebman, 1991). Many secondary symptoms are also present. Tremors are common, affecting about 75% of all patients with parkinsonism. Tremors can usually be detected in at least one arm or hand when the person is at rest. These resting tremors are in contrast to the "movement" tremors associated with long-term alcohol abuse and accordingly are caused by lesions in different areas of the brain. Whereas the basal ganglia fine-tune involuntary movement in the extrapyramidal system, the cerebellum fine-tunes voluntary movement in the pyramidal system. Alcoholism often produces cerebellar lesions.

Tremors are typically more amenable to treatment than are other symptoms. Bradykinesia is a generalized motor slowing. Masked facies (the slowing down of face movements); slowed arm swing; and difficulty initiating, maintaining, and stopping movement are several dimensions of bradykinesia. Rigidity, sometimes referred to as *lead-pipe* or *cogwheel rigidity,* impairs movement and makes the simple acts of getting out of a chair or gripping a pen so difficult that patients sometimes defer rather than attempt them. Tremor responds best to anticholinergic drugs, while rigidity and bradykinesia respond better to dopaminergic agents (Borison and Diamond, 1987).

Other important symptoms include postural difficulties, a gait disorder characterized by shuffling steps, and orthostatic hypotension. Falls are a major source of injury. Gait and postural disturbances are the most treatment-resistant symptoms and are probably caused by nondopaminergic lesions "downstream" from the dopaminergic nerve terminals. Dementia occurs in 15% to 20% of patients with parkinsonism. Depression occurs in approximately 40% of patients with parkinsonism and can be distinguished from other depressive disorders by greater anxiety and less self-punitive thinking (Cummings, 1992). Depression can be partially explained by the decreased levels of dopamine, a precursor to norepinephrine. Figure 14-5 de-

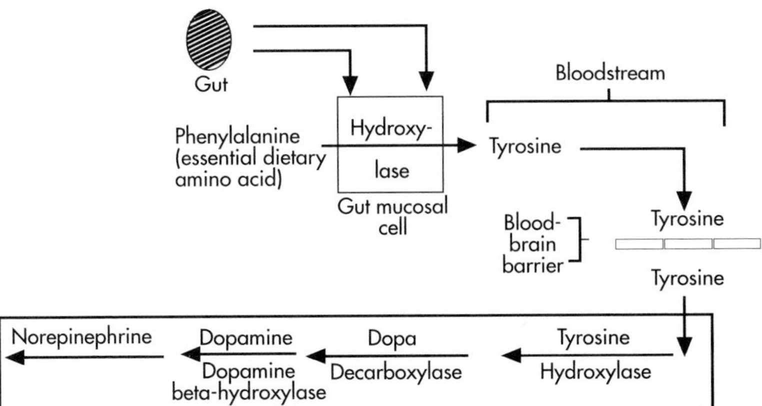

Figure 14-5 The dietary amino acid phenylalanine diffuses through mucosal cells in the GI tract and is metabolized to tyrosine. Tyrosine crosses the blood-brain barrier, enters brain neurons, and is metabolized to dihydroxyphenylalanine (Dopa, which is chemically identical to levodopa), and then to dopamine. Dopamine is converted further to norepinephrine, epinephrine, or both. In Parkinson's disease dopaminergic neurons degenerate, creating an imbalance with opposing effects of acetylcholine that is released from nearby neurons (not shown). In drug-induced parkinsonism, dopaminergic neurons may be intact, but postsynaptic dopamine receptors are blocked.

picts the synthesis of norepinephrine from dopamine. Although dopamine deficiency constitutes the bulk of parkinsonian abnormalities, other neuronal systems are also involved (Agid, 1991). Norepinephrine, serotonergic, and cholinergic systems are also disrupted and contribute to symptoms of depression and disturbed cognition.

Secondary symptoms include dysphagia, which makes eating difficult and can cause excessive accumulation of saliva leading to drool (sialorrhea). Weight loss and choking are two important consequences of dysphagia. The combined effect of bradykinesia and rigidity impair respirations (rigid, immobile respiratory muscles), bladder emptying (rigidity and retarded initiation of stream), and bowel evacuation (a rigid and immobile bowel, leading to constipation or incontinence).

EXTRAPYRAMIDAL SIDE EFFECTS

Although the previously mentioned symptoms are common among patients with idiopathic parkinsonism (referred to as *Parkinson's disease with cause unknown*), the symptoms can also be caused by a parkinson-like condition related to the use of antipsychotic drugs. High-potency agents are more likely to cause EPSEs than are low-potency agents (McEvoy, 1991). Antipsychotic drugs block dopamine receptors, frequently causing EPSEs. Many symptoms associated with Parkinson's disease, such as tremor, rigidity, and bradykinesia, are present in drug-induced parkinsonism, along with related symptoms such as akathisia, dystonic reactions, and dyskinesias. These symptoms contribute to the discomfort, anxiety, and frustration of individuals who are already suffering tremendous psychologic anguish and contribute to noncompliance (Forman, 1993). Nonneuroleptic drugs can also cause EPSEs, including antidepressants, antiemetics (many of which are directly related to antipsychotics), and lithium (Blair and Dauner, 1993). Patients taking antipsychotic drugs can experience EPSEs gradually over time or can have a sudden, dramatic onset of symptoms. The following case history illustrates the latter point:

> A 19-year-old male patient who was taking the antipsychotic drug fluphenazine (Prolixin), was brought to the nurse's station by another patient. The young man was screaming that he could not see. His eyes were rolled upward to such an extent that his vision was severely limited. He was experiencing oculogyric crisis. He was in a state of panic, and other patients began to feel very anxious and frightened. An "as needed" order for benztropine (Cogentin), 5 mg, was administered intramuscularly. The patient responded within 15 minutes.

Some clinicians think that a minimal level of EPSEs is related to a therapeutic response (Bitter, Scheurer, and Volavka, 1992).

Drugs Used to Treat Parkinsonism

If the proposed model of parkinsonism is correct (Figure 14-6), it would seem that a reasonable approach could occur in one of two ways. One could attempt to increase dopamine availability or one could attempt to decrease the availability of ACh (Figure 14-7). The two tactics basically capture the existing approaches to treating parkinsonism. Consequently two classes of antiparkinson drugs exist for treating these patients: dopaminergic antiparkinson agents (those that increase dopamine) and anticholinergic antiparkinson agents (those that block ACh). Parkinsonism caused by neuroleptic drugs is treated most often with the anticholinergic antiparkinson drugs, and much of this chapter is devoted to those agents. However, dopaminergic drugs can be used and are also discussed. Dopaminergic drugs are discussed first.

Dopaminergic antiparkinson drugs. Because parkinsonism is caused by a deficiency in dopamine, the most direct approach to treating the disorder is to give the patient dopamine. Although it would seem reasonable to give the patient dopamine, such an approach does not work. Because dopamine does not pass the blood-brain barrier easily, the large amounts needed to achieve therapeutic levels in the brain produce serious adverse peripheral nervous system (PNS) effects. There-

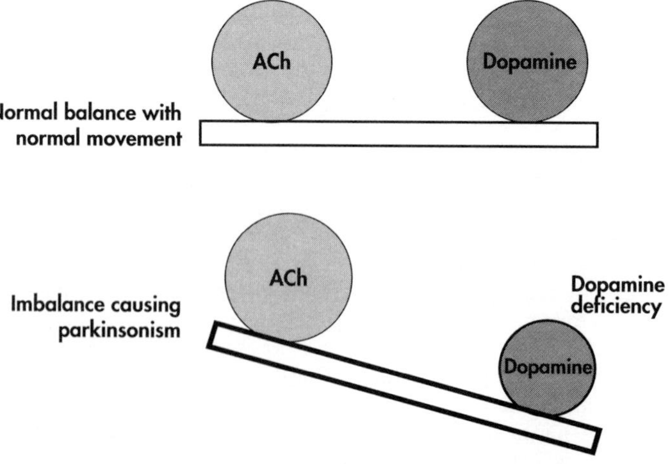

Figure 14-6 Normal and imbalanced states of acetylcholine (ACh) and dopamine.

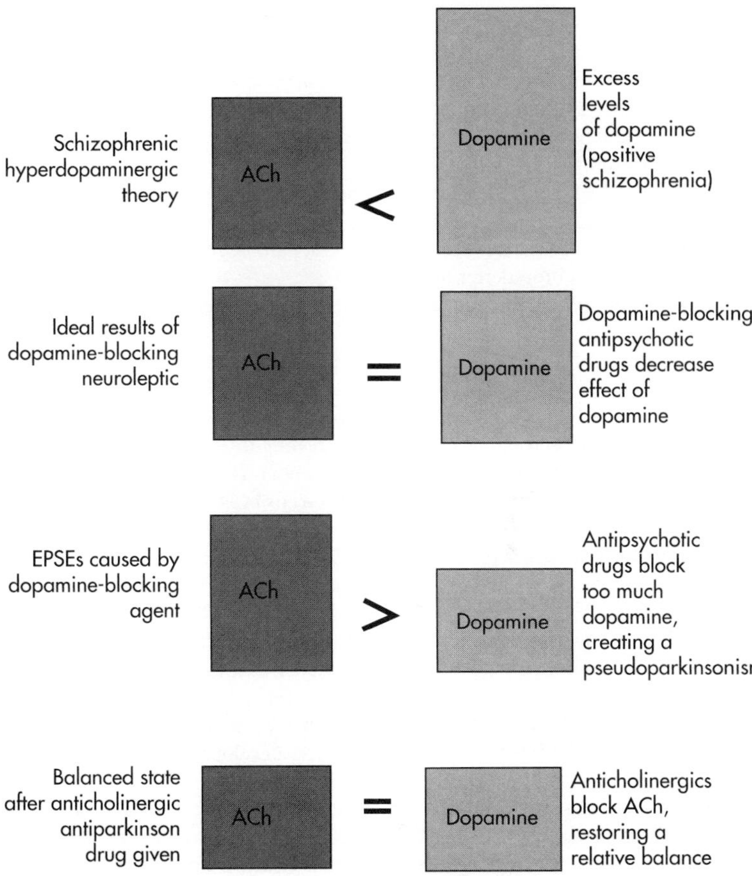

Figure 14-7 Theoretic neurochemical model of schizophrenia and chemical treatment.

fore, dopaminergic agents, which cross the blood-brain barrier easily and increase dopamine levels in the brain, have been developed to treat parkinsonism. They fall into the following categories:

1. Dopamine precursors, for example, levodopa and carbidopa-levodopa (Sinemet): These drugs *are not* prescribed for drug-induced parkinsonism and interact with most psychotropic medications. In fact, in keeping with the dopamine model of schizophrenia, a CNS side effect associated with these agents are psychotic-like symptoms, that is, hallucinations.
2. Dopamine releaser: Amantadine (Symmetrel) releases the small amounts of dopamine remaining in the dopaminergic neurons in the brain and is thought to block neuronal dopamine reuptake (Olin, 1995). Amantadine *is used* to treat drug-induced parkinsonism. However, its effect may be temporary.
3. Dopamine agonists: Bromocriptine (Parlodel) and pergolide (Permax) directly stimulate dopamine receptors. Some clinicians think bromocriptine is the best chemical approach to parkinsonism. It also *is used* to treat neuroleptic malignant syndrome.

4. Dopamine metabolism inhibitor: Selegiline (Eldepryl) blocks the metabolism of dopamine by inhibiting monoamine oxidase type B, the enzyme that breaks down dopamine. Monoamine oxidase type A breaks down serotonin and norepinephrine. The monoamine oxidase inhibitors (MAOIs) inhibit both A and B subtypes. Selegiline *is not used* for the treatment of drug-induced parkinsonism.

If this were a chapter on the treatment of parkinsonism, it would be important to discuss all the dopaminergic antiparkinson drugs; however, because the focus is primarily on drug-induced parkinsonism, only the dopamine releaser amantadine and the dopamine agonist bromocriptine are discussed.

Dopamine releaser: amantadine. Amantadine is a dopamine releaser or indirect agonist. It releases the remaining dopamine available in the otherwise dopamine-depleted dopaminergic neurons. It is also thought to inhibit the reuptake of dopamine.

Amantadine was first used as an antiviral drug; however, its application as an antiparkinson drug has been established, even in treating drug-induced parkinsonism (unlike levodopa). Because amantadine has an anticholinergic aspect, it is often used initially to treat parkinsonism and is coming to be used more often to treat drug-induced EPSEs. It is less effective than levodopa but more effective than the anticholinergics to treat parkinsonism (Olin, 1995).

Research comparing amantadine to biperiden found they both are equally effective in relieving EPSEs (Silver, Geraisy, and Schwartz, 1995).Amantadine is absorbed well from the gastrointestinal (GI) tract. Peak plasma levels occur about 4 hours after it is administered. The mean half-life is 15 hours. Amantadine is excreted unchanged by the kidneys. Impaired renal function slows the excretion of amantadine and can lead to amantadine intoxication. A protocol for prescribing amantadine in impaired renal function has been developed by Horadam et al (1981). Its excretion is hastened by acidifying the urine.

When used to treat true parkinsonism, amantadine is most effective during earlier stages of the illness because its effectiveness depends on availability of residual dopamine. In more advanced stages amantadine is effective when used adjunctively with levodopa or some other antiparkinson drug. A major drug interaction when administering amantadine is its use with other anticholinergic drugs such as antipsychotic drugs. Theoretically, amantadine is less likely to interact with high-potency antipsychotic drugs such as fluphenazine because they have fewer anticholinergic properties than do the low-potency drugs such as chlorpromazine (Thorazine).

Common side effects (5% to 10% of patients) of amantadine are nausea, dizziness, light-headedness, and insomnia (Olin, 1995). Occurring in 1% to 5% of patients are the side effects of depression, anxiety, irritability, hallucinations, confusion, anorexia, dry mouth, constipation, ataxia, peripheral edema, orthostatic hypotension, and headache (Olin, 1995). The seizure threshold is lowered, and patients with a history of seizures are at risk. A unique side effect of amantadine is the skin reaction referred to as *livedo reticularis,* in which the skin becomes purple, and localized edema develops. As with other anticholinergic agents, blurred vision can develop.

Overdose and toxic effects are treated by stopping drug absorption; that is, induced vomiting, gastric lavage, or administration of activated charcoal. An anticholinergic syndrome is manifested by excitability, delirium, hallucinations, seizures, hypotension, urinary retention, and arrhythmias. Although acidifying the urine theoretically might hasten amantadine excretion, in practice the problem of urinary retention makes this approach risky. There is no specific antidote for amantadine toxicity, but physostigmine, a drug traditionally used to treat atropine poisoning, may be beneficial (Olin, 1995).

Box 14-2 Neuroleptic Malignant Syndrome

Cause
A hypodopaminergic state

Offending agents
1. Primarily neuroleptics
2. Nonneuroleptics: withdrawal from dopaminergics (e.g. amantadine), lithium, antidepressants, antiemetics, and other dopamine blockers

Demographics*
Gender: Male/female ratio 3:1
Age: 45% between ages 20 and 39

Cardinal symptoms
Mental changes
Rigidity
Hyperthermia
Diaphoresis
Tachypnea
Autonomic dysfunction

Other signs and symptoms
Agitation, hyperreflexia, impaired breathing, muteness, pallor

Laboratory findings
Elevated CPK,† hyperkalemia, hyponatremia, metabolic acidosis, elevated WBCs

Treatment‡
Bromocriptine
2.5 to 10 mg by mouth 3 times a day initially
If no improvement in 24 hours, increase up to 20 mg by mouth 4 times a day
Dantrolene
1 to 3 mg/kg/day IV, in 4 divided doses; up to 10mg/kg/day
Oral maintenance doses range from 50 to 200 mg/day

Rechallenging with neuroleptics§
Rechallenging a patient with a neuroleptic may be warranted in cases of unremitting psychosis. About 30% will develop NMS again. A 2-week washout period should be allowed and the new neuroleptic should be a low-potency agent.

*Kellam, 1990.
†Most prominent laboratory finding.
‡Modified from Persing, 1994.
§From Buckley and Hutchinson, 1995.

Adults are usually prescribed an oral dose of 100 mg twice per day, up to 300 mg per day for EPSEs. Because the tablet is so large, many geropsychiatric patients are prescribed the syrup form for easy swallowing.

Dopamine agonist: bromocriptine, for treatment of neuroleptic malignant syndrome. Bromocriptine directly stimulates dopaminergic postsynaptic receptors, primarily in the corpus striatum, thus producing a dopamine-like effect. Technically bromocriptine does not add dopamine to the system; it adds a dopamine substitute. Bromocriptine's primary use as a drug to treat the side effects of psychotropic drugs is with neuroleptic malignant syndrome (Box 14-2). Bromocriptine is of obvious benefit in treating parkinsonism and is also used to treat endocrine disorders (it inhibits prolactin secretion by increasing dopamine availability). Pergolide, another more potent dopamine agonist, is not used to treat EPSEs.

Bromocriptine is not well absorbed from the GI tract and undergoes extensive first-pass metabolism. The drug is fully metabolized in the liver and is primarily excreted, via the bile, in the feces (85% to 98%) (Olin, 1995).

Hypotension is a major side effect of bromocriptine. Anxiety, hallucinations, depression, and confusion have been reported. Interaction with antipsychotic drugs may occur because by definition these drugs block dopamine receptors, the site of the agonistic effects of bromocriptine. If bromocriptine is needed, however, antipsychotics usually have been discontinued. When combined with other antihypertensives, bromocriptine can potentiate hypotensive effects. Other bromocriptine interactions pertain more to longer-term use than that associated with the treatment of NMS. Overdose and toxic effects intensify the side effects mentioned previously. If overdose is suspected, the drug should be discontinued and supportive, symptomatic care instituted.

Anticholinergic antiparkinson agents. Anticholinergic antiparkinson agents are most often used to treat drug-induced side effects of neuroleptics. Because of their importance, they are discussed here and from this point in the text will be identified simply as anticholinergic agents.

ANTICHOLINERGIC (ANTIPARKINSON) AGENTS

Parkinsonism, according to the model proposed in Figure 14-6, can be treated by decreasing the availability of ACh. Drugs that do this (anticholinergic drugs) have been employed for more than 100 years to treat parkinsonism (Pletscher and DaPrada, 1993). Anticholinergic agents cross the blood-brain barrier and block ACh. The most accurate term for these drugs is *antimuscarinic* because there are two basic types of ACh receptors: muscarinic and nicotinic. These agents effectively block muscarinic receptors. All of these agents are similar in function to atropine, the prototypical antimuscarinic.

Anticholinergic agents are generally less effective than levodopa but are beneficial in the early stages of parkinsonism and, in fact, are the drugs most often prescribed. As the illness progresses these agents become less beneficial and also lose appeal because of common noxious side effects related to toxicity, that is, tachycardia, dry mouth, constipation, blurred vision, and urinary retention. Further, CNS side effects such as memory problems and delirium, ("atropine poisoning") can be very troublesome and compound dementia and depression, both of which can be associated with parkinsonism (Box 14-3). Although several of these drugs are used to treat parkinsonism, only three or four are routinely used to treat drug-induced parkinsonism and the related EPSEs. A management plan for EPSEs was developed

Box 14-3 Mnemonics of the Effects of Atropine Poisoning

Dry as a bone:	Secretions of sweat and saliva and from respiratory system decrease
Red as a beet:	Atropine flush (flushing of face, neck, and upper arms) presumably because of reflex blood vessel dilation in response to increased body temperature
Blind as a bat:	Paralysis of accommodation and mydriasis have profound effect on vision
Hot as a furnace:	Decreased cutaneous heat loss with continued generation of body heat. High fever (up to 109°F rectally in poisoned children) and seizures have been documented.
Mad as a hatter:	Confusion, agitation, slurred speech, disorientation, hallucinations, and delirium

Modified from Shlafer M: *The nurse, pharmacology, and drug therapy,* ed 2, Redwood City, Calif, 1993, Addison-Wesley.

Box 14-4 Protocol for Treatment of EPSEs

If EPSEs occur the following steps can be used to reduce their intensity and length:

1. Reduce the dose of the neuroleptic if possible
2. If the dose cannot be decreased, change to a neuroleptic with less potential for causing EPSEs
3. Or add an anticholinergic based on efficacy for a particular EPSE (see Table 14-2)
4. If EPSEs continue increase amount of anticholinergic or switch to a different agent
5. If side effects of the anticholinergic become a concern, switch to another anticholinergic or use a nonanticholinergic agent.
6. Continue the anticholinergic for about 3 months, if the neuroleptic treatment is stable, and then start slowly decreasing the dosage amount until it is withdrawn.
7. If EPSEs recur, reinstitute the anticholinergic and the lowest possible effective dose. Attempt to discontinue again in a few months

Data from Bezchlibnyk-Butler KZ and Remington GJ, 1994; Boodhoo JA and Sandler M, 1991; Malhotra AK, Litman RE and Pickar D, 1993.

by Bezchlibnyk-Butler and Remington (1994). An adaptation of their protocol is provided in Box 14-4.

The anticholinergic drugs used to treat drug-induced parkinsonism and other EPSEs are trihexyphenidyl (Artane), benztropine (Cogentin), biperiden (Akineton), procyclidine (Kemadrin), and ethopropazine (Parsidol). In addition, the antihistamine diphenhydramine (Benadryl), has central anticholinergic effects and is often used substitutively for anticholinergic drugs. The antihistamines have fewer PNS side effects and may be better tolerated by elderly persons. Trihexyphenidyl is discussed as the prototypical anticholinergic drug. Table 14-1 summarizes the efficacy of these drugs for specific EPSEs.

Pharmacologic Effects

Trihexyphenidyl and the related anticholinergic drugs inhibit the actions of ACh in the brain. Acetylcholine receptors are blocked by these drugs. They may also inhibit the reuptake of dopamine (Olin, 1995). Both effects contribute to restoration of the acetylcholine-dopamine balance. When used to treat parkinsonism, trihexyphenidyl is often given adjunctively with dopaminergic drugs; when used to treat EPSEs, trihexyphenidyl is administered alone.

Pharmacokinetics

Trihexyphenidyl and the related drugs are usually given orally. Little pharmacokinetic information is available on these drugs; however, it is known that the half-lives range from 6 to 10 hours for trihexyphenidyl to up to 24 hours for biperiden (Table 14-2). The peak concentration level is achieved in about 1 hour. They are excreted by the renal system. When trihexyphenidyl is used to treat EPSEs caused by antipsychotic drugs, 1 mg is given initially, with 1 mg added every few hours until the reaction has been controlled. The usual dosage is 5 to 15 mg per day. When an oculogyric crisis or other dystonic reaction occurs, a more aggressive approach must be pursued, using intramuscular or intravascular injections with agents such as benztropine.

Side Effects

Anticholinergic drugs have the side effects associated with atropine. These drugs act both centrally and peripherally. About 19% to 30% of patients taking anticholinergics have CNS effects such as confusion, depression, delusions, and hallucinations (Olin, 1995). In addition, drowsiness and agitation are common central responses. The cholinergic system is implicated in memory and learning, and anticholinergic drugs can compromise both systems, particularly in elderly persons. PNS effects

Table 14-1 Efficacy of Antiparkinson Drugs on EPSEs

Drug	Tremor	Rigidity	Dystonia (oculogyric)	Akinesia	Akathsia
Amantadine	xx	xx	xx	xxx	xx
Benztropine	xx	xxx	xxx	xx	xx
Biperiden	xx	xx	xx	xxx	xx
Diphenhydramine	xx	x	xx	—	xxx
Ethopropazine	xxx	xx	x	x	xx
Procyclidine	xx	xx	xx	xx	xx
Trihexyphenidyl	xx	xx	xx	xxx	xx

Modified from Bezchlibnyk-Butler KZ and Remington GJ, 1994.
—: no effect; x: some effect (<20% response); xx: moderate effect (20% to 50% response); xxx: >50% response

Table 14-2 Usual Daily Dosage Range, Equivalent Dose, and Half-life of Drugs Used in the Treatment of EPSEs

	Usual daily dosage range (mg/day)	Equivalent dosage	Half-life (hrs)
Most to least potent			
Benztropine	PO: 1-8 IM/IV: 1-2 can repeat dose	2	—
Trihexyphenidyl	PO: 5-15	5	6-10
Biperiden	PO: 2-6 IM/IV: 2 can repeat in half an hour	2	18-24
Procyclidine	PO: 10 to 20	5	11-12
Ethopropazine	PO: 100-400	100	—
Diphenhydramine	PO: 75-200	25	2-7

Modified from Bezchlibnyk-Butler KZ and Remington GJ, 1994; Olin BR, 1995.

Table 14-3 Anticholinergic Effect on Cranial Nerves with Parasympathetic Function

The parasympathetic system is driven by acetylcholine. Certain cranial nerves have a parasympathetic function, and those functions are blocked by anticholinergic agents such as those discussed in this chapter. Cranial nerves III, VII, IX, and X have parasympathetic functions, and many of the side effects associated with these drugs are caused by the effect on these four cranial nerves.

Cranial nerve	Parasympathetic function	Anticholinergic effect
III	Constricts pupils	Mydriasis (dilates pupils)—blurred vision
	Alters shape of lens	Impairs accommodation
VII	Salivation	Dry mouth
	Lacrimation	Decreased tearing
	Nasal mucous secretion	Dry nasal passage
IX	Salivation	Dry mouth
	Nasal mucous secretion	Dry nasal passage
X	Slows heart rate	Tachycardia
	Promotes peristalsis	Slows peristalsis—constipation
	Constricts bronchi	Dilates bronchi

such as dry mouth, blurred vision, nausea, and nervousness occur in 30% to 50% of these patients. Constipation, a problem for many patients taking antipsychotic drugs, can be worsened by anticholinergics. Urinary hesitancy and retention, decreased sweating, tachycardia, and mydriasis are other PNS effects. Decreased sweating contributes to hyperthermia, a side effect with a potentially serious outcome. Table 14-3 outlines the effects of anticholinergic drugs on parasympathetic components of the cranial nerves. Table 14-4 summarizes common anticholinergic side effects and appropriate intervention strategies.

Table 14-4 Side Effects and Interventions for Anticholinergics

Side effects	Appropriate nursing interventions
Dry mouth	Provide sugarless hard candy and chewing gum; frequent rinses
Nasal congestion	Over-the-counter nasal decongestant (but use with caution)
Urinary hesitancy	Running water, privacy, warm water over perineum
Urinary retention	Catheterize for residual urine, encourage fluid intake and frequent voiding
Blurred vision, photophobia	Reassurance; normal vision typically returns in a few weeks; wear sunglasses; caution about driving
Constipation	Laxatives, as ordered; diet with roughage
Mydriasis	Instruct patient to report eye pain immediately
Orthostatic hypotension	Request patient to get out of bed slowly, to sit on the edge of the bed a short while, then rise slowly
Sedation	Help the patient get up early and get the day started
Decreased sweating	Can lead to fever; take reading of temperature; if fever occurs, reduce body temperature (e.g., sponge baths)

An important consideration when placing a patient on anticholinergics is the presence of glaucoma. Mydriasis, or pupil dilation, blocks the flow of aqueous humor from the anterior chamber, causing increased intraocular pressure (Shlafer, 1993). In cases of undiagnosed acute angle glaucoma, the anticholinergic effect could precipitate a very painful attack and cause blindness. Any eye pain associated with anticholinergics should be treated as an emergency. Elderly individuals are at greater risk for this complication.

Implications

Therapeutic versus toxic drug levels. The therapeutic dosage range for trihexyphenidyl is 5 to 15 mg per day for drug-induced EPSEs. Overdose may result in CNS hyperstimulation, confusion, excitement, hyperpyrexia, agitation, disorientation, delirium, and hallucinations. Convulsions, sometimes fatal, can develop related to hyperthermia associated with atropine poisoning (Box 14-3). Overdose can also result in CNS depression, drowsiness, sedation, or coma. The atropine-like effects summarized in Table 14-4 intensify. The mental symptoms of the patient receiving neuroleptics may also intensify. Circulatory collapse, cardiac arrest, and respiratory tract depression or arrest have been reported.

Treatment for anticholinergic drug overdose is similar to that for atropine overdose. The major emphasis is to prevent further absorption. Three mechanisms can be used: gastric lavage, induced vomiting, and ingestion of activated charcoal. The literature supports gastric lavage as the preferred approach, particularly when the patient is conscious. If CNS stimulation occurs, a short-acting barbiturate, for example, thiopental, may be ordered, but because stimulation could be preceding CNS depression, caution must be observed. Providing supportive care, such as airway maintenance and assisted breathing, and monitoring hyperthermia, for example, by obtaining rectal temperatures, and taking vital signs are important. PNS effects can be relieved by giving 5 mg of pilocarpine by mouth and repeating, if necessary (Olin, 1995). More serious or life-threatening situations may require advanced supportive efforts such as treating hyperthermia with a cooling blanket, tepid baths, or ice packs; treating seizures with parenteral diazepam; using physostigmine (in adults, 1 to 2 mg intramuscularly or intravenously at a rate of no more than 1 mg per minute) to reverse cardiac and CNS effects; and using fluids and vasopressors for circulatory collapse (Olin, 1995).

Use in pregnancy. Anticholinergics should be used cautiously during pregnancy. Theoretically these drugs decrease milk flow during lactation.

Side effects. Many bothersome side effects are associated with trihexyphenidyl and the other anticholinergics. Table 14-4 lists appropriate interventions. Other considerations include the following:

- Cautious use in patients with tachycardia or other arrhythmias caused by the blocking of the "braking" activity of the cholinergic system on the heart.
- Cautious use in older men with prostatic hypertrophy brought about by the inhibition of the urinary system. Anticholinergics relax the detrusor muscle of the bladder and contract the trigone muscle and sphincter, thus creating significant mechanical barriers to urination. By definition, men with prostatic hypertrophy already have significant mechanical barriers to urination, thus anticholinergics intensify those problems.
- Awareness that anticholinergics may mask the development of EPSEs because of their high anticholinergic properties.
- Cautious use when administering these drugs during hot weather, particularly in elderly persons. The major culprit is decreased sweating, which prevents the body from cooling down. Cases of fatal hyperthermia have been reported.

Interactions. Many over-the-counter drugs have anticholinergic properties and potentiate these drugs. Antihistamines, commonly a component of cold medicines, are major interactants. Other major interactants with potential for additive anticholinergic effects are amantadine, antiarrhythmics, antipsychotics, monoamine oxidase inhibitors, and tricyclic antidepressants. Elderly persons are most at risk for these additive effects.

Alcohol and other depressants can increase drowsiness and should be avoided, if possible. Antacids and antidiarrheals decrease absorption, and 1 to 2 hours should be allowed between doses of these interacting drugs. Anticholinergics may increase digoxin serum levels, decrease haloperidol levels (leading to exacerbation of schizophrenia symptoms), and reduce the efficacy of phenothiazines.

Patient Education

Patient education is an important part of the care of patients taking neuroleptics and those taking anticholinergic agents to decrease drug-induced side effects. Patients should be taught:

- To report sudden, marked changes in bowel or bladder function
- To not discontinue the drug suddenly
- To avoid driving or other hazardous activities, if drowsiness is a side effect
- To take with food if GI upset occurs
- To report eye pain immediately
- To avoid strenuous activities in hot weather

To avoid using over-the-counter and prescription drugs that contain anticholinergic properties (cold and hay fever medications)

Other patient teaching concerns for individual drugs can be reviewed in the Psychotropic Drug Profiles found in Part Two of this book.

RELATED ANTICHOLINERGIC DRUGS

Benztropine

Benztropine (Cogentin) is used to treat drug-induced EPSEs and is also prescribed on a prophylactic basis. It is the most frequently prescribed drug for EPSEs. An intramuscular form is available for noncompliant patients and for emergency intervention during an acute EPSE reaction such as oculogyric crisis. The oral form of the drug should be substituted for parenteral routes as soon as the patient's condition stabilizes. Because benztropine and trihexyphenidyl belong to different chemical classes, benztropine may be effective when trihexyphenidyl is not. Benztropine causes greater and longer-lasting muscle relaxation and sedation than does trihexyphenidyl. The more intense sedative effect may not be desirable for some patients but may make benztropine more desirable for others. Benztropine is less likely to cause a euphoric effect than is trihexyphenidyl, so benztropine is less likely to be abused. These differences notwithstanding, benztropine should be considered the equivalent of trihexyphenidyl in peripheral anticholinergic effect.

Biperiden

Biperiden (Akineton) is used occasionally to treat drug-induced EPSEs. It is chemically related to trihexyphenidyl. It is usually given orally but can be administered parenterally for acute drug-induced extrapyramidal reactions. There is some evidence that biperiden may actually ameliorate mild cases of tardive dyskinesia (Silver, Geraisy, and Schwartz, 1995).

Ethopropazine

Ethopropazine (Parsidol) is a phenothiazine derivative. Because phenothiazines block dopamine, it seems illogical to use this agent to treat neuroleptic-caused EPSEs. However, ethopropazine can be useful for drug-induced extrapyramidal disorders. The initial dose is 50 mg orally once or twice a day. The maintenance dosage range is usually 100 to 400 mg per day, but doses as high as 600 mg per day can be given.

Procyclidine

Procyclidine (Kemadrin) is used infrequently to treat drug-induced EPSEs and is particularly effective in alleviating rigidity. It is not effective in reducing tremor and may actually increase tremors early in treatment. Parenteral forms are not available. It is best given after meals.

Diphenhydramine

Diphenhydramine (Benadryl) is not a pure anticholinergic agent but is the prototypical antihistamine (H_1 antagonist). It has anticholinergic capabilities *and* appears to inhibit dopamine reuptake, providing two means of re-establishing the acetylcholine-dopamine balance. It is better tolerated in older patients who cannot tolerate the more potent anticholinergic agents. It is usually given orally but can be given parenterally.

Issues in Anticholinergic Drug Administration

A number of issues exist surrounding the use of anticholinergic agents to treat drug-induced parkinsonism and other EPSEs. These issues are presented in the form of questions and answers.

Is prophylactic anticholinergic treatment necessary and helpful?
Although it is known that these agents are therapeutic for acute EPSEs, it is not known whether they are beneficial as prophylaxis for drug-induced EPSEs. Both the prophylactic use and the duration of treatment concomitantly with neuroleptics are controversial (Double et al, 1993; Lavin and Rifkin, 1991; Tonda and Guthrie, 1994).

Arguments for prophylactic use include the following:

1. Rectifies poor assessment. Anticholinergic agents are particularly beneficial for akinesias, an extremely annoying EPSE that may contribute the most to noncompliance. Akinesia is often gradual in onset and can provoke listlessness, which, in turn, can be assessed as an exacerbation of psychosis. Prophylactic use would protect the patient from poor assessment practices.
2. Increases compliance. EPSEs are a major source of noncompliant behavior. If EPSEs can be minimized, the patient will be more likely to comply with the medication regimen.
3. Prevents frightening EPSEs. Anticholinergic agents prevent the development of frightening dystonic reactions that not only reinforce negative impressions of neuroleptic therapy but also can be health threatening. This is particularly true in young male patients.
4. High prevalence of EPSEs: An estimated 75% of all patients taking antipsychotic drugs have some level of EPSEs (Blair, 1990).
5. Depot and high-potency drugs. The extensive use of high-potency and depot drugs during the past decade increases the need for the use of anticholinergics as prophylactic agents.
6. Worsening of psychopathology. Anxiety, depression, motor agitation, and hallucinations have been reported after discontinuance of long-term anticholinergic drugs (Jellinik, Gardos and Cole, 1981).

Arguments against prophylactic use include the following:

1. Not needed. Although most patients report EPSEs, only a few have severe symptoms.
2. New problems created. Anticholinergic drugs cause additional side effects, including toxic anticholinergic psychosis, urinary retention, hyperthermia, and memory impairment
3. Unfortunate. Anticholinergic drugs unmask or worsen the development of tardive dyskinesia, which may be irreversible.
4. Questionable value. Even maintenance treatment is no guarantee that EPSEs will not occur (Comaty et al, 1990).
5. Decreased effects of neuroleptics. Anticholinergics interfere with the therapeutic effects of neuroleptics by impeding absorption.

Many clinicians think that the disadvantages of prophylactic use of anticholinergic agents for EPSEs outweigh the advantages. Hence anticholinergic drugs are often not prescribed until EPSEs occur and then are discontinued as soon as possible (4 to 8 weeks). An exception is use in young men receiving antipsychotic drugs. The rate of EPSEs among this age group is so high that many clinicians who might not consider prophylactic use in an older or female patient do order these drugs for prophylactic use in young men.

What is the potential for abuse or misuse of anticholinergic drugs, and how common is abuse or misuse?

"A review of the literature indicates that the anticholinergic drugs can be abused by some patients to achieve pleasurable effects ranging from a mild euphoria with increased sociability at the lower doses to a toxic anticholinergic psychosis with disorientation and hallucinations at higher doses." (Smith, 1980). Trihexyphenidyl may have the highest abuse potential, but this may be more a function of greater historical availability. Apparently the major effects sought by abusers are (1) a toxic confusional state accompanied by hallucinations, paranoia, and impairment of recent memory and (2) a euphoriant, antidepressant, and socially stimulating state. Abusers use several routes, such as oral, intravenous, and mixed with tobacco for smoking (Brower, 1987). Land, Pinsky, and Salzman (1991) reported that 1% to 17% of patients for whom these drugs are prescribed abuse or misuse them. Abuse of anticholinergic drugs increases as the availability of other drugs decreases.

The first case of abuse of these drugs was reported by Bolin (1960). A woman being treated for torticollis with 2 mg 4 times a day of an anticholinergic started taking up to 30 mg per day to achieve a euphoric state; eventually a full-blown toxic psychosis developed. Since that report, many other cases of anticholinergic abuse have been reported.

Misuse is different from abuse and is usually associated with a patient with negative symptoms, that is, affective blunting, who enjoys the sense of greater sociability.

Anticholinergic abuse can be deterred by the following (Land, Pinsky, and Salzman, 1991):

1. Avoid phophylactic use.
2. Do not use with low-potency antipsychotics that have high anticholinergic properties.
3. Treat EPSEs with nonanticholinergic medications (discussed elsewhere in this chapter).
4. When anticholinergic drugs are needed, prescribe the lowest dose possible while still controlling EPSEs.

Does abrupt withdrawal from anticholinergic drugs cause a significant reaction?

Anticholinergic drugs should never be abruptly discontinued, even when abuse is suspected. Abrupt withdrawal causes cholinergic rebound and withdrawal symptoms, including vomiting, malaise, sweating, excessive salivation, vivid dreams, and nightmares (Land, Pinsky, and Salzman, 1991).

What are the characteristics of toxic anticholinergic psychosis, and who is most susceptible?

Mild anticholinergic effects include those mentioned earlier in the chapter—drowsiness, dizziness, constipation, dry mouth, and nervousness. Anticholinergic psychosis or intoxication becomes evident with symptoms of agitation, visual and tactile hallucinations, nightmares, paranoid thinking, confusion, and impairment of recent memory. Toxic PNS symptoms include nausea and vomiting, diarrhea, tachycardia, arrhythmias, hypertension, and bronchospasm. Geriatric and pediatric patients are most sensitive to anticholinergic side effects (Hamdan-Allen and Nixon, 1991).

OTHER AGENTS

Although anticholinergic antiparkinson drugs are most often used to treat drug-induced side effects, several other agents with antiparkinson capabilities have been successfully administered and continue to have their own advocates.

Benzodiazepines: Treatment of EPSEs

Benzodiazepines, especially, lorazepam (Ativan) at 1.5 to 5 mg, diazepam (Valium) at 15 to 40 mg, and clonazepam (Klonopin) at 0.5 mg, have been used successfully to treat side effects (Fleischhacker, Roth, and Kane, 1990). These agents may be particularly useful for akinesia and akathisia.

Beta-Adrenergic Antagonists: Treatment of EPSEs

Propranolol (Inderal) at 20 to 100 mg and a few other beta-adrenergic antagonists have effectively reduced the side effects of neuroleptic drugs, particularly akathisia. These drugs are well tolerated and probably work through the antagonism of central beta-adrenergic receptors; however, in clinical trials these agents are combined with antiparkinson drugs, so it is difficult to interpret their precise effect on EPSEs.

Clonidine: Treatment of EPSEs

Clonidine (Catapres) is a centrally acting alpha-2 agonist. Clonidine apparently works by decreasing CNS noradrenergic neurotransmission. Dosages from 0.15 to 0.8 mg have been used successfully to treat side effects of antipsychotic drugs, but Fleischhacker, Roth, and Kane (1990) found that the alpha-2 agonists are more difficult to use and have no advantage over other agents. Tonda and Guthrie (1994) suggest clonidine as an alternative to anticholinergics in treatment-resistant akathisia.

Nifedipine and Verapamil: Treatment of Tardive Dyskinesia

Nifedipine (Procardia) at 30 to 60 mg per day and verapamil (Calan) at 80 mg 4 times a day are calcium-channel blockers that produce statistically significant improvement in patients with tardive dyskinesia (Duncan et al, 1990; Barrow and Childs, 1986). The interaction between the dopamine system in the CNS and calcium antagonists probably explains the improvement noted in patients with tardive dyskinesia.

Tardive dyskinesia, as described in Box 14-1 and in Chapter 4, Schizophrenia and Other Psychoses, is a late-appearing side effect of neuroleptic drugs. It is not satisfactorily amenable to drug therapy; however, as previously mentioned, attempts to find acceptable drug interventions continue. Prevention by careful monitoring of psychotropic medication regimens are crucial to minimizing the effects of tardive dyskinesia.

Dantrolene: Treatment of Neuroleptic Malignant Syndrome

Dantrolene (Dantrium) has been prescribed successfully in patients with neuroleptic malignant syndrome (Shader and Greenblatt, 1992) and lethal catatonia (Pennati, Sacchetti, and Calzeroni, 1991). Dantrolene interferes with the intracellular release of calcium necessary to initiate muscle contraction. Dantrolene also exerts a CNS effect (see the Psychotropic Drug Profiles in Part Two of this book for dosage information).

REFERENCES

Agid Y: Parkinson's disease: pathophysiology, *Lancet* 337:1321, 1991.

Barrow N, Childs A: An anti–tardive dyskinesia effect of verapamil, *Am J Psychiatry* 143:1485, 1986.

Bezchlibnyk-Butler KZ, Remington GJ: Antiparkinsonian drugs in the treatment of neuroleptic-induced extrapyramidal symptoms, *Can J Psychiatry,* 39(3):74, 1994.

Bitter I, Scheurer J, Volavka J: Are extrapyramidal symptoms necessary? *J Clin Psychopharmacol* 12(1):65, 1992 (letter).

Blair DT: Risk management for extrapyramidal symptoms, *Quality Assur Rev Bull* 17:116, 1990.

Blair DT, Dauner A: Nonneuroleptic etiologies of extrapyramidal symptoms, *Clin Nurs Specialist* 7($):225, 1993.

Bolin RR: Psychiatric manifestations of Artane toxicity, *J Nerv Ment Dis* 131:256, 1960.

Boodhoo JA, Sandler M: Anticholinergic antiparkinsonian drugs in psychiatry, *Br J Hosp Med* 46:167, 1991.

Borison RL, Diamond BL: Neuropharmacology of the extrapyramidal system, *J Clin Psychiatry,* 48:9 (suppl):7, 1987.

Brower KS: Smoking of prescription anticholinergic drugs, *Am J Psychiatry* 144:383, 1987.

Buckley PF, Hutchinson M: Neuroleptic malignant syndrome, *Neurosurg Psychiatry* 58:271, 1995.

Comaty JE et al: Is maintenance antiparkinsonian treatment necessary? *Psychopharmacol Bull* 26(2):267, 1990.

Cummings JL: Depression and Parkinson's disease: a review, *Am J Psychiatry* 149(4):443, 1992.

Double DB et al: Efficacy of maintenance use of anticholinergic agents, *Acta Psychiatr Scand* 88(5):381, 1993.

Duncan E et al: Nifedipine in the treatment of tardive dyskinesia, *J Clin Psychopharmacol* 10(6):414, 1990.

Fleischhacker WW, Roth SD, Kane JM: The pharmacologic treatment of neuroleptic-induced akathisia, *J Clin Psychopharmacol* 10(1):12, 1990.

Forman L: Medication: reasons and interventions for noncompliance, *J Psychosoc Nurs Ment Health Serv* 31(10):23, 1993.

Hamdan-Allen G, Nixon M: Anticholinergic psychosis in children: a case report, *Hosp Community Psychiatry* 42(2):191, 1991.

Horadam VW et al: Pharmacokinetics of amantadine HCL in subjects with normal and impaired renal function, *Ann Intern Med* 94(Part 1):454, 1981.

Jellinik T, Gardos G, Cole JO: Adverse effects of antiparkinson drug withdrawal, *Am J Psychiatry* 138:1567, 1981.

Kellam AM: The (frequently) neuroleptic (potentially) malignant syndrome, *Br J Psychiatry* 157:169, 1990.

Keltner NL, Schwecke L, Bostrom C: *Psychiatric nursing,* ed 2, St. Louis, 1995, Mosby.

Land W, Pinsky D, Salzman C: Abuse and misuse of anticholinergic medications, *Hosp Community Psychiatry* 42(6):580, 1991.

Lavin MR, Rifkin A: Psychotic patients' interpretation of neuroleptic side effects, *Am J Psychiatry* 148(11):1615, 1991 (letter).

Liebman M: *Neuroanatomy made easy and understandable.* Gaithersburg, MD, 1991, Aspen Publications.

Malhotra AK, Litman RE, Pickar D: Adverse effects of antipsychotic drugs, *Drug Saf* 9(6):429, 1993.

McEvoy GK: Central nervous system agents. In American Hospital formulary service, drug information. Bethesda, MD, 1991, American Society of Hospital Pharmacists.

Olin BR: *Drug facts and comparisons,* ed 49, St Louis, 1995, Wolters Kluwer.

Pennati A, Sacchetti E, Calzeroni A: Dantrolene in lethal catatonia, *Am J Psychiatry* 148(2):149, 1991 (letter).

Persing JS: Neuroleptic malignant syndrome: an overview, *SD J Med* 47(2):51, 1994.

Pletscher A, DaPrada M: Pharmacotherapy of Parkinson's disease: research from 1960 to 1991, *Acta Neurol Scand* 87(suppl 146):26, 1993.

Scherman D et al: Striatal dopamine deficiency in Parkinson's disease: role of aging, *Ann Neurol* 26:551, 1989.

Schwartz JT, Brotman AW: A clinical guide to antipsychotic drugs, *Drugs* 44(6):981, 1993.

Shader RI, Greenblatt DJ: A possible new approach to the treatment of neuroleptic malignant syndrome, *J Clin Psychopharmacol* 12(3):155, 1992.

Shlafer M: *The nurse, pharmacology, and drug therapy,* ed 2, Redwood City, Calif, 1993, Addison-Wesley.

Silver H, Geraisy N, Schwartz M: No difference in the effect of biperiden and amantadine on parkinsonian- and tardive dyskinesia-type involuntary movements: a double-blind crossover, placebo-controlled study in medicated chronic schizophrenic patients, *J Clin Psychiatry* 56(4):167, 1995.

Smith JM: Abuse of the antiparkinson drugs: a review of the literature, *J Clin Psychiatry* 41(10):351, 1980.

Tonda ME, Guthrie SK: Treatment of acute neuroleptic-induced movement disorders, *Pharmacotherapy* 14(5):543, 1994.

UNIT IV

Developmental Issues Related to Psychotropic Drugs

CHAPTER 15

Psychopharmacology for Children

LAWRENCE SCAHILL

Scope of the Problem

The mental illnesses of childhood are often classified according to five broad categories: disruptive behavior disorders, mood disorders, anxiety disorders, psychotic disorders, and developmental disorders. Collectively these disorders affect as many as 12% of children below age 18 (Institute of Medicine, 1989). This estimate translates into approximately 8 million children and adolescents, exacting an enormous cost to society. Increasingly, children with psychiatric disorders are being treated with medication to reduce their emotional and behavioral problems. This practice has raised concern in the popular press (Black, 1994). The empirical foundation for using psychotropic drugs in children is not as solid as it is for adults. Nonetheless, an accumulating body of evidence provides some guidance for the practitioner faced with the clinical management of children and adolescents taking psychotropic medications.

There are important differences in absorption, distribution, metabolism, and excretion of drugs (pharmacokinetics) in children compared with adults. Hence weight-based extrapolations of child dosages from adult dosages are generally inaccurate (Green, 1995a). There are also concerns about the potential effects of psychopharmacotherapeutic agents on the developing brain. As children grow, the reactions and responses to drugs begin to approximate those of adults. Consequently, this text provides separate chapters on child and adolescent psychopharmacology.

The history of pediatric psychopharmacology is brief. Box 15-1 displays important benchmarks in this chronology.

General Principles

The first principle of pediatric psychopharmacology is to *avoid drug therapy,* except when there is evidence that other treatments would be inadequate or have already failed. Accurate diagnosis is a prerequisite for initiating pharmacotherapy, but target symptoms should also be clearly identified. Diagnosis, target symptoms, and severity are discerned by careful observation and clinical history. Measurement of symptom severity can also be aided by using standardized rating scales (Scahill, Ort, 1995). Although the diagnosis does not determine medication selection, an incorrect diagnosis can result in an inappropriate medication being prescribed and that could have negative consequences.

Another issue that can affect the identification of target symptoms and therapeutic effects is that young children may not be able to describe their internal states (King and Noshpitz, 1991). Thus children may not understand words and concepts in the same way that adults do. Bearing this in mind, clinicians should thoughtfully explain relevant concepts and develop a common vocabulary for discussing symptoms with children.

Box 15-1 History of Pediatric Psychopharmacology

1937 Bradley uses benzedrine to treat behavioral disorders in children.
1950 Methylphenidate is used to treat hyperactive children.
1953 First reported use of chlorpromazine in children.
1965 Tricyclic antidepressants are used to treat children with major depressive disorder.
1969 Haloperidol is used in childhood psychosis.
1970 Lithium is used in children and adolescents with mania.
1971 First reported use of imipramine to treat school phobia.
1978 Approval for the use of haloperidol to treat tic disorders in children.
1979 First reported use of clonidine to treat tic disorders and disruptive behavior problems.
1989 Double-blind study of clomipramine to treat obsessive-compulsive disorder.
1990 First reported use of fluoxetine in children with obsessive-compulsive disorder.
1990 First reported use of fluoxetine in children with depression.
1992 Multicenter trial of clomipramine to treat obsessive-compulsive disorder.
1994 Multicenter trial for psychopharmacologic treatment of attention deficit hyperactivity disorder.
1995 First use of risperidone in children with various disorders.

The second principle in child psychopharmacology is that *children are physiologically different from adults.* Developmental immaturity not only affects dosage calculations but also may influence efficacy. Surprisingly, on a mg-per-kg basis, children often require larger doses of psychotropic drugs than adults to achieve similar drug serum levels and therapeutic effects (Green, 1995a). The reasons for this are not completely clear but are assumed to be because liver metabolism and the glomerular filtration rate are more efficient in children. Drug effects (pharmacodynamics) may be altered in children as well because of immature neural pathways. For example, the catecholamine systems, that is, norepinephrine and dopamine, are not fully developed until early adulthood (Puig-Antich et al, 1987; Green, 1995a).

Parent education is the third important principle of pediatric psychopharmacology. Because parents are ultimately responsible for compliance with dosage schedules, they are essential collaborators in determining therapeutic response and adverse effects. Parents may harbor unrealistic expectations about the potential benefits of the medication. Failure to address such expectations may contribute to noncompliance and attrition. For all these reasons, parents must be thoroughly educated about their child's medication, including any delay in positive effects, side effects, and potential for abuse and overdose. General guidelines for parent education are provided in Box 15-2.

Parents also play a key role in maintaining consistent administration of psychotropic drugs. If the drug regimen is not followed, the clinician cannot determine whether the drug is effective or make rational decisions about dosage adjustments.

Box 15-2 Parent Education for Specific Psychotropic Drugs

Stimulants

Stimulants can decrease appetite and retard growth. Hence parents should monitor appetite and weight.

Short-acting stimulants may cause rebound hyperactivity.

Stimulants can result in an increase in motor and phonic tics or stereotypic behavior.

Stimulants can improve inattention and hyperactivity but may not improve interpersonal relationships.

Drug holidays may allow the child to gain weight and recover retarded growth.

Antidepressants

Tricyclics can be fatal in overdose. Drug administration should be supervised, and the drug should be securely stored.

Other medications, including over-the-counter agents, may interact with antidepressants. Hence all medications should be reviewed with the primary clinician.

The new selective serotonin reuptake inhibitors (SSRIs) can cause motor restlessness, insomnia, and irritability.

The SSRIs alone may not be sufficient in obsessive-compulsive disorder (OCD). Additional treatments such as cognitive-behavioral therapy may be indicated.

In OCD and depression, there may be a lag between initiation of treatment and clinical response.

Antipsychotic agents

Antipsychotic drugs are only part of a comprehensive program.

Antipsychotic medications can cause dystonic reactions, especially early in treatment.

Watch for muscle rigidity, inability to remain still, and new abnormal movements.

Review the risk of tardive dyskinesia and withdrawal dyskinesia.

In treating tic disorders, the goal is to reduce tics as eradication is rarely achieveable.

Several factors can influence compliance. They include:

Parental ambivalence concerning the need for medication.

Inadequate parental surveillance of drug administration.

Parental misunderstanding of drug serum levels and the importance of consistency in drug doses.

Parental misconceptions about how drugs work, for example, that antidepressant drugs do not act as rapidly as does aspirin for a headache.

PSYCHOTROPIC MEDICATIONS USED WITH CHILDREN

STIMULANTS

Indications

Stimulants are indicated for managing attention deficit hyperactivity disorder (ADHD) and are considered the standard treatment for this disorder.

Attention deficit hyperactivity disorder (ADHD). ADHD is a relatively common psychiatric disorder of childhood, affecting approximately 6% of school-aged children (Szatmari, Offord, and Boyle, 1989). Boys are affected more often than girls. Studies of clinical populations indicate that the symptoms of ADHD are among the most common reasons children are referred to mental health agencies. ADHD is characterized by inattention, impulsiveness, and hyperactivity. The *DSM-IV* allows clinicians to distinguish between a primarily Hyperactive type and a primarily Inattentive type (American Psychiatric Association, 1994). Children with ADHD are described as overactive, restless, easily distracted, and easily frustrated. They are often socially unsuccessful because they are unable to take turns in games, tend to intrude into the affairs of others, and may misinterpret the intentions of others. Children with ADHD are also at greater risk for conduct disorder, depression, and learning disabilities.

The stimulants used to treat ADHD include methylphenidate (Ritalin), dextroamphetamine (Dexedrine)—both of which also come in sustained release forms—and pemoline (Cylert) (see Chapter 13, Drugs Used to Stimulate the Central Nervous System, for an explanation of these drugs). Each of these stimulants has shown short-term efficacy in placebo-controlled trials. Recently another preparation, Adderal, which contains a mixture of amphetamine and d-amphetamine salts, has been introduced, but to date this preparation has not been well studied (Popper, 1994). Of the stimulant medications, methylphenidate is used most often and is prescribed in as many as 6% of school-aged children (Safer and Krager, 1988). The clear preference for methylphenidate over the other stimulants cannot be attributed to greater effectiveness but may be because of its better side effect profile (Greenhill, 1995).

Empirical Support

Placebo-controlled trials have shown that stimulants improve sustained attention, impulse control, and overactivity (Pelham et al, 1990; Porrino et al, 1983 a,b). These effects can also result in decreased disruption in the classroom and better academic performance (Cunningham, Siegel, and Offord, 1991). Some studies also suggest that stimulants can improve parent-child interactions and peer relationships (DuPaul and Barkley, 1990).

Mechanism of Action

Although stimulants have become the standard treatment for ADHD, the mechanism of action is not clearly understood. It is clear that stimulants cause a release of dopamine. In addition, stimulants block the reuptake of both norepinephrine and dopamine by presynaptic neurons. These effects are proposed to enhance inhibitory output in the frontal lobe, resulting in better concentration, and impulse control, as well as decrease motor activity (Greenhill, 1995).

Pharmacokinetics, side effects, and interactions of CNS stimulants are discussed in Chapter 13, Drugs Used to Stimulate Central Nervous System. Only information specific to pediatric usage is provided here.

Clinical Management

Table 15-1 provides information about dosages for dextroamphetamine, methylphenidate, and pemoline. Before initiating a trial of a stimulant, it may be useful to obtain behavior ratings such as Conners Parent and Teacher Rating scales at baseline and then again after the medication has been stabilized (Barkley, 1990; Scahill, Lynch, and Ort, 1995). Also, if there are unanswered questions about the child's capacity to learn, a psychologic evaluation should be considered.

Methylphenidate (Ritalin). Methylphenidate is not approved for use in children under age 6 and is rarely used in children under age 5. In children over age 5, the medication is often introduced with a single 5-mg dose just before breakfast. The dosage may be increased by increments of 5 to 10 mg every 5 to 7 days and given in 2 or 3 doses 4 hours apart.

The optimal daily dose of methylphenidate has been disputed by some researchers, who argue that high doses impair cognitive performance (King and Noshpitz, 1991; Greenhill, 1995). These disparate views may be due to differences in outcome measures used and heterogeneity within ADHD (DuPaul and Barkley, 1990; Cunningham, Siegel, and Offord, 1991). Current dosage recommendations for methylphenidate range between 0.6 to 1.5 mg per kg of body weight per day in 2 or 3 divided doses, that is, approximately 0.3 to 0.7 mg per kg per dose. Doses above 60 mg per day are not recommended. A single daily dose of the sustained-release form (Ritalin-SR) can be used instead of divided doses of the regular product.

Dextroamphetamine (d-amphetamine) (Dexedrine). Dextroamphetamine is not commonly used in children under age 5. The initial dosage may be a single 2.5-mg dose in younger children or a 5-mg dose in older children. After 5 to 7 days, the medication may be raised 2.5 mg per day (5 mg in older children) and given in 2 doses. Thereafter the dosage may be raised every 5 to 7 days to a total of 15 to 20 mg per day in younger children and 40 mg per day in older children. The medication is typically given with meals or immediately before to prevent loss of appetite. The total dose is usually between 0.3 mg and 1.0 mg per kg of body weight (Dulcan, 1990). If the slow-release preparation is used, the same total dose would be given once daily in the morning.

Table 15-1 Dosing Guidelines for Commonly Used Stimulants

Drug name	Typical starting dose	Typical dose range	Doses per day
MPH	5 mg	10-60 mg	2-3
DEX	2.5 mg	5-40 mg	2
Pemoline	18.75 mg	37.5-112.5 mg	1
MPH-SR	20 mg	20-60	1
DEX-S	10 mg	5-30	1

MPH = methylphenidate; DEX = dextroamphetamine; MPH-SR = methylphenidate sustained release; DEX-S = DEX-Spansule.

Pemoline (Cylert). Pemoline differs chemically from the amphetamines and methylphenidate. It is used exclusively for ADHD, whereas amphetamines and methylphenidate are occasionally prescribed for narcolepsy. Pemoline is well absorbed and has a 12-hour half-life. A total of 50% of the agent is excreted unchanged in the urine.

Pemoline causes less cerebral stimulation than do the other two CNS stimulants. Its side effects are similar to those of the amphetamines and methylphenidate. However, several cases of choreoathetoid movements have been reported with pemoline. In addition, liver toxicity occurs in 1% to 3% of children treated with pemoline. Hence liver function should be checked every 6 months when a child is maintained on pemoline. Because of the 12-hour half-life, pemoline can be given once per day. The daily dose may be increased by 18.75 mg weekly, up to a maximum of 112.5 mg per day. The usual maintenance dose in children is 37.25 to 75 mg per day (Green, 1995a).

Side Effects of Central Nervous System Stimulants

Growth retardation is a major concern when anorexia-causing CNS stimulants are administered. Research indicates that slowed growth may be temporary and that children will eventually "catch up" (Greenhill, 1995). Appetite suppression can be reduced by giving these drugs immediately before or immediately after meals. Insomnia is reduced by giving the last dose at least 6 hours before bedtime. It may also be helpful to lower the last dose of the day to minimize the rebound effect.

Several incidents of de novo emergence or increased number of tics have been reported following exposure to stimulant medication (Riddle et al, 1995). Other investigators, however, have reported on children with tic disorders who are taking stimulants and are not experiencing a significant increase in tics (Gadow et al, 1995). Although it appears that not all children with tic disorders will exhibit a worsening of their tics when treated with stimulants, close monitoring is warranted when using these medications for such children.

Toxic Effects

Dextroamphetamine overdose can be fatal. In overdose the child appears hyperalert; is talkative; and may have tremors, exaggerated startle reflex, paranoia, hallucinations, confusion, and tachyarrhythmias. A child with this clinical presentation requires hospitalization. Overdose procedures enumerated in Chapter 13, Drugs Used to Stimulate Central Nervous System, should be followed.

Substance Abuse

The abuse potential of methylphenidate and dextroamphetamine and pemoline are low. Nonetheless, the FDA classifies methylphenidate and dextroamphetamine as Schedule II drugs. In many states, dextroamphetamine and methylphenidate require a new prescription for refills.

ANTIDEPRESSANTS

Indications

Antidepressant medications are approved for use in individuals with depression who are over age 12. Three chemically unrelated antidepressants—clomipramine (Anafranil), fluoxetine (Prozac), and fluvoxamine (Luvox)—are approved for treating OCD in patients ages 12 and older. The tricyclic medication imipramine (Tofranil) is approved for treating children with enuresis.

Antidepressant drugs include a long list of chemically diverse compounds that have all been effective in treating adults with depression. Common sense categories include the tricyclic antidepressants (TCAs), so named because of their characteristic three-ring structure; monoamine oxidase inhibitors (MAOIs), which are rarely used in children or adolescents; selective serotonin reuptake inhibitors (SSRIs), a group of chemically unrelated compounds that are grouped together because of their common mechanism; and novel antidepressants such as buproprion (Wellbutrin), venlafaxine (Effexor), and nefazodone (Serzone).

Depression. Depression is characterized by profound sadness, loss of interest in usual activities, loss of appetite with weight loss, sleep disturbance, loss of energy, feelings of worthlessness or guilt, irritability, tearfulness, and recurrent thoughts of death or suicide. To meet *DSM-IV* criteria, at least some of these symptoms must be present daily and persist for at least 2 weeks. Depression in childhood is similar in presentation to depression in adulthood. One important difference is that children may be less able to describe their feelings.

The prevalence of depression in children and adolescents is estimated to range from 1% to 5%, with adolescents being at the higher end of this range and school-age children at the lower end. Boys appear to be at higher risk for depression until adolescence, when it becomes more common in girls.

Separation Anxiety. Separation anxiety disorder is a disorder of childhood characterized by extraordinary distress when faced with routine separations from the mother (or primary caretaker) such as going to school. In most cases, children with separation anxiety disorder express worry about harm or permanent loss of their mother. The *DSM-IV* specifies childhood onset of excessive anxiety upon separation from home or major attachment figure as evidenced by acute distress, frequent nightmares about separation, and reluctance or refusal to separate. These symptoms must be present for at least a month and cause clinically significant impairment in social or academic functioning.

The prevalence of separation anxiety disorder is estimated at 4% of school-aged children and is equally common among boys and girls. The most common manifestation of separation anxiety disorder is school refusal. However, school refusal may be part of general anxiety, social phobia, obsessive-compulsive disorder, depression, or conduct disorder. Cases of school phobia have also been reported as a side effect of haloperidol. Thus school refusal warrants careful assessment.

TRICYCLIC ANTIDEPRESSANTS

Empirical Support

Tricyclic antidepressants have been used in child and adolescent psychiatry for more than 30 years. TCAs used to treat several psychiatric disorders of childhood—including depression (Puig-Antich et al, 1987), ADHD (Biederman et al, 1989; Spencer et al, 1993), obsessive-compulsive disorder (DeVeaugh-Geiss et al, 1992), separation anxiety (Klein, Koplewicz, and Kanner, 1992), and enuresis (Klein et al, 1980).

Although TCAs are frequently used in clinical practice, evidence for their efficacy in treating children with depression is unconvincing (Ambrosini et al, 1993). Geller et al (1986, 1992) have conducted several studies with nortriptyline (Pamelor) and have shown that some children and adolescents do have a positive response to nortriptyline; however, clear superiority of active drug over placebo has yet to be demonstrated. Nonetheless, it appears that at least some children with depression do benefit from nortriptyline. For example, in the study by Geller et al, 1986 approximately 60% of the patients (ages 6 to 12) responded favorably. Responders had a daily dosage range of 0.64 to 1.57 mg per kg.

In contrast, double-blind, placebo-controlled studies have demonstrated the effectiveness of desipramine for treating ADHD (Biederman et al, 1989; Singer et al, 1995) and clomipramine for treating children and adolescents with obsessive-compulsive disorder (Leonard et al, 1989; DeVeaugh-Geiss et al, 1992). The evidence supporting the use of TCAs in separation anxiety is modest, and treatment appears to be bolstered by behavioral therapy (Klein, Kopelwicz, and Kanner, 1992).

Mechanism of Action

The primary mechanism of action of the TCAs is to block the reuptake of norepinephrine and serotonin. Precisely how this known pharmacologic property brings about positive effects in depression or ADHD is unclear. In addition to blocking the reuptake of norepinephrine, clomipramine also potently blocks the reuptake of serotonin. The positive effect of imipramine on enuresis is probably due to its anticholinergic properties.

Pharmacokinetics

Children can show tremendous variation in serum level at the same dose. Thus even though therapeutic ranges for TCAs in children are not well established, serum levels can be useful in regulating the dose of the agents and to identify slow metabolizers. Suggested ranges for parent compounds are: imipramine at 150 to 240 ng per ml, desipramine at 115 ng per ml, nortriptyline at 60 to 100 ng per ml, and, for the combined level of clomipramine and desmethylclomipramine, 150 to 550 ng per ml (Green, 1995a).

Clinical Management

Table 15-2 provides dosing guidelines for the most commonly used TCAs in children. As shown in the table, dosing instructions are somewhat different across these TCAs. Imipramine is typically begun with a dosage of 25 mg and increased every fourth day to a range of 2 to 5 mg per kg per day, but usual doses are less than this maximum (Puig-Antich et al, 1987; Klein et al, 1992). In younger children, nortriptyline may be introduced with a 10-mg dose, with increases every 4 to 6 days to a range of 50 to 75 mg per day in divided doses. Clomipramine is usually given initially at a dose of 25 mg, with gradual increases every 4 or 5 days to a maximum of

Table 15-2 Dosing Guidelines for TCAs Commonly Used in Children

Drug name	Typical starting dose	Typical daily dose range	Doses per day
Imipramine	25 mg	25-150 mg	1-2
Desipramine	10-25 mg	25-125 mg	1-2
Nortriptyline	10-25 mg	20-100 mg	1-2
Clomipramine	25 mg	50-100 mg	1-2

100 mg per day in younger children. The use of desipramine in children is declining in the wake of reports of sudden death in a few children (see below).

Side Effects

Side effects of the TCAs include fatigue, dizziness, dry mouth, sweating, weight gain, urinary retention, tremor, and agitation. These anticholinergic side effects can sometimes be addressed by lowering the dose or changing the dose schedule.

Of greater concern is the potential for these medications, especially desipramine, to alter electrical conduction through the heart (Riddle, Geller, and Ryan, 1993). Although evidence from one controlled study shows that the cardiac effects of desipramine are minimal (Biederman et al, 1993), many clinicians have avoided using desipramine in children because of a report of the sudden deaths of four children who had been taking the drug. Currently most attention is focused on the potential of TCAs, especially desipramine, to prolong the QT interval, which is believed to increase the risk of fatal ventricular tachycardia in susceptible individuals (Riddle, Geller, and Ryan, 1993). Accepted guidelines for monitoring cardiac effects of TCAs include PR interval less than 210 ms, QRS interval within 30% of baseline, QT interval less than 450 ms, and heart rate less than 130 beats per minute (Green, 1995a).

Before initiating treatment with a TCA, a child should have an electrocardiogram (ECG). The ECG should be repeated during the dose adjustment phase and semi-annually during maintenance therapy (Green, 1995a). The baseline assessment should also include vital signs both lying and standing, a thorough review of medical and family history, and evidence of a recent normal physical examination. Discussion with the family should also include a review of the potential cardiac effects.

Interactions

Tricyclic antidepressants interact with many other drugs, and these interactions are reviewed in Chapter 5, Mood Disorders, and the Psychotropic Drug Profiles found in Part Two of this book.

Toxic Effects

Children are thought to be more sensitive to overdoses of TCAs than adults. Although deaths of children for whom TCAs were prescribed have been reported, TCA poisoning in children may be caused by taking another family member's (usually a parents) medication. The long-acting preparation imipramine pamoate (Tofranil-PM) is not recommended for children because the smallest available unit dose is 75 mg. Because TCAs have a narrow therapeutic index, compliance with the dose regimen warrants close monitoring, and these drugs must be made inaccessible to children. Treatment for TCA overdose is found in Chapter 5, Mood Disorders.

SELECTIVE SEROTONIN REUPTAKE INHIBITORS

The selective serotonin reuptake inhibitors (SSRIs) are a new class of antidepressants that has been introduced in recent years. The current SSRIs marketed in the United States include fluoxetine (Prozac), sertraline (Zoloft), paroxetine (Paxil), and fluvoxamine (Luvox). As noted earlier, clomipramine is a tricyclic antidepressant that acts similarly to the SSRIs. The newer SSRIs (fluoxetine, sertraline, paroxetine, and fluvoxamine) are not chemically related to one another nor are they chemically related to the older TCAs. As a group they are also more specific in their action and, consequently, they are called selective serotonin reuptake inhibitors (SSRIs).

Indications

All of the SSRIs in current use have shown efficacy for treating depression in adults. In controlled trials fluoxetine, sertraline, and fluvoxamine have also been effective for OCD.

Obsessive-Compulsive Disorder

Obsessive-compulsive disorder is now recognized as far more common than previously believed, affecting approximately 3% of the general population. It is defined by the presence of recurrent thoughts or images (obsessions) that are difficult to dislodge and repetitive habits that the person feels a strong urge to perform (compulsions). In children obsessive thoughts often involve contamination, for example, with dirt, germs, or chemicals, and fears of harm to self or close family members (Swedo et al, 1989; Riddle et al, 1990). Compulsions may involve behaviors or mental acts such as washing, checking, or counting. These habits may be performed to remove contaminants, prevent harm, or simply to reduce discomfort.

Obsessions and compulsions may be closely connected for some children, while in other cases the link is more remote. For example, perceived contamination may lead to handwashing in some children. For other children, complex touching rituals are carried out to prevent harm to themselves or a parent. Still other children may report that their rituals are performed to get it "just right" and are not related to a thought or worry.

The *DSM-IV* criteria for OCD requires that either compulsions or obsessions consume more than an hour per day, cause distress, and interfere with adaptive functioning (American Psychiatric Association, 1994). Recognition that the obsessions and compulsions are senseless and efforts to resist them must be present in adults but may not always be present in children.

Empirical Support

Several recent controlled studies have shown that these newer, more specific SSRIs are effective in reducing the intensity of OCD symptoms in adults (McDougle et al, 1993; Greist et al, 1995). The evidence supporting the use of these agents in children is not as strong (March, Leonard, and Swedo, 1995; Scahill, 1996). In a double-blind, placebo-controlled study of 14 children and adolescents, Riddle et al, (1992) reported an average of 44% improvement with fluoxetine. Large, multisite trials have recently been completed with sertraline and fluvoxamine in children and adolescents with OCD, but the results have not yet been reported. There are no published studies of paroxetine in pediatric populations.

Mechanism of Action

The SSRIs inhibit the return of serotonin into the presynaptic neuron. Although the precise mechanism is not completely understood, blocking the reuptake of serotonin produces a cascade of events that ultimately enhances serotonergic function. Moreover, available evidence suggests that this action accounts for the effectiveness of these agents in treating OCD.

Table 15-3 Dosing Guidelines for SSRIs in Children

Drug name	Typical starting dose	Typical daily dose range	Half-life*
Fluoxetine	5-10 mg	5-40 mg	2-4 days
Sertraline	25 mg	25-150 mg	1 day
Fluvoxamine	25 mg	50-150 mg	1 day
Paroxetine	10 mg	10-30 mg	1 day

* Long half-life allows single dose per day. Does not include active metabolite.

Pharmacokinetics

All four of the newer SSRIs have relatively long half-lives, permitting single daily dosing. The half-lives of sertraline, fluvoxamine, and paroxetine are each about 24 hours. Fluoxetine, which has a half-life of 2 to 4 days, also has an active metabolite with an even longer half-life (up to 9 days or more). In addition, fluoxetine and paroxetine inhibit their own breakdown, resulting in nonlinear kinetics at higher doses. Table 15-3 presents dosing guidelines for SSRIs in children.

Clinical Management

Fluoxetine (Prozac). Fluoxetine comes in a 10- or 20-mg capsule and as a liquid. The typical starting dose is 5 to 10 mg per day. Because of its long half-life, fluoxetine should be increased slowly to avoid overshooting the optimal dose. The dose range for children and adolescents is 5 to 60 mg per day, but most children will fall between 10 and 40 mg per day.

Side effects of fluoxetine. The most common side effects of fluoxetine include behavioral activation, which is characterized by motor restlessness, insomnia, and disinhibition. This side effect is especially prevalent early in treatment but may also be seen with dose increases (Riddle et al, 1991). Other side effects include abdominal pain, heartburn, diarrhea, and decreased appetite. There have also been reports of suicidal ideation and self-injurious behavior (King et al, 1991). Currently, it is unclear whether fluoxetine confers greater risk for suicidal ideation than the other SSRIs. Thus clinicians should be vigilant for suicidal thoughts or self-injurious behavior with all antidepressant medications.

Sertraline (Zoloft). Sertraline is available in 50- and 100-mg tablets that easily break in half. A therapeutic trial might begin with a 25-mg dose, with weekly increases to a range of 50 to 150 mg in children and slightly higher dosages in older adolescents. Evidence from adult studies suggests that some patients may respond to low doses of sertraline; hence clinicians should review symptomatic response before proceeding with additional dose increases. Sertraline can be given in a single daily dose.

Side effects of sertraline. The side effects of sertraline are similar to those of fluoxetine and include activation, insomnia, diarrhea, and sedation. In a review of 33 children and adolescents being treated for depression, Tierney et al (1995) reported 2 cases of sertraline-induced mania.

Fluvoxamine (Luvox). Fluvoxamine, which has been used in Europe for more than 10 years, has recently been introduced in the United States. The medication comes in 50- and 100-mg scored tablets. Treatment usually begins at 25 mg per day and is increased by 25 mg every 5 to 7 days as tolerated, for example, in the absence of diarrhea, sedation, or activation. The medication can be given once daily; typical dose range is 50 to 200 mg per day. The side effects are similar to those of fluoxetine and sertraline.

Paroxetine (Paxil). Paroxetine comes in 20- and 30-mg tablets that can be divided in half. Clear dosing guidelines are not currently available for children, but a reasonable starting dose would be 10 mg per day, with gradual increases as needed and as tolerated. The total daily dose of 10 and 40 mg can be administered in a single dose. Limited clinical experience indicates that paroxetine is generally well tolerated, with side effect profiles that are similar to those of the other SSRIs.

Withdrawal of SSRIs and Duration of Therapy

Although there are relatively few side effects associated with the SSRIs, several case studies have reported dizziness, nausea, vomiting, and diarrhea upon withdrawal of sertraline and paroxetine (Barr, Goodman, and Price, 1994; Louie, Lannon, and Ajari, 1994). Although fluoxetine has been used for more years than the other SSRIs, the symptoms just mentioned have not been associated with fluoxetine withdrawal. This is probably because of the longer half-life of fluoxetine and the presence of an active metabolite with a longer half-life, resulting in a gradual taper. Thus a slow withdrawal appears prudent with paroxetine, sertraline, and fluvoxamine.

A related question that is frequently raised by parents concerns the duration of treatment with an SSRI. Unfortunately, very little evidence exists on which to base a clear answer. Many clinicians suggest discontinuation after a symptom-free period of 8 to 12 months. Evidence from a recent follow-up study of 54 children and adolescents indicated that 70% (39/54) were maintained on medication for more than 2 years, suggesting that OCD can be chronic (Leonard et al, 1993). Thus children and parents should be informed that symptoms may return following discontinuation of an SSRI.

Augmentation Strategies

Although the SSRIs offer great promise for children and adolescents with OCD, not all children will have a positive response. Studies in adults show that 30% to 40% of patients with OCD will demonstrate only partial or no response to monotherapy with an SSRI. Studies by McDougle et al (1993) have shown that drugs such as lithium and buspirone, which enhance serotonergic function, are not effective as adjunctive agents. However, the addition of low-dose neuroleptics can be effective in refractory OCD, especially when there is a history of tics (McDougle et al, 1994).

Based on these findings in adults, many clinicians are beginning to explore augmentation strategies in children who do not have an optimal response to an SSRI. Before placing a child on a neuroleptic to augment ongoing treatment with an SSRI, the clinician should weigh several issues. First, although the transition can be difficult, an alternative SSRI should at least be considered.

Second, because the SSRI and the neuroleptic may compete in specific hepatic metabolic pathways, the level of each drug may be affected by the addition of the neuroleptic. The result may be a net increase in the SSRI and the neuroleptic, thereby potentially elevating the risk of adverse effects. For example, oculogyric crisis has been reported in two youngsters who were being treated with paroxetine and a neuroleptic (Horrigan and Barnhill, 1994; Lombroso et al, 1995). Furthermore, the interaction between a neuroleptic and an SSRI varies according to the SSRI. For example, the blood level of fluoxetine and norfluoxetine can increase markedly following the addition of a neuroleptic. In contrast, sertraline does not rely on the same metabolic pathway in the liver used by neuroleptics (Preskorn, 1993).

Finally, neuroleptic medications have both short-term side effects such as cognitive dulling, fatigue, weight gain, and akathisia, and long-term side effects such as tardive dyskinesia. In view of these concerns, other interventions should be considered. For example, cognitive-behavioral therapy has shown promise for treating children and adolescents with OCD (March, Mulle, and Herbel, 1994; Scahill et al, submitted).

SSRIs and Depression

Fluoxetine and sertraline have been studied for the treatment of depression in children and adolescents (Simeon et al, 1990; Emslie et al, 1995; Tierney et al, 1995). Although not uniformly positive, the findings of these studies suggest that the SSRIs are the first-line agents for depression in children. Dosing guidelines are similar to those described earlier for OCD.

OTHER ANTIDEPRESSANT MEDICATIONS

Bupropion (Wellbutrin) is not related to the TCAs or any other currently available antidepressant. It is approved for use in adults with depression. Few studies report its efficacy in treating children and adolescents with ADHD at doses ranging from 100 to 250 mg per day in three divided doses (Green, 1995b). Side effects include agitation, insomnia, skin rashes, nausea, vomiting, constipation, and tremor. Increased tics and seizures have also been reported (Green, 1995b). *Venlafaxine* (Effexor) and *nefazodone* (Serzone) are new antidepressants that have not yet been studied in children or adolescents.

ANTIPSYCHOTIC DRUGS

Antipsychotic drugs are discussed in detail in Chapter 4, Schizophrenia and Other Psychoses. In this chapter, only those antipsychotic agents that are commonly used in pediatric psychopharmacology are reviewed.

Indications

Antipsychotic agents are indicated for psychosis, severe aggression, and complex behavioral problems associated with autism and other developmental disorders in children and adolescents. Haloperidol and pimozide are also used to treat tics.

Psychotic disorders. Although rare, schizophrenia can occur in children under age 12 (McClellan and Werry, 1994). As defined in the *DSM-IV,* the prevalence of childhood schizophrenia is estimated at two cases per 100,000 and is more common in boys. Symptoms may include hallucinations, delusions, disordered thinking, and inappropriate affect. Speech idiosyncrasies such as neologisms, echolalia, and an inability to use verbal communication in an age-appropriate fashion are usually present. These symptoms cause substantial dysfunction in all domains, and affected children may also exhibit other developmental delays.

The etiology is unknown, but genetic vulnerability is assumed to play an important role. The diagnosis of childhood schizophrenia follows a careful assessment in which other disorders such as autism and neurodegenerative disorders have been ruled out (McClellan and Werry, 1994).

Pervasive developmental disorders. The pervasive developmental disorders (PDD) are a group of syndromes that are characterized by severe developmental delays in several areas of functioning, including socialization, communication, and interpersonal relationships. The *DSM-IV* describes several subtypes of PDD, including autism, Asberger's disorder, and PDD-Not Otherwise Specified (Volkmar et al, 1994).

Autism. The child with autism appears uninterested in social contact, has great difficulty with change, and exhibits both delayed and deviant language development. Autism is differentiated from schizophrenia by the earlier age of onset and the absence of hallucinations and delusions. Stereotypic behaviors such as rocking, hand flapping, and head banging are common; self-injurious behavior such as hitting and biting are frequently observed. These children tend to have a narrow range of interests and may prefer inanimate objects to social contact. Approximately half of children with autism are mentally retarded, and about 25% have seizures.

Asberger's disorder. Children with Asberger's disorder may have normal intelligence but typically exhibit higher verbal, rather than nonverbal, intelligence. Although their linguistic skills may not be as impaired when compared with children with autism, children with Asberger's disorder have profound social delays. They show deficits in initiating social interactions and reading social cues and have a predilection to be concrete in their interpretation of language. Stereotypic behaviors such as rocking and hand flapping are often present, and these children often exhibit intense preoccupation with peculiar topics such as fans, geography, train schedules, or dates of historical events.

PDD–not otherwise specified. Children with PPD–Not Otherwise Specified are probably a heterogenous group who are inflexible, intolerant of change, and prone to behavioral outbursts in response to modest environmental demands or change in routine. They are socially delayed, deficient in performing daily living tasks, often preoccupied with narrow fields of interest, and may have significant difficulty with regulating anxiety. Stereotypic behaviors may also be observed.

Tourette's syndrome. Tourette's syndrome (TS) is a movement disorder characterized by a changing repertoire of motor tics and vocalizations. The symptoms begin in childhood, exhibit a fluctuating course, and often decline in adulthood. Typical motor tics include eye blinking, head jerking, grimacing, and shrugging. Vocal tics include throat clearing, grunting, snorting, barking, hooting, and repetitive words or parts of words. Uncontrollable swearing (coprolalia) and/or obscene gestures (copropraxia) are present in a minority of patients. In addition to tics, many children also have significant problems with ADHD and obsessive-compulsive symptoms (Scahill, Lynch, and Ort, 1995).

TS is not a common disorder, but recent evidence suggests that it is not as rare as once believed. Current estimates are that TS occurs in approximately 1 case per 2000 in the general population, with a 2 to 4 times higher frequency in boys. Although the cause of TS is unknown, recent evidence converges on dysregulation of brain circuits connecting the cortex, basal ganglia, and thalamus (Leckman et al, 1992). Family genetic studies and twin studies provide compelling evidence that TS is an inherited disorder with variable expression in other family members, including chronic tic disorder, TS, and some forms of OCD. The evidence further suggests an autosomal dominant mode of inheritance, but other models may also be possible (Pauls et al, 1991; Walkup et al, 1995).

Mechanism of Action

The neuroleptics can be classified according to chemical family, that is, phenothiazines, or potency, that is, low versus high (see Chapter 4, Schizophrenia and Other Psychoses). The primary action of most antipsychotic medications is postsynaptic dopamine blockade at D-2 receptors. Exceptions to this general rule, such as clozapine and risperidone, are described later in this chapter and in Chapters 4, Schizophrenia and Other Psychoses, and 16, Psychopharmacology for Adolescents. Differences in action and side effects of the standard neuroleptics appear to be related to regional specificity of binding in the brain. For example, striatal binding is correlated with extrapyramidal side effects (EPSEs).

Antipsychotic medications also have anticholinergic and antihistaminergic effects. They block adrenergic pathways as well. The relative strength of these pharmacologic properties influences their side effect profile. Hence low-potency neuroleptics such as chlorpromazine and thioridazine cause more sedation, dry mouth, and constipation (anticholinergic effects). In contrast, the high-potency agents such as haloperidol and fluphenazine have greater EPSE liability. In this chapter representative agents from different chemical families and of different potencies are presented.

Pharmacokinetics

Most of the antipsychotic drugs have relatively long half-lives, for example, pimozide has a half-life of 55 hours and risperidone of 24 hours. Nonetheless, plasma blood levels at a given mg per kg dosage can vary substantially (Green, 1995a). This observation, coupled with the goal of averting unwanted side effects, favors a twice daily dosing schedule.

Clinical Management and Empirical Support

Chlorpromazine (Thorazine). Chlorpromazine is an aliphatic phenothiazine that was the first neuroleptic used in children. An early controlled study showed that in dose ranges between 120 to 430 mg per day, chlorpromazine was superior to a placebo on crude measures of behavioral disturbance. Despite modest improvement on the drug, the children remained severely impaired (Klein et al, 1980). With the introduction of newer agents, chlorpromazine is not used as frequently as in the past.

Chlorpromazine is usually prescribed at 10 to 25 mg on the first day and gradually increased over 2 weeks to a total of 150 to 300 mg per day in divided doses. For acutely disturbed children who require immediate treatment, an intramuscular dose of 0.5 mg per kg of body weight every 6 to 8 hours is appropriate. A 2- to 5-year-old child should not receive more than 40 mg per day, and a 5- to 12-year-old child should not receive more than 75 mg per day intramuscularly.

Thioridazine (Mellaril). Thioridazine is a piperidine phenothiazine that is also a low-potency neuroleptic. Compared with chlorpromazine, thioridazine is currently more commonly used for severe behavioral problems and psychotic symptoms. The dosage for treating psychosis in 3- to 12-year-old children is 0.5 to 3.0 mg per kg per day, which translates into 10 to 50 mg 2 or 3 times per day (Green, 1995a).

Haloperidol (Haldol). Haloperidol, a high-potency antipsychotic, is a butyrophenone and is structurally unrelated to the phenothiazines. It it used to treat children between ages 3 and 12 with psychosis, aggressive behavior, and tics, as well as behavioral dyscontrol associated with PDD.

Haloperidol is the most thoroughly studied of the neuroleptics in children, with both open and double-blind studies in autism, schizophrenia, severe aggressive behavior, and tics. These studies show that haloperidol is effective, though not free of side effects (Campbell and Cueva, 1995; Green, 1995a, Chappell, Leckman, and Riddle, 1995; Scahill, 1996). As a high-potency neuroleptic, haloperidol is more likely to cause EPSEs compared with chlorpromazine or thioridazine. On the other hand, haloperidol is less sedating. Table 15-4 shows typical doses for haloperidol by symptom cluster.

Fluphenazine (Prolixin). Fluphenazine, a commonly used piperazine in adults, is not approved for children under age 12. In one of the few studies of fluphenazine in prepubertal children, Joshi, Capozzoli, and Coyle (1988) found that low dosages, that is, 0.04 mg per kg per day, were effective in decreasing aggressive behavior, hyperactivity, and stereotypic behavior in a sample of 12 children with PDD. The initial dose might be 0.5 mg per day, with increases every 3 to 5 days as tolerated and according to clinical response. The total daily dose of 1 to 2.5 mg can be given in 2 divided doses.

Thiothixene (Navane). Thiothixene is a thioxanthene and is structurally related to phenothiazines. It is approved for treating psychosis in children over age 12. The meager evidence that is available for children under age 12 indicates that thiothixene is less sedating than are low-potency neuroleptics and may cause fewer EPSEs than the high-potency neuroleptics. The medication can be initiated with a 1- to 2-mg dose given 2 to 3 times per day. Therafter, the dosage can be increased to 5 to 40 mg per day in two or three divided doses (Green, 1995a).

Pimozide (Orap). Pimozide is a diphenylbutylpiperidine that is not related to the phenothiazines or to haloperidol. It is a potent blocker of dopamine at the D-2 postsynaptic receptors, and it is used to treat Tourette's syndrome.

In an open study of 66 children with TS, Sallee, Sethuraman, and Rock (1994)

Table 15-4 Recommended Doses of Haloperidol in Children

Clinical problem	Starting dose (mg)	Dose range (mg/day)
Psychosis	0.5	1-6
Tics (Tourette's syndrome)	0.25	0.5-2.0
Behavioral dyscontrol (pervasive developmental disorder)	0.5	0.5-3.0
Aggression	0.5	1-6

found that pimozide and haloperidol were equally effective in reducing tics at mean doses of 3.7 and 1.5 mg per day, respectively. In that study, children were randomly assigned to receive either haloperidol, pimozide, or no medication. The children treated with pimozide performed significantly better on computerized tests of attention. Haloperidol may have actually decreased performance on these tests. Unfortunately, differences in the type and frequency of side effects were not reported.

Pimozide comes in a 2-mg tablet. The typical starting dose is 0.5 mg (half a tablet every other day) to 1 mg per day, with increases every 5 to 7 days in 0.5- to 1-mg increments over a 3-week period. The total dose typically ranges from 2 to 4 mg per day. Common side effects include fatigue, cognitive dulling, dysphoria, akathisia, and dystonic reactions. An additional concern with pimozide is that it can cause cardiac conduction abnormalities such as prolonged QT interval and inverted T waves. These abnormalities are probably rare in the typical dose range for tics. Nonetheless, an ECG should be obtained at baseline, following dose adjustment and annually during maintenance therapy (Chappell, Leckman, and Riddle, 1995; Scahill, 1996).

Risperidone (Risperdal). Risperidone is a new neuroleptic medication that not only blocks dopamine postsynaptically but also acts as a serotonin antagonist at the 5-HT_2 site. The dual action is similar to that of clozapine and appears to protect against extrapyramidal side effects (Leysen et al, 1994). Although risperidone has some pharmacologic features in common with clozapine, it has not been associated with agranulocytosis. Risperidone has been extensively studied in adults with schizophrenia and appears to be safe and effective for treating psychosis, with fewer side effects than haloperidol (Marder and Meibach, 1994). However, the data supporting its use in children and adolescents are limited.

In an open study of 7 children between ages 10 and 17, Lombroso et al (1995) found that risperidone was effective in reducing tics in 5 of 7 patients. In most cases, the drug was initiated at 0.5 mg per day and increased by 0.5 mg every 5 to 7 days over a 2-week period to a range of 1 to 3.5 mg per day in 2 divided doses. It was well tolerated, with increased appetite and weight gain being the most commonly observed side effect.

Two other reports of open trials have recently been published (Mandoki, 1995; Simeon et al, 1995). These 2 studies report on a total of 17 children and adolescents (age range 7 to 17 years) with a variety of disorders including schizophrenia, psychotic depression, obsessive-compulsive disorder, pervasive developmental disorder, and severe attention deficit hyperactivity disorder. Although many of these patients had a positive clinical response, side effects including EPSEs were observed. The dosing schedule reported in both of these studies was apparently derived from studies of adults with schizophrenia and may have been too rapid, which may have contributed to the high frequency of adverse effects including EPSEs.

Side Effects

Side effects of antipsychotic drugs that are relevant to pediatric patients are discussed here. Side effects of neuroleptics are also discussed in Chapters 4, Schizophrenia and Other Psychoses, and 16, Psychopharmacology for Adolescents.

Drowsiness is a common side effect that may be especially prominent with chlorpromazine and thioridazine, that is, the low-potency antipsychotic agents. Anticholinergic side effects such as dry mouth, constipation, and blurred vision are also common. Dystonic reactions, rigidity, and akathisia, that is, extrapyramidal symptoms, are more common with the high-potency neuroleptics such as haloperidol, fluphenazine, and pimozide.

Toxic Effects

Deaths resulting from antipsychotic drug overdose are rare in any age group. Overdose causes CNS depression, hypotension, and EPSEs. Treatment for overdose is outlined in Chapter 4, Schizophrenia and Other Psychoses.

Tardive Dyskinesia

Long-term use of neuroleptics carries a small risk for tardive dyskinesia. A few cases of tardive dyskinesia in pediatric patients have been reported (Riddle et al, 1987; Campbell and Cueva, 1995). Thus children and adolescents treated with neuroleptics should be monitored for abnormal movements. In some cases it may be difficult to discriminate between dyskinesia, stereotypies, and/or tics. Referral to a consultant with expertise in movement disorders may be helpful in making this determination.

Because of the concern about withdrawal dyskinesia, the question of when and how to discontinue neuroleptic medication is a critical one. Dose reductions should be done gradually to minimize withdrawal dyskinesia and to evaluate changes in symptom severity. Attempts at discontinuation should be considered annually. If symptoms persist, the maintenance dose of the neuroleptic should be reduced to the lowest possible dose to minimize overall exposure (McClellen and Werry, 1994).

LITHIUM

Indications

Lithium is not approved for use for children under age 12. Nonetheless, several published studies document its use in prepubertal children with bipolar illness or severe aggressive behavior. A brief description of lithium will be provided here; more detailed descriptions are presented in Chapter 5, Mood Disorders, and Chapter 16, Psychopharmacology for Adolescents.

Bipolar disorder. Whether mania exists in children is a matter of controversy. In addition, questions remain concerning the presentation of bipolar illness in children. Until these questions are resolved, the frequency of bipolar illness in children cannot be estimated accurately. Available data suggest that although apparently uncommon in childhood, bipolar illness can be diagnosed in children and resembles the adult illness, though euphoria and grandiose thinking may be less common (Fristad, Weller, and Weller, 1992; Weller, Weller, and Fristad, 1995).

Severe aggressive behavior. Aggressive behavior is a feature of several child and adolescent psychiatric disorders such as ADHD, conduct disorder, and perhaps bipolar disorder as well. Significant, unprovoked aggressive behavior often leads to consultation and hospitalization in some cases. Both behavioral therapy and medication have been used to treat aggressive behavior in children.

Empirical Support

There are very few controlled studies of lithium in prepubertal children with bipolar illness. The best emipirical support comes from a large open study that showed that 39 of 59 (66%) children benefitted from lithium treatment (DeLong and Aldershof, 1987). A recent placebo-controlled study of 50 children (mean age 9.4 years) showed that lithium was effective in reducing severe aggressive behavior (Campbell et al, 1995).

Clinical Management

For children under age 12, dosages of 10 to 30 mg per kg per day are typical. Thus for a 30-kg child, the dose would be 900 mg per day in divided doses. The optimal serum level range is 0.6 to 1.2 mEq per L.

Before initiating a trial of lithium, a child should have a physical examination, screening laboratory tests such as a complete blood count, electrolytes, blood urea nitrogen, creatinine, liver function tests, thyroid indices, and an ECG. Lithium decreases free thyroxine and triiodothyronine, but increased thyroid-releasing hormone generally compensates in euthyroid patients. Nonetheless, thyroid function and renal function should be checked every 6 months. Lithium levels should be monitored several times during the dose adjustment phase and then periodically after the dose is stabilized. Levels above 1.4 mEq per L are associated with signs of toxicity.

Side Effects

Common side effects of lithium include weight gain, nausea, vomiting, polydipsia, polyuria, tremor, fatigue, and diarrhea.

ALPHA-2 ADRENERGIC AGENTS

Indications

The alpha-2 adrenergic agents (clonidine and guanfacine) are only approved for use in adults with hypertension. Beginning with the early studies of clonidine for Tourette's syndrome (Chappell, Leckman, and Riddle, 1995; Scahill, 1996), these drugs have become increasingly common in child psychiatry for treating tics, ADHD, and aggressive behavior.

Empirical Support

Clonidine (Catapres). A recent double-blind study showed that clonidine can be effective in reducing the severity of tics in some patients (Leckman et al, 1991). Other studies provide modest evidence for efficacy in ADHD (Hunt, Minderaa, and Cohen, 1985), but these findings were not replicated in a recent controlled study (Singer et al, 1995).

Guanfacine (Tenex). Guanfacine is another alpha-2 adrenergic agonist that was introduced more recently. Interest in guanfacine was prompted by its longer duration of action compared with clonidine, and it appears to be less sedating. To date only three open studies have evaluated guanfacine in children (Hunt, Arnsten, and Asbell, 1995; Chappell et al, 1995; Horrigan and Barnhill, 1995). These studies included a total of 38 children with ADHD. All three groups of investigators reported that guanfacine reduced the target symptoms of ADHD. The study by Chappell et al (1995) also included children with TS, and guanfacine appeared to have a modestly beneficial effect on tics. Although promising, these results are preliminary, and additional research using controlled designs is warranted.

Mechanism of Action

These drugs stimulate presynaptic noradrenergic receptors, resulting in decreased sympathetic output over time.

Clinical Management

Clonidine is usually introduced with a single 0.05-mg dose (half of a 0.1-mg tablet) and then increased by half-tablet increments every 3 to 4 days to a total of 0.15 to 0.2 mg per day. To ensure even blood levels across the entire day, clonidine is typically given three to four times per day. Sedation, which is most evident early in therapy, is the most common side effect. Other side effects include dry mouth, headache, irritability, and, occasionally, sleep disturbance. Blood pressure should be monitored, but it is rarely a problem. Clonidine should be tapered slowly, however, as abrupt discontinuation can cause a rebound increase in blood pressure, tics, and anxiety.

Clonidine is being used increasingly as an adjunct to other medications, especially the stimulants (Popper, 1995). Clinicians may resort to combined pharmacotherapy either to augment the positive effects of the first medication, offset the side effects caused by the primary medication, or treat another set of target symptoms (Walkup, 1995). Unfortunately, there is very little research support for combination pharmacotherapies in the pediatric age group, and clinicians must rely on experience, case reports, and extrapolation from adult studies (McDougle et al, 1994). The limitations of case reports are illustrated by the recent report of three deaths of children treated with the combination of clonidine and methylphenidate. A careful review of these cases showed that neither medication nor the combination played a role in the deaths of these children (Popper, 1995). Nonetheless, combination pharmacotherapy calls for careful reconsideration of the target symptoms, the dose and timing of the primary medication, and a thorough discussion with the family regarding treatment alternatives.

Treatment with guanfacine may be initiated with a 0.5-mg dose in the evening and increased every 3 to 5 days to 0.5 mg 3 times per day. The common dose range is 1.0 to 3.0 mg per day in 2 or 3 divided doses. Side effects include sedation, irritability, and mid-sleep awakening. These side effects can sometimes be managed by lowering the dose or adjusting the times of doses.

OTHER AGENTS USED IN THE TREATMENT OF CHILDREN WITH PSYCHIATRIC DISORDERS

Desmopressin. *Desmopressin* is a synthetic, antidiuretic hormone that inhibits the production of urine. It is administered intranasally. A recent review suggests that desmopressin helps approximately 25% of children who use it, with minimal risk of adverse effects (Thompson and Rey, 1995). Although desmopressin is usually well tolerated, the most effective treatment for enuresis is behavioral methods such as the use of a pad and buzzer. In this method the bed is equipped with a pad that sets off a buzzer when the child wets. The buzzer wakes up the child.

Carbamazepine (Tegretol). Carbamazepine is an anticonvulsant that has been used in a variety of psychiatric disorders. In adults it has been effective in treating lithium-resistant mania and impulsive behavior. The drug has been used in prepubertal children, but very few studies have been placebo-controlled. The meager evidence to date suggests that carbamazepine may be useful in severe aggressive behavior (Green, 1995a). Doses may begin with 100 mg given twice a day and then gradually increased to a total of 400 to 800 mg per day in 3 divided doses. Side effects include fatigue, dizziness, blurred vision, mild ataxia, slurred speech, skin rash and, rarely, blood dyscrasias.

Buspirone (BuSpar). Buspirone is an anxiolytic agent that is not related to the benzodiazepines. Its mechanism of action differs from the benzodiazepines and the SSRIs and appears to be a result of its affinity for a specific serotonin receptor. Buspirone does not cause physical dependence and does not cover benzodiazepine withdrawal. A recent study in 15 children with anxiety disorders showed that doses of 10 to 20 mg per day given in 2 divided doses resulted in significant improvement as measured by a global scale. This improvement was evident within 3 to 4 weeks of starting the medication. Side effects included tiredness, sleep disturbance, abdominal discomfort, and headache (Simeon et al, 1994). In prepubertal children the drug may be initiated at 2.5 to 5 mg per day and increased thereafter every 3 to 4 days to a total of 20 mg per day in 2 to 3 divided doses (Coffey, 1990).

Clonazepam (Klonopin). Clonazepam is a long-acting benzodiazepine that is approved as an anticonvulsant. In adults it is also used to treat anxiety disorders and tics. A recent study of 15 prepubertal children showed that clonazepam can be useful in anxiety disorders in some children, but side effects were common and problematic. The most common side effects were disinhibited behavior, irritability, and drowsiness (Graae et al, 1994). We recommend a gradual increase in the dosage, for example, beginning with 0.25 mg in the morning and increasing to 0.25 mg twice daily after 3 to 4 days. Thereafter the dose may be increased slowly to a maximum of 2 mg per day in divided doses. Upon discontinuation, clonazepam should be tapered gradually.

Propranolol (Inderal). Propranolol is a nonselective beta-adrenergic blocker that was originally developed for reducing hypertension and controlling cardiac arrhythmias. Beta-adrenergic blockade reduces peripheral autonomic tone and, consequently, decreases palpitations, tremors, and perspiration. In adults propranolol has been used with mixed success for generalized anxiety, performance anxiety, panic attacks, rage outbursts, and akathisia. To date there is very little information regarding its use in children. The few studies that are available indicate that propranolol may be useful in controlling severe aggressive behavior in children and adolescents who have not responded to standard treatment. Doses range from 30 to 150 mg per day in three divided doses (Green, 1995a). Propranolol should not be withdrawn abruptly.

REFERENCES

Ambrosini PJ et al: Antidepressant treatments in children and adolescents, Part I: affective disorders, *J Am Acad Child Adolesc Psychiatry* 32:1, 1993.

American Psychiatric Association: *Diagnostic and statistical manual of mental disorders,* ed 4, Washington, DC, 1994.

Barkley RA: *Attention deficit hyperactivity disorder: a handbook for diagnosis and treatment,* New York, 1990, Guilford.

Barr LC, Goodman WK, Price LH: Physical symptoms associated with paroxetine discontinuation, *Am J Psychiatry* 151:289, 1994.

Biederman J et al: A double-blind placebo-controlled study of desipramine in the treatment of ADD, Part I: efficacy, *J Am Acad Child Adolesc Psychiatry* 28:777, 1989.

Biederman J et al: A naturalistic study of 24-hour electro-cardiographic recordings and echocardiographic findings in children and adolescents treated with desipramine, *J Am Acad Child Adolesc Psychiatry* 32:805, 1993.

Black A: The drugging of America's children, *Redbook* p 41, Dec, 1994.

Boyer WF, Blumhardt CL: The safety profile of paroxetine, *J Clin Psychiatry* 53(suppl):61, 1992.

Campbell M et al: Lithium in hospitalized aggressive children with conduct disorder: a double-blind and placebo-controlled study, *J Am Acad Child Adolesc Psychiatry* 34:445, 1995.

Campbell M, Cueva JE: Psychopharmacology in child and adolescent psychiatry: a review of the past seven years, Part I. *J Am Acad Child Adolesc Psychiatry* 34:1124, 1995.

Chappell PB, Leckman JF, and Riddle MA: The pharmacologic treatment of tic disorders, *Child Adolesc Psychiatr Clin North Am* 4:197, 1995.

Chappell PB et al: Guanfacine treatment of comorbid attention deficit hyperactivity disorder and Tourette's syndrome: preliminary clinical experience, *J Am Acad Child Adolesc Psychiatry* 34:1140, 1995.

Coffey BJ: Anxiolytics for children and adolescents: traditional and new drugs, *J Child Adolesc Psychopharmacol* 1:57, 1990.

Cunningham CE, Siegel LS, Offord DR: A dose-response analysis of the effects of methylphenidate on the peer interaction and simulated classroom performance of ADD children with and without conduct problems, *J Child Psychol Psychiatry* 32(3):439, 1991.

DeLong GR, Aldershof AL: Long-term experience with lithium treatment in childhood: correlation with clinical diagnosis, *J Am Acad Child Adolesc Psychiatry* 26:389, 1987.

DeVeaugh-Geiss J et al: Clomipramine in child and adolescent obsessive-compulsive disorder: a multicenter trial. *J Am Acad Child Adolesc Psychiatry* 31:45, 1992.

Dulcan MK: Using psychostimulants to treat behavior disorders of children and adolescents, *J Child Adolesc Psychopharmacol* 1:7, 1990.

DuPaul GJ, Barkley RA: Medication therapy. In Barkley RA, editor: *Attention deficit hyperactivity disorder: a handbook for diagnosis and treatment*, New York, 1990, Guilford.

Emslie G et al: Efficacy of fluoxetine in depressed children and adolescents. Paper presented at the annual meeting of the American Academy of Child and Adolescent Psychiatry, New Orleans, Oct, 1995.

Fristad MA, Weller EB, Weller RA: The Mania Rating Scale: can it be used in children? A preliminary report, *J Am Acad Child Adolesc Psychiatry* 31:252, 1992.

Gadow KD et al: Efficacy of methylphenidate for attention-deficit hyperactivity disorder in children with tic disorder, *Arch Gen Psychiatry* 152:444, 1995.

Geller B et al: Preliminary data on the relationship between nortriptyline plasma level and response in depressed children, *Am J Psychiatry* 143:1283, 1986.

Geller B et al: Pharmacokinetically designed double-blind placebo-controlled study of nortriptyline in 6- to 12-year-olds with major depressive disorder, *J Am Acad Child Adolesc Psychiatry* 31:34, 1992.

Graae F et al: Clonazepam in childhood anxiety disorders, *J Am Acad Child Adolesc Psychiatry* 33:372, 1994.

Green WH: *Child and adolescent clinical psychopharmacology*, Baltimore, 1995a, Williams and Wilkins.

Green WH: The treatment of attention-deficit hyperactivity disorder with nonstimulant medications, *Child Adolesc Psychiatr Clin North Am* 4:169, 1995b.

Greenhill LL: Attention-deficit hyperactivity disorder: the stimulants, *Child Adolesc Psychiatr Clin North Am* 4(1):123, 1995.

Greist JH et al: Efficacy and tolerability of serotonin transport inhibitors in obsessive-compulsive disorder, *Arch Gen Psychiatry* 52:53, 1995.

Horrigan JP, Barnhill LJ: Paroxetine-pimozide drug interaction, *J Am Acad Child Adolesc Psychiatry* 33:1060, 1994 (letter).

Horrigan JP, Barnhill LJ: Guanfacine for treatment of attention-deficit hyperactivity disorder in boys, *J Child Adolesc Psychopharmacol* 5:215, 1995.

Hunt RD, Minderaa RB, Cohen DJ: Clonidine benefits children with attention deficit disorder and hyperactivity: report of a double-blind placebo-crossover therapeutic trial, *J Am Acad Child Adolesc Psychiatry* 24:617, 1985.

Hunt RD, Arnsten AFT, Asbell MD: An open trial of guanfacine in the treatment of attention deficit hyperactivity disorder, *J Am Acad Child Adolesc Psychiatry* 34:50, 1995.

Institute of Medicine: *Research on children and adolescents with mental, behavioral, and developmental disorder*, Washington, DC, 1989, National Academy Press.

Joshi PT, Capozzoli JA, Coyle JT: Low-dose neuroleptic therapy for children with childhood onset pervasive developmental disorder, *Am J Psychiatry* 145:335, 1988.

King RA, Nosphitz JD: Obsessive-compulsive disorder. In King RA, Nosphitz JD, editors: *Pathways of gowth: essentials of child psychiatry,* vol 2, New York, 1991, Wiley.

King RA et al: Emergence of self-destructive phenomena in children and adolescents during fluoxetine treatment, *J Am Academy Child Adolesc Psychiatry* 30:179, 1991.

Klein DF et al: *Diagnosis and drug treatment of psychiatric disorders: adults and children,* ed 2, Baltimore, 1980, Williams & Wilkins.

Klein RG, Koplewicz HS, Kanner A: Imipramine treatment of chilldren with separation anxiety disorder, *J Am Acad Child Adolesc Psychiatry* 31(1):21, 1992.

Leckman JF et al: Clonidine treatment of Gilles de la Tourette syndrome, *Arch Gen Psychiatry* 48:324, 1991.

Leckman JF et al: Pathogenesis of Tourette syndrome: clues from the clinical phenotype and natural history, *Adv Neurol* 58:15, 1992.

Leonard HL et al: Treatment of obsessive-compulsive disorder with clomipramine and desipramine in children and adolescents, *Arch Gen Psychiatry* 46:1088, 1989.

Leonard HL et al: Tics and Tourette's disorder: a 2- to 7-year follow-up of 54 obsessive-compulsive children, *Am J Psychiatry* 149:1244, 1993.

Leysen JE et al: Risperidone: a novel antipsychotic with balanced serotonin-dopamine antagonism, receptor occupancy profile, and pharmacologic activity, *J Clin Psychiatry* 55:5-12, 1994.

Lombroso PJ et al: Risperidone treatment of children and adolescents with chronic tic disorders: a preliminary report, *J Am Acad Child Adolesc Psychiatry* 34:1147, 1995.

Louie AK, Lannon RA, Ajari LJ: Withdrawal reaction after sertraline discontinuation, *Am J Psychiatry* 151(3):450, 1994.

Mandoki MW: Risperidone treatment of children and adolescents: increased risk of extrapyramidal side effects, *J Child Adolesc Psychopharmacol* 5:49, 1995.

March JS, Leonard HL, Swedo SE: Pharmacotherapy of obsessive-compulsive disorder, *Child Adolesc Psychiatr Clin North Am* 4:217, 1995.

March JS, Mulle K, Herbel B: Behavioral psychotherapy for children and adolescents with obsessive-compulsive disorder: an open trial with a new protocol driven treatment package, *J Am Acad Child Adolesc Psychiatry* 33:333, 1994.

Marder SR, Meibach RC: Risperidone in the treatment of schizophrenia, *Am J Psychiatry* 151:825, 1994.

McClellan J, Werry J: Practice parameters for the assessment and treatment of children and adolescents with schizophrenia, *J Am Acad Child Adolesc Psychiatry* 33:616, 1994.

McDougle CJ et al: The psychopharmacology of obsessive-compulsive disorder: implications for treatment and pathogenesis, *Psychiatr Clin North Am* 16:749, 1993.

McDougle CJ et al: Haloperidol addition in fluvoxamine-refractory obsessive-compulsive disorder: a double-blind, placebo-controlled study in patients with and without tics, *Arch Gen Psychiatry* 51:302, 1994.

Pauls DL et al: A family study of Gilles de la Tourette syndrome, *Am J Hum Genet* 48:154, 1991.

Pelham WE et al: Relative efficacy of long-acting stimulants on children with attention deficit-hyperactivity disorder: a comparison of standard methylphenidate, sustained-release methylphenidate, sustained-release dextroamphetamine, and pemoline, *Pediatrics* 86:226, 1990.

Popper CW: The story of four salts, *J Child Adolesc Psychopharmacol* 4:217, 1994.

Popper CW: Combining methylphenidate and clonidine: pharmacologic questions and news reports about sudden death, *J Child Adolesc Psychopharmacol* 5:157, 1995.

Porrino LJ et al: A naturalistic assessment of the motor activity of hyperactive boys, Part I. *Arch Gen Psychiatry* 40:681, 1983a.

Porrino LJ et al: A naturalistic assessment of the motor activity of hyperactive boys, Part II. *Arch Gen Psychiatry* 40:688, 1983b.

Preskorn SH: Pharmacokinetics of antidepressants: why and how they are relevant to treatment, *J Clin Psychiatry* 54(suppl):14, 1993.

Puig-Antich J et al: Imipramine in prepubertal major depressive disorders, *Arch Gen Psychiatry* 44:81, 1987.

Riddle MA, Geller B, Ryan N: Another sudden death in a child treated with desipramine, *J Am Acad Child Adolesc Psychiatry* 32:792, 1993.

Riddle MA et al: Tardive dyskinesia following haloperidol treatment in Tourette's syndrome, *Arch Gen Psychiatry* 44:98, 1987.

Riddle MA et al: Behavioral side effects of fluoxetine, *J Child Adolesc Psychopharmacol* 3:193, 1991.

Riddle MA et al: Double-blind, crossover trial of fluoxetine and placebo in children and adolescents with obsessive compulsive disorder, *J Am Acad Child Adoles Psychiatry* 31:1062, 1992.

Riddle MA et al: Effects of methylphenidate discontinuation and re-initiation in children with Tourette's syndrome and ADHD, *J Child Adolesc Psychopharmacol* 5:205, 1995.

Riddle MA et al: Obsessive compulsive disorder in children and adolescents: phenomenology and family history, *J Am Acad Child Adolesc Psychiatry* 29:766, 1990.

Safer DJ, Krager JM: A survey of medication treatment for hyperactive/inattentive students, *JAMA* 260:2256, 1988.

Sallee FR, Sethuraman G, Rock CM: Effects of pimozide on cognition in children with Tourette syndrome: interaction with comorbid attention-deficit hyperactivity disorder, *Acta Psychiatr Scand* 90:4, 1994.

Scahill L: Contemporary approaches to pharmacotherapy in Tourette syndrome and obsessive-compulsive disorder, *J Child Adolesc Psychiatr Nurs* 9(1):27, 1996.

Scahill L, Lynch KA, Ort SI: Tourette's syndrome: update and review, *J Sch Nurs* 11:22, 1995.

Scahill L, Ort SI: Clinical ratings in child psychiatric nursing, *J Child Adolesc Psychiatr Nurs* 8:33, 1995.

Scahill L et al: Behavioral therapy in children and adolescents with obsessive-compulsive disorder: a pilot study, *J Child Adolesc Psychopharmacol* (submitted).

Simeon JG et al: Adolescent depression: a placebo controlled treatment study and follow-up, *Prog Neuropsychopharmacol Biol Psychiatry* 14:791, 1990.

Simeon JG et al: Buspirone therapy of mixed anxiety disorders in childhood and adolescence: a pilot study, *J Child Adolesc Psychopharmacol* 4:29, 1994.

Simeon JG et al: Risperidone effects in treatment-resistant adolescents: preliminary case reports, *J Child Adolesc Psychopharmacol* 5:69, 1995.

Singer HS et al: The treatment of attention-deficit hyperactivity disorder in Tourette's syndrome: a double-blind placebo-controlled study with clonidine and desipramine, *Pediatrics* 95:74, 1995.

Spencer T et al: Nortriptyline treatment of children with attention-deficit disorder and tic disorder or Tourette's syndrome, *J Am Acad Child Adolesc Psychiatry* 32:205, 1993.

Swedo SE et al: Obsessive-compulsive disorder in children and adolescents, *Arch Gen Psychiatry* 46:335, 1989.

Szatmari P, Offord DR, Boyle MH. Ontario Child Health Study: prevalence of attention deficit disorder with hyperactivity, *J Child Psychol Psychiatr* 30:219, 1989.

Thompson S, Rey JM: Functional enuresis: is desmopressin the answer? *J Am Acad Child Adolesc Psychiatry* 34:266, 1995.

Tierney E et al: Sertraline for major depression in children and adolescents: preliminary clinical experience, *J Child Adolesc Psychopharmacol* 5:13, 1995.

Volkmar FR et al: Field trial for autistic disorder in DSM-IV, *Am J Psychiatry* 151:1361, 1994.

Walkup JT et al: Evidence for a mixed model of inheritance in Tourette's syndrome. Poster presentation at the annual meeting of the American Academy of Child and Adolescent Psychiatry, New Orleans, Oct, 1995.

Weller EB, Weller RA, Fristad MA: Bipolar disorder in children: misdiagnosis, underdiagnosis, and future directions, *J Am Acad Child Adolesc Psychiatry* 34:709, 1995.

CHAPTER 16

Psychopharmacology for Adolescents

LAWRENCE SCAHILL

SCOPE OF THE PROBLEM

Mental illness afflicts an estimated 12% (roughly 8 million) of children under age 18 in the United States (Institute of Medicine, 1989). A recent national survey indicates that nearly 500,000 of the 3 to 4 million adolescents (youths ages 13 to 18) with mental disorders actually use inpatient or outpatient mental health services (Pottick et al, 1995). This obvious discrepancy between the estimated number of adolescents with mental illness and those using services indicates that many adolescents with mental disorders are not using mental health services (Institute of Medicine, 1989). Several factors may explain this, including limited access to services for some segments of the population (Pottick et al, 1995) and use of primary health care systems for psychosocial and pharmacologic interventions such as methylphenidate (Horwitz et al, 1992; Safer and Krager, 1988). Nonetheless psychopharmacologic interventions are being used with increasing frequency in child and adolescent psychiatry, often without sufficient research data to inform practitioners (Popper, 1995). Finally, the proliferation of new medications poses an extraordinary challenge to the clinician in child and adolescent psychiatry. This chapter provides specific information about treating adolescents with psychotropic drugs. For example, medications such as lithium and valproic acid are used more commonly in adolescents compared with prepubertal children, but treatment guidelines for adolescents may not be the same as those for adults. Although some repetition of content from previous chapters is unavoidable, readers will be referred to those chapters when appropriate.

GENERAL PRINCIPLES OF ADOLESCENT PSYCHOPHARMACOLOGY

As with other age groups, psychotropic drug intervention should be viewed as one aspect of a multidimensional treatment approach. Although drug intervention may be the best studied treatment modality, drug therapy alone is unlikely to ensure optimal development in youth that have serious emotional or behavioral problems. Moreover, in addition to concerns such as the complex pharmacokinetics of the developing child, other issues such as treatment compliance, risk of drug abuse, and the emotional vicissitudes of adolescence are crucial variables for successful pharmacotherapy in this age group.

Strategies for Effective Administration

Evaluation. A careful review of presenting problems, their onset, course, and current severity, as well as any prior treatments and the adolescent's response to those interventions, is the foundation of a comprehensive evaluation. Other essential elements include the patient's medical history; developmental history; family history; and school, social, and family functioning. The collection of these data can be aided with the use of clinical ratings, parent and teacher checklists, and self-reports (Barkley, 1990; Scahill and Ort, 1995). The clinician should also ensure that the adolescent has had a recent physical examination, and, depending on the medication being considered, screening blood tests and an electrocardiogram (ECG) are often indicated as well.

Collaboration. The goal of the assessment is to identify the source of greatest impairment and define the target symptoms for any intervention. Identifying target symptoms involves careful collaboration among the clinicians, the family, and the adolescent. Failure to include the adolescent and the family in this negotiation can be a threat to the treatment alliance and perhaps the treatment plan as well.

Education. The adolescent patient and his or her parents should be thoroughly educated about the medication chosen and the reasons for its selection. This session may include a mutual identification of treatment goals, a review of common side effects, clarification of any delay in therapeutic response, for example, with antidepressants, and a review of alternative treatments. The clinician should also explore the expectations of the adolescent and the family concerning the medication trial to make certain that these expectations are appropriate.

Assessment and ongoing monitoring. Some aspects of assessment and monitoring are drug-specific. For example, adolescent males appear to be at greater risk for acute dystonic reactions to neuroleptics compared with adults (Green, 1995). To avoid alarm and promote early detection of a dystonic reaction, both the parents and the youth should be informed about this possible side effect.

In the early phase of treatment with any psychotropic agent, the adolescent should have frequent follow-ups to review body systems and to evaluate activity, appetite, sleep, elimination, and energy level. Following this initial phase of treatment, attention should be paid to both therapeutic and adverse effects.

Other Issues of Administration

Compliance. The efficacy and safety of any psychotropic medication cannot be evaluated if the patient is inconsistent in taking the drug. Although essential to treatment compliance, parents may not monitor their adolescent children as closely as they would a younger child. Thus it may be necessary to negotiate a system of reminders and medication monitoring with the adolescent patient and the parents to ensure optimal compliance with the medication schedule. This negotiation may include the clinician's pledge to adjust the dose of medication to promote therapeutic effects and minimize side effects.

Suicide and overdose. Drug-related emergencies among 6- to 17-year-olds accounted for more than 21,000 emergency room visits in 1988 (Kalogerakis, 1992). Suicide remains among the leading causes of death among adolescents. As many as 8.6% of adolescents acknowledge suicidal behavior (Kann et al, 1995). A recent national survey reports that tricyclic antidepressants (TCAs) and lithium were among the agents frequently used in intentional or accidental overdose. Both TCAs and lithium are being prescribed to adolescents more frequently than in the past, and both can be fatal. Although the relationship between suicidal ideation and medication is unclear, suicidal thought and attempt have been reported in adolescents being treated with the newer antidepressants such as fluoxetine (King et al, 1991). For these reasons, clinicians should be vigilant about suicidal thought and action in adolescents being treated with psychotropic drugs.

Toxic effects. Toxic effects occur when drug level surpasses therapeutic level. This is especially relevant for medications such as TCAs and lithium. Safe clinical management of these agents requires monitoring for signs of toxicity and informing parents (and adolescents to the extent that is developmentally appropriate) about these signs.

Abuse. Abuse of drugs is another important issue when working with adolescent patients. The patient, a friend, or a sibling may experiment with prescribed agents. In addition, the adolescent may be experimenting with or using illicit drugs while in treatment. These concerns require that a therapeutic alliance be developed with the adolescent and the family so that ongoing monitoring is perceived as helpful rather than imperious.

PSYCHOTROPIC MEDICATIONS USED WITH ADOLESCENTS

STIMULANTS

Indications

The stimulants methylphenidate, dextroamphetamine, and pemoline are the primary agents used to treat attention deficit hyperactivity disorder (ADHD) (Box 16-1).

ADHD is a heterogenous, relatively common disorder of childhood onset that is characterized by inattention, impulsiveness, and hyperactivity. The *DSM-IV* permits further subcategorization of ADHD into the primarily Inattentive type or primarily Hyperactive type (American Psychiatric Association, 1994). Depending on the definition and methods of case identification, ADHD affects an estimated 6% to 9% of the school-age population (Szatmari, Offord, and Boyle, 1989).

Until recently many clinicians and researchers believed that children "outgrow" ADHD. Although fidgeting and restlessness may be more prominent in adolescents than is hyperactivity, evidence from several prospective studies refutes the notion that children "outgrow" ADHD. These studies show that 40% to 70% of children with ADHD continue to meet criteria for diagnosis in adolescence. Moreover, adolescents with ADHD often demonstrate continued impairment across several domains, including academic, family, and interpersonal, and are at greater risk for legal trouble. Finally, those with comorbid conduct disorder have the poorest outcomes (Hechtman, 1992).

Empirical Support

The efficacy and safety of methylphenidate, dextroamphetamine, and pemoline have been replicated in numerous controlled studies (see Chapter 15, Psychopharmacology for Children, for a more detailed review). These studies show that stimulants decrease hyperactivity and motor restlessness and increase sustained attention. Stimulants may also improve antisocial behavior and interpersonal conflict. However, most studies have only considered the short-term benefit of stimulants, longer term benefits are more difficult to show (Schachar and Tannock, 1993).

Box 16-1 Stimulants Used to Treat Adolescents with ADHD

Methylphenidate (Ritalin)

Dosage: The total daily dose ranges from 0.6 to 2.1 mg per kg per day given in 2 or 3 divided doses. Methylphenidate is typically started at 5 mg once or twice a day and increased by 5 to 10 mg every 5 to 7 days. Doses above 60 mg are not recommended.

Available dose forms: 5- and 10-mg tablets; 20-mg sustained-release tablets.

Dextroamphetamine (Dexedrine)

Dosage: The total daily dose ranges from 0.3 mg to 1.5 mg per kg per day in 2, or occasionally, 3 divided doses. Dextroamphetamine is usually started at 5 mg per day and increased by 5 mg every 5 to 7 days. Doses above 40 mg per day are not recommended.

Available dose forms: 5- and 10-mg tablets; 5-, 10-, and 15-mg sustained-release tablets.

Pemoline (Cylert)

Dosage: The total daily dose ranges from 56.25 to 112.5 mg per day in a single morning dose. Treatment is initiated at 37.5 mg per day and is increased by 18.75 mg every 7 days as tolerated or until the maximum dose of 112.5 mg per day is reached.

Available dose forms: 18.75-, 37.5-, and 75-mg tablets.

Side effects related to above stimulants

Insomnia, loss of appetite, weight loss, behavioral rebound (as medication wears off), increased heart rate and blood pressure, involuntary movements, mood lability, and cognitive rigidity. Psychotic reactions can occur but are rare.

Mechanism of Action

Although the precise mechanism by which stimulants exert their positive effect is not known, it is presumed that the capacity of stimulants to increase the levels of dopamine and norepinephrine in the brain is central to this mechanism (Greenhill, 1995).

Clinical Management

Contemporary clinical management of an adolescent being treated with a stimulant includes a thorough evaluation to rule out other causes of behavioral disturbance. In addition, psychologic testing may be indicated if there are questions about intellectual functioning or learning disability. Assessment of general health status, sleep and appetite, and vital signs are also necessary. Finally, assessing the severity of the patient's symptoms and response to the medication can be aided by the use of parent and teacher checklists (Barkley, 1990; Scahill and Ort, 1995).

ANTIDEPRESSANTS

Indications

Antidepressant medications are approved for treating depression in youths over age 12. A small group of chemically unrelated antidepressants, including clomipramine (Anafranil), fluoxetine (Prozac), and fluvoxamine (Luvox), are approved for treating obsessive-compulsive disorder (OCD). Imipramine (Tofranil) is also approved for treating enuresis. Although not officially approved for use in ADHD, several antidepressants have shown benefit for treating both children and adolescents with the disorder (Table 16-1).

Empirical Support

Depression. All currently available antidepressants have demonstrated efficacy and safety in treating adults with depression. The effectiveness of these agents has been less convincing in children and adolescents with depression. To date there have been only 12 controlled trials of antidepressants in depressed children and adolescents. In a recent review of 11 of these studies Kye and Ryan (1995) noted that only one study found antidepressant medication to be of significant benefit. An additional study presented by Emslie et al (1995) showed that fluoxetine was significantly better than placebo. These predominately negative results may be partially caused by differences in neurotransmitter systems in children, adolescents, and adults (Kye and Ryan, 1995; Laraia, 1996). In addition, because of a surprisingly large percentage of placebo responders in these studies of depressed children and

Table 16-1 Antidepressants Commonly Used With Adolescents

Name of drug	Class*	Dose range (mg/day)†	Disorder(s) with empirical support
Imipramine (Tofranil)	TCA	50-150	Enuresis, depression, ADHD, separation anxiety
Desipramine (Norpramin)	TCA	50-150	Depression, ADHD
Nortriptyline (Pamelor)	TCA	50-125	Depression, ADHD
Clomipramine (Anafranil)	TCA/SRI	50-150	OCD
Fluoxetine (Prozac)	SSRI	10-60	OCD, depression
Sertraline (Zoloft)	SSRI	50-200	OCD‡, depression
Fluvoxamine (Luvox)	SSRI	50-200	OCD‡, depression
Paroxetine (Paxil)	SSRI	10-40	Depression‡
Bupropion (Wellbutrin)	Aminoketone	100-250	ADHD, depression

*TCA = tricyclic, SSRI = selective serotonin reuptake inhibitor, SRI = serotonin reuptake inhibitor.
† Administered in a single or divided dose, depending on agent.
‡ Results from large clinical trials in children and adolescents are pending.

adolescents (as high as 50% in several trials), it is difficult to show a statistically significant difference between active drug and placebo (Kye and Ryan, 1995).

Obsessive-compulsive disorder. As noted in Table 16-1, results from large clinical trials are pending for the use of sertraline, fluvoxamine, and fluoxetine to treat children and adolescents with OCD. To date, fluoxetine and clomipramine are the only SSRIs that have been effective in controlled trials for treating this disorder in children and adolescents (DeVeaugh-Geiss et al, 1992; Riddle et al, 1992). (For a more complete review of SSRIs to treat children and adolescents with OCD see Chapter 15, Psychopharmacology for Children) (March, Leonard, and Swedo, 1995; Scahill, 1996).

Attention deficit hyperactivity disorder. Several TCAs and bupropion have been studied for their effectiveness in treating ADHD. Available evidence suggests that desipramine (Biederman et al, 1989), nortriptyline (Spencer et al, 1993), and bupropion (Barrickman et al, 1995) are effective against ADHD. In general, these agents have not produced the same level of improvement as that shown by stimulants, but they do have potential advantages:

1. They have a longer duration of action.
2. They may be given as a single dose without rebound.
3. Some permit monitoring of plasma drug levels.
4. They have minimal potential for abuse.
5. TCAs have not been associated with increased tics.

Mechanism of Action

TCAs block serotonin reuptake and are potent blockers of norepinephrine reuptake, which ultimately enhances noradrenergic function. The SSRIs and clomipramine inhibit the reuptake of serotonin by presynaptic receptors, which, in turn, enhances serotonergic functioning. For both the standard TCAs and the SSRIs, however, other neurotransmitters are also involved. The precise mechanism of bupropion remains unclear, though it appears to have dopamine agonist effects.

Clinical Management

Specific guidelines for dosing the various types of antidepressants are provided in Chapter 15, Psychopharmacology for Children. General principles include starting at low doses followed by gradual increases. The upper dose limit for TCAs ranges from a low of 1.5 mg per kg per day for nortriptyline to 3 mg per kg per day for others. Daily dosages of the SSRIs vary so widely that it is difficult to provide a mg per kg formula. The average daily dose of bupropion may be as high as 5 mg per kg and is typically given in divided doses.

Side effects. The frequency and seriousness of adverse effects vary greatly among the different classes of antidepressants (see Chapter 5, Mood Disorders, and Chapter 15, Psychopharmacology for Children). TCAs are associated with anticholinergic side effects such as dry mouth, blurred vision, sweating, tremor, and urinary retention. Central nervous system (CNS) side effects include dizziness, drowsiness, agitation, and rarely, seizures. The cardiovascular side effects are of particular concern with TCAs (Riddle, Geller, and Ryan, 1993; Scahill and Lynch, 1994; Green, 1995). Although controversy continues concerning the degree of risk for cardiac arrhythmias attributable to TCAs, available evidence suggests pulse, blood pressure, and the ECG should be monitored in adolescents receiving a TCA. Vital signs and an ECG should be obtained before initiating treatment and repeated during upward dose adjustment, after reaching a stable dose, and periodically during treatment (see Chapter 15, Psychopharmacology for Children, for specific guidelines).

SSRIs appear to be better tolerated than TCAs and there is no evidence of serious cardiac effects. Common side effects include decreased appetite, diarrhea, abdominal pain, and fatigue. Perhaps the most common side effect is behavioral activation, which may be accompanied by motor restlessness, impulsiveness, and insomnia. This effect has been well documented for fluoxetine, but it clearly occurs with the other SSRIs as well (Riddle et al, 1991; Scahill, 1996). These side effects are most likely to occur early in treatment or with dose increases. There have also been reports of suicidal ideation and self-injurious behavior, but this has also been observed with other types of antidepressants (King et al, 1991).

The side effects of bupropion include skin rash, dry mouth, insomnia, agitation, headache, constipation, tremor, and tics. Although apparently rare, more serious adverse effects such as serum sickness and seizures have been reported (Sikich et al, 1995; Green, 1995).

In summary, the best available evidence suggests that fluoxetine is probably the best choice for treating depression in adolescents, with nortriptyline as the second-line agent. Until results of recent clinical trials become available, clomipramine and fluoxetine appear to be the first-line treatment for OCD. Concerns about the potential for cardiac conduction abnormalities with desipramine and increasing concern about adverse effects of bupropion suggest that nortriptyline may be the antidepressant of choice for ADHD.

ANTIPSYCHOTICS

Antipsychotic drugs are also discussed in Chapters 4, Schizophrenia and Other Psychoses, and 15, Psychopharmacology for Children. This chapter focuses on the treatment of adolescents with psychotic disorders.

Indications

Psychotic disorders such as schizophrenia are the primary indication for antipsychotic drugs. They are also used to treat aggressive behavior, tic disorders, and severe behavioral problems associated with autism and mental retardation (see Chapter 15, Psychopharmacology for Children).

Psychotic disorder. *Psychotic disorder* is a broad term that embraces a group of heterogenous conditions having multiple etiologies. The best described psychotic disorder is schizophrenia, though it, too, is probably heterogenous with respect to etiology. Schizophrenia may emerge in childhood but more often it begins in late adolescence. Symptoms include hallucinations, delusions, disordered thinking, blunted affect, idiosyncratic speech, concrete thinking, and profound social deficits. In children diagnostic uncertainty can be present between schizophrenia and autism, but this ambiguity is less problematic during adolescence when schizophrenia resembles the adult form of the disorder. However, the hallucinations, delusions, and thought disorder seen in schizophrenia can be present in psychotic depression, bipolar disorder, metabolic disorders such as Wilson's disease, or drug-induced psychosis. Thus careful assessment is essential when evaluating an adolescent with psychotic symptoms.

Schizophrenia in childhood is considered rare (approximately 2 cases per 100,000). In contrast, the prevalence of schizophrenia among older adolescents is several fold more common, affecting between 0.5% and 1% of the general population. Schizophrenia is more common in males, tends to be chronic, and is associated with significant disability.

Empirical Support

The phenothiazines were the first drugs used to treat psychoses in adolescents. Since then several other classes of antipsychotic drugs have been introduced. More than 100 randomized clinical trials with neuroleptics have been conducted in adults with schizophrenia. These studies provide a convincing body of evidence concerning the effectiveness of neuroleptics to treat adults with schizophrenia. Unfortunately, the number of controlled studies in adolescents is far fewer (Teicher and Glod, 1990; McClellan and Werry, 1994; Green, 1995). Currently there is little or no evidence to support the use of one antipsychotic agent over another. Until such evidence becomes available, deciding which antipsychotic drug to use in a given case is predicated on the experience of the clinician, the past treatment experience of the patient, and side effect profiles.

Mechanism of Action

Neuroleptics block dopamine at the postsynaptic D-2 receptor. However, to varying degrees antipsychotic agents also block histamine, norepinephrine, and acetylcholine receptors. In addition, antipsychotic drugs differ in their affinity for specific dopamine receptor subtypes. The blocking of these additional neurotransmitters and differences in affinity for dopamine receptor subtypes among the various antipsychotic agents influence their potency and side effect profiles. For example, the low-potency neuropleptics such as thioridazine are less D2-selective and more anticholinergic than haloperidol. Not surprisingly, thioridazine is used at higher doses, and more anticholinergic side effects are associated with it than with haloperidol.

The newer antipsychotic agents, clozapine and risperidone, have relatively weak affinity for D-2 receptors but are potent serotonin antagonists. The serotonin antagonism is believed to reduce the risk of extrapyramidal side effects (EPSEs) and may protect against tardive dyskinesia as well (see Chapter 4, Schizophrenia and Other Psychoses).

Clinical Management

An overview of drugs used to treat psychotic disorders is presented in Table 16-2 and Box 16-2. For additional discussion of antipsychotic drugs see Chapter 4, Schizophrenia and Other Psychoses; for information related to pediatric usage see Chapter 15, Psychopharmacology for Children.

As shown in Table 16-2, the dosages of these neuroleptics vary tremendously. In general, the low-potency neuroleptics such as chlorpromazine and thioridazine require higher doses and are more likely to be accompanied by sedation and anticholinergic effects. The high-potency compounds such as thiothixene, trifluoperazine, and haloperidol are effective at much lower doses. However, these agents are also associated with an increased risk of dystonic reactions, akathisia, and parkinsonism.

Clozapine, which is not recommended for use with children under age 16, has proved effective in treating patients with schizophrenia who have failed to

Table 16-2 Commonly Used Antipsychotic Agents for the Treatment of Psychosis and Severe Behavior Disturbance in Adolescents

Name of drug	Class	Typical dose range mg/day	Studied in adolescents
Chlorpromazine (Thorazine)	Phenothiazine	50-400	Yes
Thioridazine (Mellaril)	Phenothiazine	50-400	Yes
Trifluoperazine (Stelazine)	Phenothiazine	10-20	Yes
Fluphenazine (Prolixin)	Phenothiazine	2-8	Yes
Haloperidol (Haldol)	Butyrophenone	2-10	Yes
Thiothixene (Navane)	Thioxanthene	8-40	Yes
Loxapine (Loxitane)	Dibenzoxazepine	60-100	Yes
Clozapine (Clozaril)	Dibenzodiazepine	100-700	Yes
Risperidone (Risperdal)	Benzisoxazole	2-8	Yes

respond to standard antipsychotic medications. However, clozapine can cause life-threatening agranulocytosis and hence is generally not used unless standard antipsychotic medications have failed.

Risperidone, an even newer antipsychotic medication that shares some features in common with clozapine but without the same risk for agranulocytosis, has shown promise for treating adolescents with psychosis (Mandoki, 1995; Simeon et al, 1995). These open-label studies show that, although effective, risperidone is not free of EPSEs. For example, 6 of 10 youngsters (age range 7 to 17 years) treated by Mandoki (1995) experienced EPSEs such as dystonia, muscle rigidity, dyskinesia, and/or oculogyric crises.

LITHIUM

Indications

Lithium is a naturally occurring element that is indicated for treating bipolar disorder. A full discussion of lithium can be found in Chapter 5, Mood Disorders.

Bipolar disorder. Over the past several decades various criteria have been used to define bipolar disorder. The *DSM-IV* identifies two broad types: bipolar I and bipolar II. Bipolar I is characterized by the occurrence of a manic episode but may occur in the absence of depression. In contrast, bipolar II disorder is marked by a history of major depression and hypomanic episodes (American Psychiatric Association, 1994). A manic episode is defined by the presence of elevated or irritable mood and three or more additional clinical features (Box 16-3).

The prevalence of bipolar illness in adolescents has recently been estimated at approximately 1% (Lewinsohn, Klein, and Seeley, 1995). In this large community survey, the authors identified 18 cases of bipolar illness, 11 of which were bipolar II

Box 16-2 Guidelines for Selected Antipsychotic Drugs Used to Treat Adolescents With Psychotic Disorders

Thioridazine (Mellaril)

Start with 25 to 50 mg 2 or 3 times per day depending on severity of presenting symptoms. Dose can be gradually increased over 1 to 3 weeks as tolerated to bring about symptomatic relief. Typical dose is 200 mg per day in 2 or 3 divided doses. Common side effects include sedation, weight gain, dry mouth, and blurred vision. Extrapyramidal effects are not common.

Trifluoperazine (Stelazine)

Start with 1 to 5 mg 2 times per day, with gradual increases over 2 to 3 weeks up to 15 mg per day in 2 divided doses. Common side effects include dystonic reactions, akathisia, and drowsiness.

Thiothixene (Navane)

Start with 2 mg 3 times per day and gradually increase to 5 mg 3 times per day or higher if necessary. Typical dose is 15 to 20 mg per day in 3 divided doses. Common side effects include drowsiness, dystonic reactions, weight gain, and akathisia.

Haloperidol (Haldol)

Start with 0.5 to 2 mg 2 or 3 times daily. Higher starting doses may be required in acutely disturbed adolescents. The dose can then be adjusted upward to achieve symptomatic control or decreased to manage side effects. Average dose is about 10 mg per day in 2 or 3 divided doses. The maintenance dose can usually be given twice daily. Common side effects include muscle rigidity, dystonic reactions, akathisia, weight gain, and cognitive blunting.

Loxapine (Loxitane)

Start with 10 mg twice daily and adjust according to therapeutic and adverse effects. Typical dose is 80 mg per day. Higher doses may be required in some cases, but dose does not usually exceed 100 mg per day. Common side effects include muscle rigidity and sedation.

Clozapine (Clozaril)

Start with 25 mg once or twice a day and increase daily over a 2-week period to a target dose range of 300 to 450 mg per day. The dose is then increased more slowly as needed to achieve benefit. A dose of 700 mg per day is usually considered the maximum daily dose for adolescents. Side effects include weight gain (which can be substantial), tachycardia, orthostatic hypotension, seizures (risk appears to be dose related), and agranulocytosis, which occurs in as many as 2% of patients.

Risperidone (Risperdal)

Start with 0.5 mg twice daily and increase in 0.5-mg every 3 or 4 days to a total dose of 3 mg per day in 2 divided doses. Thereafter the dose should be increased more slowly, e.g., weekly. The average dose range is 3 to 6 mg per day. Side effects include weight gain, drowsiness, dystonic reactions (especially if the dose is increased too rapidly), dizziness, tachycardia, and anxiety.

Box 16-3 Definition of a Manic Episode

A manic episode includes three or more of the following:
Grandiosity
Pressured speech or excessive talking
Decreased need for sleep
Flight of ideas or racing thoughts
Distractibility
Hyperactivity
Excessive pleasure-seeking behavior

cases, that is, had a history of depression. Girls were affected more frequently than boys. The mean age of onset for the whole group was about 12 years, with depression being the most common feature present at onset. This finding is consistent with a prospective study of 79 children with major depression in which nearly a third went on to develop bipolar illness (Geller, Fox, and Clark, 1994).

Two other findings from the community survey by Lewinsohn et al (1995) are worth noting. First, the authors identified 97 cases of "subclinical" bipolar illness. These youngsters (55 girls and 42 boys) had past or current symptoms of mania that were not severe enough to warrant a diagnosis. Second, of the 18 bipolar cases identified, only one had been treated with lithium. These findings underscore the importance of careful assessment before initiating therapy so that subclinical cases are not treated inappropriately and true cases are not overlooked.

Empirical Support

The evidence supporting the use of lithium in adolescents with bipolar disorder derives from case reports, open trials, and a small number of controlled trials. These studies suggest that lithium is effective and safe in adolescents with bipolar illness. Nonetheless, for reasons that are not clear, lithium is not always successful in treating adolescents with bipolar illness (Alessi et al, 1994). A naturalistic study by Strober et al, 1990 showed that youngsters with bipolar illness who discontinued lithium were three times more likely to relapse compared with those who remained on maintenance therapy. This finding suggests, as shown in adults with bipolar illness, that lithium may have prophylactic value for preventing future manic episodes.

Mechanism of Action

Lithium is an alkali metal and is in the same chemical family as sodium and potassium. Although it has been used to treat psychiatric disorders for more than four decades, only recently have its complex neurophysiologic effects begun to be understood. Lithium is known to enhance several neurotransmitter systems, including serotonin, norepinephrine, and dopamine. In addition, lithium has other neurobiologic effects on ion channels and other cellular activity (Alessi et al, 1994).

Clinical Management

Before starting a trial of lithium, the adolescent with bipolar illness should have a thorough medical evaluation, including a physical examination and careful medical history. Laboratory screening measures to assess thyroid and renal function, as well as an ECG and complete blood count, should also be obtained. Lithium is excreted by the kidneys, thus renal impairment could affect dosing and drug level. Lithium can decrease free thyroxine and triiodothyronine, but increased thyroid-releasing hormone typically compensates in euthyroid patients. Cardiac complications of lithium are not common, but it has been reported to alter cardiac conduction in some cases. Occasionally, lithium also causes elevated white blood cell and platelet counts. Thus renal function, thyroid function, ECG, and blood count should be monitored every 6 months or so during maintenance therapy. Girls of child-bearing age should be counseled about the importance of preventing pregnancy while taking lithium because of the elevated risk for birth defects related to fetal exposure.

Healthy adolescents usually tolerate lithium well, and the dose can be increased rapidly to therapeutic level (between 0.6 and 1.2 mEq per L). The initial dose of 300 to 600 mg may be given after a meal to decrease gastrointestinal (GI) side effects. Thereafter the dose can be increased by 300 to 600 mg every 4 to 5 days to the typical dose range of 1500 to 1800 mg per day in 2 divided doses. Levels should be checked 3 to 4 days after dose increases and after the typical dose range has been reached. The maintenance dose of lithium is usually lower, for example, 900 to 1200 mg per day, than the initial dose required to achieve therapeutic blood levels (Green, 1995; Botteron and Geller, 1995). How long an adolescent patient should remain on lithium following the resolution of a manic episode is unclear. Some researchers recommend years of stability before withdrawal of the drug (Botteron and Geller, 1995).

Side effects. Lithium can have serious side effects, but children and adolescents appear to tolerate it well. Common side effects include weight gain, tremor, headache, and GI upset (nausea, vomiting, and diarrhea). The stomach upset can often be reduced by administering the medication after meals. Other side effects include polydipsia, polyuria, ataxia, weakness, dysarthria, and mental confusion. Lithium may also exacerbate acne.

Interactions. Drugs with the ability to interact with lithium are discussed in Chapter 5, Mood Disorders.

Toxic effects. Lithium has a low therapeutic index, necessitating frequent serum level analysis. Adolescents should be advised that they may be required to measure lithium blood levels frequently. Lithium levels can be determined from saliva specimens, though saliva-to-serum ratios show tremendous individual variation. Because dehydration can lead to toxic levels of lithium, parents and adolescents should also be advised to maintain adequate hydration. Parents should be instructed to hold the medication if the child has a GI illness accompanied by frequent vomiting or diarrhea. Other toxic effects of lithium are discussed in Chapter 5, Mood Disorders.

OTHER DRUGS USED IN THE TREATMENT OF BIPOLAR DISORDER

Carbamazepine (Tegretol)

Lithium is the drug of choice for bipolar disorder in adolescents, but a substantial minority of patients do not respond to lithium (Alessi et al, 1994). Carbamazepine is an anticonvulsant that has been used in children and adolescents with seizure disorders for many years. It has also been shown to be an effective alternative for mood stabilization in adults. Unfortunately, there are very few studies demonstrating its efficacy in adolescents with bipolar illness (Green, 1995). The mechanism of action is not clear, but it is believed to reduce firing from the amygdala and turn down the limbic system (Botteron and Geller, 1995).

The medical assessments just described for lithium are also appropriate before initiating a trial of carbamazepine. The starting dose for adolescents is usually 200 mg twice daily and is gradually increased weekly by 200 mg to reach a blood level of 5 to 12 μg per mL. This blood level has not been established as the therapeutic range for adolescents with bipolar illness; however, experience with adult patients who have bipolar illness and children with seizure disorders suggests that levels above this range can result in toxicity. The usual maintenance dose is 800 to 1200 mg per day in divided doses.

Side effects include dizziness, sedation, irritability, nausea and vomiting, and diplopia. These side effects are most likely to occur early in treatment, epecially if the dose is increased too rapidly. Skin rashes occur in 10% to 15% of patients. Carbamazepine has also been reported to cause reversible agranulocytosis in 2% to 3% of patients. Aplastic anemia is a rare adverse effect.

Valproate (Depakote)

Valproate is another anticonvulsant medication that has been effective in treating adults with acute mania. To date there have been only a few case reports in adolescents (West et al, 1994; West, Keck, and McElroy, 1995). In these 2 studies West et al treated a total of 16 adolescents with bipolar illness, all of whom had failed on standard treatment. Of these 16 patients, 13 responded positively to valproate and with a minimum of adverse effects. In the second of these open trials (West, Keck, and McElroy, 1995), the investigators used a relatively large initial dose (20 mg per kg) in the hope of achieving more rapid stabilization. This strategy achieved clinically meaningful response in four of the five patients within several days as opposed to several weeks with more conservative dose increases. However, these findings should be regarded with caution because of the small sample size and the non-blinded design of the study.

Following a careful workup as just described for lithium, the medication may be initiated at 100 mg twice daily and gradually increased to reach serum levels of 50 to 100 μg per mL. Side effects include GI upset, tremor, and skin eruptions. In children being treated for seizure disorders there have been reports of cognitive dulling and a few cases of fatal liver toxicity. These cases had an acute onset and occurred in children under age 10. Safety monitoring during maintenance therapy should include complete blood counts, liver function tests, and drug levels.

DRUGS USED IN THE TREATMENT OF AGGRESSIVE BEHAVIOR

A substantial percentage of children and adolescents referred for emotional or behavioral problems exhibit aggressive behavior. Indeed, aggressive behavior is associated with several different psychiatric diagnoses, including ADHD, schizophrenia, bipolar disorder, conduct disorder, paranoid thinking, and seizure disorders (Marohn, 1992). Control of aggressive behavior is also a critically important clinical management issue for adolescent inpatient psychiatric units.

Several different classes of psychopharmacologic agents have been used to treat aggressive states. Information presented in Chapter 9, Acute Psychoses and the Violent Patient, is appropriate for older adolescents. A brief review is provided here as additional guidance to managing younger adolescents.

Neuroleptics

Neuroleptics are used for managing acute aggressive behavior and as an ongoing treatment approach. Youths who require immediate treatment can be given an intramuscular dosage of chlorpromazine at 0.5 mg per kg every 6 to 8 hours, as needed. For severely agitated adolescents an intramuscular dose of 25 mg may be given and repeated in 1 hour. Thereafter injections should be spaced at least 4 to 6 hours apart. A 12-year-old child should not receive more than 75 mg intramuscularly per day.

For the longer term treatment of aggressive behavior several studies have shown that chlorpromazine, thioridazine, and haloperidol are useful, with haloperidol being the most effective of the three. Doses tend to be less than those used for psychosis. Side effects are similar to those described earlier in the section on psychotic disorders.

Lithium

A series of double-blind studies showed that lithium was as effective as chlorpromazine and haloperidol, though better tolerated, for treating aggressive behavior (Campbell, Cohen, and Small, 1982; Campbell et al, 1984). More recently, lithium was examined in a double-blind study of 50 children and adolescents and was found to be superior to placebo (Campbell et al, 1995). The clinical management of lithium for aggression is essentially the same as that described earlier in the section on bipolar disorders.

Anticonvulsants

Carbamazepine has been used to treat aggression and outbursts of rage (Green, 1995). However, there are very few open studies and no controlled studies of carbamazepine for aggressive behavior in children and adolescents on which to base rational treatment. Valproate has not been studied in children and adolescents for aggressive behavior.

Alpha-2 Adrenergic Agents

The alpha-2 adrenergic drugs clonidine and guanfacine were developed as antihypertensive agents. Beginning with the early studies of clonidine for Tourette's syndrome, these drugs have become increasingly common in child psychiatry for tics, ADHD, and aggressive behavior (see Chapter 15, Psychopharmacology for Children, and Chappell, Leckman, and Riddle, 1995; Scahill, 1996).

In an open study of 17 youngsters, clonidine showed some promise for reducing aggressive behavior, but the drug has not been well studied in double-blind trials (Green, 1995). The typical starting dose of clonidine is 0.05 mg at bedtime; then it is increased by 0.05 mg every 3 to 4 days to a total of of 0.15 to 0.2 mg per day in three or four divided doses.

Guanfacine is a newer alpha-adrenergic medication that has a slightly longer duration of action than clonidine. To date it has shown promise in three open studies in children with ADHD, many of whom also had tics (see Chapter 15, Psychopharmacology for Children). It has not been studied for effectiveness in treating aggressive behavior.

TIC DISORDERS

The treatment of tic disorders is reviewed in detail in Chapter 15, Psychopharmacology for Children.

USE OF COMBINED DRUG THERAPIES

Another trend in pediatric psychopharmacology that warrants mention concerns the increasing use of combined drug therapies (Walkup, 1995; Popper, 1995). Concern about this trend has provoked controversy with the recent report of the deaths of three children who had been treated with methylphenidate and clonidine. A careful review ruled out a causal role for either the combination or the individual medications in these deaths. Nonetheless, because the combination of methylphenidate and clonidine is fairly common, many clinicians and parents were shocked by these reports (Popper, 1995).

There are various reasons for adding a second medication to treat children and adolescents with psychiatric disorders. First, a second agent may diminsh the severity of unwanted side effects produced by the primary therapeutic agent. The addition of benztropine for side effects from neuroleptic medications is an example of this type of combined treatment.

Second, an additional medication is sometimes administered because clinically important symptoms remain that are not addressed by the first medication. For example, some clinicians recommend clonidine at bedtime to reduce the sleep problems associated with ADHD that may even be amplified by stimulant medication.

Third, the second medication may be selected in the hope of boosting the treatment benefit of a partially effective medication for the target symptoms. The addition of a neuroleptic to ongoing treatment with an SSRI in refractory OCD or the addition of lithium to an antidepressant for a partial response depression are examples of this line of reasoning.

Unfortunately, there are very few studies on which to base such difficult clinical decisions. What little information that is available comes primarily from adult studies. As emphasized by Walkup (1995), in lieu of clear evidence on how to proceed with additional strategies, it is essential to be thorough in gathering history and systematic in approaching rational polypharmacy. Consulting with colleagues also can be helpful.

REFERENCES

Alessi N et al: Update on lithium carbonate therapy in children and adolescents, *J Am Acad Child Adolesc Psychiatry* 33:291, 1994.

American Psychiatric Association: *Diagnostic and statistical manual of mental disorders,* ed 4, Washington, DC, 1994, The Association.

Barkley RA: *Attention deficit hyperactivity disorder: a handbook for diagnosis and treatment,* New York, 1990, Guilford.

Barrickman LL et al: Bupropion versus methylphenidate in the treatment of attention-deficit hyperactivity disorder, *J Am Acad Child Adolesc Psychiatry* 34:649, 1995.

Biederman J et al: A double-blind placebo controlled study of desipramine in the treatment of ADD, Part I: efficacy, *J Am Acad Child Adolesc Psychiatry* 28:777, 1989.

Botteron KN, Geller B: Pharmacologic treatment of childhood and adolescent mania, *Child Adolesc Psychiatr Clin North Am* 4:283, 1995.

Campbell M, Cohen I, Small AM: Drugs in aggressive behavior, *J Am Acad Child Adolesc Psychiatry* 21:107, 1982.

Campbell M et al: Behavioral efficacy of haloperidol and lithium carbonate, *Arch Gen Psychiatry* 41:650, 1984.

Campbell M et al: Lithium in hospitalized aggressive children with conduct disorder: a double-blind and placebo-controlled study, *J Am Acad Child Adolesc Psychiatry* 34:445, 1995.

Chappell PB, Leckman JF, Riddle MA: The pharmacologic treatment of tic disorders, *Child Adolesc Psychiatr Clin North Am* 4:197, 1995.

DeVaugh-Geiss J et al: Clomipramine in child and adolescent obsessive-compulsive disorder: a multicenter trial, *J Am Acad Child Adolesc Psychiatry* 31:45, 1992.

Emslie G et al: Efficacy of fluoxetine in depressed children and adolescents. Paper presented at the annual meeting of the American Academy of Child and Adolescent Psychiatry, New Orleans, Oct, 1995.

Geller B, Fox LW, Clark KA: Rate and predictors of prepubertal bipolarity during follow-up of 6- to 12-year-old depressed children, *J Am Acad Child Adolesc Psychiatry* 33:461, 1994.

Green WH: *Child and adolescent clinical psychopharmacology,* Baltimore, 1995, Williams & Wilkins.

Greenhill LL: Attention-deficit hyperactivity disorder: the stimulants, *Child Adolesc Psychiatr Clin* 4(1):123, 1995.

Hechtman L: Long-term outcome in attention-deficit hyperactivity disorder, *Child Adolesc Psychiatr Clin North Am* 1:553, 1992.

Horwitz SM et al: Identification and management of psychosocial and developmental problems in community-based primary care pediatric practices, *Pediatrics* 89:480, 1992.

Institute of Medicine: *Research on children and adolescents with mental, behavioral, and developmental disorder,* Washington, DC, 1989, National Academy Press.

Kalogerakis MG: Emergency evaluation of adolescents, *Hosp Community Psychiatry* 43(6):617, 1992.

Kann L et al: Youth risk behavior surveillance: United States, 1993, *J Sch Health* 65:163, 1995.

King RA et al: Emergence of self-destructive phenomena in children and adolescents during fluoxetine treatment, *J Am Acad Child and Adolesc Psychiatry* 30:179, 1991.

Kye C, Ryan N: Pharmacologic treatment of child and adolescent depression, *Child Adolesc Psychiatr Clin North Am* 4:261, 1995.

Laraia, MT: Current approaches to the psychopharmacologic treatment of depression in children and adolescents, *J Child Adolesc Psychiatr Nurs* 9:15, 1996.

Leckman JF et al: Clonidine treatment of Gilles de la Tourette syndrome, *Arch Gen Psychiatry* 48:324, 1991.

Lewinsohn PM, Klein DN, Seeley JR: Bipolar disorders in a community sample of older adolescents: prevalence, phenomenology, comorbidity, and course, *J Am Acad Child Adolesc Psychiatry* 34:454, 1995.

Mandoki MW: Risperidone treatment of children and adolescents: increased risk of extrapyramidal side effects, *J Child Adolesc Psychopharmacol* 5:49, 1995.

Marohn RC: Management of the assaultive adolescent, *Hosp Community Psychiatry* 43(6):622, 1992.

McClellan J, Werry J: Practice parameters for the assessment and treatment of children and adolescents with schizophrenia, *J Amer Acad Child Adolesc Psychiatry* 33:616, 1994.

Popper CW: Combining methylphenidate and clonidine: pharmacologic questions and news reports about sudden death, *J Child Adolesc Psychopharmacol* 5:157, 1995.

Pottick K et al: Factors associated with inpatient and outpatient treatment for children and adolescents with serious mental illness, *J Am Acad Child Adolesc Psychiatry* 34:425, 1995.

Riddle MA, Geller B, Ryan N: Another sudden death in a child treated with desipramine, *J Am Acad Child Adolesc Psychiatry* 32:792, 1993.

Riddle MA et al: Behavioral side effects of fluoxetine, *J Child Adolesc Psychopharmacol* 3:193, 1991.

Riddle MA et al: Double-blind, crossover trial of fluoxetine and placebo in children and adolescents with obsessive compulsive disorder, *J Am Acad Child Adolesc Psychiatry* 31:1062, 1992.

Safer DJ, Krager JM: A survey of medication treatments for hyperactive/inattentive students, *JAMA* 260:2256, 1988.

Scahill L: Contemporary approaches to pharmacotherapy in Tourette syndrome and obsessive-compulsive disorder, *J Child Adolesc Psychiatr Nurs* 9(1):27, 1996.

Scahill L, Lynch KA: Tricyclic antidepressants: cardiac effects and clinical implications, *J Child Adolesc Psychiatr Nurs* 7:37, 1994.

Scahill L, Ort SJ: Clinical ratings in child psychiatric nursing, *J Child Adolesc Psychiatr Nurs* 8:33, 1995.

Schachar R, Tannock R: Childhood hyperactivity and psychostimulants: a review of extended treatment studies, *J Child Adolesc Psychopharmacol* 3:81, 1993.

Sikich LM et al: Allergic reactions to bupropion in child psychiatric inpatients: a case series. Poster presentation at the annual meeting of the American Academy of Child and Adolescent Psychiatry, New Orleans, Oct 1995.

Simeon JG et al: Risperidone effects in treatment-resistant adolescents: preliminary case reports, *J Child Adolesc Psychopharmacol* 5:69, 1995.

Spencer T et al: Nortriptyline treatment of children with attention-deficit hyperactivity disorder and tic disorder or Tourette's syndrome, *J Am Acad Child Adolesc Psychiatry* 32:205, 1993.

Strober M et al: Relapse following discontinuation of lithium maintenance therapy in adolescents with bipolar-I illness: a naturalistic study, *Am J Psychiatry* 147:457, 1990.

Szatmari P, Offord DR, Boyle MH. Ontario Child Health Study: prevalence of attention deficit disorder with hyperactivity. *J Child Psychol Psychiatr* 30:219, 1989.

Teicher MH, Glod CA: Neuroleptic drugs: indications and guidelines for their rational use in children and adolescents, *J Child Adolesc Psychopharmacol* 1:33, 1990.

Volkmar FR: Autism and the pervasive developmental disorders, *Hosp Community Psychiatry* 42(1):33, 1991.

Walkup JT: Clinical decision making in child and adolescent psychopharmacology, *Child Adolesc Psychiatr Clin North Am* 4:23, 1995.

West SA et al: Open trial of valproate in the treatment of adolescent mania, *J Child Adolesc Psychopharmacol* 4:263, 1994.

West SA, Keck PE, McElroy SL: Oral loading doses in the valproate treatment of adolescents with mixed bipolar disorder, *J Child Adolesc Psychopharmacol* 5:225, 1995.

CHAPTER 17

Psychopharmacology for Elderly Persons

Psychotropics are the second most frequently prescribed class of drugs for older patients (Folks, 1990). Two thirds of elderly persons take 5 to 12 medications each day (Wantanabe and Davis, 1990). Ninety-two percent of patients in long-term care facilities take psychotropic drugs. Regarding single-drug prescriptions, more sedative-hypnotics are prescribed to older patients than is any other single drug (Balter and Bauer, 1975). The segment of the population that is older than age 65 accounts for about 25% of the total drug expenditures in developed countries (Williams and Lowenthal, 1992). This figure is predicted to reach 40% by 2030 (Vestal, 1982).

Pharmacotherapy in an older patient may be complicated by many factors. Reduced life expectancy and functional capacity, the relative physiologic effects of aging, pharmacokinetic and pharmacodynamic influences, polypharmacy, drug interactions, treatment setting, coexisting medical conditions, cognitive impairment, and issues pertinent to compliance are all important considerations in the effective pharmacologic approach to the geriatric patient (Folks, 1990). When pharmacologic treatment is indicated for an older patient, specific knowledge of drug actions and effects are especially pertinent. Ultimately the primary goal of psychotropic drug therapy for a geriatric patient is to improve quality of life. By enhancing communication and understanding between an older patient and the clinician, the overall quality of care can often be significantly improved.

The psychopharmacologic approach to treating a geriatric patient requires knowledge of psychiatric and nonpsychiatric conditions that are more prevalent in these patients. An appreciation of comorbid medical conditions is sometimes critical to safe and effective drug treatment. Also, the health care provider who is familiar with the bioepidemiologic differences among older adults will be better prepared to individualize treatment plans and evaluate the response to drug intervention (Montamat, Cusack, and Vestal, 1989). Most data on older populations report that elderly individuals are either taking drugs that are unnecessary (Wilcox et al 1994) or that drug dosage can be decreased or a safer alternative drug can be substituted (Avorn et al, 1992; Gurwitz, 1994).

SCOPE OF THE PROBLEM

The geriatric population is growing at a remarkable rate. Several factors are chiefly responsible for the disproportionate rate of growth that is occurring in this segment of the population: decreased infant mortality, declining birth rates, increased life expectancy, and declining death rates for those over age 65. As depicted in Figure 17-1, the significant rate of growth among elderly persons has occurred steadily since the turn of the century, when about 3.1 million people, or 4% of the population in the United States, were over age 65. Currently approximately 13% of the population, or 31 million individuals, have reached their sixty-fifth birthday. This age group accounts for 20% to 40% of a primary care physician's caseload (Cadieux

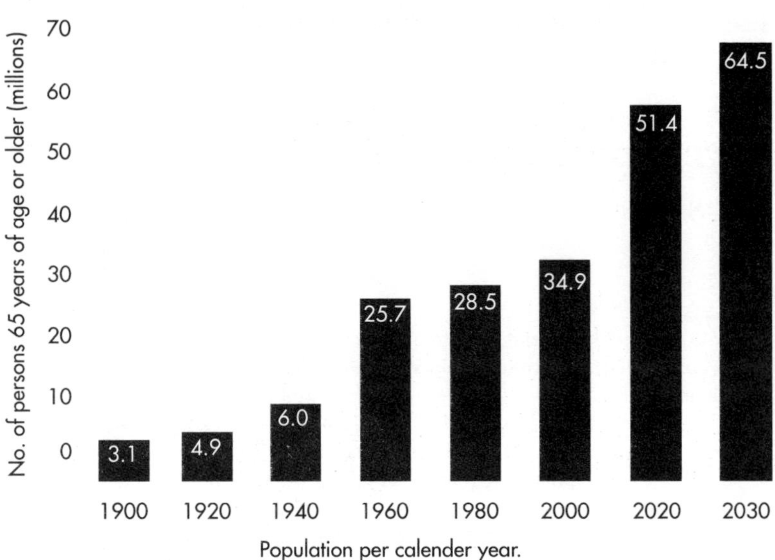

Figure 17-1 Geriatric population demographics through the year 2030. The disproportionate growth rate for the geriatric population in the United States is evident. (From Folks DG: Clinical approaches to anxiety in the medically ill elderly, *Drug Ther Suppl* August 1990, p 72.)

et al, 1993). The so-called baby boomers will begin to reach their sixty-fifth birthdays after 2010. An estimated 65 million people, or approximately 20% to 25% of the U.S. population, will be over age 65 by 2030 (Gaitz, Niederehe, and Wilson, 1985). The declining death rate for those over age 65 is primarily responsible for the rapid growth of the "true elderly segment," that is, those over age 85. This subsegment is indeed the most rapidly growing of all age groups. It is staggering to realize that the elderly subsegment of the population will more than double in the next decade, with a growth rate approximately 22 times that of the adolescent subsegment of our population.

Psychiatric disorders are not generally encountered in isolation in geriatric patients (Masoro, 1987). Acute, life-threatening illness and prevalent chronic conditions require careful consideration with respect to psychiatric intervention. Multiple disease processes, common environmental influences, and genetic variation often combine with the physiologic or psychobiologic effects of aging, significantly influencing pharmacologic treatment outcome (Boxes 17-1, 17-2, and 17-3). Of course, physiologic aging does not necessarily parallel chronologic aging; apart from the prominent effects of overt disease states, physiologic aging more often underlies the age-related differences in the action of psychotropic drugs (Rowe and Kahn, 1987). Thus understanding the pharmacologic consequences of the physiologic effects of aging is also critical to safe and effective pharmacotherapeutics.

GENERAL FACTORS PERTINENT TO PSYCHOTROPIC DRUG THERAPY

This section outlines the pharmacokinetic, pharmacodynamic, and nontherapeutic effects of drugs as they relate to psychotropics used to treat geriatric patients. Additionally, issues relating to compliance are outlined with respect to the clinical ap-

Box 17-1 Diseases Causing Death in Individuals 65 Years of Age and Older

Heart disease
Cancer, malignant neoplasms
Stroke, cerebrovascular disease
Alzheimer's disease, related disorders
Influenza, pneumonia
Accidents: falls and motor-pedestrian
Suicide

Box 17-2 Chronic Medical Conditions in Individuals 65 Years of Age and Older

Arthritis and rheumatologic disease
Neurosensory loss: hearing disturbance, visual disturbance
Cardiovascular disease: congestive heart failure, ischemic heart disease, hypertension, peripheral vascular disease
Gastrointestinal disorders
Chronic sinusitis and upper respiratory disturbances
Genitourinary tract problems
Chronic obstructive pulmonary disease
Adult-onset diabetes mellitus
Thyroid disease, endocrinopathy
Dermatologic disturbances

Box 17-3 Targets of Psychobiologic Effects of Aging

Autonomic nervous system
Behavioral and personality function
Bone density
Body composition
Cognitive function
Glucose tolerance
Hearing and vision
Immune function
Pulmonary function
Renal function
Skin
Systolic blood pressure

proach. These factors determine many of the general principles that are useful in the clinical approach to common psychiatric syndromes encountered in late life.

Pharmacokinetics

Pharmacokinetics refers to what the body does to a drug with respect to absorption, distribution, metabolism, and elimination. Altered pharmacokinetics in elderly individuals is due in part to physiologic changes that accompany aging. The predictable age-related changes in body composition and organ function in older adults also result in altered pharmacokinetics. These changes include diminished renal function, diminished hepatic blood flow, decreased serum albumin level and lean-muscle mass, decreased total body water, and increased alpha-1 acid glycoprotein (AGP). Thus age-related differences and drug disposition are multifactorial and are significantly influenced by environmental, genetic, physiologic, and pathologic factors.

Most studies of older populations and pharmacokinetics are cross-sectional and merely provide information about the average age-related differences. Because of the difficulties in design, administration, and cost of longitudinal studies, few studies have provided a precise picture of the changes in pharmacokinetics that occur within an aging cohort (Williams and Lowenthal, 1992). Whereas some age-related physiologic changes profoundly affect drug kinetics, for example, renal function, others, such as gastrointestinal (GI) absorption, do not appear to alter pharmacokinetic values consistently.

Absorption. Despite several age-related alterations that occur with age in the GI tract, such as increased gastric pH, delayed gastric emptying, diminished blood flow, and impaired intestinal motility, few psychotropic drugs actually show any delayed rates of GI tract absorption after oral administration (Montamat, Cusack, and Vestal, 1989). Thus the anatomic and physiologic changes that occur with aging in the GI tract have little effect on drug metabolism.

The term *bioavailability* refers to the relative amount of drug reaching the systemic circulation after absorption. The bioavailability of a drug is determined not only by the extent of absorption through the GI tract but also by the presystemic drug elimination in the liver as the drug passes from the portal circulation. The bioavailability of drugs is generally unchanged in older adults, except in the case of those drugs that are abstracted at a high rate by the liver (Cusack and Vestal, 1986). Decreased presystemic hepatic extraction leads to modest increases in the bioavailability of certain drugs, for example, beta blockers. However, these findings have no real clinical significance. In contrast, pathologic and surgical alterations in the GI tract and interactions between psychotropics and drugs such as laxatives, antacids, and agents that decrease gastric emptying may alter absorption.

Distribution. Changes in body composition (Figure 17-2) and blood flow may profoundly affect drug distribution in an older adult (Greenblatt, Sellers, and Shader, 1982). A decrease in total body water and lean-body mass, combined with a proportional increase in body fat, undoubtedly affects the volume of distribution of many drugs. Water-soluble drugs, for example, ethanol and lithium, have a reduced volume of distribution in elderly individuals, with increased initial concentrations in the central compartment and resultant higher plasma concentrations. Lipid-soluble drugs, for example, the benzodiazepines, tend to have a much greater distribution in older persons because of the average increase in body fat. Interestingly, some lipophilic drugs, most notably lorazepam (Ativan) and amobarbital (Amytal), do not have significantly different volumes of distribution with increased

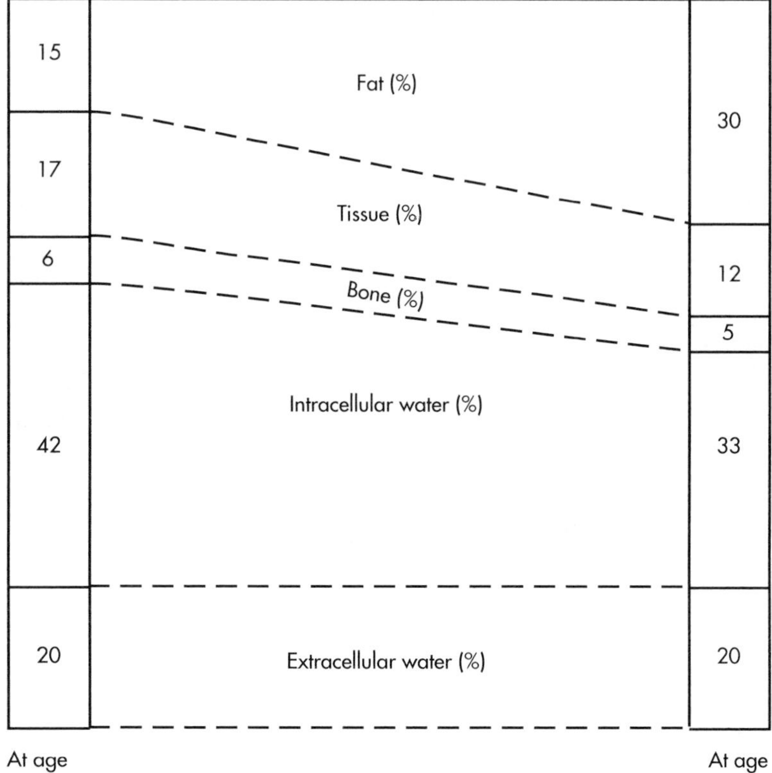

Figure 17-2 Representation of changes in body composition in the "average" individual, comparing body composition at 25 and 75 years of age. (From Folks DG: Clinical approaches to anxiety in the medically ill elderly, *Drug Ther Suppl* August 1990, p 92.)

age. When the volume of distribution is increased for an anxiolytic or another psychotropic, as is the case with diazepam (Valium), the result may be a prolonged action because of an even longer elimination half-life, as discussed in Chapter 6, Anxiety Disorders.

Free and unbound drug concentrations are important determinants of both drug distribution and elimination. Thus alterations in binding of drugs to plasma proteins, red blood cells, and metabolic organs can and do alter pharmacokinetic properties in elderly persons. The tendency is toward lower protein binding of drugs related to the average decline in serum albumin concentration or alteration in albumin receptor configuration, or both, related to age and disease. In fact, however, epidemiologic studies indicate that decreases in albumin concentrations are minimal in healthy elderly persons and not likely to be of clinical significance (Folks and Fuller, in press; Greenblatt, 1979). In contrast, chronic diseases may be associated with substantial reductions in serum albumin levels. In this case it is important to note that weakly acidic drugs, for example, barbiturates and phenytoin (Dilantin), bind primarily to plasma albumin. Weak bases such as propranolol (Inderal) are bound basically to AGP; thus some degree of variability exists in the concentration of this specific agent, especially because the concentration of AGP tends to increase with age (Abernathy and Kerznel, 1984). Thus in elderly persons the decrease in albumin and the increase in AGP concentrations may be associated with both reduced and increased protein bindings of drugs, respectively (Wallace and Verbeeck, 1987).

Hepatic metabolism. Metabolism of drugs by the liver depends on the activity of enzymes, which carry out biotransformation and are influenced by the extent of hepatic blood flow that determines the rate of delivery of drugs to the liver. Drugs that are metabolized slowly and have a low intrinsic clearance are processed proportionately to the rate of hepatic metabolism. Because hepatic mass decreases with age in absolute terms and in proportion to body weight, the metabolism of drugs with low intrinsic clearance is reduced. Generally this includes drugs that to a great extent depend on oxidation, that is, those that use oxidative pathways of drug metabolism (Wynne et al, 1989).

Drugs with a rapid rate of metabolism and high intrinsic clearance are extracted rapidly by the liver. The rate-limiting step in this case is hepatic blood flow. This relationship is particularly pertinent to drugs that are administered intravenously, for example, diazepam. Advancing age is associated with reduction in the presystemic metabolism of drugs that have a relatively higher rate of extraction (Castleden and George, 1979). Thus the bioavailability of certain drugs such as beta blockers is increased, and accordingly other drugs with high rates of hepatic extraction, for example, antipsychotics or tricyclic antidepressants (TCAs), should be administered with great caution and careful monitoring for side effects.

Liver metabolism may be classified based on biotransformation reactions as *phase 1,* with oxidation, reduction, and hydrolysis; and *phase 2,* with conjugation reactions that include glucuronidation, acetylation, and sulfation. Microsomal and nonmicrosomal enzymes are involved in both processes. Phase 1 pathways of metabolism are either reduced or unchanged in elderly persons, whereas phase 2 pathways are not altered and are more predictable. Benzodiazepines undergo both types of metabolism (Bellatuono et al, 1980). For example, chlordiazepoxide (Librium), diazepam, clorazepate (Tranxene), and prazepam (Centrax) all undergo oxidative metabolism and therefore their elimination is prolonged in elderly persons. These drugs are converted to an active metabolite, for example, desmethyldiazepam, which, in turn, has other active metabolites for which the half-life is substantially longer than in the parent compound, that is, up to 220 hours in elderly patients. Other benzodiazepines, oxazepam (Serax), lorazepam, and temazepam (Restoril), undergo conjugation reactions; the metabolism of these agents remains unaltered by age. Thus these compounds do not give rise to active metabolites and represent safer compounds within the benzodiazepine class for use with elderly persons (Folks, 1990).

Age is only one of many factors that potentially affect drug metabolism. For example, cigarette smoking, alcohol intake, dietary considerations, drugs, illness, and caffeine consumption may all affect the rate of drug metabolism. Enzyme induction through smoking and alcohol consumption and hepatic enzyme inhibition through decreased drug clearance by other drugs such as cimetidine (Tagamet) may also affect drug metabolism in older individuals. In short, hepatic metabolism is a complex process and psychotropic agents that are more easily metabolized, for example, the benzodiazepine lorazepam or the secondary amine TCA nortriptyline (Pamelor, Aventyl) are generally preferred for older patients.

Elimination. Perhaps the best documented and the most predictable alteration in pharmacokinetics with advancing age is the reduction in the rate of renal elimination or excretion (Rowe et al, 1976). This reduction is caused by a decline in both the glomerular filtration rate (GFR) and the tubular secretion rate, which accounts for the decreased creatinine clearance that results from aging. Beginning with the fourth decade of life a 6% to 10% reduction in GFR and renal plasma occurs every 10 years. Thus by age 70 an individual may have as much as a 50% decrease in renal function in the absence of renal disease.

Drug elimination in patients who have normal serum creatinine concentrations is affected because creatinine production decreases with age. Thus measuring creatinine clearance is useful in determining a dosage. Direct measurement can be difficult to achieve, but an estimate for men may be derived from the following formula: Creatinine clearance equals 140 minus age and multiplied by the body weight in kilograms, then divided by 72 and multiplied by the serum creatinine (Cockcroft and Gault, 1976). For women this result should be multiplied by 0.85. As a caveat, this formula has been shown to be less than accurate in estimating creatinine clearance among nursing home patients (Drusano et al, 1988). Thus this method of assessment may provide only a crude estimate of dosage requirements.

Drugs that are eliminated predominantly by the kidneys and have untoward pharmacologic effects are even more potentially serious with respect to toxic effects in elderly persons. Amantadine (Symmetrel), lithium, beta blockers, clonidine (Catapres), and several nonpsychotropic drugs, that is, aminoglycosides, digoxin, antiarrhythmics, diuretics, nonsteroidal antiinflammatory drugs, and angiotensin-converting enzyme inhibitors are noteworthy examples (Williams and Lowenthal, 1992). The discussion of lithium excretion in kidney function, as noted in Chapter 5, Mood Disorders, is of particular concern in elderly persons.

Drug interactions. The pharmacokinetic effects outlined in this section prominently affect interactions with other drugs. Absorption may be affected significantly by antacids. Distribution of drugs may be affected by the competition for binding proteins among various drugs. Metabolism of drugs that use the oxidative cytochrome P-450 enzyme system—for example, barbiturates, anticonvulsants, and oral hypoglycemics—may induce drug metabolism. Other compounds may inhibit metabolism, for example, cimetidine, neuroleptics, TCAs, selective serotonin reuptake inhibitors (SSRIs), beta blockers, and methylphenidate (Ritalin). Excretion of psychotropic agents may be significantly affected by proximal-loop and potassium-sparing diuretics, especially lithium. Nonsteroidal antiinflammatory agents may also be responsible for disrupting excretions of lithium and other psychotropic agents. In short, GI tract diseases may affect absorption; diseases affecting volume of distribution may result from altered concentrations of binding protein; hepatic disease may affect metabolism; and renal disease may affect excretion.

Pharmacodynamics

Pharmacodynamics refers to what a drug does to the system and to the study of effects of drugs on the target site; more broadly, *pharmacodynamics* reflects the physiologic or psychologic response to a drug or combination of drugs. Pharmacodynamics has been examined less extensively in elderly persons than has pharmacokinetics, largely because of the difficulty of such investigation. Older patients are generally more responsive to the effects of psychotropic agents, perhaps because of changes in neurotransmitter systems or receptor site sensitivity.

Geriatric patients can be exquisitely sensitive to the effects of psychotropic drugs but less so to nonpsychotropic agents such as cardiovascular preparations. This is in part caused by changes with respect to beta-receptor functioning and resultant vulnerability to side effects, for example, orthostatic hypotension. Beta-receptor density and affinity for antagonists on human lymphocytes are not altered with age (Abrass and Scarpace, 1981). Lower levels of cyclic adenosine monophosphate (AMP) and adenylate cyclase activity after beta-adrenergic stimulation have been noted in the lymphocytes of elderly persons (Scarpace, 1986). Receptor affinity for antagonists is lessened in association with reduced ability to form a high affinity state for agonists, and this reduction may result in an age-related alteration in the interaction between the beta-adrenergic receptors and regulatory proteins. In contrast, studies of alpha-adrenergic receptors have revealed either no change or a decrease in the relative affinities for receptors with increasing age (Buckley et al, 1986). Thus receptor changes result in a differential (and sometimes exaggerated or diminished) response in older individuals.

Other significant age-related neurophysiologic changes include cholinergic degeneration that is known to occur in older adults and can affect memory function and presumably predispose patients to the effects of drugs that potentially exacerbate disorders of cognitive impairment. For example, the patient with Alzheimer's disease is vulnerable to drugs that exert anticholinergic effects. The degeneration of the nigrostriatal pathways may also result in an older individual's predisposition to extrapyramidal side effects (EPSEs) or to the development of tardive dyskinesia with use of a neuroleptic. Moreover, the sedation threshold and unfavorable effects on memory in response to benzodiazepines may be exaggerated in older patients. The effects of TCAs on cardiac conduction in patients with cardiac disease and neuroleptics in patients with Parkinson's disease may also be accentuated. It is thought there is a greater potential for TCAs to interact with antihypertensive agents, antiarrhythmics, and other agents that possess anticholinergic properties. Similarly, low-potency neuroleptics may affect response to antihypertensives; specifically, alpha-receptor blockade may also be accentuated as a result of the pharmacodynamic interactions with the nonpsychiatric medication.

Drug Reactions

Nontherapeutic drug reactions are commonly encountered in older adults who receive psychotropic medications. As mentioned previously, many side effects are related to sedation, which can result in excessive drowsiness, cognitive impairment, or motor impairment or simply can compound the sedation resulting from other drugs interacting with sedative-hypnotic agents, including alcohol. The high prevalence of dizziness reported in elderly persons in association with certain psychotropics, that is, benzodiazepines, TCAs and newer antidepressants, and antipsychotic agents, may also predispose these individuals to falls that may result in hip fracture (Ray et al, 1987; Sloane, Blazer, and George, 1989).

Many psychotropic agents used safely in younger patients require closer attention when prescribed for older individuals because of clinically important adverse drug reactions. Risk factors for adverse drug reactions include multiple medications, increased number of illnesses, severe illness, or increased sensitivity to drug effects. The incidence of adverse drug reactions or nontherapeutic effects ranges between 10% and 20% among inpatients (Cusack, 1989). Patients taking nonsteroidal antiinflammatory drugs have an increased risk of hyperkalemia, renal failure, or death resulting from GI hemorrhage. Patients receiving diuretic therapy are more susceptible to fluid and electrolyte disorders, including volume depletion, hypokalemia, hyponatremia, and hypomagnesemia. As mentioned previously, disease states may also alter the disposition or effect of a drug, and because in geriatric patients often more than one disease is involved, careful attention should be given when prescribing any medication (Folks, 1990; Montamat, Cusack, and Vestal, 1989).

Compliance

Noncompliance with drug therapy is reported to occur in one third to half of geriatric patients (Morrow, Leirer, and Sheikh, 1988). Causes of noncompliance include poor communication with the health care professional, decline in cognitive function, and complicated dosing regimens. Using the fewest possible drugs at low doses and in convenient combinations usually enhances compliance. Once a therapeutic goal has been achieved, a dosage of a particular drug should be reduced and therapy discontinued whenever possible. Of course, continuation therapy should be followed by maintenance throughout the period in which the patient may be most susceptible to recurrence or relapse.

Dosage schedules should be kept simple and multiple drug regimens minimized. If a geriatric patient is unable to read or comprehend directions, family members or caregivers should be given simple written instructions. Containers that are easy to open should be provided. Liquid formulations should be used for those individuals who have difficulty with swallowing. Various aids and devices can be improvised or obtained to assist patients and their families with accurate self-administration.

PSYCHIATRIC DISTURBANCES PREVALENT IN LATE LIFE

Psychotropic drugs are prescribed for geriatric patients with disabling or debilitating target symptoms, clinically significant syndromes, or bona fide psychiatric disorders, as defined within the nomenclature. Symptoms that become a focus of treatment include anxiety, insomnia, agitation, and aggression. Syndromes commonly treated include mixed anxiety-depression, psychosis, and agitation or confusion that complicate disorders of cognitive impairment, in particular, dementia and delirium. Psychiatric disturbances that are commonly encountered in late life include anxiety, mood, and sleep disorders, and disorders of cognitive impairment, for example, Alzheimer's disease. Of course, chronic psychotic disorders, personality disorders, and other significant disturbances may have extended into later life. As with younger patients, these symptoms, syndromes, and disorders are ideally treated with a combination of interventions. Pharmacologic treatment is best combined with psychotherapeutic interventions or behavioral techniques. It would be unthinkable to prescribe a psychotropic drug to an older patient without first providing an adequate assessment that seeks to optimize the patient's medical and physiologic condition while providing some documentation of the patient's baseline mental and psychosocial status. Generally this assessment should seek to answer the following questions:

1. What is the patient's medical status?
2. What is the patient's mental status?
3. What is the patient's functional status and capacity to carry out daily activities?
4. What is the patient's psychosocial status and ability to function socially and occupationally, and to maintain interpersonal and relationship functioning?
5. What is the patient's or caregiver's potential to comply with a medical regimen, including recommendations for nonpharmacologic interventions or adjunctive interventions that may serve to enhance compliance?

Mood Disorders

Mood disorders are frequently encountered among geriatric patients. Epidemiologic data suggest that about half of all major depression is encountered initially by an individual over age 65 (Kalayam and Shamoian, 1990). Of community-dwelling elderly persons, 13% are found to have clinically significant symptoms within the depressive spectrum (Blazer et al, 1988). Medical illnesses are frequently associated with depression; for example, 20% to 35% of patients within medical-surgical settings are found to have coexisting symptoms of depression (Folks and Ford, 1985). Mortality rates are increased for geriatric patients with depression, and the suicide rate among elderly individuals is disproportionate (Folks, 1990). The current geriatric population accounts for at least 25% of all completed suicides, but elderly persons attempt suicide at least 3 times less frequently than do nongeriatric patients, that is, suicide attempts made by older adults are more often successfully completed (Folks and Ford, 1994). Thus effective drug treatment of depression, careful monitoring of response, and an appreciation of potential suicide risk are imperative for depressed geriatric patients.

Depression. Among the antidepressants and mood stabilizers, SSRIs are most frequently prescribed for older patients. Geriatric patients may require lower doses of SSRIs.

Regarding other new-generation antidepressants, venlafaxine (Effexor), is well tolerated by geriatric patients and has fewer side effects than do TCAs (as discussed in Chapter 5, Mood Disorders). Bupropion (Wellbutrin) may be beneficial, particularly for those patients who are not responsive to SSRIs. Bupropion has been touted as being useful in patients with a history of bipolar disorder or in those who require maintenance antidepressant therapy after electroconvulsive therapy (Jenike, 1988). Bupropion has virtually no anticholinergic or cardiotoxic effects and lacks sedative properties that may contribute to daytime drowsiness. Nefazodone (Serzone) appears to be another drug that is well tolerated in the geriatric patient. As discussed in Chapter 5, Mood Disorders, nefazodone enhances sleep, rapidly reduces anxiety, and lacks significant potential for orthostatic or anticholinergic symptoms. Few drug-drug interactions occur with nefazodone other than with astemizole, terfenadine, and other agents metabolized by the P450-IIIA4 enzyme system, for example, alprazolam and triazolam (see Chapter 5, Mood Disorders).

When TCAs are selected, the secondary amine tricyclics desipramine (Norpramin) and nortriptyline (Pamelor) are generally preferred because of their more favorable side effect profile, as discussed in Chapter 5, Mood Disorders. Acute antidepressant drug treatment with resultant remission of symptoms and continuation therapy for at least 6 to 12 months is recommended, because more than 50% of successfully treated patients either have a relapse or recurrence in the first year (Rubin, Kinscherf, and Wehrman, 1991).

MAOIs may be found to be effective for those depressed elderly patients who are refractory to SSRIs or other antidepressant intervention (Jenike, 1989). Moreover, because monoamine oxidase enzyme activity increases with increasing age, a special niche for these agents in the geriatric population is implied, particularly for those individuals with dementia complicated by depression. However, orthostatic hypotension or other adverse reactions, as outlined in Chapter 5, Mood Disorders, may emerge; geriatric patients may also be potentially at risk for noncompliance with the necessary dietary precautions.

Although activating antidepressants, for example, desipramine, fluoxetine, or bupropion, are useful in geriatric patients who may be abulic, motor retarded, or cognitively impaired, psychostimulants have gained popularity as being useful in the initial or sustained treatment of depression among geriatric patients (Jenike, 1988). Psychostimulants may be used safely for initial or sustained treatment of major depression, for treatment of organic affective disorders, for treatment of apathy, or for depressive symptoms in patients with Alzheimer's disease and related dementias.

Surprisingly these agents have few adverse or nontherapeutic effects, as noted in Chapter 13, Drugs Used to Stimulate the Central Nervous System. The use of methylphenidate in doses of 5 to 30 mg is generally preferred both as a short-term agent with or without concomitant administration of a conventional antidepressant and as an adjunct in the long-term treatment of treatment-refractory cases (Chiarello et al, 1987). The stimulant challenge test, in which a test dose of a stimulant is given before conventional antidepressant intervention is begun, has also been reported as a useful way of predicting potential responses to antidepressant drug therapy (Goff, 1986).

Bipolar disorder. Using lithium carbonate to treat bipolar disorder in geriatric patients is well documented. Lithium has also been useful for augmenting antidepressant agents (Price, Charney, and Heninger, 1986). The dose-response relationship for using lithium in bipolar illness in geriatric cases can result in a response or maintenance prophylaxis with low therapeutic plasma levels, that is, 0.4 to 0.8 mEq per L. Low-dose treatment is preferred, because side effects and adverse reactions are much more commonly encountered among older adult patients, including a great potential for neurotoxic effects and dyskinesia. Interestingly many older patients who seek medical attention with an apparent agitated depression may actually have mixed bipolar disorder that is ultimately responsive to lithium or other mood-stabilizing agents in concert with antidepressant therapy (Folks and Ford, 1994; Stone and Folks, 1992). For the 30% to 50% of patients who are either nonresponders to lithium or intolerant of its side effects, carbamazepine (Tegretol), valproate (Depakote), or other mood stabilizers may be used alternatively. Valproate is well tolerated, especially in the form of divalproex (Depakote), and is gaining popularity as a first-line agent for this age group. Carbamazepine and valproate, as discussed in Chapter 5, Mood Disorders, possess similar dose-response relationships for psychotropic uses in older patients (Keltner and Folks, 1991; Lerer et al, 1987). Because these alternative mood-stabilizing compounds do not lower the seizure threshold or significantly interfere with cognitive function, they may also be useful in cognitively impaired patients who have prominent symptoms of mood instability or aggression, both of which will be discussed later in this chapter.

Psychotic Disorders

Psychotic syndromes in older patients may include schizophrenia or other syndromes that are potentially treatable or manageable with antipsychotic or neuroleptic agents (as they are in younger patients). The choice of drug often entails selection of a high-potency agent or a low-potency agent, as discussed in Chapter 4, Schizophrenia and Other Psychoses. The relative efficacy versus the side-effect profile generally includes consideration of whether the patient has any pre-existing conditions that might result in greater risk for side effects of either the high-potency or low-potency agent. In general, high-potency agents in low doses, for example, haloperidol (Haldol), are preferred as initial drugs for treating psychotic symptoms (Peabody et al, 1987). However, EPSEs, akinesia, and akathisia are frequent problems in the geriatric population as is the emergence of tardive dyskinesia over time, which occurs most frequently in elderly persons. For some patients sedation associated with a low-potency neuroleptic may represent a "therapeutic fringe benefit," and the relative risk is low for nontherapeutic effects using lower doses, that is, anticholinergic effects, orthostatic effects, or adverse influence on cardiac conduction time. In general, low doses of a compound such as thioridazine (Mellaril) at 10 to 50 mg 2 to 4 times daily may be quite effective. Likewise the low-potency novel antipsychotic agent clozapine (Clozaril) may be beneficial for geriatric conditions that are treatment refractory, as discussed in Chapter 4, Schizophrenia and Other Psychoses (Small et al, 1987). Clozapine may be particularly beneficial in elderly persons with Parkinson's disease. Risperidone has also been used with significant benefit to older patients (Bernstein, 1995). This drug is well tolerated, with minimal sedation, low cholinergic effect, limited hypotension, and minimal EPSEs at low doses, for example, initial dose of 0.5 mg daily or twice a day.

Older patients with schizophrenia, delusional disorder, or other psychoses constitute one of several groups for whom depot neuroleptics have a special role. Both fluphenazine (Prolixin) decanoate and haloperidol decanoate have proved to be useful, particularly because elderly noncompliant patients in the community can be treated effectively with periodic home visits. Moreover, for patients in institutional settings, lower doses of depot rather than oral neuroleptic agents may ultimately be required to maintain the antipsychotic effect. Antipsychotic agents may also be generally useful for patients with sundowning, confusional episodes, delirium, transient psychosis, agitation, or behavioral disturbances secondary to dementia. Further, patients who may be at risk for harm to themselves or others or for those individuals who are simply unable to carry out essential daily activities without some degree of tranquilization are helped by antipsychotics.

Anxiety Disorders and Acute Insomnia

As mentioned previously, anxiety disorders represent one of the common syndromes encountered in later life and represent symptoms for which patients readily seek treatment. Using anxiolytics primarily involves choosing a benzodiazepine, an antidepressant for treating specific anxiety subtypes, or buspirone (as noted in Chapter 6, Anxiety Disorders). Benzodiazepines, sedatives, trazodone, or a short-term regimen of chloral hydrate is also useful for treating acute insomnia.

The pharmacology and pharmacologic properties of anxiolytics and sedatives have been discussed in preceding chapters with respect to neurobiology and basic science. Differential drug effects related to drug metabolism and pharmacokinetics in elderly persons may be exaggerated, as outlined generally in this chapter with respect to plasma protein-binding, increased volume of distribution, diminished hepatic biotransformation, and impaired renal clearance. However, as mentioned previously, the clinical impact resulting from alteration of plasma proteins is not thought to be marked. In fact, the equilibrium between bound and unbound drug is not changed significantly in the vast majority of elderly patients. Thus the amount of psychotropic drug available to produce clinical effects often remains unchanged, although the total amount of protein binding is diminished.

Hepatic biotransformation and renal clearance are significant pharmacokinetic considerations that often do account for differences in drug response. For example, reduced hepatic biotransformation and reduced renal clearance in elderly persons both lead to metabolic accumulation, diminished clearing of the drug, and a resultant higher blood level of drug or active metabolite, or both. This is, indeed, why short-acting benzodiazepines that undergo metabolism through conjugation pathways in the liver, that is, oxazepam, lorazepam, and temazepam, are preferred.

A number of treatment issues and guidelines must be considered with the use of anxiolytics and sedatives in geriatric patients. These primarily relate to the potential for nontherapeutic effects of the drugs in relation to the effects of aging per se, as outlined in Chapter 8, Sleep Disorders. Diazepam and other benzodiazepines, that is, alprazolam (Xanax), oxazepam, and lorazepam, are known to result in disinhibition; this phenomenon is characterized by an episode of violence or increasing agitation that is clearly drug induced (Hall and Zisook, 1981). Thus the loss of behavioral control and explosive or violent behavior may also occur during the course of benzodiazepine treatment (Folks, 1990; Gardos et al, 1968). Triazolam (Halcion) occasionally has shown this effect but more often produces other significant side effects in older patients, for example, amnestic episodes. Benzodiazepines have well-known amnestic properties, which are prominent in elderly persons (Kumar et al, 1987; Wolkowitz et al, 1987). The potential for lorazepam, alprazolam, and triazolam to produce amnestic effects has been discussed in Chapter 8, Sleep Disorders.

Drug accumulation with long-acting benzodiazepines is thought to explain the higher incidence of falls in elderly persons (Ray et al, 1987; Sloane, Blazer, and George, 1989). Moreover, the benzodiazepines with long half-lives pose the greatest risk for resultant falls that may be complicated by hip fracture or head injury, or both (Ray, Griffin, and Downey, 1989). The potential adverse effects of sedation and negative direct influence on cognition are also compounded in elderly patients with pre-existing dementia, creating additional risk for accidents (Folks, 1990).

The clinical approach to sedative treatment of acute insomnia requires careful selection of a specific drug with the most suitable pharmacologic profile in relatively low doses. The dose should preserve normal sleep architecture to the extent possible during ingestion and after withdrawal The pharmacokinetic profile should meet the clinical requirement to shorten sleep onset, to reduce nocturnal wakefulness, or to provide the anxiolytic effect required during the following day. This approach should result in the patient being as free as possible from untoward effects on daytime functioning. The utility and clinical appropriateness of any hypnotic must depend to some extent on whether the therapeutic profile solves the clinical problems.

Benzodiazepines used as hypnotics are likely to have some side effects. However, unnecessarily high doses for long periods are the major problem, essentially resulting in adverse effects. Impaired daytime performance, anterograde amnesia, and other adverse effects associated with several of the anxiolytics are especially problematic for elderly persons (Nicholson and Ward, 1984). Anterograde amnesia can also be associated with rage or psychosis. A 20% incidence of amnesia is associated with triazolam, but approximately 45% of patients with insomnia who do not receive treatment also complain of memory problems, making it difficult to establish the clinical significance of triazolam's effect on memory (Mendelson, 1992). Also, on cessation of sedative treatment, insomnia may arise as a rebound phenomenon, particularly when short-acting agents are withdrawn suddenly. Rebound insomnia occurs more often when a relatively high dose of a rapidly eliminated drug is prescribed and used nightly. Generally this phenomenon is not observed when these drugs are used in recommended doses for limited periods (Roehrs et al, 1986).

Benzodiazepine hypnotics remain effective as sleeping agents for approximately 6 months of continued use (Oswald et al, 1982); however, they do produce adaption and tolerance (Greenblatt and Shader, 1978). For example, the patient may have fewer sedating effects (tolerance) over time and achieve physiologic homeostasis with loss of hypnotic effect. Drug dependence is also a possible consequence with the use of hypnotics, as it is with the anxiolytics. The possibility of dependence can be minimized by intermittent use of low doses together with limited duration of prescription and gradual withdrawal in the event that continuous treatment has been given for more than 1 month (Ladewig, 1983). Indeed, withdrawal of hypnotics after long-term use may lead to a recrudescence of the original symptoms, as well as to rebound insomnia (Nicholson, 1980). Zolpidem (Ambien) is an ideal hypnotic for elderly individuals, especially in low doses of 5 mg and for short courses. However, long-term use seems to result in little accumulation. Minimal daytime drowsiness and lack of drug interaction makes this drug a choice agent among elderly persons.

Mixed Anxiety-Depression

Mixed anxiety-depression is frequently diagnosed in older adults who receive treatment in primary care settings. Clinical presentations may not meet the full syndromal criteria for a mood or anxiety disorder, and anxiety or depression may not always be distinguishable as the overriding disorder. Elderly individuals may also come to medical attention with clinical symptoms for which diagnostic criteria are not clearly identifiable or for which the clinical setting or brief nature of the assessment may not lend itself to a definitive diagnosis, for example, the nursing home or emergency department. Nonetheless these patients come to medical attention with clinically significant symptoms that are potentially responsive to anxiolytics (Feigner, Merideth, and Hendrickson, 1982; Rakel, 1990; Rickels et al, 1982; Sussman, 1988).

The pharmacotherapy of mixed anxiety-depression is perhaps best accomplished with a broad-spectrum, first-line agent such as an SSRI, buspirone, or alprazolam. Mixed anxiety-depression is perhaps better treated with a benzodiazepine when anxiety is associated with an acute stressor or overwhelming situational factors. Buspirone or the SSRIs represent an ideal drug in patients requiring long-term therapy and may ultimately alleviate several target symptoms of anxiety-depression, diminishing agitation, improving concentration, and enhancing functional ability (Folks, 1990; Preskorn, 1990). A full discussion of these agents may be found in Chapters 5, Mood Disorders, and 6, Anxiety Disorders.

Agitation and Aggression

Older patients, particularly those who may be cognitively impaired or institutionalized, often receive treatment with an anxiolytic or sedative drug for agitation or aggression. In many cases, when the agitation is the result of psychosis or delirium, the best treatment choice is an antipsychotic or neuroleptic, for example, haloperidol. However, the anxiolytics, for example, buspirone; or the benzodiazepines, for example, oxazepam and lorazepam; offer certain advantages with reduced potential for side effects such as EPSEs and oversedation. Moreover, in long-term care settings the Omnibus Budget Reconciliation Act of 1987 (OBRA) guidelines restrict the prescription of antipsychotic medications, and further restrictions are being developed for the "tranquilizing" anxiolytics. These guidelines require that nursing home patients be appropriately diagnosed. Patients can then receive treatment in adherence to federal guidelines, which mandate that specific psychiatric conditions be appropriately treated with a selected psychotropic agent (Domantay and Napoliello, 1989; Keltner and Folks, 1995).

OBRA guidelines require both a rationale and a justification for using a psychotropic drug, including documentation and monitoring. Additionally, drug selection, dosage, duration of therapy, and discontinuation of prescription when potential dependency and addiction are present are addressed by OBRA guidelines. Thus anxiolytic drug therapy with benzodiazepines and antipsychotics in long-term care settings is subject to OBRA guidelines. Also, as a result of the OBRA legislation the incidental use of anxiolytics or antipsychotics in long-term care settings will be discouraged and may even be prohibited. Buspirone, SSRIs, valproate, and trazodone are agents that have great utility in the long-term setting, especially because these agents are not subject to the drug holidays, tapering, and monitoring required with tranquilizing agents. Further discussion of this topic is found in both Chapters 4, Schizophrenia and Other Psychoses, and 8, Sleep Disorders.

Antipsychotic or neuroleptic drugs have been both vigorously recommended and condemned for treating chronically agitated or anxious elderly patients in any clinical setting. Although high-potency neuroleptics such as haloperidol are often used for this purpose, drugs with strongly sedating properties may be preferred. For example, thioridazine may be prescribed at low doses, as mentioned previously, in the range of 10 to 50 mg 1 to 4 times per day. Although using a neuroleptic agent avoids the risk of drug dependency, the risk of tardive dyskinesia and the emergence of other equally problematic side effects are concerns. Thus neuroleptics are *not* recommended for simple anxiety or agitation.

The availability of newly developed anxiolytics, for example, short-acting benzodiazepines or buspirone, should also be considered as therapeutic in the context of risks versus benefits for treating agitation and aggression. Buspirone; low doses of short-acting benzodiazepines such as alprazolam, lorazepam, and oxazepam; and other agents may be useful alone or as adjuncts for treating agitation. Trazodone, lithium, valproate, carbamazepine, and the beta blockers have been reported most often to be potentially useful (see Chapter 9, Acute Psychoses and the Violent Patient). One or more of these alternative agents may be necessary for long-term treatment when persistent agitation, aggression, or suicidality poses a significant risk.

Short-acting benzodiazepines have been useful primarily for the acute treatment of agitation associated with underlying anxiety or depression. Interestingly severe agitation not amenable to a neuroleptic may sometimes be more likely to respond to a benzodiazepine. Lorazepam is particularly useful in this regard because it may be given intramuscularly. Lenox et al (1992) have advocated using lorazepam as an adjunct to the neuroleptics in violent or aggressive patients at a ratio of 1 mg of lorazepam for every 5 mg of haloperidol. Similarly clonazepam (Klonopin) is useful for patients with mania who are agitated (Rosenbaum, 1989). Buspirone is likely to reduce agitation and aggression in elderly patients with mental retardation (Ratey et al, 1989) or who are cognitively impaired (Eison, 1989). Moreover, the long-term use of buspirone avoids the problem of addiction or dependency and is not likely to impair the older patient's cognition or motor function. However, aggressive patients who do not respond or remit with neuroleptic or anxiolytic intervention may require long-term use of lithium, carbamazepine, or a beta-adrenergic blocking agent, as outlined in Chapter 9, Acute Psychoses and the Violent Patient.

Delirium, "Sundowning," and Confusion Associated with Dementia

A variety of psychotropic agents may be useful in treating agitation, confusion, or aggression in patients with disturbed cognition. In many cases the patient has some degree of delirium. See Box 17-4 for diagnostic measures for delirium. Effective

Box 17-4 Delirium: Diagnostic Measures

- Serum chemical survey
- Complete blood cell count
- Arterial blood gas levels
- Urinalysis
- Serum and urine drug screen
- Serum B_{12} and folate levels
- Thyroid functions
- Serum test for syphilis
- Chest radiograph
- Electrocardiogram (Holter monitor)
- Electroencephalogram
- Computed tomography scan of head
- Cerebral spinal fluid examination

management of delirium may require any of three therapeutic tasks. The first fundamental task is assessment to determine the underlying physiologic or anatomic disturbances thought to be causal. Generally this phase of treatment requires a diligent clinical evaluation using any or all of the diagnostic tests listed in Box 17-4. Medications must also be assiduously evaluated, in particular, their accumulative doses and temporal relationship to the onset of the delirium. A high index of suspicion is warranted for any of the classes of medications listed in Box 17-5.

The second therapeutic task is to provide general supportive measures, including both environmental measures and physiologic stabilization (Box 17-6). Ideally these therapeutic principles obviate the need for pharmacologic intervention or prolonged physical restraint. However, the effective use of psychotropic drugs is indi-

Box 17-5 Classes and Examples of Medications that Induce Delirium

Anticholinergics:	Benztropine, trihexyphenidyl
Anticonvulsants:	Barbiturates, phenytoin
Antidiabetics:	Insulin, oral hypoglycemics
Antihypertensives:	Clonidine, methyldopa
Antiparkinsons:	Levodopa, carbidopa
Cancer chemotherapeutics:	Procarbazine, nitrogen mustard
Cardiovascular agents:	Digoxin, lidocaine
Corticosteroids:	Prednisone, prednisolone
Gastrointestinal agents:	Cimetidine, belladona
Narcotic analgesics:	Opiates, synthetic narcotics
Nonnarcotic analgesics:	Salicylates, propoxyphene
Psychotropics:	Anxiolytics, antidepressants

Box 17-6 Nonpharmacologic Treatment of Delirium

Environmental manipulation
Arrange consistent, supportive nursing care
Minimize personnel
Place family member or significant other at bedside
Utilize orienting remarks and devices such as calendars or clocks
Place in a well-lighted room with window
Provide familiar objects such as personal belongings and photos

Supportive measures
Effect fluid and electrolyte balance
Maintain nutritional and vitamin status
Obtain visual or hearing aids
Provide moderate sensory input
Encourage physical activity or ambulation
Apply physical restraints as necessary

cated when behavioral disturbances, psychomotor agitation, or psychosis predominates the clinical picture.

The third therapeutic task involves selecting one or more pharmacologic agents that will result in symptomatic relief or effectively treat the underlying cause, or both. Box 17-7 outlines pharmacologic considerations and lists specific medications for each of the three categories of delirium. Cases categorized as induced by withdrawal from alcohol, sedative-hypnotic agents, or a similar agent are best treated with the judicious use of a benzodiazepine. However, delirium precipitated by anticholinergic drugs requires withdrawal of the offending agents, and urgent cases may also benefit from using an anticholinesterase agent such as physostigmine (Antilirium). Antipsychotic drug treatment should be avoided or minimized in cases of anticholinergic delirium because of the potential for additional anticholinergic effects and the possible lowering of the seizure threshold. Most cases that represent delirium either are multifactorial or result from a nonspecific cause and simply require a drug regimen that is designed to normalize sleep or control psychomotor agitation, psychosis, or disruptive behavior. Although employing a short-acting sedative may be useful for sleep enhancement, behavioral symptoms of motor agitation, aggression, or psychosis are more effectively treated with a low-dose antipsychotic agent such as haloperidol, as discussed in Chapter 9, Acute Psychoses and the Violent Patient. These potent antipsychotic medications possess minimal anticholinergic effects and rarely result in an adverse drug interaction or contribute to the delirium;

Box 17-7 Pharmacologic Treatment of Delirium

Sedative hypnotic, similar agent, or alcohol withdrawal

1. Careful maintenance of fluid and electrolyte balance
2. Careful replacement or provision of nutritional and vitamin requirements
3. Effective sedation with a benzodiazepine agent: Chlordiazepoxide (Librium) 25 to 50 mg orally or intramuscularly every 4 to 6 hours or lorazepam (Ativan) 1 to 2 mg orally or intramuscularly every 6 to 8 hours

Anticholinergic-induced delirium

1. Withdraw offending anticholinergic agent(s)
2. Counteract severe cases with physostigmine (Antilirium) 1 to 2 mg slowly intravenously; may be repeated every 30 to 60 minutes

Multifactorial or miscellaneous variables

1. Withdraw offending agent(s) or treat underlying cause(s)
2. Enhance sleep with short–half-life hypnotic*†: Triazolam (Halcion) 0.25 to 0.5 mg; zolpidem (Ambien) 0.5 to 10 mg; temazepam (Restoril) 15 to 30 mg orally at bedtime; or chloral hydrate 500 to 1000 mg orally at bedtime
3. Treat "sundowning" or disruptive behavior with high-potency antipsychotic†: Haloperidol (Haldol) or fluphenazine (Prolixin) hydrochloride 1 to 2 mg orally (concentrate) or intramuscularly, 2 to 4 times daily

*Hypnotics can potentially worsen the clinical course and diminish cognition.
†Dosage must be adjusted individually; geriatric patients may be started on a regimen of half doses.

furthermore, serious hypotension or cardiotoxic effects are unlikely to occur. However, EPSEs, for example, dystonic reactions, akathisia, or parkinsonian symptoms, should be monitored and counteracted, preferably with amantadine (Symmetrel) at 100 mg orally once or twice daily. As a corollary psychotropic drugs are unnecessary in the absence of psychotic or behavioral disturbances except in drug or alcohol withdrawal states, which are notorious for intensifying if the patient is not adequately sedated (Folks, 1988).

Alzheimer's Disease and Related Disorders

As shown in Box 17-8 and in Figure 17-3 management of disorders characterized by other cognitive impairment requires careful assessment to consider possible underlying problems. Individuals are diagnosed with dementia if irreversible intellectual loss occurs of sufficient degree to cause social, occupational, or daily disturbance of function, together with memory loss and other cognitive deficits. The Mini-Mental State Examination can be very useful in screening for Alzheimer's disease (Figure 17-4).

Alzheimer's disease is the most prevalent type of dementia and accounts for up to three fourths of such cases. Vascular, or multiinfarct, dementia is the second most common type. Multiinfarct dementia is frequently associated with depression or lability of affect or other behavioral disturbance (Cummings, 1987). Alzheimer's disease can be divided into three stages—early, middle and late—as shown in Box 17-9. Alzheimer's disease affects 4 million people in the United States and is the most frequent cause of long-term care (Katzman, 1986). This age-related disease results from a degenerative process characterized by deposits of amyloid and other abnormal proteins in the brain (Bondareff, 1987). Inflammatory and immune mechanisms are involved in neuronal destruction (Aisen and Davis, 1994). Further, complementary components are known to attack and are found around neurons and neurofibrillary tangles. Thus antiinflammatory and immunosuppressive drugs are being investigated as possible treatments of Alzheimer's disease.

Although numerous changes in various neurotransmitter systems have been documented in the brains of patients with Alzheimer's disease, accumulating evidence suggests dysfunction of the cholinergic system is crucial in the development of memory loss and related cognitive problems. This has been termed the *cholinergic hypothesis of memory dysfunction* (Bartus et al, 1985). In the hippocampus and cortex, two brain areas associated with memory and cognitive function, there is an excellent congruence between the neurochemical alterations and the pathologic

Box 17-8 Underlying Causes of Cognitive Impairment

D Drug toxicity
E Eyes/ears, sensory impairment
M Metabolic disturbance or endocrinopathy
E Emotional disturbances, especially depression
N Normal pressure hydrocephalus or nutritional deficiency
T Toxins, tumors, trauma to the head
I Infection
A Atherosclerosis in vascular disease

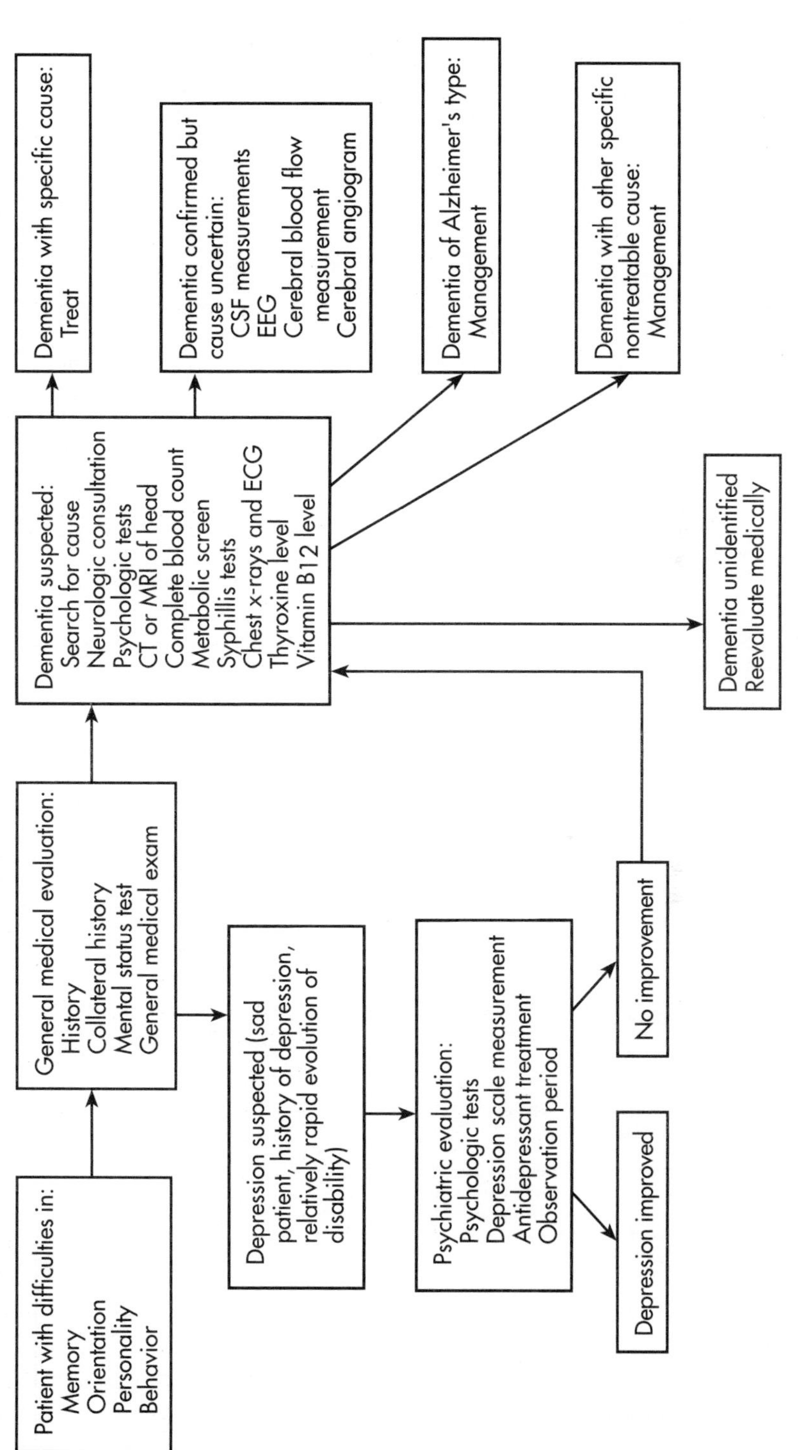

Figure 17-3 Assessment of cognitive impairment.

I. Orientation (Maximum score 10)

Ask "What is today's date?" Then ask specifically for parts omitted: eg, "Can you also tell me what season it is?"

- Date (eg, January 21) ... 1 ___
- Year ... 2 ___
- Month ... 3 ___
- Day (eg, Monday) ... 4 ___
- Season ... 5 ___

Ask "Can you tell me the name of this hospital?" "What floor are we on?" "What town (or city) are we in?" "What county are we in?" "What state are we in?"

- Hospital ... 6 ___
- Floor ... 7 ___
- Town/City ... 8 ___
- County ... 9 ___
- State ... 10 ___

II. Registration (Maximum score 3)

Ask the subject if you may test his/her memory. Then say "ball," "flag," "tree" clearly and slowly, about one second for each. After you have said all 3 words, ask subject to repeat them. This first repetition determines the score (0-3), but keep saying them (up to 6 trials) until the subject can repeat all 3 words. If (s)he does not eventually learn all three, recall cannot be meaningfully tested.

- "ball" ... 11 ___
- "flag" ... 12 ___
- "tree" ... 13 ___

Record number of trials: ___

III. Attention and calculation (Maximum score 5)

Ask the subject to begin at 100 and count backward by 7. Stop after 5 subtractions (93, 86, 79, 72, 65). Score one point for each correct number.

- "93" ... 14 ___
- "86" ... 15 ___
- "79" ... 16 ___
- "72" ... 17 ___
- "65" ... 18 ___

OR

If the subject cannot or will not perform this task, ask him/her to spell the word "world" backwards (D, L, R, O, W). The score is one point for each correctly placed letter, eg, DLROW = 5: DLORW = 3. Record how the subject spelled "world" backwards: ___
DLROW

- Number of correctly placed letters ... 19 ___

IV. Recall (Maximum score 3)

Ask the subject to recall the three words you previously asked him/her to remember (learned in Registration)

- "ball" ... 20 ___
- "flag" ... 21 ___
- "tree" ... 22 ___

V. Language (Maximum score 9)

Naming: Show the subject a wrist watch and ask "What is this?" Repeat for pencil. Score one point for each item named correctly.

- Watch ... 23 ___
- Pencil ... 24 ___

Repetition: Ask the subject to repeat, "No ifs, ands, or buts." Score one point for correct repetition.

- Repetition ... 25 ___

3-Stage Command: Give the subject a piece of blank paper and say, "Take the paper in your right hand, fold it in half and put it on the floor." Score one point for each action performed correctly.

- Takes in right hand ... 26 ___
- Folds in half ... 27 ___
- Puts on floor ... 28 ___

Reading: On a blank piece of paper, print the sentence "Close your eyes" in letters large enough for the subject to see clearly. Ask subject to read it and do what it says. Score correct only if s(he) actually closes his/her eyes.

- Closes eyes ... 29 ___

Writing: Give the subject a blank piece of paper and ask him/her to write a sentence. It is to be written spontaneously. It must contain a subject and verb and make sense. Correct grammar and punctuation are not necessary.

- Writes sentence ... 30 ___

Copying: On a clean piece of paper, draw intersecting pentagons, each side about 1 inch, and ask subject to copy it exactly as it is. All 10 angles must be present and two must intersect to score 1 point. Tremor and rotation are ignored. Eg,

- Draws pentagons ... 31 ___

Score: Add number of correct responses. In section III, include items 14-18 or item 19, not both. (Maximum total score 30) Total score ___

Rate subject's level of consciousness: ___ (a) coma, (b) stupor, (c) drowsy, (d) alert

Figure 17-4 The Mini-Mental State Examination: a tool for cognitive screening of patients with suspected Alzheimer's disease. (From Folstein MF, Folstein SE, McHugh PR: Mini-mental state: a practical method of grading the cognitive state of patients for the clinician, *J Psychiatr Res* 12:189, 1975.)

Box 17-9 Cognitive Symptoms of Early, Middle, and Late Stages of Alzheimer's Disease

Early Stage

Forgetfulness for faces, names, and conversations

Subtle decline in performing work or activities of daily living (trouble learning new routines, slowing of work performance, and decreased output)

Subtle personality changes (decline in social graces and withdrawal from social contacts)

Early language problems (difficulty expressing complex ideas, shortening of phraseology)

Repetitiveness

Anxiety, worry, and depression concerning the decline of these abilities

Early-Middle Stage

Pervasive memory problems (forgetting major, important items and "forgetting to remember")

Inability to work in one's customary job

Paranoia, apathy, or delusions

Need for supervision in household chores

Difficulties in naming objects

Disorientation outdoors, especially in relatively unfamiliar places

Definite decline in personal grooming

Occasional incontinence

Needing reminders to bathe and assistance in dressing

Late-Middle Stage

Frequent disorientation indoors

Needing supervision in bathroom

Very limited vocabulary and comprehension

Disorders of sleep-wakefulness cycle

Extremes of emotional reactivity

General withdrawal from all social contacts

State of "living in the past"

Purposeless hyperactivity or energy

Late Stage

Dissolution of personality

Lack of recognition

Severe language impairment

Inability to feed oneself

Incontinence

Severe motor deficits

The order, intensity, and duration of symptoms varies considerably among patients. Seizures, myoclonus, or gait disturbance may predominate in some subsets of patients.

Modified from Kokmen E: Etiology, diagnosis, and management of dementia, *Compr Ther* 15(9):59-69, 1989.

changes found. For example, the degeneration of cholinergic neurons that originate in the basal nucleus of Meynert and project into the hippocampus and cortex correlates well with the decrease (40% to 90%) found in levels of choline acetyltransferase (CAT), the biosynthetic enzyme for the neurotransmitter acetylcholine (Katzman, 1986; Bartus et al, 1985).

The relationship between memory loss and a cholinergic deficit has been demonstrated repeatedly in both preclinical and clinical studies. Partial amelioration of these deficits can be achieved by the anticholinesterase inhibitor physostigmine (Bartus et al, 1985). It has also been demonstrated that injections of the anticholinergic drug scopolamine into healthy young subjects cause confusion and memory loss similar to the symptoms of early Alzheimer's disease (Katzman, 1986; Bartus et al, 1982). It is also noteworthy that cortical cholinergic deficits are found in a variety of degenerative conditions of the central nervous system that cause memory loss, including parkinson's disease, in association with dementia (Perry, 1988).

MANAGEMENT OF DELIRIUM, DEMENTIA, AND ALZHEIMER'S DISEASE

Supportive Care

The principal goals of supportive care for dementias of all types are to maintain the patient's socialization in a safe but stimulating environment and to counsel the family (Cooper, 1991). Agitation, paranoid thinking, and irrational behavior can be avoided to some degree by providing patients with nonstressful, familiar, and constant surroundings; as well as schedules that are both regular and structured to encourage patients to continue physical and mental activities within their capacity (Winograd and Jarvik, 1986). Measures that can help patients orient themselves within their home environment include prominently displaying clocks and calendars, supplying nightlights, posting a bulletin board with a schedule of daily activities, pictures of family members, and the like (Skelton and Skelton, 1991); putting labels on commonly used items; and addressing notes to patients about simple safety measures. Activities that may help preserve cognitive function include listening to the radio or looking at newspapers or television, doing chores, engaging in physical exercise, attending structured social events, and participating in discussion and reminiscences (Winograd and Jarvik, 1986). A patient can cope better when household activities—meals, walks, chores—occur at the same time every day (Skelton and Skelton, 1991). Familiarity with an environment can make a patient's life less stressful; thus a patient should be surrounded with familiar furniture and objects. Discouraging naps can lessen the chances of night wandering.

Patients who have progressed beyond the earliest stages of Alzheimer's disease should not be permitted to drive, because of disease-associated disorientation and impairment of judgment, reaction time, and visual perception (Kokmen, 1989). This recommendation is substantiated by study results that show that 30% of 72 patients with dementia had experienced at least one accident since the onset of dementia, and an additional 11% were said by caregivers to have been responsible for accidents (Lucas-Blaustein et al, 1988).

Most patients, especially those in the last stages of Alzheimer's disease, will eventually require institutional care. Incontinence and disruptive behavior are the most common factors that influence families' decisions to seek a long-term care facility (Besdine et al, 1992). What constitutes appropriate care for people with dementia is still an evolving body of knowledge.

Drug Therapy Options

Pharmacologic treatment of patients with Alzheimer's disease primarily involves using drugs that are directed at the psychiatric symptoms that commonly occur with the disease (Cooper, 1991) and that help improve cognitive function and the memory loss associated with the disease. The drugs used to treat the concurrent behavioral disorders, for example, neuroleptics and antidepressants, are those that have been and are currently used to treat those disorders when they occur in the absence of Alzheimer's disease. Additional therapies are needed to effectively treat deficits in memory and cognitive function. To date, only one approved therapy exists; a list of drugs that may be of potential benefit is given in Box 17-10.

Psychiatric Symptoms Concurrent with Alzheimer's Disease

Depression. Depression occurs in approximately 20% to 25% of patients with Alzheimer's disease, with a higher prevalence among those with mild to moderate,

Box 17-10 Drugs of Potential Benefit in Improving Cognitive Function or Slowing the Progression of Alzheimer's Disease

Augmenting acetylcholine
Cholinesterase inhibitors
Physostigmine
Tacrine hydrochloride
Velnacrine maleate
E-2020

Increasing precursors
Lecithin

Nootropics*
Piracetam
Oxiracetam

Vascular system
Vasodilators†
Ergoloid mesylates
Nicergoline
Captopril
Calcium channel blockers
Nimodipine

Miscellaneous
Monoamine oxidase B inhibitors
Selegiline (Deprenyl)
Nerve growth factor
Cell membrane stabilizers
Phosphatidylserine

*These are drugs otherwise affecting neuron function.
† Nominally vasodilators, the mechanism of action in treating Alzheimer's disease may be different.

rather than severe, cognitive impairment (Reifler et al, 1982). The treatment of depression, however, may be complicated by the questionable efficacy and side effects of antidepressant drugs in patients with Alzheimer's disease (Winograd and Jarvik, 1986). Patients with Alzheimer's disease, because of their cholinergic deficit, may be more vulnerable to the anticholinergic side effects of TCAs (Winograd and Jarvik, 1986). The agent selected should produce minimal anticholinergic activity to avoid further decreases in cognitive function. Newer agents, SSRIs including venlafaxine, bupropion, and nefazodone, are preferred. For patients who do not respond to these newer agents, tricyclics or MAOIs may be used, provided attention is paid to dietary and drug precautions. MAOIs have virtually no anticholinergic effect and are less sedating than tricyclics; the most problematic side effects in elderly persons are hypotension and insomnia. A maxim is to start antidepressant therapy at the lowest dose possible in elderly patients and slowly increase the dose until improvement is seen.

Agitation. Agitated or aggressive behavior may mandate therapy with a neuroleptic agent, although these drugs should be prescribed in low doses and only when necessary. In addition, periodic attempts should be made to reduce the dosage or discontinue the drug. As for TCAs, neuroleptics may cause anticholinergic side effects. In addition, these agents may cause EPSEs. However, neuroleptics may produce substantial improvement in as many as one third of patients with Alzheimer's disease who have delusions, hallucinations, and aggressive agitation. Neuroleptics should be reserved for use with those individuals whose behavior constitutes a danger and is not appropriate in cases of insomnia, fidgeting, or uncooperativeness (Cooper, 1991). As previously mentioned, buspirone, propranolol, lithium, valproate, carbamazepine, and SSRIs, for example, fluoxetine and sertraline, have also been used successfully to treat aggressive agitation in patients with dementia similar to other patients who are agitated or aggressive, as discussed in Chapter 9, Acute Psychoses and the Violent Patient.

Anxiety. Benzodiazepines may be helpful in treating less severe agitation in patients with Alzheimer's disease, although OBRA regulations restrict their use. These drugs do not carry the risk of EPSEs, although they may increase the chances of falling (Cooper, 1991). Buspirone is another therapeutic option not subject to OBRA restrictions that has a very safe drug profile (see Chapter 6, Anxiety Disorder).

Treatment of Cognitive Impairment. Successful management by pharmacologic agents of cognitive function in patients with Alzheimer's disease is limited. Our understanding of the pathogenesis and pathophysiology of the disease is incomplete, consequently impeding the design of appropriate therapy. None of the drugs now being used for treatment has proved to be efficacious in a large percentage of patients. The fact that the disease appears to include several subtypes may partly explain this. Following is a discussion of classes of drugs that have been studied for use in treating Alzheimer's disease.

Metabolic Enhancers/Vasodilators. Hydergine, a compound of ergoloid mesylates previously termed a *vasodilator* but now classified a *metabolic enhancer,* is approved by the FDA for treating dementia; however, its mechanism of action is currently unknown, and a recent well-controlled trial has found this agent to be of no benefit (Cooper, 1991). The peripheral vasodilator nicergoline, another ergot drug, ameliorated disorientation in 30% of patients in a multicenter, double-blind placebo trial, but this drug is not available in the United States. The calcium channel blocker nimodipine, which is specific for the brain vasculature, is currently under investigation in patients with Alzheimer's disease (Cooper, 1991). Its potential benefit in treating Alzheimer's disease may reside in its ability to reduce focal ischemia.

Nootropics. *Nootropics* are drugs that enhance neuronal metabolic activity. One avenue of research has focused on increasing nerve cell function so that neurotransmitter synthesis is increased. The mechanisms of action of nootropics responsible for improving memory are uncertain but are thought to include stimulation of phospholipid turnover and protein synthesis and subsequently enhance cholinergic transmission. Potentially beneficial nootropics include piracetam and the related drug oxiracetam (Cooper, 1991). As previously stated, disruption of other neurotransmitter systems such as the serotonergic and noradrenergic systems has been documented in patients with Alzheimer's disease. Attempts to increase their synthesis and thus improve symptoms by using an MAOI or the SSRI imipramine have yielded only mild or nonsignificant improvements.

Cholinergic Enhancers. The documented deficiency in cholinergic function in patients with Alzheimer's disease and the probable role of this deficit in contributing to memory loss and cognitive dysfunction have inspired therapeutic trials of cholinergic enhancers in an attempt to improve symptoms in these patients. Numerous attempts to improve memory through the use of choline or lecithin (both precursors to the neurotransmitter acetylcholine) have failed to definitively demonstrate a beneficial effect on cognitive function in either demented or nondemented aged patients (Davidson et al, 1991).

Studies with cholinergic agonists have yielded equivocal results. For example, early preclinical and clinical trials with the muscarinic agonist, arecoline have demonstrated a significant improvement in delayed recall tasks in aged monkeys and normal volunteers; results in trials with patients with Alzheimer's disease, however, have been inconsistent (Bartus et al, 1985; Davidson et al, 1991). Studies with bethanecol, oxotremorine, and RS-86 have not been encouraging (Davidson et al, 1991).

The results with cholinesterase inhibitors have been more promising. A number of small clinical trials have demonstrated minimal to modest improvement in memory in about one third of patients treated with physostigmine, compared with those treated with placebo. However, no other improvements in other areas of cognition during treatment with physostigmine were observed (Mohs et al, 1985). Tacrine (Cognex), a longer-acting cholinesterase inhibitor, has recently been approved by the FDA for treating mild to moderate dementia of the Alzheimer's type. In patients with mild to moderate Alzheimer's disease, tacrine has demonstrated improvement compared with placebo as measured by the Alzheimer's Disease Assessment Scale, the clinician-rated Clinical Global Impression of Change (CGIC), and the caregiver-rated CGIC (Gauthier, 1990). Dosing of tacrine in protocols has ranged from 40 to 160 mg per day, in 4 divided doses usually given between meals. Higher doses are not recommended because of concerns about hepatotoxicity and adverse effects. Blood monitoring is required every other week for the first 18 weeks after initiation of tacrine therapy to monitor alanine aminotransferase levels (ALT) and for 6 weeks after each successive dosage increase. Common side effects include GI upset and agitation. Approximately 25% to 30% of cases will show ALT elevations that require withdrawal from the drug. Interestingly about two thirds of patients who show elevated enzymes, therefore requiring drug discontinuation, are able to resume treatment after a rechallenge. The recommended modifications with ALT elevations are shown in Box 17-11. Overall, 30% to 60% of cases show improvement in cognitive function and/or maintain their present level of cognitive function for extended periods of time.

Other cholinergic enhancers are now being investigated. E-2020 or donezepil shows the most promise. It is a cholinesterase inhibitor that in preliminary studies

Box 17-11 Recommended Dose Regimen Modification in Response to Transaminase Elevation with Tacrine Therapy

Transaminase Level	Treatment Regimen
$\leq 3 \times$ ULN	Continue treatment according to recommended titration.
> 3 to $\leq 5 \times$ ULN	Reduce the daily dose of tacrine (Cognex) by 40 mg per day. Resume dose titration when transaminases return to within normal limits.
$> 5 \times$ ULN	Stop tacrine treatment. Monitor transaminase levels until within normal limits. See information on rechallenging below.
	Experience is limited with patients who have an alanine aminotransferase level $> 10 \times$ ULN. The risk of rechallenge must be considered against demonstrated clinical benefit.
	Patients with clinical jaundice confirmed by a significant elevation in total bilirubin ($>$ 3 mg per dL) should permanently discontinue tacrine and not be rechallenged.

From package insert for Cognex, Parke-Davis, Morris Plains, NJ.
ULN = Upper limit of normal.

shows similar efficacy to tacrine but without the hepatotoxicity and degree of adverse effect. This drug is currently under FDA consideration for approval. This agent has been shown to be comparable to tacrine in reversing scopolamine-induced dementia in animal models while causing less liver toxicity. It is dosed at 5 or 10 mg daily, with a half-life of approximately 60 hours. Initial clinical results show that approximately half of patients with Alzheimer's disease who tolerate the therapy experience improvement in cognitive function.

A new avenue of therapeutic investigation is the pharmacologic application of nerve growth factor (NGF) to treat Alzheimer's disease (Hefti and Schneider, 1991). Intraventricular administration of NGF in adult rats and primates has been shown to produce trophic actions on cholinergic neurons and prevent age-related neuronal atrophy. It is suggested that exogenously administering human NGF could cause the magnocellular cholinergic neurons of the basal forebrain to hypertrophy, synthesize more choline acetyltransferase, and sprout new nerve fibers (Goedert, 1989).

Clearly there is currently no pharmacologic "magic bullet" with which to treat Alzheimer's disease. Drawbacks to drugs under study include unclear benefits, the presence of side effects (serious and otherwise), and inefficacious bioavailability. The search for effective therapy is made more difficult by a still murky understanding of the etiology and progression of the disease. Continued research should provide insights to both arms of inquiry.

Remarks

The primary goal of psychotropic drug therapy in elderly patients is improvement in the quality of life. Often a psychiatric disturbance is not curable; this is particularly true for disorders of cognitive impairment such as Alzheimer's disease. Thus the goal of drug therapy can be alleviation of secondary psychiatric symptoms or maintenance. The therapeutic goal may sometimes be accomplished with simple behavioral or environmental measures, often without using drugs. The potential effects of aging and disease with respect to pharmacokinetics and pharmacodynamics and the possible ramifications of adverse drug reaction or interaction must be considered carefully. Increased knowledge of the action and effects of drugs in older patients and enhanced communication between the patient and treatment team can significantly improve the overall quality of care.

Using a psychotropic agent in a geriatric patient must be carefully planned. Psychotropics should not be used merely for the convenience of staff or family and should not be used without appropriate evaluation. Diagnostic uncertainty regarding symptoms of anxiety, insomnia, and agitation should lead to assessment for underlying psychiatric conditions such as major depression, delusional disorder, or dementia. Symptomatic treatment without diagnostic clarification should not be undertaken. A clear rationale for using a drug must be based on a sound risk-benefit analysis that should be carefully developed and documented, especially in settings where federal guidelines or reimbursement mechanisms are strict.

In general, using benzodiazepines and antipsychotic agents is justified when drug therapy results in improvement in the patient's functional status. Benzodiazepines and antipsychotics may be used as a primary treatment for major psychiatric conditions, for example, panic, generalized anxiety, mood disorder, dementia, or delirium. In using anxiolytics, sedatives, or antipsychotic agents, frequent attempts should be made to reduce the dosage or discontinue the medication, or both. These efforts should take place at intervals no longer than 4 months. Alternative pharmacologic intervention should be considered when appropriate or indicated.

The geriatric patient is more sensitive to the nontherapeutic effects of anxiolytics, sedatives, and antipsychotics than is the younger patient; initial dose regulation should be low and titrated perhaps at one fourth to half of the usual adult dosage. Short-acting benzodiazepines are preferred because of their pharmacokinetic properties and because of reduced potential for metabolic accumulation. Furthermore, drugs requiring only phase 2 hepatic metabolism have more predictable effects. Drugs that meet these criteria, that is, oxazepam, lorazepam, and temazepam, are preferred for older patients. High-potency antipsychotic agents in low doses may be better tolerated in geriatric patients, although the potential for EPSEs and oversedation exists. Subtle nontherapeutic effects of anxiolytics, sedatives, and antipsychotic agents may not be evident immediately after starting drug treatment. Thus geriatric patients receiving these drugs must be monitored carefully. Cognitive impairment, confusion, concentration difficulties, conceptual defects, and motor dysfunction, including incoordination and ataxia, should be identified promptly.

Alternative agents, that is, low-potency neuroleptics or antihistamines, are sometimes prescribed simply to sedate geriatric patients. However, this practice is generally not effective, and these drugs are not as well tolerated as are the benzodiazepines. Occasionally a barbiturate such as phenobarbital is used as an anxiolytic; again, however, these older agents are not as effective as a short-acting benzodiazepine or the newer anxiolytic agents. In abandoning older agents, it is important to recognize the potential risk of dependency associated with their long-term use, as well as the superior safety profile of benzodiazepines.

Using antidepressants or newer anxiolytic agents should be considered for treating both anxiety and insomnia, as well as in cases involving depression. Low-dose antipsychotics, lithium, valproate, or carbamazepine may be indicated for treating severely agitated elderly patients who do not respond to buspirone, trazodone, or a benzodiazepine. Patients with symptoms that are frankly psychotic, that is, delusions, hallucinations, or conceptual disorganization, are best treated with an antipsychotic drug.

Caution is the hallmark for drug treatment in elderly persons. Diagnosis, drug selection, and evaluation of the clinical effectiveness of the pharmacologic agent over time are important management considerations. Ideally drug treatment should be combined with other nonpharmacologic approaches, which may also enhance compliance and improve the likelihood of an initial or sustained response.

REFERENCES

Abernathy DR, Kerznel L: Age effects on alpha-1 acid glycoprotein concentrations and imipramine plasma protein binding, *J Am Geriatr Soc* 32:705, 1984.

Abrass IB, Scarpace PJ: Human lymphocyte beta-adrenergic receptors are unaltered with age, *J Gerontol* 36:298, 1981.

Aisen PS, Davis KL: Inflammatory mechanisms in Alzheimer's disease: implications for therapy, *Am J Psychiatry* 151:1105-13, 1994.

Avorn J et al: A randomized trial of a program to reduce the use of psychoactive drugs in nursing homes, *N Engl J Med* 327:168-73, 1992.

Balter MB, Bauer ML: Patterns of prescribing and use of hypnotic drugs in the United States. In Clift AD, editor: *Sleep disturbances and hypnotic drug dependence,* Amsterdam, 1975, *Excerpta Medica.*

Bartus RT et al: The cholinergic hypothesis: a historical overview, current perspective and future directions, *Ann NY Acad Sci* 444:332-58, 1985.

Bartus RT et al: The cholinergic hypothesis of geriatric memory dysfunction, *Science* 217:408-17, 1982.

Bellatuono C et al: Benzodiazepines: clinical pharmacology and therapeutic use, *Drugs* 19:195, 1980.

Bernstein JG: *Drug therapy in psychiatry,* ed 3, Littleton, Mass, 1995, PSG Publishing.

Besdine RW, Lissy JF, Tangalos EG: Managing advanced Alzheimer's disease, *Patient Care* 25(18):75-90, 1992.

Blazer D et al: Depressive symptoms and depressive diagnoses in a community population: use of a new procedure for analysis of psychiatric classification, *Arch Gen Psychiatry* 45:1078, 1988.

Bondareff W et al: Age and histopathologic heterogeneity in Alzheimer's disease: evidence for subtypes, *Arch Gen Psychiatry* 44:412-8, 1987.

Buckley C et al: Aging and platelet alpha$_2$-adrenoreceptors, *Br J Clin Pharmacol* 21:721, 1986.

Cadieux RJ: Geriatric psychopharmacology: a primary care challenge, *Geriatr Psychopharmacol* 83(4):281-301, March 1993.

Castleden CM, George CF: The effect of aging on the hepatic clearance of propranolol, *Br J Clin Pharmacol* 7:49, 1979.

Chiarello RJ, Cole JO: The use of psychostimulants in general psychiatry, *Arch Gen Psychiatry* 44:286-95, 1987.

Cockcroft DW, Gault MH: Prediction of creatinine clearance from serum creatinine, *Nephron* 16:31, 1976.

Cooper JK: Drug treatment of Alzheimer's disease, *Arch Intern Med* 151:245-9, 1991.

Cummings JL: Multi-infarct dementia: diagnosis and management, *Psychosomatics* 28:117-26, 1987.

Cusack BJ: Polypharmacy and clinical pharmacology. In Beck J, editor: *Geriatrics review syllabus: a core in geriatric medicine,* New York, 1989, American Geriatrics Society.

Cusack B, Vestal RE: Clinical pharmacology: special considerations in the elderly. In Calkins E, editor: *The practice of geriatrics,* Philadelphia, 1986, WB Saunders.

Davidson M et al: Cholinergic strategies in the treatment of Alzheimer's disease, *Acta Psychiatr Scand* 366:47-51, 1991.

Domantay AG, Napoliello MJ: Buspirone for elderly anxious patients, *Int Med Certif* 3:1, 1989.

Drusano GL et al: Commonly used methods of estimating creatinine clearance are inadequate for elderly debilitated nursing home patients, *J Am Geriatr Soc* 36:437, 1988.

Eison MS: The new generation of serotonergic anxiolytics: possible clinical roles, *Psychopathology* 22(suppl 1):13, 1989.

Feighner JP, Merideth CH, Hendrickson RM: A double-blind comparison of buspirone and diazepam in outpatients with generalized anxiety disorder, *J Clin Psychiatry* 43:102, 1982.

Folks DG: Delirium. In Rakel RE, editor: *Conn's current therapy*, Philadelphia, 1988, WB Saunders.

Folks DG: Clinical approaches to anxiety in the medically ill elderly, *Drug Ther Suppl* p 72, Aug 1990.

Folks DG, Ford CV: Psychiatric disorders in geriatric medical-surgical patient, part I: report of 195 consecutive consultations, *South Med J* 78:239, 1985.

Folks DG, Ford CV: Clinical features of depression and dysthymia in older adults. In Blazer D, editor: *Principles and practice of geriatric psychiatry*, West Sussex, England, 1994, John Wiley & Sons.

Folks DG, Fuller WC: Uses of anxiolytics and sedatives in geriatric practice: clinical selection and treatment considerations, *Psychiatr Clin North Am* (in press).

Folstein MF, Folstein SE, McHugh PR: Mini-mental state: a practical method of grading the cognitive state of patients for the clinician, *J Psychiatr Res* 12:189, 1975.

Gaitz CM, Niederehe G, Wilson NL: *Aging 2000: our health care destiny: psychosocial and policy issues*, vol 2, New York, 1985, Springer-Verlag.

Gardos G et al: Differential actions of chlordiazepoxide and oxazepam on hostility, *Arch Gen Psychiatry* 18:757, 1968.

Gautheir S et al: Tetrahydroaminoacridine-lecithin combination treatment in patients with intermediate-stage Alzheimer's disease, *New Engl J Med* 322:1271-6, 1990.

Goedert M et al: Nerve growth factor receptor mRNA distribution in human brain: normal levels in basal forebrain in Alzheimer's disease, *Mol Brain Res* 5:1-7, 1989.

Goff DC: The stimulant challenge test in depression, *J Clin Psychiatry* 47:538, 1986.

Greenblatt DJ: Reduced serum albumin concentration in the elderly: a report from the Boston Collaborative Drug Surveillance Program, *J Am Geriatr Soc* 27:20, 1979.

Greenblatt DJ, Sellers EM, Shader RI: Drug disposition in old age, *N Engl J Med* 306:1081-8, 1982.

Greenblatt DJ, Shader RI: Dependence, tolerance and addiction to benzodiazepines: clinical and pharmacokinetic considerations, *Drug Metab Rev* 8:13, 1978.

Gurwitz JH: Suboptimal medication use in the elderly: the tip of the iceberg, *JAMA* 272:316-7, 1994 (editorial).

Hall RCW, Zisook S: Paradoxical reactions to benzodiazepines, *Br J Clin Pharmacol* 11:995, 1981.

Hefti F, Schneider LS: Nerve growth factor and Alzheimer's disease, *Clin Neuropharmacol* 14(suppl):S62-S76, 1991.

Jenike MA: Assessment and treatment of affective illness in the elderly, *J Geriatr Psychiatry Neurol* 1:89, 1988.

Jenike MA: *Geriatric psychiatry and psychopharmacology: a clinical approach*, St Louis, 1989, Mosby.

Kalayam B, Shamoian CA: Geriatric psychiatry: an update, *J Clin Psychiatry* 51(5):177, 1990.

Katzman R: Alzheimer's disease, *N Engl J Med* 314:964-73, 1986.

Keltner NL, Folks DG: Alternatives to lithium in the treatment of bipolar disorder, *Perspect Psychiatr Care* 27:36, 1991.

Keltner NL, Folks DG: The Omnibus Budget Reconciliation Act: impact on psychotropic drug use in long-term care facilities, *Perspect Psychiatr Care* 31:30, 1995.

Kokmen E: Etiology, diagnosis, and management of dementia, *Compr Ther* 15(9):59-69, 1989.

Kumar R et al: Anxiolytics and memory: a comparison of lorazepam and alprazolam, *J Clin Psychiatry* 48:158, 1987.

Ladewig D: Abuse of benzodiazepines in Western European society: incidence and prevalence, motives, drug acquisition, *Pharmacopsychiatry* 16:103, 1983.

Lenox RH et al: Adjunctive treatment of manic agitation with lorazepam versus haloperidol: a double-blind study, *J Clin Psychiatry* 53:47, 1992.

Lerer B et al: Carbamazepine versus lithium in mania: a double-blind study, *J Clin Psychiatry* 48(3):89, 1987.

Lucas-Blaustein MJ et al: Driving in patients with dementia, *J Am Geriatr Soc* 36:987-1091, 1988.

Maletta GJ: Pharmacologic treatment and management of the aggressive demented patient, *Psychiatr Ann* 20(8):454, 1990.

Masoro EJ: Biology of aging: current state of knowledge, *Arch Intern Med* 147:166, 1987.

Mendelson W: Pharmacologic treatment of insomnia. In Pies R, editor: Advances in psychiatric medicine, *Psychiatr Times* (suppl), p 2, 1992.

Mohs RC et al: Oral physostigmine treatment of patients with Alzheimer's disease, *Am J Psychiatry* 142:28-33, 1985.

Montamat S, Cusack B, Vestal RE: Management of drug therapy in the elderly, *New Engl J Med* 321:303, 1989.

Morrow D, Leirer V, Sheikh J: Adherence and medication instructions: review and recommendations, *J Am Geriatr Soc* 36:1147, 1988.

Nicholson AN: Hypnotics: rebound insomnia and residual sequelae, *Br J Clin Pharmacol* 9:223, 1980.

Nicholson AN, Ward J, editors: Psychomotor drugs and performance, *Br J Clin Pharmacol* 18(suppl 1):1S-139S, 1984.

Oswald I et al: Benzodiazepine hypnotics remain effective for 24 weeks, *Br Med J* 284:860, 1982.

Peabody CA et al: Neuroleptics and the elderly, *J Am Geriatr Soc* 35:233, 1987.

Perry E: Acetylcholine and Alzheimer's disease, *Br J Psychiatry* 153:737-40, 1988.

Preskorn SH: The future and psychopharmacology: potentials and needs, *Psychiatr Ann* 20(11):625, 1990.

Price LH, Charney DS, Heninger GR: Variability of response to lithium augmentation in refractory depression, *Am J Psychiatry* 143:1387, 1986.

Rakel RE: Mixed anxiety/depression, *Drug Ther Suppl* p 137, Aug 1990.

Ratey JJ et al: Buspirone therapy for maladaptive behavior and anxiety in developmentally disabled persons, *J Clin Psychiatry* 50:382, 1989.

Ray WA, Griffin MR, Downey W: Benzodiazepines of long and short elimination half-life and the risk of hip fracture, *JAMA* 262(23):3303, 1989.

Ray WA et al: Psychotropic drug use and the risk of hip fracture, *New Engl J Med* 316:363, 1987.

Reifler B, Larson E, Hanley R: Coexistence of cognitive impairment and depression in geriatric outpatients, *Am J Psychiatry* 139:623-6, 1982.

Rickels K et al: Buspirone and diazepam in anxiety: a controlled study, *J Clin Psychiatry* 43:81, 1982.

Risse SC, Barnes R: Pharmacologic treatment of agitation associated with dementia, *J Am Geriatr Soc* 34:368-76, 1986.

Roehrs TA et al: Dose determinants of rebound insomnia, *Br J Clin Pharmacol* 22:143, 1986.

Rosenbaum JF, editor: *Clonazepam update: a review of the literature*, vol 1, Bellemead, NJ, 1989, *Excerpta Medica*, Elsevier.

Rowe JW, Kahn RL: Human aging: usual and successful, *Science* 237:143, 1987.

Rowe JW et al: The effect of age on creatinine clearance in men: a cross-sectional and longitudinal study, *J Gerontol* 31:155, 1976.

Rubin EH, Kinscherf BA, Wehrman SA: Response to treatment of depression in the old and very old, *J Geriatr Psychiatry Neurol* 4:65, 1991.

Scarpace PJ: Decreased beta-adrenergic responsiveness during senescence, *Fed Proc* 45:51, 1986.

Skelton WP III, Skelton NK: Alzheimer's disease: recognizing and treating a frustrating condition, *Postgrad Med* 90(4):33-41, 1991.

Sloane P, Blazer D, George LK: Dizziness in a community elderly population, *J Am Geriatr Soc* 37:101, 1989.

Small JG et al: Treatment outcome with clozapine in tardive dyskinesia, neuroleptic sensitivity, and treatment-resistant psychosis, *J Clin Psychiatry* 48:263, 1987.

Stone T, Folks DG: Somatization in the elderly, *Psychiatr Med* 10(3):25, 1992.

Sussman N: Diagnosis and drug treatment of anxiety in the elderly, *Geriatr Med Today* 7(10):1, 1988.

Vestal RE: Pharmacology and aging, *J Am Geriatr Soc* 30:191, 1982.

Wallace SM, Verbeeck RK: Plasma protein binding of drugs in the elderly, *Clin Pharmacokinet* 12:41, 1987.

Watanabe M, Davis JM: Overview: pharmacotherapeutic considerations in the elderly psychiatric patient, *Am Fam Physician* 31(5):105, 1990.

Williams L, Lowenthal DT: Drug therapy in the elderly, *South Med* 85(2):127, 1992.

Winograd CH, Jarvik LF: Physician management of the demented patient, *J Am Geriatr Soc* 34:295-308, 1986.

Wolkowitz OM et al: Diazepam-induced amnesia: a neuropharmacological model of an "organic amnestic syndrome," *Am J Psychiatry* 144:25, 1987.

Wynne HA et al: The effect of age upon liver volume and apparent liver blood flow in healthy men, *Hepatology* 9:297, 1989.

PART TWO

PSYCHOTROPIC DRUG PROFILES

Acetazolamide

DIAMOX, AK-ZOL, DAZAMIDE
(a-set-a-zolé-a-mide) (Chapter 7)

Functional classifications: Diuretic, anticonvulsant
Chemical classification: Carbonic anhydrase inhibitor
FDA pregnancy category: C

Indications: *Diuretic* indications are not discussed here, e.g., edema related to CHF, glaucoma; *Anticonvulsant:* Especially petit mal and tonic-clonic seizures, particularly in children

Contraindications: Known hypersensitivity to acetazolamide; depressed sodium or potassium levels; kidney and liver disease or dysfunction; suprarenal gland failure

Pharmacologic Effects: Inhibition of carbonic anhydrase apparently slows abnormal firing of CNS neurons. However, anticonvulsant effect not truly understood

Pharmacokinetics: Absorbed from GI tract; distributed to body tissues and CNS; eliminated unchanged in urine

Side Effects: *CNS:* Convulsions, weakness, malaise, fatigue, nervousness, sedation, depression; *Peripheral:* Nausea, vomiting, constipation, hematuria, urinary frequency, hepatic insufficiency, blood dyscrasias, skin problems, weight loss, fever, acidosis

Interactions
- Amphetamines: Because it alkalinizes urine, may increase effect of amphetamines (and ephedrine, pseudoephedrine, flecainide, and quinidine)
- Digitalis: May sensitize patient to digitalis toxicity r/t hypokalemia
- Primidone: May delay primidone absorption
- Salicylates: Together may cause metabolic acidosis

Implications
Assess
- Weight, I&O for fluid loss, respirations, B/P
- Check potassium, sodium, and other electrolyte levels

Teaching
- To increase fluid, if indicated
- To rise slowly when orthostatic hypotension is a problem
- To notify clinician when symptoms of blood dyscrasias occur, i.e., sore throat, bruising, etc

Evaluate
- For seizure activity, CNS side effects, confusion in elderly, signs of metabolic acidosis, signs of hypokalemia

Lab Test Interference: May interfere with tests for urinary protein, i.e., false positive

Treatment of Overdose: Lavage for oral doses, monitor electrolytes and fluid profile, assess renal function, give dextrose in saline, give bicarbonate for acidosis

Administration
- Epilepsy: 8-30 mg/kg/day in divided doses; optimum range 375-1000 mg/day
- Concomitant antiepileptic dosage: start with 250 mg/day and increase to levels for epilepsy
- Available forms include: Tabs 125, 250 mg; caps sus-rel 500 mg; inj 500 mg/vial

Acetophenazine*

TINDAL
(a-set-oh-feń-a-zeen) (Chapter 4)

Functional classification: Antipsychotic
Chemical classification: Piperazine phenothiazine
FDA pregnancy category: C

Indications: Management of psychotic disorders

Contraindications: See trifluoperazine

Pharmacologic Effects: See trifluoperazine

Pharmacokinetics: See trifluoperazine

Side Effects: *CNS:* See trifluoperazine; *Peripheral:* See trifluoperazine

Interactions: See trifluoperazine

Implications: See trifluoperazine

Treatment of Overdose: See trifluoperazine

*Infrequently used.

Administration

- 20 mg tid; if insomnia present, give last tablet 1 hr before bedtime; usual daily dosage 40-80 mg
- Hospitalized patients: Optimally 80-120 mg/day in divided doses
- Severe schizophrenia: Up to 400-600 mg/day
- Available forms: Tabs 20 mg

Alprazolam

XANAX

(al-praý-zoe-lam) (Chapter 6)

Functional classification: Antianxiety
Chemical classification: Benzodiazepine
Controlled substance schedule IV
FDA pregnancy category: D

Indications: Anxiety, panic disorders

Contraindications: Hypersensitivity to benzodiazepines; narrow-angle glaucoma; psychosis; nursing women; child <18 yr
Cautious use: Elderly or debilitated patients; hepatic or renal disease

Pharmacologic Effects: Apparently potentiates effects of GABA and other inhibitory transmitters by binding to specific benzodiazepine receptor sites; depresses subcortical levels of CNS, including limbic system and reticular formation

Pharmacokinetics

- Speed of onset: intermediate
- PO: Onset 30 min, peak 1-2 hr, duration 4-6 hr, therapeutic response 2-3 days; metabolized by liver; excreted by kidneys; crosses placenta, breast milk; half-life 12-15 hr

Side Effects: *CNS:* **Drowsiness, dizziness, confusion, headache,** anxiety, tremor, stimulation, fatigue, **depression, insomnia;** paradoxic agitation can occur
Peripheral: Photophobia caused by mydriasis, **blurred vision** caused by cycloplegia; sleeplike slowing of respirations with therapeutic doses; cough; **orthostatic hypotension; tachycardia;** hypotension; **constipation, dry mouth**

Interactions

- Alcohol and other CNS depressants: Increased risk of excessive CNS depression
- Cimetidine: Potentiation of CNS depression
- Digoxin: Increased risk of cardiac side effects
- Levodopa: Decreased antiparkinson effect
- Phenytoin: Increased phenytoin serum levels

Implications

Assess

- Patient's level of anxiety and method of coping
- B/P, VS
- Establish baseline physical assessment data before medications are started
- Periodically perform CBC, UA
- Reassess need for treatment q 4 mo

Planning/Implementation

- Monitor patient's response to medication
- Observe elderly, very young, and debilitated patients for paradoxic excitement
- Reduce dose of other depressant drugs
- Observe for signs of withdrawal when discontinuing antianxiety medication; discontinue by decreasing daily dose no more than 0.5 mg q 3 days

Teaching

- To avoid operating dangerous machinery and other tasks requiring good reflexes
- To report ocular pain at once, and any other visual disturbances
- Drug may be taken with food

Evaluate

- Whether patient achieves lower levels of anxiety without undue sedation
- Whether patient can follow prescribed regimen
- For physical dependence: withdrawal symptoms include headache, nausea, vomiting, muscle pain, and weakness after long-term use

Lab Test Interferences

- Increase: AST/ALT, serum bilirubin
- False increase: 17-OHCS
- Decrease: RAIU

Treatment of Overdose: Lavage, VS, supportive care. There have been few deaths, if any, from benzodiazepine overdose alone. Deaths occur when benzodiazepines are mixed with other drugs, i.e., alcohol

Administration *Adult:* PO 0.25-0.5 mg tid, not to exceed 4 mg/day in divided doses; *geriatric:* PO 0.25 mg bid-tid

- Available forms include: Tabs 0.25, 0.5, 1 mg

Amantadine HCl

SYMMETREL

(a-mań-ta-deen) (Chapter 14)

Functional classification: Antiparkinson agent, antiviral

Chemical classification: Tricyclic amine

FDA pregnancy category: C

Indications: Extrapyramidal reactions, parkinsonism, antiviral (A)

Contraindications: Hypersensitivity, lactation, child <1 yr

Cautious use: Epilepsy, CHF, orthostatic hypotension, psychiatric disorders, hepatic or renal disease

Pharmacologic Effect: Causes release of dopamine from neurons

Pharmacokinetics: PO: Onset 48 hr, peak 4 hr, half-life 15 hr in normal renal function, not metabolized, excreted in urine (90%) unchanged, crosses placenta, excreted in breast milk

Side effects: *CNS:* **Confusion,** headache, **dizziness, drowsiness,** fatigue, anxiety, psychosis, depression, **hallucinations,** tremors, convulsions, insomnia; *Peripheral:* **Orthostatic hypotension,** CHF, photosensitivity, dermatitis, livedo reticularis, **blurred vision,** leukopenia, **nausea, vomiting,** constipation, **dry mouth,** urinary frequency, retention

Interactions

- Atropine, other anticholinergics: Increased anticholinergic responses
- CNS stimulants: Increased CNS stimulation

Implications

Assess

- EPSEs; urinary frequency
- Mental alertness
- History of seizure activity; may increase seizure activity

Planning/Implementation

- Give at least 4 hr before bedtime to prevent insomnia
- Give after meals for better absorption to decrease GI symptoms
- Give in divided doses to prevent CNS disturbances: headache, dizziness, fatigue, drowsiness

Teaching

- To change body position slowly to prevent orthostatic hypotension
- To report dyspnea, weight gain, dizziness, poor concentration, behavioral changes
- To avoid hazardous activities when dizziness occurs
- To take drug exactly as prescribed; if drug is discontinued abruptly, parkinsonian crisis may occur

Evaluate

- Therapeutic response: Decrease in EPSEs
- Bowel pattern before and during treatment
- Skin eruptions, photosensitivity after administration of drugs
- Respiratory status: Breathing rate and character, wheezing, tightness in chest

Treatment of Overdose: Withdraw drug, empty stomach, maintain airway, administer O_2, IV corticosteroids; use appropriate antiarrhythmic and vasopressor therapy as needed

Administration

- Extrapyramidal reaction and parkinsonism: *Adult:* PO 100 mg bid, up to 300 mg/day for EPSEs in divided doses; *geriatric:* 100 mg/day
- Influenza type A: Not addressed here
- Available forms include: Caps 100 mg; syr 50 mg/5 mL
- A suggested dosing guideline for patients with impaired renal function is available

Amitriptyline HCl

ELAVIL, ENDEP, ENOVIL, LEVATE,† MERAVIL,† NOVOTRIPTYN,† ROLAVIL†
(a-mee-triṕ-ti-leen) (Chapter 5)

Functional classification: TCA
Chemical classification: Dibenzocycloheptadiene, tertiary amine
FDA pregnancy category: C

Indications: Depression

Contraindications: Hypersensitivity to TCAs, recovery phase of myocardial infarction

Cautious use: Suicidal patients, convulsive disorders, prostatic hypertrophy, schizophrenia, psychosis, severe depression, increased intraocular pressure, narrow-angle glaucoma, urinary retention, cardiac disease, hepatic or renal disease, hyperthyroidism, ECT, elective surgery, child <12 yr, MAOI therapy

Pharmacologic Effects: Blocks reuptake of norepinephrine, serotonin into nerve endings, increasing action of norepinephrine, serotonin in nerve cells; also r/t changes in receptor sensitivity; therapeutic plasma levels 110-250 ng/mL

Pharmacokinetics: PO/IM onset 45 min, peak 2-12 hr, therapeutic response 2-3 wk; metabolized by liver; excreted in urine and feces; crosses placenta; excreted in breast milk; half-life 31-46 hr

Side Effects: *CNS:* **Sedation,** ataxia; confusion, delirium; *Peripheral:* **Blurred vision,** photophobia, increased intraocular pressure, decreased tearing, orthostatic hypotension, arrhythmias, tachycardia, palpitations, dry mouth, constipation, diarrhea, decreased sweating, **urinary retention, hesitancy**

Interactions

- Anticholinergic agents: Additive anticholinergic effects
  - Atropine
  - Antihistamines (H_1 blocker)
  - Antiparkinson drugs
  - Antipsychotics
  - OTC cold and allergy drugs
- CNS depressants: Additive depressant effect
- Guanethidine, clonidine: Decreased antihypertensive effect
- MAOIs: Hypertensive crisis; atropine-like poisoning
- Oral contraceptives: Inhibit metabolism of TCAs
- Phenothiazines: May increase TCA serum level
- Quinidine: Additive effect, heart block possible
- Sympathomimetics: Potentiates sympathomimetic effects
- Thyroid preparations: Tachycardia, arrhythmias; may increase TCA effect

Implications

Assess

- Establish baseline data to aid recognition of adverse responses to medication, e.g., liver enzyme levels, VS, renal function, mental status, speech patterns, affect, weight
- Assess for signs of noncompliance, e.g., poor therapeutic response
- Observe for major symptoms of depression: apathy, sadness, sleep disturbances, hopelessness, guilt, decreased libido, spontaneous crying
- Review history for contraindicated conditions, e.g., glaucoma, CV disease, GI conditions, urologic conditions, seizures, pregnancy

Planning/Implementation

- Monitor for "cheeking" or hoarding; check drug dosage carefully—a small overdose may cause toxicity
- Monitor for suicidal ideations; suicidal thought content may increase as antidepressants begin to "energize" patient
- Monitor vital signs; withhold TCAs when hypotension, tachycardia, or arrhythmias occur
- Give most TCAs in a single dose hs
- Observe for early signs of toxicity, e.g., drowsiness, tachycardia, mydriasis, hypotension, agitation, vomiting, confusion, fever, restlessness, sweating
- Discontinue drug when CNS overstimulation occurs, e.g., hypomania, delirium

Teaching

- That these drugs have a lag time of up to 1 month
- To adhere to drug regimen

†Available in Canada only.

- To avoid OTC drugs, particularly those containing sympathomimetics or anticholinergics
- To avoid drugs listed in section on interactions
- About ways to deal with minor side effects, as follows: dry mouth: with hard candies, sips of water, mouth rinses; visual disturbances: with artificial tears, sunglasses, assistance with ambulation; constipation: with bulk-forming foods, increased fluids; urinary hesitancy: with adequate fluids, privacy; decreased perspiration: with appropriate clothing, avoidance of unnecessary exercise; orthostatic hypotension: with slow positional changes, avoidance of hot baths and showers; drowsiness: take single dose hs with physician approval, avoid driving
- That abrupt discontinuance may result in cholinergic rebound, e.g., nausea, vomiting, insomnia, headache

Evaluate

- Desired therapeutic serum level
- Verbalize decrease in subjective symptoms
- Observe decrease in objective symptoms
- Minimal to no adverse drug effects
- Stable VS
- Less anxiety; sleep, talk, and feel better

Lab Test Interferences

- Increase: Serum bilirubin, blood glucose, and alkaline phosphatase levels
- Decrease: VMA, 5-HIAA
- False increase: Urinary catecholamines

Treatment of Overdose: ECG monitoring, induce emesis, lavage, activated charcoal, treat anticholinergic effects, administer anticonvulsants if needed

Administration

Adult: PO 40-100 mg hs, may increase to 200 mg qd, not to exceed 300 mg/day; IM 20-30 mg qid

Adolescent/geriatric: PO 30 mg/day in divided doses, may add 20 mg hs

- Available forms include: Tabs 10, 25, 50, 75, 100, 150 mg; IM 10 mg/mL

Amobarbital/Amobarbital Sodium

AMYTAL, ISOBEC, AMYTAL SODIUM

(am-oh-bar´-bi-tal) (Chapter 8)

Functional classifications: Sedative, hypnotic

Chemical classification: Amylobarbitone

Controlled substance schedule II

FDA pregnancy category: B

Indications: Sedation, preanesthetic sedation, anticonvulsant

Contraindications: Hypersensitivity to barbiturates, respiratory depression, addiction to barbiturates, severe liver dysfunction, porphyria

Pharmacologic Effects: Depresses activity in reticular activating system; when used as anticonvulsant, inhibits CNS neural firing.

Pharmacokinetics: Onset within 45-60 min after PO dose, with duration of action of 6-8 hr; metabolized by liver, excreted by kidneys; highly protein bound; Half-life 16-40 hr; excreted in breast milk; onset in 5 min when given IV, e.g., for seizures

Side Effects: *CNS:* Lethargy, drowsiness, barbiturate hangover, dizziness, paradoxic stimulation of children and elderly patients on occasion, CNS depression, slurred speech, physical dependence; *Peripheral:* Nausea, vomiting, diarrhea, constipation, skin eruptions, e.g., rashes; hypotension, bradycardia, respiratory depression, apnea, blood dyscrasias

Interactions

- CNS depressants: Increased CNS depression
- MAOIs: CNS depression
- Valproic acid: decreased half-life of valproic acid
- Oral anticoagulants, corticosteroids, quinidine, oral contraceptives: Decreased effect of these drugs
- Phenytoin: Unpredictable effect

Implications

Assess

- If given parenterally, check VS q 30 min for 2 hr
- Assess blood values because of potential for blood dyscrasias
- Check prothrombin time when patient is on anticoagulant regimen
- Hepatic studies to determine liver status

Planning/Implementation

- Have staff assist patient in walking after dose is given, to prevent falls
- Maintain safety

Teaching

- Physical dependence potential with long-term use
- To avoid alcohol and other CNS depressants
- To notify other prescribers about amobarbital

Evaluate

- Therapeutic responses
- Mental status
- Tendencies toward dependence
- Toxic effects
- Respiratory depression
- Blood dyscrasias

Treatment of Overdose: In general, 1 g causes serious poisoning in adults; lavage if taken orally, alkalinize urine; warm with blankets if needed; supportive measures, including monitoring VS; hemodialysis may be required

Administration

- Sedation: *Adult:* PO 30-50 mg bid or tid; range from 15-120 mg bid-qid; *child:* PO 2 mg/kg/day in 4 divided doses
- Anticonvulsant: *Adult:* Give IV 65-500 mg over several minutes, should not exceed 100 mg/min, do not exceed 1 g; *child:* < 6 yr: IV/IM 3-5 mg/kg over several minutes
- Available forms: Tabs 30, 50, 100 mg; caps 65, 200 mg; powder for inj IM, IV 250, 500 mg/vial

Amoxapine

ASENDIN

(a-mox̆-a-peen) (Chapter 5)

Functional classification: TCA
Chemical classification: Dibenzoxazepine-derivative secondary amine
FDA pregnancy category: C

Indications: Depression

Contraindications: Hypersensitivity to TCAs, recovery phase of myocardial infarction

Cautious use: Seizure disorders, suicidal patients, severe depression, increased intraocular pressure, narrow-angle glaucoma, urinary retention, CV disease, hepatic disease, hyperthyroidism, ECT, elective surgery, elderly patients, patients receiving MAOI therapy, NMS, child < 16 yr

Pharmacologic Effects: Blocks reuptake of norepinephrine, serotonin into nerve endings, increasing action of norepinephrine, serotonin in nerve cells; also blocks dopamine receptors and can produce EPSEs; therapeutic plasma levels 200-500 ng/mL

Pharmacokinetics: PO: Steady state 2-7 days, metabolized by liver, excreted by kidneys, crosses placenta, half-life 8-30 hr

Side Effects: *CNS:* **Sedation,** ataxia; confusion, delirium, tardive dyskinesia, NMS; *Peripheral effects:* **Blurred vision,** photophobia, increased intraocular pressure; decreased tearing; orthostatic hypotension, arrhythmias, tachycardia, palpitations, **dry mouth, constipation,** diarrhea, decreased sweating, **urinary retention, hesitancy, nausea**

Interactions

- Anticholinergic agents: Additive anticholinergic effects with atropine, antihistamines (H_1 blockers), antiparkinson drugs, antipsychotics, OTC cold and allergy drugs
- CNS depressants: Additive depressant effect
- Guanethidine, clonidine: Decreased antihypertensive effect
- MAOIs: Hypertensive crisis, atropine-like poisoning

- Oral contraceptives: Inhibit effects of TCAs
- Phenothiazines: May increase TCA serum level, EPSEs
- Quinidine: Additive effect, heart block possible
- Sympathomimetics: Potentiates sympathomimetic effects
- Thyroid preparations: Tachycardia, arrhythmias; may increase TCA effect

Implications

Assess

- Establish baseline data to aid recognition of adverse responses to medication, e.g., liver enzyme levels, VS, renal function, mental status, speech patterns, affect, weight
- Assess for signs of noncompliance, e.g., poor therapeutic response
- Observe for major symptoms of depression: apathy, sadness, sleep disturbances, hopelessness, guilt, decreased libido, spontaneous crying
- Review history for contraindicated conditions, e.g., glaucoma, CV disease, GI conditions, urologic conditions, seizures, pregnancy

Planning/Implementation

- Monitor for "cheeking" or hoarding; check drug dosage carefully, because a small overdose may cause toxicity
- Monitor for suicidal ideations; suicidal thought content may increase as antidepressants begin to "energize" patient
- Monitor VS; withhold TCAs when hypotension, tachycardia, or arrhythmias occur
- Give most TCAs in a single dose hs
- Observe for early signs of toxicity, e.g., drowsiness, tachycardia, mydriasis, hypotension, agitation, vomiting, confusion, fever, restlessness, sweating
- Discontinue drug when CNS overstimulation occurs, e.g., hypomania, delirium

Teaching

- That amoxapine has a shorter lag time (4-7 days) than other TCAs
- To adhere to drug regimen
- To avoid OTC drugs, particularly those containing sympathomimetics or anticholinergics
- To avoid drugs listed in section on interactions
- About ways to deal with minor side effects, as follows: dry mouth: with sugarless hard candies, sips of water, mouth rinses; visual disturbances: with artificial tears, sunglasses, assistance with ambulation; constipation: with bulk-forming foods, increased fluids; urinary hesitancy: with adequate fluids, privacy; decreased perspiration: with appropriate clothing, avoidance of unnecessary exercise; orthostatic hypotension: with slow positional changes, avoidance of hot baths and showers; drowsiness: take single dose hs with physician approval, avoid driving
- That abrupt discontinuance may result in cholinergic rebound, e.g., nausea, vomiting, insomnia

Evaluate

- Desired therapeutic serum level
- Verbalize decrease in subjective symptoms
- Observe decrease in objective symptoms
- Minimal to no adverse drug effects
- Stable VS
- Less anxiety: sleep, talk, and feel better
- For EPSEs

Lab Test Interferences

- Increase: Serum bilirubin, blood glucose, alkaline phosphatase levels
- False increase: Urinary catecholamines
- Decrease: VMA, 5-HIAA

Treatment of Overdose: ECG monitoring, induce emesis, lavage; consider prophylactic antiepileptics; support respirations

Administration

Adult >16 yr: PO 100-150 mg/day in divided doses, may increase to 300 mg/day or may give daily dose hs

Geriatric: PO 50-75 mg/day, may increase to 150 mg/day

- Available forms include: Tabs 25, 50, 100, 150 mg

A

Amphetamine Sulfate

AMPHETAMINE SULFATE (am-fet́-a-meen) (Chapters 12, 13, 15, 16)

Functional classification: Cerebral stimulant
Chemical classification: Amphetamine
Controlled substance schedule II
FDA pregnancy category: X

Indications: Narcolepsy, exogenous obesity, ADHD

Contraindications: Hypersensitive to sympathomimetic amines, hyperthyroidism, hypertension, glaucoma, severe arteriosclerosis, nephritis, angina pectoris, parkinsonism, drug abuse, CV disease, anxiety, MAOI use

Cautious use: Tourette's syndrome, lactation, child <3 yr, diabetes mellitus, elderly patients

Pharmacologic Effects: Stimulates release of norepinephrine in cerebral cortex, brain stem, and reticular activating system and dopamine in the mesolimbic system; therapeutic plasma levels 5-10 μg/dl

Pharmacokinetics: PO: Onset 30 min, peak 1-3 hr, duration 4-20 hr, metabolized by liver, excreted by kidneys, crosses placenta, enters breast milk, half-life 10-30 hr

Side Effects: *CNS:* **Hyperactivity, insomnia, restlessness, talkativeness,** dizziness, headache, chills, stimulation, dysphoria, irritability, aggressiveness; *Peripheral:* Nausea, vomiting, anorexia, dry mouth, diarrhea, constipation, weight loss, metallic taste, cramps, impotence, change in libido, **palpitations, tachycardia,** hypertension, hypotension

Interactions

- MAOIs or within 14 days of MAOIs: Hypertensive crisis
- Acetazolamide, antacids, sodium bicarbonate, ascorbic acid, ammonium chloride, phenothiazines, haloperidol: Increase half-life of amphetamine
- Urinary acidifiers: decreased half-life of amphetamines
- Guanethidine, other antihypertensives: Decreased effects of these drugs

Implications

Assess

- VS, B/P because this drug may reverse antihypertensives; check patients with cardiac disease more often
- CBC, urinalysis; in diabetes: blood and urine glucose levels, insulin changes may need to be made because eating decreases
- **Height, growth rate in children (growth rate may be decreased)**

Planning/Implementation

- Give at least 6 hr before bedtime to avoid sleeplessness
- **Give with meals or immediately after to avoid loss of appetite**
- For obesity only when patient is on weight-reduction program that includes dietary changes, exercise; tolerance develops, and weight loss will not occur without additional methods
- Sugarless gum, hard candies, frequent sips of water for dry mouth
- If drug is for obesity, 30-60 min before meals
- Dispense least amount feasible to minimize risk of overdose

Teaching

- To decrease caffeine consumption (coffee, tea, cola, chocolate), which may increase irritability, stimulation
- Avoid OTC preparations unless approved by physician
- To taper off drug over several weeks, or depression, increased sleeping, lethargy may occur
- To avoid alcohol ingestion
- To avoid hazardous activities until patient's condition is stabilized on medication regimen
- To get needed rest; patients feel more tired than usual at end of day
- Check to see that PO medication has been swallowed

Evaluate

- Mental status: mood, sensorium, affect, stimulation, insomnia; aggressiveness may occur
- Physical dependency; should not be used for extended time; drug should be discontinued gradually

- **Withdrawal symptoms: headache, nausea, vomiting, muscle pain, weakness**
- Drug tolerance develops after long-term use
- If tolerance develops, dosage should not be increased

Treatment of Overdose: Gastric evacuation if overdose < 4 hr old; otherwise, acidify urine, administer fluids until urine flow is 3-6 mL/kg/hr; hemodialysis, peritoneal dialysis may be helpful; antihypertensives for increased B/P; ammonium chloride for increased excretion; chlorpromazine for CNS stimulation

Administration
- Narcolepsy: PO 5-60 mg qd in divided doses; *adult and adolescent >12 yr:* PO 10 mg qd, increasing by 10 mg/day at weekly intervals; *child* 6-12 yr: PO 5 mg qd, increasing by 5 mg/wk, maximum dose, 60 mg/day
- ADHD: *Child >6 yr:* PO 5 mg qd-bid, increasing by 5 mg/wk; *child 3-6 yr:* PO 2.5 mg qd, increasing by 2.5 mg/day at weekly intervals
- Obesity in adult: PO 5-30 mg in divided doses 30-60 min before meals
- Available forms include: Tabs 5, 10 mg

Benztropine

COGENTIN
(Benź-troe-peen) (Chapter 14)

Functional classification: Anticholinergic
Chemical classification: Tertiary amine
FDA pregnancy category: C

Indications: Parkinsonism, EPSEs

Contraindications: Hypersensitivity, narrow-angle glaucoma, duodenal obstruction, peptic ulcer, prostatic hypertrophy, myasthenia gravis, megacolon

Pharmacologic Effects: Block cholinergic receptors, may inhibit the reuptake and storage of dopamine

Pharmacokinetics: Little pharmacokinetic information is known

Side Effects: *CNS:* Depression develops in 19% to 30% of patients; disorientation, confusion, memory loss, hallucinations, psychoses, agitation, delusions, nervousness; *Peripheral:* **Tachycardia,** palpitations, hypotension, **orthostatic hypotension, dry mouth,** nausea, vomiting, constipation, paralytic ileus, **blurred vision,** mydriasis, diplopia, urinary retention and hesitancy, elevated temperature

Interactions
- Amantadine: Increased anticholinergic effect
- Digoxin: Digoxin serum levels increased
- Haloperidol: Worsening of schizophrenia, decreased haloperidol serum levels
- Levodopa: Possible reduction of levodopa efficacy
- Phenothiazines: increased anticholinergic effect, decreased antipsychotic effect

Implications
Assess
- VS, B/P
- For glaucoma
- Mental status

Planning/Implementation
- Provide instructions for anticholinergic responses, i.e., dry mouth, constipation, urinary hesitancy, decreased sweating, and the like

Teaching
- Give with meals
- May cause drowsiness, blurred vision, dizziness: Emphasize safety
- Avoidance of alcohol and other CNS depressants
- Notify physician for rapid or pounding heartbeat
- Use caution in hot weather

Evaluate
- EPSE improvement
- For adverse effects
- Mental status: Confusion, delirium, memory

Treatment of Overdose: Emesis, lavage, activated charcoal, treat respiratory depression, hyperpyrexia

Administration
- EPSEs: *Adult:* PO/IM 1-4 mg qd-bid
- Acute EPSEs: *Adult:* IM/IV 1-2 mg, followed by 1-2 mg PO, taken twice to prevent recurrences
- Prophylactic: *Adult* PO 1-2 mg bid-tid

Biperiden

AKINETON
(bye-peŕ-i-den) (Chapter 14)

Functional classification: Anticholinergic
FDA pregnancy category: C

Indications: Parkinsonism, EPSEs

Contraindications: Hypersensitivity, narrow-angle glaucoma, duodenal obstruction, peptic ulcer, prostatic hypertrophy, myasthenia gravis, megacolon

Pharmacologic Effects: Block cholinergic receptors, may inhibit reuptake and storage of dopamine

Pharmacokinetics: Peak 1-1½ hr, half-life 18.4-24.3 hr; little pharmacokinetic information is known

Side Effects: *CNS:* Depression develops in 19% to 30% of patients; disorientation, confusion, memory loss, hallucinations, psychoses, agitation, delusions, nervousness; *Peripheral:* **Tachycardia,** palpitations, hypotension, **orthostatic hypotension, dry mouth,** nausea, vomiting, constipation, paralytic ileus, **blurred vision,** mydriasis, diplopia, urinary retention and hesitancy, elevated temperature

Interactions

- Amantadine: Increased anticholinergic effect
- Digoxin: Digoxin serum levels increased
- Haloperidol: Worsening of schizophrenia, decreased haloperidol serum levels
- Levodopa: Possible reduction of levodopa efficacy
- Phenothiazines: Increased anticholinergic effect, decreased antipsychotic effect

Implications

Assess

- VS, B/P
- For glaucoma
- Mental status

Planning/Implementation

- Provide instructions for anticholinergic responses, i.e., dry mouth, constipation, urinary hesitancy, decreased sweating, and the like

Teaching

- Give with meals
- May cause drowsiness, blurred vision, dizziness: Emphasize safety
- Avoidance of alcohol and other CNS depressants
- Notify physician for rapid or pounding heartbeat
- Use caution in hot weather

Evaluate

- EPSE improvement
- For adverse effects
- Mental status: Confusion, delirium, memory

Treatment of Overdose: Emesis, lavage, activated charcoal, treat respiratory depression, hyperpyrexia

Administration

- EPSEs: *Adult:* PO 2 mg qd-tid
- Acute EPSEs: *Adult:* IM/IV 2 mg q 30 min prn, up to 4 doses in 24 hr

Bromocriptine Mesylate

PARLODEL
(broe-moe-kriṕ-teen)
(Chapter 14)

Functional classification: Dopamine receptor agonist
Chemical classification: Ergot alkaloid derivative
FDA pregnancy category: C

Indications: Female infertility, Parkinson's disease, prevention of postpartum lactation, amenorrhea, galactorrhea caused by hyperprolactinemia, acromegaly, treatment of NMS, cocaine withdrawal and craving

Contraindications: Hypersensitivity to ergot, severe ischemic disease, pregnancy
Cautious use: Lactation, hepatic or renal disease, hypotension, acromegalic patients

Pharmacologic Effects: Stimulates prolactin release by activating postsynaptic dopamine receptors; activation of dopamine receptors is the reason for improvement in Parkinson's disease and NMS (symptom of primary interest in this text)

Pharmacokinetics: PO: Peak 1-3 hr, duration 4-8 hr, 90% to 96% protein bound, half-life 3-8 hr, metabolized by liver (inactive metabolites), excreted in feces (85% to 98%) and urine (2.5% to 5.5%)

Side Effects: *CNS:* **Headache, abnormal involuntary movements,** depression, restlessness, anxiety, nervousness, confusion, **convulsions,** hallucinations; *Peripheral:* Frequency, retention, incontinence, diuresis, blurred vision, diplopia, burning eyes, **nausea, vomiting, anorexia,** cramps, constipation, diarrhea, dry mouth, rash on face or arms, alopecia, orthostatic hypotension, decreased B/P, palpitation, shock, arrhythmias, **shortness of breath**

Interactions:
- Phenothiazines, haloperidol, droperidol, oral contraceptives: Decrease action of bromocriptine, thus increasing likelihood of conception in women taking birth control pills
- Antihypertensives, levodopa: Increase effect of these drugs

Implications (for NMS treatment only)
Assess
- B/P; this drug decreases B/P

Planning/Implementation
- With meals to prevent GI symptoms
- Administer hs so that dizziness, orthostatic hypotension are not problems

Teaching
- To prevent orthostatic hypotension, change position slowly
- To use barrier contraceptives during treatment with this drug; pregnancy may occur
- To avoid hazardous activity when dizziness occurs

Evaluate
- Therapeutic response (NMS): Decreased fever, sweating, rigidity, decreased slow movements, drooling

Lab Test Interferences: Increase: BUN, SGOT, CPK, alkaline phosphatase

Administration:
- Parkinson's disease: *Adult:* PO 1.25 mg bid with meals, may increase q 2-4 wk, not to exceed 100 mg qd
- NMS: Although standardized dose not established for this unlabeled use, doses of 2.5-10 mg 3 times a day *have been reported* to be effective. If no improvement in 24 hr, increase to 20 mg po 4 times a day (for other uses see *PDR*)
- Cocaine withdrawal: 1.25 mg tid for 7 days, then discontinue
- Available forms include: caps 5 mg; tabs 2.5 mg (must be cut in half for 1.25-mg dose)

Bupropion HCl

WELLBUTRIN

(byoo-proé-pee-on) (Chapter 5)

Functional classification: Unicyclic antidepressant
Chemical classification: Aminoketone
FDA pregnancy category: B

Indications: Depression

Contraindications: Hypersensitivity, concomitant use of MAOIs, seizure history, children <18 yr, patients with prior diagnosis of bulimia or anorexia (high incidence of seizures in these patients)
Cautious use: Psychoses, suicidal patients, CV disorders, hepatic or renal disorders, elderly patients

Pharmacologic Effects: Not clear; *does not* block reuptake of serotonin or norepinephrine well; *does not* inhibit monoamine oxidase

Pharmacokinetics: Peak levels 2 hr; metabolized in liver, excreted in urine (87%) and feces (10%), half-life 15 hr

Side Effects: *CNS:* **Seizures** that are dose related (doses below 450 mg/day reduce risk of seizures); **agitation, confusion,** insomnia, **headache, sedation,** tremor; *Peripheral:* Blurred vision, **dizziness, tachycardia,** arrhythmias, **dry mouth, constipation, weight loss or gain, nausea and vomiting,** anorexia; **excessive sweating,** menstrual complaints, **rash,** impotence, upper respiratory tract complaints

Interactions
- Carbamazepine, phenytoin, cimetidine, phenobarbital: Slow metabolism of bupropion
- Levodopa: Increased incidence of adverse effects of bupropion

- MAOIs and alcohol: Increased toxicity of bupropion and seizures (alcohol)
- Drugs that lower seizure threshold (phenothiazines, TCAs): Increased risk of seizures

Implications

Assess

- Blood studies: CBC, leukocyte count, cardiac enzyme levels
- Liver function tests before and during therapy: bilirubin level, AST, ALT
- ECG: Flattening of T wave; bundle branch block; AV block; arrhythmias in cardiac patients

Planning/Implementation

- Treat constipation and dry mouth
- Give with food or milk for GI upset
- Assist with ambulation
- Give last dose no later than 4 PM to minimize effects on sleep

Teaching

- Therapeutic effects take 2-4 wks
- Use caution in driving or other hazardous activities
- To avoid alcohol; when alcohol is consumed, to wait until next morning to take bupropion
- Not to discontinue use abruptly

Evaluate

- Therapeutic response: Level of depression; ability to perform activities of daily living, ability to sleep
- Mental status: Mood, suicidal ideation

Treatment of Overdose: Hospitalization; give emetic, if patient is conscious; activated charcoal, provide adequate fluids, treat seizures with IV benzodiazepines

Administration

Adult: 100 mg bid to start (morning and evening); based on clinical response, may be increased to 300 mg/day in divided doses no sooner than 3 days after beginning therapy; maximum dose 450 mg/day, with never more than 150 mg given in single dose

- Available forms: Tabs 75, 100 mg

Buspirone HCl

BUSPAR

(byoo-spear-own) (Chapter 6)

Functional classification: Antianxiety agent

Chemical classification: Azaspirodecanedione

FDA pregnancy category: B

Indications: Management and short-term relief of anxiety disorders

Contraindications: Hypersensitivity, psychosis

Cautious use: Lactation, child <18 yr, elderly patients, impaired hepatic or renal function

Pharmacologic Effects: Unknown; not related to benzodiazepines; may act by binding to serotonin receptors in brain

Pharmacokinetics: Rapidly absorbed and undergoes extensive first-pass metabolism, peak serum levels within 90 min, excreted in urine and feces, half-life 2-11 hr

Side Effects: *CNS:* **Dizziness, headache,** depression, **stimulation,** insomnia, nervousness, light-headedness, numbness, paresthesia, incoordination, tremors, excitement, involuntary movements, confusion, akathisia; *Peripheral:* **Nausea, dry mouth,** diarrhea, constipation; tachycardia, palpitations, hypotension; sore throat, tinnitus, blurred vision, nasal congestion; frequency, hesitancy; muscle cramps; hyperventilation, chest congestion, shortness of breath; rash, edema, pruritus, alopecia, dry skin

Interactions

- MAOIs: Increase B/P
- Alcohol: Do not mix, even though serious interactions have not been documented
- Trazodone: Increases ALT
- Haloperidol: Increased haloperidol serum levels

Implications

Assess

- B/P, pulse; if systolic B/P drops 20 mm Hg, withhold drug

- Hepatic studies: AST, ALT, bilirubin, creatinine, LDH, alkaline phosphatase levels
- Mental status
- Give with food or milk for GI symptoms; food may decrease absorption but increase bioavailability

Planning/Implementation
- Assistance with ambulation during beginning of therapy; drowsiness, dizziness occur
- Safety measures, including side rails, when drowsiness occurs

Teaching
- Optimum results may take 3 to 6 weeks; some improvement within 7 to 10 days
- Take with food
- To avoid driving and activities requiring alertness because drowsiness may occur
- To avoid alcohol or other CNS depressant medications, unless prescribed by physician
- Not to discontinue medication abruptly after long-term use
- To rise slowly, or fainting may occur
- To notify physician if chronic abnormal movements occur (restlessness, involuntary movements)

Evaluate
- Therapeutic response: Decreased anxiety
- Physical dependency, withdrawal symptoms, headache, nausea, vomiting, muscle pain, weakness after long-term use
- Suicidal tendencies

Treatment of Overdose: Gastic lavage, VS, supportive care; no deaths from overdose have been reported

Administration

Adult: PO 5 mg tid, may increase 5 mg/day q 2-3 days, not to exceed 60 mg/day
- Available forms include: Tabs 5, 10 mg

Butabarbital/Butabarbital Sodium*

BUTISOL, MEDARSED, BUTATRAN, BUTICAPS, BUTISOL SODIUM
(byoo-ta-bar΄-bi-tal) (Chapter 8)

Functional classifications: Sedative, hypnotic
Chemical classification: Barbitone
Controlled substance schedule II
FDA pregnancy category: D

Indications: Sedation, insomnia

Contraindications: See amobarbital

Pharmacologic Effects: See amobarbital

Pharmacokinetics: Onset 45-60 min, duration 6-8 hr; metabolized by liver, excreted in urine; half-life 66-140 hr

Side Effects: *CNS:* See amobarbital; *Peripheral:* See amobarbital

Interactions: See amobarbital

Implications: See amobarbital

Treatment of Overdose: See amobarbital

Administration
- Insomnia: PO 50-100 mg hs
- Available forms: Tabs 15, 30, 50, 100 mg; caps 15, 30 mg; elix 30, 33.3 mg/5 mL

Caffeine

NO DOZ, TIREND, VIVARIN
(kaf-een) (Chapter 13)

Functional classification: Cerebral stimulant
Chemical classification: Xanthine
FDA pregnancy category: C

Indications: Mild CNS stimulation to stay awake or increase mental alertness, used with analgesics

Contraindications: Gastric or duodenal hypersensitivity

*Infrequently used.

Cautious use: Arrhythmias, lactation

Pharmacologic Effects: Promotes accumulation of cyclic AMP by increasing calcium permeability and causes CNS stimulation; constricts cerebral blood vessels and relaxes smooth muscles in blood vessels to bronchi

Pharmacokinetics: PO: Readily absorbed, onset 15 min, peak 1/2 -1 hr, metabolized by liver, excreted by kidneys, crosses placenta, enters breast milk, half-life 3-4 hr

Side Effects: *CNS:* **Hyperactivity, insomnia, restlessness, talkativeness,** dizziness, headache, **stimulation,** irritability, aggressiveness, tremors, twitching; *Peripheral:* Nausea, vomiting, anorexia, diuresis, **tachycardia**

Interactions: Oral contraceptives, cimetidine: Increased effects of caffeine
Smoking: Enhances caffeine elimination

Implications

Assess

- VS, B/P

Planning/Implementation

- Do not give to patient with peptic ulcer disease

Teaching

- To decrease other caffeine consumption (coffee, tea, cola, chocolate), which may increase irritability, stimulation
- To taper off drug over several weeks after long-term use
- To not use as a substitute for regular sleep

Evaluate

- Therapeutic response; increased CNS stimulation, decreased drowsiness
- Mental status; stimulation, insomnia, irritability
- Tolerance or dependency; an increased amount may be used to get same effect
- Overdose: Pain, fever, dehydration, insomnia, hyperactivity

Treatment of Overdose: Lavage, activated charcoal, monitor electrolyte levels, VS, administer anticonvulsants if needed

Administration

Adult: PO 100-200 mg q4h prn; *infant or child:* 8 mg/kg, not to exceed 500 mg

- Available forms include: Tabs 100, 200 mg; time-rel caps 200, 250 mg

Carbamazepine

MAZEPINE,† TEGRETOL
(kar-ba-maź-e-peen) (Chapters 4, 5, 7, 15, 16)

C

Functional classification: Antiepileptic
Chemical classification: Iminostilbene derivative
FDA pregnancy category: C

Indications: Tonic-clonic, psychomotor, mixed seizures; pain-associated trigeminal neuralgia
Unlabeled uses: bipolar illness, schizoaffective illness, resistant schizophrenia; PTSD

Contraindications: History of bone marrow depression; hypersensitivity to carbamazepine and TCAs; concomitant use of MAOIs
Cautious use: History of hematologic reaction to any drug, glaucoma, psychosis history, child <6 yr, lactation

Pharmacologic Effects: Unrelated to other antiepileptics; mechanism of action unknown but might act by reducing polysynaptic responses, blocking post-tetanic potentiation, and modifying Na^{++}, Ca^{++} conductances; therapeutic serum levels 4-12 μg/mL

Pharmacokinetics: PO peak serum in 4-5 hr, metabolized in liver, excreted in urine (72%) and feces (28%), half-life 12-17 hr with repeated doses, protein binding 76%

Side Effects: *CNS:* **Drowsiness, dizziness, unsteadiness,** confusion, fatigue, paralysis, headache, hallucinations; *Peripheral:* **Nausea, vomiting, diarrhea,** blood dyscrasias that lead to fatalities, i.e., aplastic anemia, leukopenia, agranulocytosis, thrombocytopenia, bone marrow depression; hepatitis; urinary frequency and retention; pulmonary hypersensitivity; fever, dyspnea; CHF, **hypertension,** hypotension, transient diplopia, fever and chills; rash

Interactions

- Cimetidine, danazol, diltiazem, erythromycin, isoniazid, nicotinamide,

†Available in Canada only.

propoxyphene, verapamil: Drugs that elevate carbamazepine serum levels
- Carbamazepine: Increases the metabolism of acetaminophen and oral anticoagulants
- Barbiturates; primidone: Lower serum level of carbamazepine
- Doxycycline: Reduces half-life of doxycycline
- Haloperidol: Decreases effect of haloperidol
- Hydantoins: Decreases carbamazepine levels; both increases and decreases hydantoin serum levels
- Lithium: Increases CNS intoxication or enhanced antimanic effects
- Nondepolarizing muscle relaxants: Resist or reverse muscle relaxants
- Succinimides: Reduces succinimide levels
- Theophylline: Both drugs decrease effects
- Valproic acid: Decreases serum levels of valproic acid

Implications

Assess
- Renal studies, blood studies, hepatic studies for baseline data and to determine whether carbamazepine therapy is appropriate

Planning/Implementation
- Give with food or milk to decrease GI upset (may enhance absorption)
- Chewable tabs to be chewed, not swallowed
- Assist with ambulation, if patient is dizzy

Teaching
- To avoid driving or operating hazardous machinery when dizzy, drowsy, or having blurred vision
- To notify physician of unusual bleeding or bruising, jaundice, abdominal pain, pale stools, darkened urine, impotence, CNS disturbances, edema, fever, chills, sore throat, or ulcer in mouth
- MedicAlert* identification bracelet
- That abrupt discontinuance can cause seizures

Evaluate
- Therapeutic responses, decreased seizure activity, decreased flashbacks, and the like
- Mental status
- Blood dyscrasias: Fever, sore throat, rash, bruising
- Toxic effects: Bone marrow depression, nausea and vomiting

Treatment of Overdose *Symptoms:* Neuromuscular disturbances, irregular breathing, hypotension or hypertension, respiratory depression; treat symptoms with lavage, charcoal; maintain airway; elevate legs and administer plasma volume expander for hypotension; monitor breathing, heart rate (ECG), B/P, kidney function

Administration
- Seizures: *Adults and children >12 yr:* Initially 200 mg bid; increase at weekly intervals by up to 200 mg/day in 3 to 4 doses; not to exceed 1000 mg/day in children 12-15 yr; not to exceed 1200 mg/day in children >15 yr; maintenance usually 800 to 1200 mg/day; *children 6-12 yr:* Initially 100 mg bid; increase at weekly intervals by adding 100 mg/day in 3 to 4 doses; do not exceed 1000 mg/day; maintenance dose usually 400-800 mg/day
- Available forms: Tabs, chewable 100 mg; tabs 200 mg, suspension 100 mg/5 mL

Carbidopa-levodopa

SINEMET
(kar-bi-doé-pa lee-voe-doé-pa)
(Chapter 14)

Functional classification: Antiparkinson drug
Chemical classification: Catecholamine
FDA pregnancy category: C

Indications: Parkinsonism

Contraindications: Narrow-angle glaucoma, hypersensitivity, undiagnosed skin lesions, MAOI therapy

Pharmacologic Effects: Carbidopa prevents metabolism of levodopa to dopamine (dopamine cannot cross blood-brain barrier in significant amounts), so more levodopa enters CNS

Pharmacokinetics: Peak blood level 1-3 hr; excreted in urine

*MedicAlert, Turlock, Calif.

Side Effects: *CNS:* Tremors of hand, fatigue, involuntary movements, headache, anxiety, twitching, confusion, agitation, insomnia, nightmares, hallucinations; *Peripheral:* **Nausea,** vomiting, GI symptoms, gas, dysphagia, skin eruptions, orthostatic hypotension, tachycardia, palpitations, blurred vision, dilated pupils, dark urine, urinary retention

Interactions
- MAOIs: Hypertensive crisis
- Anticholinergics, hydantoins, papaverine, pyridoxine, haloperidol: Decreased effect of levodopa
- Antihypertensives: Orthostatic hypotension
- Antacids, metoclopramide: Increased effects of levodopa
- TCAs: Hypertension
- Consult *PDR* for the many other interactions

Implications
Assess
- B/P, respirations, mental status

Planning/Implementation
- Assist patient with ambulation until condition is stabilized on drug regimen

Teaching
- Change positions slowly
- To not discontinue use abruptly, since parkinsonian crisis can occur
- To not be alarmed by dark urine or sweat
- That a therapeutic effect may take 3 to 4 mo

Evaluate
- Mental status, therapeutic response

Lab Test Interferences
- False positive: urine ketones
- False negative: urine glucose
- False increase: uric acid, urine protein
- Decrease: VMA, BUN, creatinine levels

Treatment of Overdose: There are no reports of overdosage with carbidopa; for levodopa, provide supportive care with immediate gastric lavage; monitor for airway, development of arrhythmias

Administration
Adults: PO 3-6 tabs of 25 mg carbidopa/250 mg levodopa per day in divided doses; maximum dose should not exceed 8 tabs/day
- Available forms: Tabs 10 mg (carbidopa)/100 mg (levodopa), 25/100, 25/250 mg

Chloral Hydrate

AQUACHLORAL SUPPRETTES, NOCTEC, NOVOCHLORHYDRATE†
(klor-al hyédrate) (Chapter 8)

Functional classifications: Sedative, hypnotic
Chemical classification: Chloral derivative
Controlled substance schedule IV
FDA pregnancy category: C

Indications: Sedation, insomnia

Contraindications: Hypersensitivity to chloral hydrate, severe renal and hepatic disease, GI problems

Pharmacologic Effects: Mechanism of action not clear; hypnotic dose causes mild CNS depression

Pharmacokinetics: Metabolized to trichloroethanol, an active metabolite that has a half-life of 7-10 hr; protein binding is 35% to 41%; trichloroethanol is metabolized to trichloroacetic acid, an inactive metabolite; trichloroacetic acid is excreted in urine and bile and has a protein binding capacity of 71% to 88%; it can displace other acidic drugs from protein binding sites

Side Effects: *CNS:* Somnabulism, disorientation, incoherence, paradoxic excitement, delirium, drowsiness, ataxia; *Peripheral:* Nausea and vomiting; other GI disturbances; blood dyscrasias; skin eruptions, e.g., rashes, hives

Interactions
- Alcohol: Synergistic effect with disulfiram-like reactions, i.e., tachycardia, flushing
- CNS depressants: Additive effect
- Oral anticoagulants: Slight increased effect
- Furosemide: Sweating, hot flashes, tachycardia

†Available in Canada only.

- Hydantoins: Reduced effect of hydantoin

Implications
Assess
- Blood studies

Planning/Implementation
- Maintain safety, e.g., prevent falls, keep side rails up, etc
- Give ½-1 hr before bedtime for insomnia
- Give after meals to decrease GI effect

Teaching
- To **avoid driving and use of alcohol** and other CNS depressants
- Potential for dependence
- Do not discontinue use abruptly
- Do not chew capsules

Evaluate
- Therapeutic response, mental status, respiratory difficulties, monitor for blood dyscrasias

Lab Test Interferences: Interferes with urine catecholamines and urinary 17-OHCS determinations; false-positive result for urinary glucose when using copper sulfate test

Treatment of Overdose: Symptoms are similar to those for barbiturate overdose; doses >2 g may produce intoxication; deaths have occurred with doses as low as 1.25 to 3 g; doses as high as 36 g have been tolerated; treatment is gastric lavage or induced emesis; activated charcoal may retard absorption; hemodialysis may be helpful; other supportive care as needed

Administration
- Insomnia: *Adult:* PO/rec 500 mg-1 g ½-1 hr before bedtime; *child:* PO/rec 25-50 mg/kg in one dose, up to 1 g (hypnotic) or 500 mg (sedative)
- Available forms: Caps 250, 500 mg; syr 250, 500 mg/5 mL, supp 324, 500, 648 mg

Chlordiazepoxide HCl

A-POXIDE, CHLORDIAZEPOXIDE HCL, LIBRITABS, LIBRIUM, MEDILIUM,† NOVOPOXIDE,† SOLIUM†
(klor-dye-az-e-pox́-ide)
(Chapters 6 and 10)

Functional classification: Antianxiety
Chemical classification: Benzodiazepine
Controlled substance schedule IV
FDA pregnancy category: D

Indications: Short-term management of anxiety, acute alcohol withdrawal, preoperatively for relaxation

Contraindications: Hypersensitivity to benzodiazepines, narrow-angle glaucoma, psychosis, child <6 yr (oral), child <12 yr (inj)

Cautious use: Elderly or debilitated patients, hepatic or renal disease

Pharmacologic Effects: Apparently potentiates effects of GABA and other inhibitory transmitters by binding to specific benzodiazepine receptor sites; depresses subcortical levels of CNS, including limbic system and reticular formation

Pharmacokinetics
- Speed of onset: Intermediate
- PO: Onset 30 min, peak 0.5-4 hr, duration 4-6 hr, metabolized by liver, excreted by kidneys, crosses placenta, enters breast milk, half-life 5-30 hr (average 18 hr)

Side Effects: *CNS:* **Drowsiness, dizziness,** confusion, headache, anxiety, tremor, stimulation, fatigue, depression, insomnia; *Peripheral:* Photophobia caused by mydriasis, **blurred vision** caused by cycloplegia; sleep-like slowing of respirations with therapeutic doses, cough; **orthostatic hypotension, tachycardia,** hypotension; constipation, dry mouth

Interactions
- Alcohol and other CNS depressants: Increased risk of excessive CNS depression

†Available in Canada only.

- Cimetidine: Potentiation of CNS depression
- Digoxin: Increased risk of cardiac side effects from digoxin
- Levodopa: Decreased antiparkinson effect
- Phenytoin: Increased phenytoin serum levels
- Oral anticoagulants: Increases or decreases anticoagulant effect

Implications

Assess

- Patient's level of anxiety and method of coping
- B/P, VS
- Establish baseline physical assessment data before medications are started

Planning/Implementation

- Monitor patient's response to medication
- Observe elderly, very young, and debilitated patients for paradoxic excitement
- Reduce dose of other depressant drugs
- Observe for signs of withdrawal when discontinuing antianxiety drug regimen

Teaching

- To avoid operating dangerous machinery and performing other tasks requiring good reflexes
- To report ocular pain at once, as well as other visual disturbances
- That drug may be taken with food

Evaluate

- Whether patient achieves lower levels of anxiety without undue sedation
- Whether patient can follow prescribed regimen
- For physical dependence: withdrawal symptoms of headache, nausea, vomiting, muscle pain, weakness after long-term use

Lab Test Interferences

Increase: AST/ALT, serum bilirubin level
False increase: 17-OHCS
Decrease: RAIU

Treatment of Overdose: Lavage, VS, supportive care; there have been few deaths, if any, resulting from benzodiazepine overdose alone; deaths occur when benzodiazepines are mixed with other drugs, especially alcohol

Administration

- Mild anxiety: *Adult:* PO 5-10 mg tid or qid; *child* >6 yr: 5 mg bid-qid, not to exceed 10 mg bid-tid
- Severe anxiety: *Adult:* PO 20-25 mg tid-qid
- Alcohol withdrawal: *Adult:* PO/IM/IV 50-100 mg, not to exceed 300 mg/day; is poorly absorbed
- Available forms include: Caps 5, 10, 25 mg; tabs 5, 10, 25 mg; powder for IM inj 100-mg ampule

Chlorpromazine HCl

THORAZINE, CHLORPROMANYL, ORMAZINE (klor-proé-ma-zeen) (Chapter 4)

Functional classifications: Antipsychotic, neuroleptic
Chemical classification: Phenothiazine, aliphatic
FDA pregnancy category: D

Indications: *Psychiatric:* Psychotic disorders, mania, schizophrenia. *Other:* Intractable hiccups, nausea, vomiting, preoperatively for relaxation, acute intermittent porphyria

Contraindications: Hypersensitivity, liver damage, cerebral arteriosclerosis, coronary disease, severe hypertension or hypotension, blood dyscrasias, coma, child <6 mo, brain damage, bone marrow depression, presence of alcohol and barbiturate

Cautious use: Lactation, seizure disorders, hypertension, hepatic disease, cardiac disease, respiratory impairment, especially in children

Pharmacologic Effects: Antipsychotic drugs produce a neuroleptic effect characterized by sedation, emotional quieting, psychomotor slowing, and affective indifference; exact mode of action is not fully understood; antipsychotics primarily block dopamine D_2 receptors in the basal ganglia, hypothalamus, limbic system, brain stem, and medulla; they are also thought to depress certain components of the reticular activating system that partially control body temperature, wakefulness, vasomotor tone, emesis, and hormonal balance; additionally, antipsychotics have significant anticholinergic and alpha-adrenergic blocking effects. Therapeutic plasma levels are 30-500 ng/mL

Pharmacokinetics

- PO: Onset erratic, peak 2-4 hr, duration may be detected for up to 6 mo after last dose
- IM: Onset 15-30 min, peak 15-20 min, duration may be detected for up to 6 mo after last dose; IM provides 4 to 10 times more active drug than do oral doses
- IV: Onset 5 min, peak 10 min, duration may be detected for up to 6 mo after last dose
- REC: Onset erratic, peak 3 hr
- Metabolized by liver, excreted in urine (metabolites), crosses placenta, enters breast milk; 95% bound to plasma proteins; elimination half-life 10-30 hr

Side Effects: *CNS:* Parkinsonism, akathisias, dystonias, tardive dyskinesia, oculogyric crisis *Peripheral:* Blurred vision (cycloplegia or paralysis of accommodation), ocular pain, photophobia, mydriasis, impaired vision; intolerance of extreme heat or cold, possible heat stroke or fatal hyperthermia; nasal congestion, wheezing, dyspnea; **hypotension, especially orthostatic,** leading to dizziness, syncope, **tachycardia,** irregular pulse, arrhythmias; **dry mouth, constipation,** jaundice, abdominal pain, urinary retention; urinary hesitancy, galactorrhea, gynecomastia, impaired ejaculation, amenorrhea

Interactions

- Alcohol and other CNS depressants (barbiturates, antihistamines, antianxiety or antidepressant drugs): Increased CNS depression; increased risk of EPSEs
- Amphetamines: Possible decreased antipsychotic effect
- Antacids (magnesium and aluminum products): Possible decreased antipsychotic effect
- Anticholinergics (atropine, H_1-type antihistamines, antidepressants, etc.): Increased risk of excessive atropine-like side effects or toxic effects
- Benztropine: Possible decreased antipsychotic effect, increased risk of severity of peripheral anticholinergic side effects
- Diazoxide: Possible severe hyperglycemia, prediabetic coma
- Guanethidine: Poor control of hypertension by guanethidine
- Hypoglycemia drugs (insulin, oral hypoglycemia agents): Poor diabetic control
- Lithium: Poor control of psychosis with combined therapy; can mask lithium intoxication; neurotoxic effects with confusion, delirium, seizures, encephalopathy
- Meperidine, morphine: Increased risk of severe CNS depression, respiratory depression, hypotension
- Propranolol: Increased pharmacologic effects of either drug

Implications

Assess

- Establish baseline VS, laboratory values to aid in assessing side effects, allergic or hypersensitivity reactions
- Physiologic and psychologic status before therapy, to determine needs and evaluate progress
- For early stages of tardive dyskinesia by use of Abnormal Involuntary Movement Scale
- Identify concurrent symptoms that may be aggravated by antipsychotics, e.g., glaucoma, diabetes

Planning/Implementation

- Ensure that drug has been taken; check mouth for "cheeking"
- When giving liquid antipsychotics, use at least 60 mL of compatible beverage to mask taste; dilute and give immediately; take drug with food to minimize GI upset; give IM injections in lateral thigh
- Keep patient quiet after injection to prevent falls associated with postural hypotension
- For dry mouth, give chewing gum, hard candies, lip balm, monitor urinary output, check for bladder distention in inactive patients, older men, and patients receiving high doses
- Assist patient with ambulation when blurred vision occurs; dim room lights for photosensitivity
- Ensure safety with hypotension; sit on side of bed before rising, head-low position for dizziness, avoid hot showers, wear elastic stockings

- Check B/P (supine, sitting, standing) and pulse before and after each dose when possible; observe for side effects
- Monitor body temperature for indications of muscle rigidity, fever, depressed neurologic status; ensure adequate hydration, nutrition, and ventilation
- Protect patient from exposure to extreme heat or cold
- Recognize impending hypersensitivity: pruritus or jaundice with hepatitis, flu or coldlike symptoms, evidence of bleeding with blood dyscrasia
- Observe for involuntary movements

Teaching

- About benefits and potential harm of antipsychotic drugs; weigh need to know against causing apprehension
- To comply with drug treatment
- To avoid activities requiring clear vision for a few weeks after treatment starts; to report eye pain immediately
- About importance of exercise, fluids, and fiber in the diet
- To watch for symptoms of heart failure: weight gain, dyspnea, distended neck veins, tachycardia
- Possible male sexual performance failure; suggest relaxed, stress-free environment
- To avoid conception; women should practice effective contraception; phenothiazines may cause false-positive results in pregnancy tests
- To avoid exposure to sunlight; keep skin covered but with temperature-appropriate clothing
- That patient cannot become addicted to antipsychotic drugs

Evaluate

- Whether patient follows prescribed regimen, takes medications as ordered
- Avoids injury; reports dizziness or need for assistance
- Verbalizes reduced anxiety
- Experiences minimal or no adverse responses
- Uses appropriate interventions to minimize side effects
- Achieves improved mental status; most problems occur during first 2 weeks of therapy
- For agranulocytosis, especially within 4 to 10 weeks after initiation of chlorpromazine therapy

Lab Test Interferences

- Increase: Liver function tests; determinations of cardiac enzymes, cholesterol, blood glucose, prolactin, bilirubin, PBI, cholinesterase, I-131
- Decrease: Hormones (blood and urine)
- False positive: Pregnancy tests, PKU
- False negative: Urinary steroids, 17-OHCS

Treatment of Overdose: Lavage, if orally ingested; provide an airway; do not induce vomiting; control EPSEs and hypotension

Administration: (Psychiatric Indications)

- Psychiatry: *Adult:* PO 10-50 mg q1-4h initially, then increase up to 800 mg/day or more (up to 2000 mg/day): *adult:* IM 10-50 mg q1-4h; *child:* PO 0.25 mg/lb q4-6h or 0.5 mg/kg; *child:* IM 0.25 mg/lb q6-8h or 0.5 mg/kg; *child:* REC 0.5 mg/lb q6-8h or 1 mg/kg; *other uses:* See *PDR*
- Available forms include: Tabs 10, 25, 50, 100, 200 mg; time-rel caps 30, 75, 150, 200, 300 mg; syr 10 mg/5 mL; conc 30, 100 mg/mL; supp 25, 100 mg; inj IM, IV 25 mg/mL

Chlorprothixene

TARACTAN

(klor-proe-thix́-een) (Chapter 4)

Functional classifications: Antipsychotic, neuroleptic

Chemical classification: Thioxanthene

FDA pregnancy category: C

Indications: Psychotic disorders, schizophrenia

Contraindications: Hypersensitivity, liver damage, cerebral arteriosclerosis, coronary disease, severe hypertension or hypotension, blood dyscrasias, coma, child <6 yr (PO), child <12 yr (IM), brain damage, bone marrow depression, alcohol and barbiturate withdrawal states

Cautious use: Lactation, seizure disorders, hypertension, hepatic disease, cardiac disease

Pharmacologic Effects: Antipsychotic drugs produce a neuroleptic effect characterized by sedation, emotional quieting, psychomotor slowing, and affective indifference; exact mode of action is not fully understood; antipsychotics primarily block dopamine D_2 receptors in the basal ganglia, hypothalamus, limbic system, brain stem, and medulla; antipsychotics are also thought to depress certain components of the reticular activating system that partially control body temperature, wakefulness, vasomotor tone, emesis, and hormonal balance; additionally, antipsychotics have significant anticholinergic and alpha-adrenergic blocking effects

Pharmacokinetics: PO: Onset erratic, peak 2-4 hr; duration may be detected for up to 6 mo after last dose; metabolized by liver, excreted in urine (metabolites), crosses placenta, enters breast milk

Side Effects: *CNS:* Parkinsonism, akathisias, dystonias, tardive dyskinesia, oculogyric crisis; *Peripheral:* Blurred vision (cycloplegia or paralysis of accommodation); ocular pain, photophobia, mydriasis, impaired vision; intolerance of extreme heat or cold, possible heat stroke or fatal hyperthermia; nasal congestion, wheezing, dyspnea; **hypotension, especially orthostatic,** leading to dizziness, syncope; **tachycardia,** irregular pulse, arrhythmias; **dry mouth, constipation,** jaundice, abdominal pain; urinary retention, urinary hesitancy, galactorrhea, gynecomastia, impaired ejaculation, amenorrhea

Interactions

- Alcohol and other CNS depressants (barbiturates, antihistamines, antianxiety or antidepressant drugs): Increased CNS depression; increased risk of EPSEs
- Amphetamines: Possible decreased antipsychotic effect
- Antacids (magnesium and aluminum products): Possible decreased antipsychotic effect
- Anticholinergics (atropine, H_1-type antihistamines, antidepressants, etc): Increased risk of excessive atropine-like side effects or toxic effects
- Benztropine: Possible decreased antipsychotic effect, increased risk of severity of peripheral anticholinergic side effects
- Diazoxide: Possible severe hyperglycemia, prediabetic coma
- Guanethidine: Poor control of hypertension by guanethidine
- Hypoglycemia drugs (insulin, oral hypoglycemia agents): Poor diabetic control
- Lithium: Poor control of psychosis with combined therapy; can mask lithium intoxication; neurotoxic effects with confusion, delirium, seizures, encephalopathy
- Meperidine, morphine: Increased risk of severe CNS depression, respiratory depression, hypotension
- Propranolol: Increased pharmacologic effects of either drug

Implications

Assess

- Establish baseline VS, laboratory values, to aid recognition of side effects, allergic or hypersensitivity reactions
- Assess physiologic and psychologic status before therapy, to determine needs and evaluate progress
- Assess for early stages of tardive dyskinesia by use of Abnormal Involuntary Movement Scale
- Identify concurrent symptoms that may be aggravated by antipsychotics, e.g., glaucoma, diabetes

Planning/Implementation

- Ensure that drug has been taken; check mouth for "cheeking"
- When giving liquid, dilute in milk, water, fruit juice, coffee, or soft drink; take drug with food to minimize GI upset; give IM injections in lateral thigh
- Keep patient quiet after injection to prevent falls associated with postural hypotension
- For dry mouth, give chewing gum, hard candies, lip balm, monitor urinary output; check for bladder distention in inactive patients, older men, and patients receiving high doses
- Assist with ambulation when patient has blurred vision; dim room lights for photosensitivity
- Ensure safety with hypotension; sit on side of bed before rising, head-low position for dizziness, avoid hot showers, wear elastic stockings
- Check B/P (supine, sitting, standing) and pulse before and after each dose when possible; observe for side effects
- Monitor body temperature for indications of NMS, e.g., muscle rigidity,

fever, depressed neurologic status; ensure adequate hydration, nutrition, and ventilation
- Protect patient from exposure to extreme heat or cold
- Recognize impending hypersensitivity: pruritus or jaundice with hepatitis, flu or coldlike symptoms, evidence of bleeding with blood dyscrasia
- Observe for involuntary movements

Teaching
- About benefits and potential harm of antipsychotic drugs; weigh need to know against causing apprehension
- To comply with drug treatment
- To avoid activities requiring clear vision for a few weeks after treatment starts; to report eye pain immediately
- About importance of exercise, fluids, and fiber in diet
- To watch for symptoms of heart failure: weight gain, dyspnea, distended neck veins, tachycardia
- Possible male sexual performance failure; suggest relaxed, stress-free environment
- To avoid conception; women should practice effective contraception
- To avoid exposure to sunlight; keep skin covered but with temperature-appropriate clothing
- That patient cannot become addicted to antipsychotic drugs

Evaluate
- Whether patient follows prescribed regimen, takes medications as ordered
- Avoids injury; reports dizziness or need for assistance
- Verbalizes reduced anxiety
- Experiences minimal or no adverse responses
- Uses appropriate interventions to minimize side effects
- Achieves improved mental status

Lab Test Interferences
- Increase: Liver function tests; determinations of cardiac enzymes, cholesterol, blood glucose, prolactin, bilirubin, PBI, cholinesterase, I-131
- Decrease: Hormones (blood and urine)
- False positive: Pregnancy tests, PKU
- False negative: Urinary steroids, 17-OHCS

Treatment of Overdose: Lavage, if orally ingested; provide an airway; do not induce vomiting

Administration

Adult: PO 25-50 mg tid or qid, increased to desired response, maximum dosage 600 mg/qd

Geriatric: Start at 10-25 mg tid or qid; IM 25-50 mg tid or qid

Child >6 yr: PO 10-25 mg tid or qid; IM not recommended for children <12 yr

- Available forms include: Tabs 10, 25, 50, 100 mg; conc 100 mg/5 mL; inj IM 12.5 mg/mL

C

Clomipramine

ANAFRANIL

(kloe-mí-pra-meen) (Chapter 5)

Functional classification: TCA
Chemical classification: Tertiary amine, serotonin reuptake inhibitor
FDA pregnancy category: C

Indications: Obsessive-compulsive disorder

Contraindications: Hypersensitivity to TCAs; acute recovery phase following MI; concomitant use with MAOIs; children <10 yr

Cautious use: Seizure disorders, glaucoma, urinary retention, hepatic and renal disorders, psychosis, ECT, elective surgery

Pharmacologic Effects: Blocks serotonin reuptake while the active metabolite desmethylclomipramine blocks norepinephrine reuptake; therapeutic plasma level 150-300 ng/mL

Pharmacokinetics: Metabolized by liver, excreted in urine; half-life 19-37 hr

Side Effects: *CNS:* **Sedation, headache** (52%), **insomnia** (25%), **libido change** (21%), **nervousness** (18%), **myoclonus** (13%), **increased appetite** (11%), ataxia; confusion, delirium; *Peripheral:* **Blurred vision,** photophobia, increased intraocular pressure; decreased tearing; **orthostatic hypotension;** arrythmias, tachycardia, palpitations; **dry mouth** (84%), **constipation** (47%), **diarrhea; increased sweating; urinary retention, hesitancy, ejaculation failure** (42%), **impotence** (20%), **fatigue** (39%), **weight gain** (18%)

Interactions
- Alcohol and other CNS depressants: Increased CNS depression
- Anticholinergics: Increased anticholinergic effect
- Sympathomimetics: Increased risk of sympathomimetic effect
- Haloperidol, cimetidine: Toxic effects r/t increased plasma levels of clomipramine
- Estrogens: Decreased or increased effects of clomipramine
- MAOIs: Hypertensive crisis, convulsions
- Phenytoin, phenobarbital: Decreased seizure threshold
- Ethchlorvynol: Delirium

Implications
Assess
- Establish baseline data to aid recognition of adverse responses to medication, e.g., liver enzyme levels, VS, renal function, mental status, speech patterns, affect, weight
- Assess for signs of noncompliance, e.g., poor therapeutic response
- Observe for major symptoms of depression: apathy, sadness, sleep disturbances, hopelessness, guilt, decreased libido, spontaneous crying
- Review history for contraindicated conditions, e.g., glaucoma, CV disease, GI conditions, urologic conditions, seizures, pregnancy

Planning/Implementation
- Monitor for "cheeking" or hoarding; check drug dosage carefully, because a small overdose may cause toxic effects
- Monitor for suicidal ideations; suicidal thought content is associated with obsessive-compulsive disorder
- Monitor VS; withhold when hypotension, tachycardia, or arrhythmias occur
- After titration, may give in a single dose hs
- Observe for early signs of toxicity, e.g., drowsiness, tachycardia, mydriasis, hypotension, agitation, vomiting, confusion, fever, restlessness, sweating
- Discontinue drug when CNS overstimulation occurs, e.g., hypomania, delirium

Teaching
- That these drugs have a lag time of up to 1 month
- Warn males of high incidence of sexual dysfunction
- To adhere to drug regimen
- To avoid OTC drugs, particularly those containing sympathomimetics or anticholinergics
- To avoid drugs listed in section on interactions
- About ways to deal with minor side effects, as follows: dry mouth: with sugarless hard candies, sips of water, mouth rinse; visual disturbances: with artificial tears, sunglasses, assistance with ambulation; constipation: with bulk-forming foods, increased fluids; urinary hesitancy: with adequate fluids, privacy; decreased perspiration: with appropriate clothing, avoidance of unnecessary exercise; orthostatic hypotension: with slow positional changes, avoidance of hot baths and showers; for drowsiness, take large dose at bedtime with physician approval, avoid driving
- That abrupt discontinuance may result in dizziness, nausea, vomiting, insomnia

Evaluate
- For therapeutic serum level
- For decrease in subjective symptoms
- For decrease in objective symptoms
- For mental impairment
- Stable VS
- Level of anxiety; should sleep, talk, and feel better

Administration

Adult: 25 mg/day to start, gradually increase to 100-200 mg/day during first 2 wk; give in divided doses and with food to reduce GI upset; maximum dose is 250 mg/day; eventually total doses can be given hs

Children and adolescents: 25 mg/day to start, gradually increase in first 2 wk to 3 mg/kg or 200 mg, whichever is smaller; can be given once a day hs

- Available forms include: Caps 25, 50, 75 mg

Clonazepam

KLONOPIN
(kloe-ná-zi-pam) (Chapters 6, 7)

Functional classification: Anticonvulsant
Chemical classification: Benzodiazepine
Controlled substance schedule IV
FDA pregnancy category: C

Indications: Absence, Lennox-Gastaut syndrome, atypical absence, akinetic, myoclonic seizures

Unlabeled use: panic attacks, benzodiazepine withdrawal

Contraindications: Hypersensitivity to benzodiazepines, acute narrow-angle glaucoma

Cautious use: Open-angle glaucoma, chronic respiratory disease, impaired hepatic and renal function

Pharmacologic Effects: Inhibits spike and wave formation in absence seizures (petit mal), decreases amplitude, frequency, duration, and spread of discharge in minor motor seizures

Pharmacokinetics: PO: Peak 1-2 hr, metabolized by liver, excreted in urine, half-life 18-60 hr; therapeutic plasma level is 20 to 80 ng/mL

Side Effects: *CNS:* **Drowsiness** (50%), **ataxia** (30%), dizziness, confusion, **behavioral changes,** tremors, insomnia, headache, suicidal tendencies; *Peripheral:* Nausea, constipation, polyphagia, anorexia, xerostomia, diarrhea, rash, alopecia, hirsutism, increased salivation, nystagmus, diplopia, abnormal eye movements, sore gums, respiratory depression, dyspnea, congestion (from increased salivation), palpitations, bradycardia, thrombocytopenia, leukocytosis, eosinophilia

Interactions
- Alcohol, CNS depressants, and other anticonvulsants: Increased CNS depression
- Carbamazepine: Increased carbamazepine serum level
- Valproic acid: Increased potential for seizures

Implications

Assess
- Renal studies: urinalysis, BUN and urine creatinine levels
- Blood studies: RBC, hematocrit, hemoglobin level, reticulocyte counts q wk for 4 wk, then q mo
- Hepatic studies: ALT, AST, bilirubin and creatinine levels
- Drug serum levels during initial treatment

Planning/Implementation
- Give with milk or food, to decrease GI symptoms
- Hard candy, frequent rinsing of mouth, gums for dry mouth
- Assistance with ambulation during early part of treatment; dizziness occurs

Teaching
- To carry MedicAlert identification bracelet
- To avoid driving, other activities that require alertness
- To avoid ingestion of alcohol or CNS depressants; increased sedation may occur
- Not to discontinue medication quickly after long-term use; taper off over several weeks (can precipitate status epilepticus)

Evaluate
- Therapeutic response: Decreased seizure activity, document on patient's chart
- Mental status
- Eye problems: Need for ophthalmic examinations before, during, and after treatment
- Allergic reaction: Red raised rash; if rash occurs, drug should be discontinued
- Blood dyscrasias: Fever, sore throat, bruising, rash, jaundice
- Toxic effects: Ataxia, hypotension, hypotonia

Lab Test Interferences: Increase: AST, alkaline phosphatase

Treatment of Overdose: Lavage, activated charcoal, monitor electrolyte levels, VS, administer vasopressors

Administration

Adult: PO: First start with 1.5 mg/day in 3 divided doses; may be increased 0.5-1 mg q 3 days until desired response, not to exceed 20 mg/day; *infant or child <10*

yr or 30 kg: PO 0.01-0.03 mg/kg/day in divided doses q8h, not to exceed 0.05 mg/kg/day; may be increased 0.25-0.5 mg q 3 days until desired response, not to exceed 0.1-0.2 mg/kg/day
- Available forms include: Tabs 0.5, 1, 2 mg

Clorazepate Dipotassium

TRANXENE
(klor-aź-e-pate) (Chapter 6)

Functional classification: Antianxiety
Chemical classification: Benzodiazepine
Controlled substance schedule IV
FDA pregnancy category: D

Indications: Anxiety, acute alcohol withdrawal, adjunct in partial seizure treatment

Contraindications: Hypersensitivity to benzodiazepines, narrow-angle glaucoma, psychosis, child <9 yr
Cautious use: Elderly or debilitated patients, hepatic or renal disease, lactation

Pharmacologic Effects: Apparently potentiates effects of GABA and other inhibitory transmitters by binding to specific benzodiazepine receptor sites; depresses subcortical levels of CNS, including limbic system and reticular formation

Pharmacokinetics: Speed of onset: Fast PO: Onset 15 min, peak 1-2 hr, duration 4-6 hr, metabolized by liver, excreted by kidneys, crosses placenta, enters breast milk, half-life 30-100 hr

Side Effects: *CNS:* **Drowsiness, dizziness,** confusion, headache, anxiety, tremor, stimulation, fatigue, depression, insomnia; *Peripheral:* Photophobia caused by mydriasis, blurred vision caused by cycloplegia; sleeplike slowing of respirations with therapeutic doses, cough; orthostatic hypotension, tachycardia, hypotension; constipation, dry mouth, decreased hematocrit, transient skin rash

Interactions
- Alcohol and other CNS depressants: Increased risk of excessive CNS depression
- Cimetidine: Decreased clearance of clorazepate
- Digoxin: Increased risk of cardiac side effects from digoxin
- Levodopa: Decreased antiparkinson effect
- Phenytoin: Increased phenytoin serum levels

Implications
Assess
- Patient's level of anxiety and method of coping
- B/P, VS
- Establish baseline physical assessment data before medications are started

Planning/Implementation
- Monitor patient's response to medication
- Observe elderly, very young, and debilitated patients for paradoxic excitement
- Reduce dose of other depressant drugs
- Observe for signs of withdrawal when discontinuing antianxiety medication

Teaching
- To avoid operating dangerous machinery and other tasks requiring good reflexes
- To report ocular pain at once, as well as other visual disturbances
- Drug may be taken with food

Evaluate
- Whether patient achieves lower levels of anxiety without undue sedation
- Whether patient can follow prescribed regimen
- For physical dependence: withdrawal symptoms of headache, nausea, vomiting, muscle pain, weakness after long-term use.

Lab Test Interferences
- Increase: AST/ALT, serum bilirubin level
- Decrease: RAIU
- False increase: 17-OHCS

Treatment of Overdose: Lavage, VS, supportive care; there have been few deaths, if any, from benzodiazepine overdose alone; deaths occur when benzodiazepines are mixed with other drugs, especially alcohol

Administration
- Anxiety: *Adult:* PO 15-60 mg/day; *geriatric:* 7.5-15 mg/day
- Alcohol withdrawal: *Adult:* PO 30 mg, then 30-60 mg in divided doses; day 2,

45-90 mg in divided doses; day 3, 22.5-45 mg in divided doses; day 4, 15-30 mg in divided doses; then reduce daily dose to 7.5-15 mg
- Seizure disorders: *Adult and child >12 yr:* PO 7.5 mg tid, may increase by 7.5 mg/wk or less, not to exceed 90 mg/day *Children 9-12 yr:* PO 7.5 mg bid; increase by 7.5 mg/wk, not to exceed 60 mg/day
- Available forms: Caps 3.75, 7.5, 15 mg; tabs 3.75, 7.5, 11.25, 15, 22.5 mg

Clozapine

CLOZARIL

(kloź-a-peen) (Chapter 4)

Functional classifications: Antipsychotic, neuroleptic, serotonin/dopamine antagonist

Chemical classification: Dibenzodiazepine

FDA pregnancy category: B

Indications: Management of schizophrenia refractory to other antipsychotics

Contraindications: History of clozapine-induced agranulocytosis; myeloproliferative disorders; concomitant use with other agents that can depress bone marrow function, severe CNS depression, coma, child <16 yr, lactation

Cautious use: Patients with hepatic, renal, or cardiac disease

Pharmacologic Effects: Interferes with binding of dopamine at D_1 and D_4 receptors and serotonin at $5HT_2$ receptors; preferentially more active at limbic than at striatal dopamine receptors, probably accounting for the relative lack of EPSEs. Weakly blocks D_2 receptors

Pharmacokinetics: Metabolized in liver, excreted in urine and feces, half-life 4-12 hr

Side Effects: Clozapine has relatively few EPSEs; *CNS:* Drowsiness (39%), dizziness or vertigo (19%), headache (7%), tremor (6%), syncope (6%), disturbed sleep or nightmares (4%), restlessness (4%), akinesia (4%), agitation (4%), dose-related seizures (3%), ridigity (3%), akathisia (3%), confusion (3%); *Peripheral:* Salivation (31%), sweating (6%), dry mouth (6%), visual disturbances (5%), tachycardia (25%), hypotension (9%), hypertension (4%), constipation (14%), nausea (5%), fever (5%), agranulocytosis (1%); fatalities have occurred often enough to necessitate a special monitoring system

Interactions
- Anticholinergics: Increased anticholinergic effect
- Antihypertensives: Increased hypotensive effect
- CNS depressants: Additive effect
- Agents that suppress bone marrow function: Agranulocytosis
- Protein binding drugs: Potentiation of clozapine or the other drug
- Antiepileptics: May diminish efficacy of clozapine
- Epinephrine: Severe hypotension

Implications

Assess
- Blood studies
- Concomitant illness
- Fever; flulike symptoms may indicate agranulocytosis

Planning/Implementation
- Monitor WBC and granulocyte count weekly
- Monitor ECG
- Monitor B/P (standing and sitting) for hypotension

Teaching
- Warn about risk of agranulocytosis and need for weekly blood tests
- Inform about significant risk of seizures
- To avoid driving or operating hazardous machinery
- Advise about risk of orthostatic hypotension
- Not to become pregnant
- Not to breast-feed

Evaluate
- Blood values
- Mental status
- Seizure activity

Treatment of Overdose: Symptoms of altered states of consciousness, i.e., drowsiness, delirium, coma, tachycardia, respiratory depression: Establish and maintain airway, ensure adequate ventilation and oxygenation; activated charcoal; supportive care. **Do not use epinephrine or its derivatives for hypotension**

Administration *Adult:* PO: 25 mg qd or bid, then increase by 25 to 50 mg/day; target dose is 300 to 450 mg/day by the end of 2 wk, if tolerated; some patients may require 600-900 mg/day

- Available forms: Tabs 25, 100 mg

Dantrolene Sodium

DANTRIUM, DANTRIUM IV
(dań-troe-leen) (Chapter 14)

Functional classification: Skeletal muscle relaxant, direct acting
Chemical classification: Hydantoin
FDA pregnancy category: C

Indications: Spasticity caused by upper motor neuron disorders, **malignant hyperthermia** and NMS

Contraindications: Hypersensitivity, active hepatic disease, impaired myocardial function, lactation, children < 5 yr
Cautious use: Peptic ulcer disease, renal or hepatic disease, stroke, seizure disorder, diabetes mellitus, impaired pulmonary function

Pharmacologic Effect: Produces skeletal muscle relaxation by affecting the muscle directly. Probably this effect is associated with interference with the release of calcium

Pharmacokinetics: PO: Peak 5 hr, half-life 8 hr, metabolized in liver, excreted in urine (metabolites)

Side Effects: *CNS:* **Dizziness, weakness, fatigue, drowsiness,** headache, disorientation, insomnia, paresthesias, tremors, decreased seizure threshold; *Peripheral:* Nasal congestion, blurred vision, mydriasis, eosinophilia, hypotension, chest pain, palpitations, **nausea,** constipation, vomiting, abdominal pain, dry mouth, anorexia, urinary frequency, rash, pruritus

Interactions

- Alcohol and CNS depressants: CNS depression
- Warfarin and clofibrate: Reduce plasma protein binding of dantrolene

Implications (for treatment of neuroleptic malignant syndrome)

Assess

- For increased seizure activity in patient with epilepsy
- Hepatic function by frequent determination of AST, ALT

Planning/Implementation

- With meals for GI symptoms
- Sugarless gum, frequent sips of water for dry mouth
- Assistance with ambulation when dizziness or drowsiness occurs

Teaching

- Not to discontinue medication quickly, because hallucinations, spasticity, tachycardia may occur; drug should be tapered off over 1-2 wk
- Not to take with alcohol or other CNS depressants
- To avoid altering activities while taking this drug
- To avoid hazardous activities when drowsiness or dizziness occurs
- To avoid using OTC medication such as cough preparations and antihistamines unless directed by physician

Evaluate

- Therapeutic response: For neuroleptic malignant syndrome, decreased fever, sweating, rigidity
- Allergic reactions: Rash, fever, respiratory distress
- Severe weakness, numbness in extremities
- CNS depression: Dizziness, drowsiness, psychiatric symptoms

Treatment of Overdose: Induce emesis in conscious patient, lavage, dialysis

Administration

- Spasticity: *Adult:* PO 25 mg/day; may increase by 25-100 mg bid-qid, not to exceed 400 mg/day; *child:* PO 0.5 mg/kg/day bid; may increase gradually, not to exceed 100 mg qid
- Malignant hyperthermia: *Adult and child:* IV 1 mg/kg, may repeat to total dose of 10 mg/kg; PO 4-8 mg/kg/day in 4 divided doses for 1-3 days to prevent further hyperthermia
- NMS: 1-3 mg/kg/day in 4 divided doses, up to 10mg/kg/day
- Available forms include: Caps 25, 50, 100 mg; powder for inj IV 20 mg/vial

Desipramine HCl

NORPRAMIN, PERTOFRANE
(dess-iṕ-ra-meen) (Chapter 5)

Functional classification: TCA
Chemical classifications: Dibenzazepine, secondary amine
FDA pregnancy category: C

Indications: Depression
Unlabeled use: Cocaine withdrawal

Contraindications: Hypersensitivity to TCAs, recovery phase of myocardial infarction, narrow-angle glaucoma
Cautious use: Convulsive disorders, prostatic hypertrophy, child < 12 yr; suicidal patients, severe depression, increased intraocular pressure, narrow-angle glaucoma, elderly patients, thyroid disease, MAOI therapy, ECT

Pharmacologic Effects: Blocks uptake of norepinephrine, serotonin in nerve cells; therapeutic plasma level 125-300 ng/mL

Pharmacokinetics: PO: Steady state 2-11 days; metabolized by liver, excreted by kidneys, crosses placenta, half-life 12-24 hr

Side Effects: *CNS:* **Sedation,** ataxia; confusion, delirium; *Peripheral:* **Blurred vision,** photophobia, increased intraocular pressure, decreased tearing, orthostatic hypotension, arrhythmias, tachycardia, palpitations, dry mouth, constipation, diarrhea, decreased sweating, **urinary retention, hesitancy**

Interactions
- Anticholinergic agents: Additive anticholinergic effects with atropine, antihistamines (H_1 blocker), antiparkinson drugs, antipsychotics, OTC cold and allergy drugs
- CNS depressants: Additive depressant effect
- Guanethidine, clonidine: Decreases antihypertensive effect
- MAOIs: Hypertensive crisis, atropine-like poisoning
- Oral contraceptives: Inhibit metabolism of TCAs
- Phenothiazines: May increase tricyclic serum level
- Quinidine: Additive effect, heart block possible
- Sympathomimetics: Potentiates sympathomimetic effects
- Thyroid preparations: Tachycardia, arrhythmias; may increase TCA effect

Implications
Assess
- Establish baseline data to aid recognition of adverse responses to medication, e.g., liver enzyme levels, VS, renal function, mental status, speech patterns, affect, weight
- For signs of noncompliance, e.g., poor therapeutic response
- Observe for major symptoms of depression: apathy, sadness, sleep disturbances, hopelessness, guilt, decreased libido, spontaneous crying
- Review history for contraindicated conditions, e.g., glaucoma, CV disease, GI conditions, urologic conditions, seizures, pregnancy

Planning/Implementation
- Monitor for "cheeking" or hoarding; check drug dosage carefully, because a small overdose may cause toxic effects
- Monitor for suicidal ideations; suicidal thought content may increase as antidepressants begin to "energize" patient
- Monitor VS, withhold TCAs when hypotension, tachycardia, or arrhythmias occur
- Give most TCAs in a single dose hs
- Observe for early signs of toxic effects, e.g., drowsiness, tachycardia, mydriasis, hypotension, agitation, vomiting, confusion, fever, restlessness, sweating
- Discontinue drug when CNS overstimulation occurs, e.g., hypomania, delirium

Teaching
- That these drugs have a lag time of up to 1 month
- To adhere to drug regimen
- To avoid OTC drugs, particularly those containing sympathomimetics or anticholinergics
- To avoid drugs listed in section on interactions
- About ways to deal with minor side effects, as follows: dry mouth, with sugarless hard candies, sips of water, mouth rinses; visual disturbances, with artificial tears, sunglasses, assistance with ambulation; constipation, with bulk-

forming foods, increased fluids; urinary hesitancy, with adequate fluids, privacy; decreased perspiration, with appropriate clothing, avoidance of unnecessary exercise; orthostatic hypotension, with slow positional changes, avoidance of hot baths and showers; for drowsiness, take single dose hs with physician approval, avoid driving
- That abrupt discontinuance may result in cholinergic rebound, e.g., nausea, vomiting, insomnia, headache

Evaluate
- Desired therapeutic serum level
- Verbalize decrease in subjective symptoms
- Observe decrease in objective symptoms
- Minimal to no adverse drug effects
- Stable VS
- Less anxiety: sleep, talk, and feel better

Lab Test Interferences
- Increase: Serum bilirubin, blood glucose, alkaline phosphatase levels
- False increase: Urinary catecholamines
- Decrease: VMA, 5-HIAA

Treatment of Overdose: Hospitalization, ECG monitoring, monitor cardiac function for at least 5 days, induce emesis, lavage, support airway

Administration

Adult: PO 100-200 mg/day in divided doses, may increase to 300 mg/day or may give daily dose; *adolescent/geriatric:* PO 25-100 mg/day, may increase to 150 mg/day
- Available forms include: Tabs 10, 25, 50, 75, 100, 150 mg; caps 25, 50 mg

Dextroamphetamine Sulfate

DEXEDRINE, FERNDEX, OXYDESS II, SPANCAP NO. 1
(dex-troe-am-fet́-a-meen)
(Chapters 12, 13, 15, 16)

Functional classification: Cerebral stimulant
Chemical classification: Amphetamine
Controlled substance schedule II
FDA pregnancy category: C

Indications: Narcolepsy, exogenous obesity, ADHD

Contraindications: Hypersensitivity to sympathomimetic amines, glaucoma, severe arteriosclerosis, drug abuse, CV disease, anxiety, hyperthyroidism, MAOI use
Cautious use: Tourette's syndrome, lactation, child <3 yr

Pharmacologic Effects: Increases release of norepinephrine, dopamine in cerebral cortex, brain stem, and reticular activating system; therapeutic plasma level 5-10 μg/dL

Pharmacokinetics: PO: Onset 30 min, peak 1-3 hr, duration 4-20 hr, metabolized by liver, excreted by kidneys, crosses placenta, enters breast milk, half-life 10-30 hr

Side Effects: *CNS:* **Hyperactivity, insomnia, restlessness, talkativeness,** dizziness, headache, chills, stimulation, dysphoria, irritability, aggressiveness; *Peripheral:* Nausea, vomiting, anorexia, dry mouth, diarrhea, constipation, weight loss, metallic taste, cramps, impotence, change in libido, **palpitations, tachycardia,** hypertension, hypotension

Interactions
- MAOIs or within 14 days of MAOIs: Hypertensive crisis
- Acetazolamide, antacids, sodium bicarbonate, ascorbic acid, ammonium chloride, phenothiazines, haloperidol: Increases half-life of amphetamine
- Barbiturates: Decreased effects of this drug
- Guanethidine, other antihypertensives: Decreased effects of these drugs

Implications

Assess

- VS, B/P because this drug may reverse antihypertensives; check patients with cardiac disease more often
- CBC, urinalysis; in diabetes, blood and urine sugar levels, insulin changes may be necessary because eating decreases
- **Height, growth rate in children (growth rate may be decreased)**

Planning/Implementation

- Give at least 6 hr before bedtime to avoid sleeplessness
- Give with meals to reduce appetite suppression
- For obesity, only when patient is on weight reduction program that includes dietary changes, exercise; patient tolerance develops, and weight loss will not occur without additional methods
- Gum, hard candies, frequent sips of water for dry mouth
- If drug is for obesity, 30-60 min before meals
- Dispense least amount feasible, to minimize risk of overdose

Teaching

- To decrease caffeine consumption (coffee, tea, cola, chocolate) that may increase irritability, stimulation
- Avoid OTC preparations unless approved by physician
- To taper off drug over several weeks, or depression, increased sleeping, lethargy may occur
- To avoid alcohol ingestion
- To avoid hazardous activities until condition is stabilized on medication
- To get needed rest; patients feel more tired at end of day
- Check to see that PO medication has been swallowed

Evaluate

- Mental status: mood, sensorium, affect, stimulation, insomnia; aggressiveness may occur
- Physical dependency; should not be used for extended time; dosage should be discontinued gradually
- **Withdrawal symptoms: headache, nausea, vomiting, muscle pain, weakness**
- Drug tolerance develops after long-term use
- If tolerance develops, dosage should not be increased

Treatment of Overdose: Administer fluids, hemodialysis or peritoneal dialysis; antihypertensive for increased B/P, ammonium chloride for increased excretion, chlorpromazine for CNS stimulation

Administration

- Narcolepsy: PO 5-60 mg qd in divided doses; *adult and adolescents >12 yr:* PO 10 mg qd, increasing by 10 mg/day at weekly intervals; *child 6-12 yr:* PO 5 mg qd, increasing by 5 mg/day at weekly intervals, up to 60 mg/day
- ADHD: *Child >6 yr:* PO 5 mg qd-bid, increasing by 5 mg/wk; *child 3-6 yr:* PO 2.5 mg qd, increasing by 2.5 mg/wk
- Obesity: *Adult:* PO 5-30 mg qd in divided doses 30-60 min before meals
- Available forms: Tabs 5, 10 mg; caps time-rel 5, 10, 15 mg; elix 5 mg/5 mL

Diazepam

D-TRAN,† E-PAM,† MEVAL,† NOVODIPAM,† STRESS-PAM,† VALIUM, VALRELEASE, VIVOL† (dye-aź-e-pam) (Chapters 6, 7, 9, 14)

Functional classification: Antianxiety
Chemical classification: Benzodiazepine
Controlled substance schedule IV
FDA pregnancy category: D

Indications: Anxiety, acute alcohol withdrawal, status epilepticus

Contraindications: Hypersensitivity to benzodiazepines, narrow-angle glaucoma, psychosis, child <6 mo (oral)
Cautious use: Elderly or debilitated patients, hepatic or renal disease

Pharmacologic Effects: Apparently potentiates effects of GABA and other inhibitory transmitters by binding to specific benzodiazepine receptor sites; depresses subcortical levels of CNS, including limbic system and reticular formation

Pharmacokinetics: Speed of onset: Very fast
PO: Onset ½ hr, duration 2-3 hr; IM: Onset 15-30 min, duration 1-1½ hr; IV: Onset 1-5 min, duration 15 min; metabolized by liver, excreted by kidneys, crosses

†Available in Canada only.

placenta, enters breast milk, half-life 20-80 hr

Side Effects: *CNS:* **Drowsiness, dizziness,** confusion, headache, anxiety, tremor, stimulation, fatigue, depression, insomnia; *Peripheral:* Photophobia caused by mydriasis, **blurred vision** caused by cycloplegia; sleeplike slowing of respirations with therapeutic doses, cough; **orthostatic hypotension, tachycardia,** hypotension; constipation, dry mouth

Interactions
- Alcohol and other CNS depressants: Increased risk of excessive CNS depression
- Cimetidine: Potentiation of CNS depression
- Digoxin: Increased risk of cardiac side effects from digoxin
- Levodopa: Decreased antiparkinson effect
- Phenytoin: Increased phenytoin serum levels
- Oral anticoagulants: Increases or decreases anticoagulant effect

Implications

Assess
- Patient's level of anxiety and method of coping
- B/P, VS
- Establish baseline physical assessment data before medications are started

Planning/Implementation
- Monitor patient's response to medication
- Observe elderly, very young, and debilitated patients for paradoxic excitement
- Reduce dose of other depressant drugs
- Observe for signs of withdrawal when discontinuing antianxiety agent

Teaching
- To avoid operating dangerous machinery and performing other tasks requiring good reflexes
- To report ocular pain at once, as well as other visual disturbances
- Drug may be taken with food

Evaluate
- Whether patient achieves lower levels of anxiety without undue sedation
- Whether patient can follow prescribed regimen
- For physical dependence: withdrawal symptoms of headache, nausea, vomiting, muscle pain, weakness after long-term use

Lab Test Interferences
Increase: AST/ALT, serum bilirubin levels
- False increase: 17-OHCS
- Decrease: RAIU

Treatment of Overdose: Lavage, VS, supportive care; there have been few deaths, if any, from benzodiazepine overdose alone; deaths occur when benzodiazepines are mixed with other drugs, especially alcohol

Administration
- Anxiety: *Adult:* PO 2-10 mg tid-qid or time-rel 15-30 mg qd; *child >6 mo:* PO 1-2.5 mg tid-qid
- Acute alcohol withdrawal: 10 mg tid-qid during first 24 hr; then reduce to 5 mg tid-qid PRN
- Status epilepticus: *Adult:* IV bolus 5-10 mg, 5 mg/min, may repeat q 10-15 min, not to exceed 30 mg, may repeat in 2-4 hr, if seizures reappear; *child > 5 yr:* IV bolus 0.1-0.3 mg/kg (1 mg/min q 2-5 min), up to a maximum of 10 mg; repeat in 2-4 hr if necessary; *child 30 days to 5 yr:* 0.2-0.5 mg slowly q 2-5 min, to a maximum of 5 mg
- Available forms include: Tabs 2, 5, 10 mg; caps time-rel 15 mg, IM/IV inj 5 mg/mL; oral solution 5 mg/5 mL, 5 mg/mL

Diphenhydramine

ALLERDRYL, BARAMINE, BAX, BENACHLOR, BENADRYL, BENAHIST, BENTRACT, COMPŌZ, DIPHENACEN, FENYLHIST, NORDRYL, ROHYORA, SPANLANIN, VAIDRENE, WEHDRYL
(dye-fen-hyé-dra-meen) (Chapter 14)

Functional classification: Antihistamine
Chemical classifications: H_1-receptor antagonist, ethanolamine
FDA pregnancy category: C

Indications: Parkinsonism, EPSEs, motion sickness, allergies and allergic reactions, sedation, other nonpsychiatric uses

Contraindications: Hypersensitivity, acute asthma attacks, lower respiratory tract disease

Pharmacologic Effects: Competes with histamine for H_1-receptor sites; blocks allergic responses by blocking histamine

Pharmacokinetics: Absorbed readily in GI tract; PO peaks in 1-3 hr; duration of action 4-7 hr; IM onset ½ hr, peak 1-4 hr, duration 4-7 hr; IV onset immediate, duration 4-7 hr; metabolized in liver, excreted in urine, crosses placenta, excreted in breast milk, half-life 2-7 hr

Side Effects: *CNS:* Drowsiness (usually transient), sedation, dizziness, disturbed coordination; *Less frequent:* Fatigue, confusion, restlessness, nervousness; *Peripheral:* Nausea and vomiting; dry mouth, blood dyscrasias, urinary retention, blurred vision, nasal stuffiness, dry throat and nose

Interactions

- CNS depressants: Increased depression
- Heparin: Decreased effect of heparin
- MAOIs: Increased anticholinergic effect

Implications

Assess

- For urinary retention
- Blood studies with long-term use

Planning/Implementation

- Give with meals to decrease GI upset
- Give IV at 25 mg/min
- Give IM in large muscle

Teaching

- Hard candies, gum for dry mouth
- To avoid driving
- To avoid CNS depressants, e.g., alcohol

Evaluate

- For EPSEs: Therapeutic responses
- For congestion: Ability to breathe
- Insomnia: Sleep
- For wheezing and chest tightness

Lab Test Interference
False negative: Skin allergy tests

Treatment of Overdose: Anticholinergic toxicity includes flushing, dry mouth, hyperthermia (up to 107° F), gastric lavage or induced emesis, diazepam, vasopressors, and short-acting barbiturates

Administration

- Parkinsonism and EPSEs: *PO adults:* 25-50 mg tid to qid daily; *PO children >20 lb:* 12.5 to 25 mg tid or qid daily or 5 mg/kg/day, not to exceed 300 mg/day; *IM or IV adult:* 10-50 mg, 100 mg if required, maximum daily dosage is 400 mg; *children:* 5 mg/kg/day divided into 4 doses, maximum daily dosage is 300 mg
- Available forms: Caps 25, 50 mg; tabs 25, 50 mg; elixir 12.5 mg/5 mL; syr 12.5 mg/5 mL; IM, IV 10, 50 mg/mL

Disulfiram

ANTABUSE
(dye-suĺ-fi-ram) (Chapter 10)

Functional classification: Alcohol deterrent
Chemical classification: Aldehyde dehydrogenase inhibitor
FDA pregnancy category: X

Indications: Treatment of chronic alcoholism

Contraindications: Hypersensitivity, patients who have received paraldehyde, alcohol intoxication, psychoses, CV disease

Cautious use: Hypothyroidism, hepatic disease, diabetes mellitus, seizure disorders, nephritis

Pharmacologic Effects: Blocks oxidation of alcohol at acetaldehyde stage by inhibiting aldehyde dehydrogenase

Pharmacokinetics: PO: Onset 12 hr, oxidized by liver, excreted in urine

Side Effects: *CNS:* **Headache, drowsiness,** restlessness, dizziness, fatigue, tremors, psychosis, neuritis, **sweating, convulsions, death;** *Peripheral:* Nausea, vomiting, anorexia, severe thirst, hepatoxicity; rash, dermatitis, urticaria; respiratory depression, hyperventilation; tachycardia, chest pain, hypotension, arrhythmia

Interactions

- Alcohol: Violent symptoms of sweating, throbbing headache, nausea and profuse vomiting, flushed face and neck, palpitations, tightness of chest, tremor, dyspnea
- TCAs, diazepam, hydantoins, oral anticoagulants, paraldehyde, phenytoin, chlordiazepoxide: Increased effects of these drugs
- Metronidazole, isoniazid: Psychosis

Implications

Assess

- Liver function studies q 2 wk during therapy; AST, ALT, CBC, SMA-12 q 3-6 mo to detect any abnormality

Planning/Implementation

- If drowsiness occurs, give once per day in morning or hs
- Give only after patient has not been drinking for >12 hr

Teaching

- Effect of this drug when alcohol is taken; written consent for disulfiram therapy should be obtained
- That shaving lotions, creams, cough preparations, skin products must be checked for alcohol content; even in small amount, alcohol can produce a reaction
- That tolerance does not develop when treatment is prolonged
- That reaction may occur for 14 days after last dose
- That tabs can be crushed, mixed with beverage
- To carry identification that lists disulfiram therapy and physician phone number
- To avoid driving or hazardous tasks when drowsiness occurs
- That disulfiram reaction can be fatal and occurs 15 min after drinking

Evaluate

- Mental status: Ability to abstain from alcohol

Treatment of Overdose: IV vitamin C, ephedrine sulfate, antihistamines, O_2

Administration

Adult: PO 250-500 mg qd for 1-2 wk, then 125-500 mg qd until desired response

- Available forms include: Tabs 250, 500 mg

Doxepin HCl

ADAPIN, SINEQUAN

(doẋ-e-pin) (Chapter 5)

Functional classification: TCA

Chemical classifications: Dibenzoxepin, tertiary amine

FDA pregnancy category: C

Indications: Depression, anxiety

Contraindications: Hypersensitivity to TCAs, urinary retention, narrow-angle glaucoma, prostatic hypertrophy

Cautious use: Suicidal or elderly patients, lactation, MAOI therapy, children < 12 yr

Pharmacologic Effects: Blocks reuptake of norepinephrine, serotonin into nerve endings, increasing action of norepinephrine, serotonin in nerve cells; also r/t changes in receptor sensitivity; therapeutic plasma levels 100-200 ng/mL

Pharmacokinetics: PO: Steady state 2-8 days; metabolized by liver, excreted in kidneys, crosses placenta, excreted in breast milk, half-life 8-24 hr

Side Effects: *CNS:* **Sedation,** ataxia; confusion, delirium; *Peripheral:* **Blurred vision,** photophobia, increased intraocular pressure, decreased tearing, orthostatic hypotension, arrhythmias, tachycardia, palpitations, dry mouth, constipation, diarrhea, decreased sweating, **urinary retention, hesitancy**

Interactions

- Anticholinergic agents: Additive anticholinergic effects with atropine, antihistamines (H_1 blocker), antiparkinson drugs, antipsychotics, OTC cold and allergy drugs
- CNS depressants: Additive depressant effect
- Guanethidine, clonidine: Decreased antihypertensive effect
- MAOIs: Hypertensive crisis, atropine-like poisoning
- Oral contraceptives: Inhibits metabolism of tricyclics
- Phenothiazines: May increase TCA serum level
- Quinidine: Additive effect, heart block possible
- Sympathomimetics: Potentiates sympathomimetic effects
- Thyroid preparations: Tachycardia, arrhythmias; may increase TCA effect

Implications

Assess

- Establish baseline data to aid recognition of adverse responses to medication, e.g., liver enzyme levels, VS, renal function, mental status, speech patterns, affect, weight
- For signs of noncompliance, e.g., poor therapeutic response
- For major symptoms of depression: Apathy, sadness, sleep disturbances, hopelessness, guilt, decreased libido, spontaneous crying
- History for contraindicated conditions, e.g., glaucoma, CV disease, GI conditions, urologic conditions, seizures, pregnancy

Planning/Implementation

- Monitor for "cheeking" or hoarding; check drug dosage carefully, because a small overdose may cause toxic effects
- Monitor for suicidal ideations; suicidal thought content may increase as antidepressants begin to "energize" patient
- Monitor VS; if hypotension, tachycardia, or arrhythmias occur, withhold TCAs
- Give most TCAs in a single dose hs
- Observe for early signs of toxic effects, e.g., drowsiness, tachycardia, mydriasis, hypotension, agitation, vomiting, confusion, fever, restlessness, sweating
- If CNS overstimulation occurs, e.g., hypomania, delirium, discontinue drug
- Dilute oral concentrate with 120 mL of water, milk, or fruit juice

Teaching

- That these drugs have a lag time of up to 1 month
- To adhere to drug regimen
- To avoid OTC drugs, particularly those containing sympathomimetics or anticholinergics
- To avoid drugs listed in section on interactions
- About ways to deal with minor side effects, as follows: dry mouth, with hard candies, sips of water, mouth rinses; visual disturbances, with artificial tears, sunglasses, assistance with ambulation; constipation, with bulk-forming foods, increased fluids; urinary hesitancy, with adequate fluids, privacy; decreased perspiration, with appropriate clothing, avoidance of unnecessary exercise; orthostatic hypotension, with slow positional changes, avoidance of hot baths and showers; for drowsiness, take single dose hs with physician approval, avoid driving
- That abrupt discontinuance may result in cholinergic rebound, e.g., nausea, vomiting, insomnia, headache

Evaluate

- Desired therapeutic serum level
- Verbalize decrease in subjective symptoms
- Observe decrease in objective symptoms
- Minimal to no adverse drug effects
- Stable VS
- Less anxiety; sleep, talk, and feel better

Lab Test Interferences

- Increase: Serum bilirubin, blood glucose, alkaline phosphatase levels
- False increase: Urinary catecholamines
- Decrease: VMA, 5-HIAA

Treatment of Overdose: ECG monitoring, induce emesis, lavage, activated charcoal, administer anticonvulsant

Administration

Adult: PO 10-25 mg tid to start, may increase to 300 mg/day or may give daily dose hs

- Available forms include: Caps 10, 25, 50, 75, 100, 150 mg; oral conc 10 mg/mL

Estazolam

PROSOM

(esś-ta-zoe-lam) (Chapter 8)

Functional classifications: Sedative, hypnotic
Chemical classification: Benzodiazepine
Controlled substance schedule IV
FDA pregnancy category: X

Indications: Insomnia

Contraindications: Hypersensitivity, sleep apnea

Pharmacologic Effects: Believed to potentiate GABA receptors, which are inhibitory, causing CNS depression; may affect BZ_1 (sleep) receptors

Pharmacokinetics: Peak levels 2 hr, half-life 10-24 hr, protein binding 93%, less than 5% excreted unchanged in urine, metabolized in liver

Side Effects: *CNS:* Somnolence (42%), asthenia (11%), hypokinesia (8%), hangover (3%), headache, nervousness, talkativeness, drowsiness, dizziness, confusion; see diazepam for other benzodiazepine side effects; *Peripheral:* Nausea and vomiting, other GI upsets, constipation, skin eruptions, blood dyscrasias

Interactions

- Cimetidine, disulfiram, isoniazid, probenecid: Estazolam effects increased
- CNS depressants and alcohol: Additive CNS depression
- Theophylline, rifampin: Decreased effect of estazolam

Implications

Assess

- B/P
- Blood studies, if indicated

Planning/Implementation

- Give ½-1 hr before bedtime
- Give with food for GI upset
- Maintain safety

Teaching

- To avoid driving
- To avoid alcohol

Evaluate

- Therapeutic response, sleeping
- Mental status

Lab Test Interference
Increase: AST, ALT

Treatment of Overdose: Deaths caused by benzodiazepine overdose alone have not been recorded; lavage, monitor VS, provide supportive care

Administration

- Insomnia: *Adult:* 1 mg hs, up to 2 mg; *elderly:* If healthy, 1 mg hs; if small or debilitated, 0.5 mg hs (effectiveness not clear)
- Available forms: Tabs 1, 2 mg

Ethchlorvynol*

PLACIDYL

(eth-klor-ví-nole) (Chapter 8)

Functional classifications: Sedative, hypnotic
Chemical classification: Tertiary acetylenic alcohol
Controlled substance schedule IV
FDA pregnancy category: C

Indications: Sedation, insomnia

Contraindications: Hypersensitivity, severe pain, porphyria, lactation
Cautious use: Pain

Pharmacologic Effects: Mechanism of action not known, produces CNS depression

Pharmacokinetics: Rapidly absorbed from GI tract; onset 15-30 min, peak level 2 hr, duration 5 hr, metabolized in liver, excreted in urine, half-life 10-20 hr for parent compound

Side Effects: *CNS:* Dizziness, facial numbness, giddiness; *Peripheral:* Nausea and vomiting; GI upset, blood dyscrasias, blurred vision, hypotension, rash

Interactions

- Alcohol and other CNS depressants: Additive depressive effect
- Oral anticoagulants: Decreased thrombin time
- TCAs: Transient delirium
- MAOIs: Increased CNS depression

*Infrequently used.

Implications
Assess
- Blood studies may be indicated

Planning/Implementation
- Give with food ½-1 hr before bedtime for sleeplessness, to decrease dizziness and giddiness; maintain safety, i.e., protect from falls, keep bed rails up, etc

Teaching
- To avoid driving
- To avoid alcohol and other CNS depressants

Evaluate
- Ability to sleep through night
- Mental status
- Decreased respiration (if below 10/min, withhold drug)

Lab Test Interference: Interferes with Clinitest

Treatment of Overdose: Overdose is characterized by deep coma, severe respiratory depression, hypothermia, hypotension, bradycardia; death has been reported at doses of 6 g but doses as high as 50 g have been survived; lavage or other approaches to gastric evacuation should be performed immediately; provide supportive care; forced diuresis with high urinary output is helpful

Administration
- Do not prescribe for more than 1 wk
- Sedation: *Adult:* PO 100-200 mg bid or tid
- Insomnia: *Adult:* PO 500-1000 mg ½ hr before bedtime, may repeat 200 mg, if original dose was 500-750 mg
- Available forms: Caps 200, 500, 750 mg

Ethopropazine HCl*

HCL PARSIDOL
(eth-oh-proé-pa-zeen) (Chapter 14)

Functional classification: Anticholinergic
Chemical classification: Phenothiazine
FDA pregnancy category: C

Indications: For parkinsonism and EPSEs but not frequently prescribed

Contraindications: See trihexyphenidyl

Pharmacologic Effects: See trihexyphenidyl

Pharmacokinetics: See trihexyphenidyl

Side Effects: *CNS:* See trihexyphenidyl; *Peripheral:* See trihexyphenidyl

Interactions: See trihexyphenidyl

Implications: See trihexyphenidyl

Lab Test Interference: See trihexyphenidyl

Treatment of Overdose: See trihexyphenidyl

Administration
- Parkinsonism and EPSEs: PO *adult:* Begin with 50 mg qd or bid, increase gradually, if necessary; *for mild to moderate symptoms:* 100 to 400 mg/day; *severe cases:* Gradually increase to 500 to 600 mg/day or more
- Available forms: Tabs 10, 50 mg

*Infrequently used.

Ethosuximide

ZARONTIN
(eth-oh-sux́-i-mide) (Chapter 7)

Functional classification: Antiepileptic
Chemical classification: Succinimide
FDA pregnancy category: C

Indications: Absence seizures (petit mal)

Contraindications: Hypersensitivity to succinimide derivatives
Cautious use: Lactation, hepatic or renal disease

Pharmacologic Effect: Inhibits spike and wave formation in absence seizures; therapeutic serum level 40-100 μg/mL

Pharmacokinetics: PO peak 3-7 hr; steady state 5-10 days; metabolized by liver; excreted in urine, bile, feces; half-life 40-60 hr (adult), 30 hr (child)

Side Effects: *CNS:* **Drowsiness, dizziness, fatigue, euphoria, lethargy;** anxiety, aggressiveness, irritability, depression, insomnia; *Peripheral:* **Nausea, vomiting, heartburn, anorexia, diarrhea, abdominal pain, cramps, constipation,** vaginal bleeding, hematuria, renal damage, urticaria, pruritic erythema, hirsutism, Stevens-Johnson syndrome, myopia, gum hypertrophy, tongue swelling, blurred vision, agranulocytosis, aplastic anemia, thrombocytopenia, leukocytosis, eosinophilia, pancytopenia (some blood dyscrasias have been fatal)

Interactions
- TCAs: Antagonist effect (imipramine, doxepin); also, lower seizure threshold
- Estrogens: Decreased effects of oral contraceptives

Implications
Assess
- Mental status: mood, sensorium, affect
- CNS depressants: Increased CNS depression

Implications
Assess
- Renal studies: Urinalysis, BUN, and urine creatinine levels
- Blood studies: CBC, hematocrit, hemoglobin level
- Hepatic studies: AST, ALT, bilirubin and creatinine levels
- Drug levels during initial treatment, therapeutic range (40-100 μg/mL)

Planning/Implementation
- Take with milk or food to decrease GI symptoms
- Assistance with ambulation during early part of treatment; dizziness occurs

Teaching
- To carry identification card or MedicAlert bracelet stating drugs taken, condition, physician's name and phone number
- To avoid driving, other activities that require alertness
- To avoid alcohol ingestion, CNS depressants; increased sedation may occur
- Not to discontinue medication quickly after long-term use

Evaluate
- Therapeutic response: decreased seizure activity, document on patient's chart
- Mental status
- Allergic reaction: red raised rash, exfoliative dermatitis; if these occur, drug should be discontinued
- Blood dyscrasias: fever, sore throat, bruising, rash, jaundice
- Toxic effects: Bone marrow depression, lupus have been reported

Lab Test Interferences
- Increase: Coomb's test

Treatment of Overdose: Lavage, activated charcoal, monitor electrolyte levels, VS

Administration
Adult and child >6 yr: PO 500 mg/day or 250 mg bid initially; may increase by 250 mg q 4-7 days, not to exceed 1.5 g/day; *child 3-6 yr:* PO 250 mg/day or 125 mg bid; may increase by 250 mg q 4-7 days, no one should exceed 1.5 g/day; optimal dose 20 mg/kg/day
- Available forms include: Caps 250 mg, syr 250 mg/5 mL

Ethotoin*

PEGANONE
(eth́-oh-toyin) (Chapter 7)

Functional classification: Antiepileptic
Chemical classification: Hydantoin derivative
FDA pregnancy category: D

Indications: Generalized tonic-clonic or psychomotor seizures

Contraindications: Hypersensitivity to hydantoins, blood dyscrasias, **hematologic disease, hepatic disease,** lactation
Cautious use: Renal disorders

Pharmacologic Effect: Inhibits spread of seizure activity in motor cortex; therapeutic plasma level 15-50 μg/mL

Pharmacokinetics: Metabolized by liver, excreted in urine, half-life 3-9 hr

Side Effects: *CNS:* Drowsiness, dizziness, insomnia, paresthesias, depression, suicidal tendencies, aggression, headache; *Peripheral:* **Nausea, vomiting, constipation,** anorexia, weight loss, hepatitis, jaundice, nephritis, albuminuria, rash, agranulocytosis, leukopenia, aplastic anemia

Interactions
- Allopurinol, cimetidine, diazepam, disulfiram, alcohol (acute ingestion), phenacemide, succinimides, valproic acid: Increased effect of hydantoins
- Barbiturates, carbamazepine, alcohol (chronic use) theophylline, antacids, dietary calcium: Decreased effects of hydantoins
- Corticosteroids, dicumarol, digitoxin, doxycycline, haloperidol, methadone, oral contraceptives, dopamine, furosemide, levodopa: Decreased effects of these drugs
- Phenacemide: Causes paranoid syndrome

Implications
Assess
- Blood studies: CBC, platelets q mo until stabilized, discontinue if marked depression of blood cell count occurs

*Infrequently used.

Planning/Implementation
- Describe seizures accurately

Teaching
- All aspects of drug administration, i.e., route, action, dose
- To report side effects
- To avoid driving or operating dangerous equipment
- To practice good oral hygiene
- Not to discontinue abruptly
- To wear MedicAlert identification bracelet

Evaluate
- Mental status: Mood, sensorium, affect, memory (long-term, short-term)
- Respiratory depression
- Blood dyscrasias: Fever, sore throat, bruising, rash, jaundice

Treatment of Overdose: Mean lethal dose in adults is thought to be 2-5 g; initial symptoms are nystagmus, ataxia; death is due to respiratory and circulatory depression; lavage, emesis, activated charcoal

Administration
Adult: PO 250 mg qid (1000 mg/day) or less initially, may increase over several days to 3 g/day in divided doses; *child:* PO 250 mg tid, may increase to 250 mg qid (1000 mg/day)
- Available forms: Tabs 250, 500 mg

Flumazenil

ROMAZICON
(floo-maź-eh-nill) (Chapter 6)

Functional classifications: Benzodiazepine receptor antagonist, antidote
Chemical classification: Imidazobenzodiazepine derivative
FDA pregnancy category: C

Indications: Complete or partial reversal of the sedative effects of benzodiazepines in cases where general anesthesia has been induced or maintained with benzodiazepines. Management of benzodiazepine overdose

Contraindications: Hypersensitivity to flumazenil or to benzodiazepines; in patients administered benzodiazepines for potentially life-threatening disorders; patients showing signs of serious cyclic antidepressant overdose

Cautious use: History of seizure; hepatic dysfunction; lactation

Pharmacologic Effects: Antagonizes the actions of benzodiazepines on the CNS and inhibits activity of GABA/benzodiazepine receptor sites

Pharmacokinetics: Initial distribution half-life 7-15 min, then a terminal half-life of 41-79 min; protein binding 50%; elimination is through the renal system and is essentially complete within 72 hr

Side Effects: *CNS:* Dizziness (10%), agitation, emotional lability, confusion; *Peripheral:* Nausea, vomiting (11%), headache, blurred vision, parasthesia

Interactions
- CNS depressants: theoretically possible interaction
- Benzodiazepines: pharmacokinetics unaltered in presence of flumazenil
- Food: increases clearance of flumazenil

Implications
Assess
- Hypersensitivity to flumazenil or benzodiazepines

Planning/Implementation
- Administer by IV only
- Ensure that emergency equipment is available
- Secure airway during administration
- Monitor clinical response to drug
- Inject into running IV

Teaching
- Explain flumazepine does not consistently reverse amnesia
- Explain that although patient feels alert at time of discharge, the effects of benzodiazepines may recur
- Avoid activities requiring alertness
- Refuse alcohol and do not take nonprescription drugs for 18 to 24 hr after flumazenil given

Evaluate
- Hepatic status
- Emergence of withdrawal symptoms

Lab Test Interferences
- None reported

Treatment of Overdose: No serious adverse reactions or clinically significant test abnormalities have been reported. Most adverse responses are extensions of pharmacologic effects of the drug because it reverses a benzodiazepine

Administration
- Benzodiazepine overdose: *Adult:* IV: Initially 0.2 mg (2 mL) over 30 seconds. If desired level of consciousness is not obtained, wait 30 seconds and give 0.3 (3 mL) over 30 seconds. Further doses of 0.5 mg (5 mL) can be administered over 30 seconds at 1-min intervals up to a total cumulative dose of 3 mg

  IV compatibility: Flumazenil is compatible with 5% dextrose in water, lactated Ringer's solution, and normal saline solutions. Discard after 24 hours. Do not remove from vial until ready for use
- Available forms: Inj 0.1 mg/mL in 5- and 10-mL vials

Fluoxetine

PROZAC
(floo-óx-e-teen) (Chapter 5)

Functional classification: Selective serotonin reuptake inhibitor, antidepressant
FDA pregnancy category: B

Indications: Depression

Contraindications: Hypersensitivity; use with MAO inhibitors because of the possibility of causing the sometimes fatal serotonin syndrome
Cautious use: Anxiety, insomnia, lactation, children, elderly patients, MAOI therapy

Pharmacologic Effects: Inhibits CNS neuron uptake of serotonin but only slightly inhibits that of norepinephrine

Pharmacokinetics: PO: Peak 6-8 hr; metabolized in liver, excreted in urine; half-life 48-216 hr (including metabolite)

Side Effects: *CNS:* Anxiety (9.4%), nervousness (14.9%), insomnia (13.8%), drowsiness, headache (20.3%), tremor, dizziness, fatigue; *Peripheral:* Nausea (21.1%), diarrhea (12.3%), dry mouth (9.5%), anorexia (8.7%), dyspepsia, constipation, cramps, vomiting, taste changes, flatulence, sweating (8.4%), rash, pruritus, acne, alopecia, urticaria, infection (7.6%), nasal congestion, hot flashes (1.8%), palpitations, dysmenorrhea (2%), decreased libido, urinary frequency, urinary tract infection, visual changes (2.8%), ear or eye pain, photophobia, tinnitus, asthenia (4.4%), viral infection (3.4%)

Interactions

- Do not use with MAOIs; may precipitate a serotonin syndrome
- L-tryptophan: agitation
- Highly protein bound drugs, i.e., digitoxin: Increased side effects
- Diazepam: Half-life of diazepam increases
- TCAs: Toxic effects of tricyclics increased, suicidal tendencies, increase in psychiatric symptoms, depression, panic
- B/P (lying, standing), pulse q4h; if systolic B/P drops 20 mm Hg, withhold drug, notify physician; VS q4h in patients with CV disease
- Blood studies: CBC, leukocyte count, differential blood cell count; cardiac enzyme level when patient is receiving long-term therapy
- Hepatic studies: AST, ALT, bilirubin and creatinine levels
- Weigh q wk, appetite may increase
- ECG for flattening of T wave, bundle branch or AV block, arrhythmias in cardiac disease

Planning/Implementation

- If constipation, urinary retention occur, increase fluids, bulk in diet
- **Do not give with MAO inhibitors. If switching from MAOI to fluoxetine, wait at least 14 days. If switching from fluoxetine to an MAOI, wait at least 6 weeks**
- With food or milk for GI symptoms
- Empty pulvule if patient is unable to swallow medication whole
- Give dose at hs if oversedation occurs during day; may take entire dose hs; elderly patients may not tolerate once-per-day dosage
- Sugarless gum, hard candy, frequent sips of water for dry mouth
- Store at room temperature, do not freeze
- Assistance with ambulation during therapy because drowsiness, dizziness occur
- Safety measures, including side rails, primarily with elderly patients
- Check to see that PO medication is swallowed

Teaching

- That therapeutic effect may take several days to weeks
- Use caution when driving or performing other activities requiring alertness because of drowsiness, dizziness, or blurred vision
- Not to discontinue medication suddenly after long-term use, because abrupt discontinuance may cause nausea, headache, malaise
- To avoid ingesting alcohol or other CNS depressants
- To notify physician when pregnant or when planning to become pregnant or to breast-feed

Evaluate

- EPSEs, primarily in elderly; rigidity, dystonia, akathisia
- Urinary retention, constipation
- Withdrawal symptoms: Headache, nausea, vomiting, muscle pain, weakness; do not usually occur unless drug is discontinued abruptly
- Alcohol consumption: If alcohol is consumed, withhold dose until morning

Lab Test Interferences

- Increase: Serum bilirubin, blood glucose, alkaline phosphatase levels
- Decrease: VMA, 5-HIAA
- False increase: Urinary catecholamines

Treatment of Overdose: There are no antidotes; establish and maintain airway; ensure adequate oxygenation and ventilation; activated charcoal may be more effective than emesis or lavage

Administration

Adult: PO 20 mg qd in morning; after several weeks, if no clinical improvement is noted, dose may be increased to 20 mg bid in morning, noon, not to exceed 80 mg/day

- Available forms include: Pulvules 20 mg

F

Fluphenazine Decanoate, Fluphenazine Enanthate, Fluphenazine HCl

MODECATE DECANOATE,† PROLIXIN DECANOATE/MODITEN ENANTHATE,† PROXLIN ENANTHATE/MODITEN HCL,† PERMITIL HCL, PROLIXIN HCL†
(floo-feń-a-zeen) (Chapter 4)

Functional classifications: Antipsychotic, neuroleptic
Chemical classifications: Phenothiazine, piperazine
FDA pregnancy category: C

Indications: Psychotic disorders, schizophrenia

Contraindications: Hypersensitivity to sesame seeds or fluphenazine, liver damage, CV disease, severe hypertension or hypotension, blood dyscrasias, coma, child <12 yr, brain damage, bone marrow depression, alcohol and barbiturate withdrawal states
Cautious use: Lactation, seizure disorders, hypertension, hepatic disease, cardiac disease, extreme heat

Pharmacologic Effects: Antipsychotic drugs produce a neuroleptic effect characterized by sedation, emotional quieting, psychomotor slowing, and affective indifference; exact mode of action is not fully understood; antipsychotics primarily block dopamine D_2 receptors in the basal ganglia, hypothalamus, limbic system, brain stem, and medulla; antipsychotics are also thought to depress certain components of the reticular activating system that partially control body temperature, wakefulness, vasomotor tone, emesis, and hormonal balance; additionally, antipsychotics have significant anticholinergic and alpha-adrenergic blocking effects; therapeutic plasma levels 0.13-2.8 ng/mL

†Available in Canada only.

Pharmacokinetics: PO/IM (HCl): Onset 1 hr, peak 2-4 hr, duration 6-8 hr; Decanoate: onset 1-3 days, peak 1-2 days, duration over 4 wk, half-life (single dose) 6.8-9.6 days, (multiple dose) 14.3 days; metabolized by liver, excreted in urine (metabolites), crosses placenta, enters breast milk

Side Effects: *CNS:* Parkinsonism, akathisias, dystonias, tardive dyskinesis, oculogyric crisis; neuroleptic malignant syndrome; *Peripheral:* Blurred vision (cycloplegia or paralysis of accommodation); ocular pain, photophobia, mydriasis, impaired vision; intolerance of extreme heat or cold, possible heat stroke or fatal hyperthermia; nasal congestion, wheezing, dyspnea; **hypotension, especially orthostatic,** leading to dizziness, syncope; **tachycardia,** irregular pulse, arrhythmias; **dry mouth, constipation,** jaundice, abdominal pain; urinary retention, urinary hesitancy, galactorrhea, gynecomastia, impaired ejaculation, amenorrhea

Interactions

- Alcohol and other CNS depressants (barbiturates, antihistamines, antianxiety, or antidepressant drugs): Increased CNS depression, increased risk of EPSEs
- Amphetamines: Possible decreased antipsychotic effect
- Antacids (magnesium and aluminum products): Possible decreased antipsychotic effect
- Anticholinergics (atropine, H_1-type antihistamines, antidepressants, etc): Increased risk of excessive atropine-like side effects or toxic effects
- Anticonvulsants: Increased risk of seizures
- Benztropine: Possible decreased antipsychotic effect, increased risk of severity of peripheral anticholinergic side effects
- Diazoxide: Possible severe hyperglycemia, prediabetic coma
- Guanethidine: Poor control of hypertension by guanethidine
- Hypoglycemia drugs (insulin, oral hypoglycemia agents): Poor diabetic control
- Lithium: Poor control of psychosis with combined therapy, encephalopathy
- Meperidine, morphine: Increased risk

of severe CNS depression, respiratory depression, hypotension

- Propranolol: Increased pharmacologic effects of either drug

Implications

Assess

- Establish baseline VS, laboratory values, to assess side effects, allergic or hypersensitivity reactions
- Use test dose SC to check for hypersensitivity
- Physiologic and psychologic status before therapy, to determine needs and evaluate progress
- For early stages of tardive dyskinesia by use of Abnormal Involuntary Movement Scale
- Identify concurrent symptoms that may be aggravated by antipsychotics, e.g., glaucoma, diabetes

Planning/Implementation

- Ensure that drug has been taken; check mouth for "cheeking"
- If giving liquid, use water, clear soda, milk, fruit juice; *do not* mix with caffeine, tannics (tea), or pectinates (apple juice); take drug with food to minimize GI upset; give IM injections in lateral thigh
- Keep patient quiet after injection to prevent falls associated with postural hypotension
- For dry mouth, give chewing gum, hard candies, lip balm
- Monitor urinary output; check for bladder distention in inactive patients, older men, and patients on high doses
- Assist with ambulation, if patient is having blurred vision; dim room lights for photosensitivity
- Ensure safety with hypotension; sit on side of bed before rising, head-low position for dizziness, avoid hot showers, wear elastic stockings
- Check B/P (supine, sitting, standing) and pulse before and after each dose when possible; observe for side effects
- Monitor body temperature for indications of neuroleptic malignant syndrome, e.g., muscle rigidity, fever, depressed neurologic status; ensure adequate hydration, nutrition, and ventilation
- Protect patient from exposure to extreme heat or cold
- Recognize impending hypersensitivity: pruritus or jaundice with hepatitis; flu or coldlike symptoms, evidence of bleeding with blood dyscrasia
- Observe for involuntary movements

Teaching

- About benefits and potential harm of antipsychotic drugs; weigh need to know against causing apprehension
- To comply with drug treatment
- To avoid activities requiring clear vision for a few weeks after treatment starts; to report eye pain immediately
- About the importance of exercise, fluids, and fiber in diet
- To watch for symptoms of heart failure: weight gain, dyspnea, distended neck veins, tachycardia
- Possible male sexual performance failure; suggest relaxed, stress-free environment
- To avoid conception; women should practice effective contraception; phenothiazines may cause false-positive result in pregnancy tests
- To avoid exposure to sunlight; keep skin covered but with temperature-appropriate clothing
- That patient cannot become addicted to antipsychotic drugs

Evaluate

- Whether patient follows prescribed regimen, takes medications as ordered
- Avoids injury; reports dizziness or need for assistance
- Verbalizes reduced anxiety
- Experiences minimal or no adverse responses
- Uses appropriate interventions to minimize side effects
- Achieves improved mental status

Lab Test Interferences

- Increase: Liver function tests, determinations of cardiac enzymes, cholesterol, blood glucose, prolactin, bilirubin, PBI, cholinesterase, I-131
- Decrease: Hormones (blood and urine)
- False positive: Pregnancy test, PKU
- False negative: Urinary steroids, 17-OHCS

Treatment of Overdose: Lavage; if orally ingested, provide an airway, do not induce vomiting, control EPSEs and hypotension

Administration

- Decanoate: *Adult and child >12 yr:* IM or SC 12.5-25 mg q 1-3 wk HCl; *adult:*

PO 0.5-10 mg in divided doses q6-8h, typically not to exceed 20 mg qd; *geriatrics:* Start with 1-2.5 mg/day, adjust according to response; IM initially 1.25 mg, then 2.5-10 mg in divided doses q6-8h

- Concentrate *should not* be mixed with caffeine, tannics, or pectinates
- Available forms include: HCl tabs 1, 2.5, 5, 10 mg; elixir 2.5 mg/5 mL; concentrate 5 mg/mL; inj IM, 2.5 mg/mL; decanoate, inj SC, IM 25 mg/mL

Flurazepam

DALMANE, SOMNOL†
(flure-aź-e-pam) (Chapter 8)

Functional classifications: Sedative, hypnotic
Chemical classification: Benzodiazepine derivative
Controlled substance schedule IV
FDA pregnancy category: NR

Indications: Insomnia

Contraindications: Hypersensitivity to benzodiazepines, pregnancy, lactation, intermittent porphyria
Cautious use: Anemia, hepatic or renal disease, suicidal patients, drug abuse, elderly patients, child $<$15 yr, psychosis

Pharmacologic Effects: Produces CNS depression

Pharmacokinetics: PO onset 0.5-1 hr, duration 7-8 hr; active metabolite peak plasma level 1-3 hr; metabolized by liver, excreted by kidneys, crosses placenta, excreted in breast milk; half-life 47-100 hr

Side Effects: *CNS:* Lethargy, drowsiness, daytime sedation, dizziness, confusion, light-headedness, headache, anxiety, irritability; *Peripheral:* Nausea, vomiting, diarrhea, heartburn, abdominal pain, constipation, chest pain, pulse changes, palpitations

Interactions
- Cimetidine, disulfiram: Prolong half-life of flurazepam
- Alcohol, CNS depressants: CNS depression
- Antacids: Decrease effects of flurazepam

†Available in Canada only.

Implications
Assess
- Blood studies: Hematocrit, hemoglobin level, RBCs (if on long-term therapy regimen)
- Suicide potential: Use with caution in suicidal patients

Planning/Implementation
- ½-1 hr before bedtime for sleeplessness
- Fast onset on empty stomach, but if GI symptoms occur, may be taken with food
- Assistance with ambulation after receiving dose
- Safety measure: side rails, night light, call bell within easy reach
- Checking to see that PO medication has been swallowed

Teaching
- To avoid driving or other activities requiring alertness until drug regimen is stabilized
- To avoid alcohol ingestion or CNS depressants because serious CNS depression may result
- That may take 2 nights for clinical effect
- Alternate measures to improve sleep: reading, exercise several hours before bedtime, warm bath, warm milk, television, self-hypnosis, deep breathing
- That hangover is common in elderly patients but less common than with barbiturates

Evaluate
- Therapeutic response: Ability to sleep at night, decreased amount of early-morning awakening when taking drug for insomnia
- Mental status: Mood, sensorium, affect, memory (long-term, short-term)
- Blood dyscrasias (rare): Fever, sore throat, bruising, rash, jaundice, epistaxis
- Type of sleep problem: Falling asleep, staying asleep

Lab Test Interferences
- Increase: ALT/AST, serum bilirubin level
- Decrease: RAIU
- False increase: Urinary 17-OHCS

Treatment of Overdose: Lavage, activated charcoal, monitor electrolyte levels, VS

Administration

Adult: PO 15-30 mg hs, may repeat dose once, if needed; *geriatric:* PO 15 mg hs, may increase, if needed

- Available forms include: Caps 15, 30 mg

Fluvoxamine maleate

LUVOX

(floo-vox́-a-meen) (Chapter 5)

Functional classification: Antidepressant
Chemical classification: Selective serotonin reuptake inhibitor
FDA pregnancy category: C

Indications: Obsessive-compulsive disorder

Contraindications: Co-administration with terfenadine or astemizole; history of hypersensitivity to fluvoxamine

Cautious use: Mania, hypomania, history of seizures, pregnancy, lactation

Pharmacologic Effect: Inhibits CNS neuronal uptake of serotonin

Pharmacokinetics: Peak levels 3 to 8 hr; half-life 15-19 hr; extensive metabolism; excreted in urine; protein binding 80%

Side Effects: *CNS:* Somnolence (22%), headache (22%), insomnia (21%), nervousness (12%), dizziness (11%); *Peripheral:* Nausea (40%), asthenia (14%), dry mouth (14%), diarrhea (11%), constipation (10%), dyspepsia (10%)

Interactions:

- MAO inhibitors, tryptophan: Possible enhancement of serotonin effect (serotonin syndrome) leading to fatal outcomes
- Terfenadine, astemizole: Fatal reactions may occur
- Theophylline: Theophylline clearance decreased significantly
- Increased effects of triazolam, alprazolam, warfarin, carbamazepine, methadone, clozapine, TCAs, beta blockers, diltiazem
- Smoking: a 25% increase in fluvoxamine metabolism occurs
- Haloperidol: Haloperidol serum levels may double; negative and positive symptoms may increase

Implications

Assess

- For history of hypersensitivity to fluvoxamine; impaired hepatic or renal function; suicidal tendencies
- B/P, VS
- Urinary output, CBC
- Activation of mania

Planning/Implementation

- Maintain safety
- Closely supervise patients at high risk for suicide because there may be a relationship between suicide and alterations in serotonin levels

Teaching

- Caution about driving (though problems in this area are not established)
- To avoid alcohol
- Caution about the use of OTC products
- If dose more than 100 mg/day, divide in 2 and give larger dose at bedtime

Evaluate

- Evaluate for therapeutic effect, e.g., improvement of OCD
- Mental status
- Take drug at bedtime
- Report rash, mania, seizures

Lab Test Interference: None known

Treatment of Overdose: Some fatalities have occurred in conjunction with fluvoxamine overdose. Treatment includes: airway maintenance; close observation, including VS and ECG; activated charcoal or emesis; be aware of possibility of multiple drug overdose. No known antidote for fluvoxamine

Administration

Adult: PO 50 mg at bedtime to start. Increase by 50 mg/day every 4 to 7 days until therapeutic response acheived. Therapeutic dose typically 100 to 300 mg/day. Maximum dose 300 mg/day. If dose more than 100 mg/day, divide in 2 and give larger dose at bedtime; *elderly and hepatically impaired:* Give reduced dose and titrate more slowly; *children and adolescents:* Not approved for children $<$ 18 yr

- Available forms: Tabs 50, 100 mg

F

Gabapentin

NEURONTIN

(gab-ah-peń-tin) (Chapter 7)

Functional classification: Antiepileptic
Chemical classification: Structurally related to GABA
FDA pregnancy category: C

Indications: Adjunctive therapy in the treatment of partial seizures with and without secondary generalization in adults with epilepsy

Contraindications: Hypersensitivity to gabapentin, lactation

Pharmacologic Effects: Therapeutic actions are not understood

Pharmacokinetics: Absorption is dose-dependent, and food does not alter absorption. Half-life 5-8 hr; protein binding <3%. Gabapentin is not metabolized and is excreted unchanged in the urine

Side Effects: *CNS:* Somnolence (19%), dizziness (17%), ataxia (12%); *Peripheral:* Fatigue (11%)

Interactions
- Gabapentin does not interact with other antiepileptics
- Antacids: Reduce bioavailability of gabapentin by 20%
- Cimetidine: Increases bioavailability of gabapentin
- Oral contraceptives: Increased serum levels of oral contraceptives

Implications

Assess
- History of hypersensitivity to gabapentin
- Baseline physical data

Planning/Implementation
- Give with food to prevent GI distress

Teaching
- Take gabapentin as prescribed
- Advise that gabapentin may cause dizziness and/or somnolence so care should be taken with hazardous machinery
- To not discontinue gabapentin abruptly because of the possibility of withdrawal-precipitated seizures
- Wear MedicAlert bracelet to alert others to seizure disorder

Evaluate
- Absence of epilepsy
- Minimal side effects

Lab Test Interference: Urinary protein should be checked by the sulfosalicylic acid precipitation procedure

Treatment of Overdose: No reported fatalities have occurred with gabapentin to date (1995). Although not necessary to this point, hemodialysis will remove gabapentin from the system

Administration

Adults and children >12 yr: PO 300 mg on day 1, 300 mg twice a day on day 2, and 300 mg 3 times a day on day 3. The dose on day 1 should be given at bedtime to reduce somnolence or daytime dizziness. Dosage can be increased up to 1800 mg/day. Dosage spacing should not exceed 12 hours between doses
- Available forms: Caps 100, 300, 400 mg

Glutethimide*

DORIDEN

(gloo-teth́-i-mide) (Chapter 8)

Functional classifications: Sedative, hypnotic
Chemical classification: Piperidine derivative
Controlled substance schedule III
FDA pregnancy category: C

Indications: Insomnia

Contraindications: Hypersensitivity, porphyria

Pharmacologic Effects: Produces CNS depression

Pharmacokinetics: Is erratically absorbed from GI tract; average half-life 10-12 hr; 50% bound to plasma proteins; conjugant excreted in urine

Side Effects: *CNS:* Hangover (1.1%), drowsiness (1%); *Peripheral:* Skin rash (8.6%), nausea (2.7%), blood dyscrasias are rare

*Infrequently used.

Interactions
- Alcohol and CNS depressants: Additive depressant effect
- Oral anticoagulants: Decreased effect of anticoagulant

Implications
Assess
- Blood studies for rare individual with blood dyscrasias

Planning/Implementation
- Give ½-1 hr before bedtime
- Maintain safety

Teaching
- To avoid driving
- To avoid alcohol and other CNS depressants
- To taper drug discontinuance, to avoid withdrawal syndrome

Evaluate
- Ability to sleep through night
- Mental status
- Blood dyscrasias (rare)

Lab Test Interference: Interferes with 17-OHCS

Treatment of Overdose: Lethal dose ranges from 10 to 20 g; a low dose of 5 g has killed a patient and a high dose of 35 g has been survived; symptoms same as barbiturate intoxication; maintain airway, monitor VS, gastric lavage (induce emesis only in alert patient); lavage in all cases, regardless of elapsed time, with a 1:1 mixture of castor oil and water; charcoal delays absorption

Administration
- Insomnia: *Adult* PO 250-500 mg hs, may repeat dose if more than 4 hr before usual awakening; *do not* exceed 1 g
- Available forms: Tablets 250, 500 mg, caps 500 mg

Halazepam

PAXIPAM
(hal-aź-e-pam) (Chapter 6)

Functional classification: Antianxiety
Chemical classification: Benzodiazepine
Controlled substance schedule IV
FDA pregnancy category: D

Indications: Anxiety

Contraindications: Hypersensitivity, psychosis, narrow-angle glaucoma, child <18 yr

Pharmacologic Effects: Depresses CNS, i.e., limbic and reticular formation

Pharmacokinetics: Speed of onset: Intermediate to slow; PO peak level 1-3 hr, duration 3-6 hr, metabolized by liver, excreted by kidneys, crosses placenta and breast milk, half-life 14 hr

Side Effects: *CNS:* See diazepam; *Peripheral:* See diazepam

Interactions: See diazepam

Implications: See diazepam

Lab Test Interference: See diazepam

Treatment of Overdose: See diazepam

Administration
Adult: PO 60-160 mg/day in divided doses; *geriatric:* PO 20 mg qd to bid
- Available forms: Tabs 20, 40 mg

Haloperidol, Haloperidol Decanoate

HALDOL, HALDOL DECANOATE
(ha-loe-peŕ-i-dole) (Chapter 4)

Functional classifications: Antipsychotic, neuroleptic
Chemical classification: Butyrophenone
FDA pregnancy category: C

Indications: Psychotic disorders, control of tics and vocal utterances in Tourette's syndrome, short-term treatment of hyperactive children with excessive motor activity, severe behavioral problems in children

Contraindications: Hypersensitivity, blood dyscrasias, coma, child <3 yr, brain damage, bone marrow depression, alcohol and barbiturate withdrawal states, parkinsonism

Cautious use: Lactation, seizure disorders, hypertension, hepatic disease, cardiac disease, breast cancer

Pharmacologic Effects: Antipsychotic drugs produce a neuroleptic effect characterized by sedation, emotional quieting, psychomotor slowing, and affective indifference; exact mode of action is not fully understood; antipsychotics primarily block dopamine D_2 receptors in the basal ganglia, hypothalamus, limbic system, brain stem, and medulla; antipsychotics are also thought to depress certain components of the reticular activating system that partially control body temperature, wakefulness, vasomotor tone, emesis, and hormonal balance; additionally, antipsychotics have significant anticholinergic and alpha-adrenergic blocking effects; therapeutic plasma levels 5-20 ng/mL

Pharmacokinetics: PO: Onset erratic, peak 3-5 hr, half-life 24 hr; IM: Onset 15-30 min, peak 15-20 min, half-life 21 hr; IM (decanoate): Peak 4-11 days, half-life 3 wk; metabolized by liver, excreted in urine (40%) and bile (15%), crosses placenta, enters breast milk

Side Effects: *CNS:* **Parkinsonism, akathisias, dystonias,** tardive dyskinesia, oculogyric crisis, neuroleptic malignant syndrome; *Peripheral:* Blurred vision (cycloplegia or paralysis of accommodation), ocular pain, photophobia, mydriasis, impaired vision; intolerance of extreme heat or cold, possible heat stroke or fatal hyperthermia; nasal congestion; wheezing, dyspnea; hypotension, especially orthostatic, leading to dizziness, syncope; **tachycardia,** irregular pulse, arrhythmias; dry mouth, constipation, jaundice, abdominal pain; urinary retention, urinary hesitancy, galactorrhea, gynecomastia, impaired ejaculation, amenorrhea

Interactions

- Alcohol and other CNS depressants (barbiturates, antihistamines, antianxiety, or antidepressant drugs): Increased CNS depression, increased risk of EPSEs
- Amphetamines: Possible decreased antipsychotic effect
- Antacids (magnesium and aluminum products): Possible decreased antipsychotic effect
- Anticholinergics (atropine, H_1-type antihistamines, antidepressants, etc): Increased risk of excessive atropine-like side effects or toxic effects
- Benztropine: Possible decreased antipsychotic effect, increased risk of severity of peripheral anticholinergic side effects
- Diazoxide: Possible severe hyperglycemia, prediabetic coma
- Fluoxetine: EPSEs
- Fluvoxamine: May double haloperidol serum levels, leading to increase in both negative and positive symptoms
- Guanethidine: Poor control of hypertension by guanethidine
- Hypoglycemia drugs (insulin, oral hypoglycemia agents): Poor diabetic control
- Lithium: Disorientation, unconsciousness, EPSEs, and potentially neurotoxic effects
- Meperidine, morphine: Increased risk of severe CNS depression, respiratory depression, hypotension
- Propranolol: Increased pharmacologic effects of either drug

Implications

Assess

- Establish baseline VS, laboratory values, to assess side effects, allergic or hypersensitivity reactions
- Physiologic and psychologic status before therapy, to determine needs and evaluate progress
- For early stages of tardive dyskinesia by use of Abnormal Involuntary Movement Scale
- Identify concurrent symptoms that may be aggravated by antipsychotics, e.g., glaucoma, diabetes

Planning/Implementation

- Ensure that drug has been taken; check mouth for "cheeking"
- If giving liquid haloperidol, use at least 60 mL of compatible beverage to mask taste; dilute and give immediately; take drug with food to minimize GI upset; give IM injections in lateral thigh
- Keep patient quiet after injection to

prevent falls associated with postural hypotension
- For dry mouth, give chewing gum, hard candies, lip balm; monitor urinary output; check for bladder distention in inactive patients, older men, and patients on high doses
- Assist with ambulation, if patient is having blurred vision; dim room lights for photosensitivity
- Ensure safety with hypotension; sit on side of bed before rising, head-low position for dizziness, avoid hot showers, wear elastic stockings
- Check B/P (supine, sitting, standing) and pulse before and after each dose when possible; observe for side effects
- Monitor body temperature for indications of neuroleptic malignant syndrome, e.g., muscle rigidity, fever, depressed neurologic status; ensure adequate hydration, nutrition, and ventilation
- Protect patient from exposure to extreme heat or cold
- Recognize impending hypersensitivity, i.e., to pruritus or jaundice with hepatitis; flu or coldlike symptoms, evidence of bleeding with blood dyscrasia
- Observe for involuntary movements

Teaching
- About benefits and potential harm of antipsychotic drugs; weigh need to know against causing apprehension
- To comply with drug treatment
- To avoid activities requiring clear vision for a few weeks after treatment starts; to report eye pain immediately
- About importance of exercise, fluids, and fiber in diet
- To watch for symptoms of heart failure: weight gain, dyspnea, distended neck veins, tachycardia
- Possible male sexual performance failure; suggest relaxed, stress-free environment
- To avoid conception; women should practice effective contraception
- To avoid exposure to sunlight; keep skin covered but with temperature-appropriate clothing
- That patient cannot become addicted to antipsychotic drugs

Evaluate
- Whether patient follows prescribed regimen, takes medications as ordered
- Avoids injury; reports dizziness or need for assistance
- Verbalizes reduced anxiety
- Experiences minimal or no adverse responses
- Uses appropriate interventions to minimize side effects
- Achieves improved mental status

Lab Test Interferences
- Increase: Liver function test, determinations of cardiac enzymes, cholesterol, blood glucose, prolactin, bilirubin, PBI, cholinesterase, I-131
- Decrease: Hormones (blood urine)
- False positive: Pregnancy tests, PKU
- False negative: Urinary steroids

Treatment of Overdose: Lavage; if orally ingested, provide an airway; do not induce vomiting

Administration
- Psychosis: *Adult:* PO 0.5-5 mg bid or tid initially depending on severity of condition; dose is increased to desired dose, max 100 mg/day; IM 2-5 mg q1-8h; *child 3-12 yr:* PO/IM 0.05-0.15 mg/kg/day; Decanoate: Initial dose IM is 10-15 times the daily oral dose at 4-wk intervals; do not administer IV
- Tourette's syndrome: *Adult:* PO 0.5-5 mg bid or tid, increased until desired response occurs; *child 3-12 yr:* PO 0.05-0.075 mg/kg/day (0.5-2.0 mg/day)
- Hyperactive children: *child 3-12 yr:* PO 0.05-0.075 mg/kg/day
- Available forms include: Tabs 0.5, 1, 2, 5, 10, 20 mg; conc 2 mg/mL; inj IM 5 mg/mL; decanoate IM 50, 100 mg/mL

Hydroxyzine*

ATARAX QUIESS, VISTARIL/VISTARIL IM
(hye-drox́-i-zeen) (Chapter 6)

Functional classification: Antianxiety
Chemical classification: Piperazine
FDA pregnancy category: C

Indications: Anxiety, often used preoperatively to prevent nausea; IM form for hysterical patients

Contraindications: Hypersensitivity, early pregnancy

Pharmacologic Effects: Depresses subcortical CNS, i.e., limbic and reticular areas

Pharmacokinetics: Rapidly absorbed from gut; clinical effect in 15-30 min; half-life 3 hr but longer in elderly patients; metabolized by liver

Side Effects: *CNS:* Drowsiness (transient); rarely reported: tremor and seizures; *Peripheral:* Dry mouth; respiratory problems have occurred

Interactions

- CNS depressants: Additive effect
- Phenothiazines: Decreased antipsychotic effect

Implications

Assess

- B/P

Planning/Implementation

- Give with food or milk
- Assist with ambulation
- Maintain safety

Teaching

- To take hard candies, gum, etc, for dry mouth
- To avoid alcohol, CNS depressants
- To avoid driving

Evaluate

- Mental status

Lab Test Interference False increase: 17-OHCS

Treatment of Overdose: Oversedation most common problem; induce vomiting, gastric lavage; if hypotension occurs, give IV fluids and norepinephrine (do not use epinephrine)

*Infrequently used.

Administration

- Anxiety: *Adult:* PO 50-100 mg qid; *child* >6 *yr:* 50-100 mg/day in divided doses; *child* <6 *yr:* 50 mg/day in divided doses
- Available forms: Tabs 10, 25, 50, 100 mg; caps 25, 50, 100 mg; syr 10 mg/5 mL; oral suspension 25 mg/5 mL; IM inj 25, 50 mg/mL

Imipramine HCl

JANIMINE, NOVOPRAMINE,† TOFRANIL
(im-iṕ-ra-meen) (Chapter 5)

Functional classification: TCA
Chemical classifications: Dibenzazepine, tertiary amine
FDA pregnancy category: C

Indications: Depression, enuresis in children
Unlabeled use: Panic disorder

Contraindications: Hypersensitivity to TCAs, recovery phase of myocardial infarction
Cautious use: Suicidal patients, severe depression, increased intraocular pressure, narrow-angle glaucoma, urinary retention, cardiac disease, hepatic disease, hyperthyroidism, ECT, elective surgery, elderly patients, MAOI therapy, convulsive disorders, prostatic hypertrophy

Pharmacologic Effects: Blocks reuptake of norepinephrine, serotonin into nerve endings, increasing action of norepinephrine, serotonin in nerve cells; also r/t changes in receptor sensitivity; therapeutic plasma levels 200-350 ng/mL

Pharmacokinetics: PO: Steady state 2-5 days, metabolized by liver, excreted by kidneys and feces, crosses placenta, excreted in breast milk, half-life 11-25 hr; desipramine is a metabolite

Side Effects: *CNS:* **Sedation,** ataxia, confusion, delirium; *Peripheral:* **Blurred vision,** photophobia, increased intraocular pressure, decreased tearing, orthosta-

†Available in Canada only.

tic hypotension, arrhythmias, tachycardia, palpitations, dry mouth, constipation, diarrhea, decreased sweating, **urinary retention, hesitancy**

Interactions

- Anticholinergic agents: Additive anticholinergic effects with atropine, antihistamines (H_1 blocker), antiparkinson drugs, antipsychotics, OTC cold and allergy drugs
- CNS depressants: Additive depressant effect
- Guanethidine, clonidine: Decreased antihypertensive effect
- MAOIs: Hypertensive crisis, atropine-like poisoning
- Oral contraceptives: Inhibit effects of TCAs
- Haloperidol: May increase TCA serum level
- Quinidine: Additive effect, heart block possible
- Sympathomimetics: Potentiates sympathomimetic effects
- Thyroid preparations: Tachycardia, arrhythmias; may increase TCA effect

Implications

Assess

- Establish baseline data to aid recognition of adverse responses to medication, e.g., liver enzyme levels, VS, renal function, mental status, speech patterns, affect, weight
- For signs of noncompliance, e.g., poor therapeutic response
- For major symptoms of depression: apathy, sadness, sleep disturbances, hopelessness, guilt, decreased libido, spontaneous crying
- Review history for contraindicated conditions, e.g., glaucoma, CV disease, GI conditions, urologic conditions, seizures, pregnancy

Planning/Implementation

- Monitor for "cheeking" or hoarding; check drug dosage carefully, because a small overdose may cause toxic effects
- Monitor for suicidal ideations; suicidal thought content may increase as antidepressants begin to "energize" patient
- Monitor VS; if hypotension, tachycardia, or arrhythmias occur, withhold TCAs
- Give most TCAs in a single dose hs
- Observe for early signs of toxic effects, e.g., drowsiness, tachycardia, mydriasis, hypotension, agitation, vomiting, confusion, fever, restlessness, sweating
- If CNS overstimulation occurs, e.g., hypomania, delirium, discontinue drug

Teaching

- That these drugs have a lag time of up to 1 month
- To adhere to drug regimen
- To avoid OTC drugs, particularly those containing sympathomimetics or anticholinergics
- To avoid drugs listed in section on interactions
- About ways to deal with minor side effects, as follows: dry mouth, with sugarless hard candies, sips of water, mouth rinse; visual disturbances, with artificial tears, sunglasses, assistance with ambulation; constipation, with bulk-forming foods, increased fluids; urinary hesitancy, with adequate fluids, privacy; decreased perspiration, with appropriate clothing, avoidance of unnecessary exercise; orthostatic hypotension, with slow positional changes, avoid hot baths and showers; for drowsiness, take single dose hs with physician approval, avoid driving
- That abrupt discontinuance may result in cholinergic rebound, e.g., nausea, vomiting, insomnia, headache

Evaluate

- Desired therapeutic serum level
- Verbalize decrease in subjective symptoms
- Observe decrease in objective symptoms
- Minimal to no adverse drug effects
- Stable VS
- Less anxiety; sleep, talk, and feel better

Lab Test Interferences

- Increase: Serum bilirubin, alkaline phosphatase, blood glucose levels
- Decrease: 5-HIAA, VMA, urinary catecholamines

Treatment of Overdose: ECG monitoring, induce emesis, lavage, activated charcoal, administer anticonvulsant, if needed; treat anticholinergic effects

Administration

- Depression: *Adult:* PO/IM 75-100 mg/day in divided doses, may gradually increase to 200 mg, not to exceed 300

I

mg/day; may give daily dose hs; *child:* 1.5 mg/kg/day in 3 divided doses to start; may increase by 1-1.5 mg/kg/day q 3-5 days; maximum dose 5 mg/kg/day; *adolescent and geriatric:* 10 mg tid-qid, typically not necessary to exceed 100 mg/day

- Enuresis: *Child 6-12 yr:* 25 mg/day 1 hr before bedtime; if no improvement in 1 wk, may increase to 50 mg/night; *adolescent:* may give up to 75 mg/night
- Available forms: Tabs 10, 25, 50, mg; inj IM 25 mg/2 mL; Pamoate salt (slow-release capsules) 75, 100, 125, 150 mg

Isocarboxazid*

MARPLAN
(eye-soe-kar-bóx-a-zid)
(Chapter 5)

Functional classifications: Antidepressant, MAOI
Chemical classification: Hydrazine
FDA pregnancy category: C

Indications: Depression in patients refractory to TCAs and ECT

Contraindications: Hypersensitivity to MAOIs, elderly patients (>60 yr), children <16 yr, hypertension, CHF, severe hepatic disease, pheochromocytoma, severe renal disease, severe cardiac disease, paranoid schizophrenia

Cautious use: Suicidal patients, convulsive disorders, schizophrenia, hyperactivity, diabetes mellitus, hypomania, agitation, hyperthyroidism, lactation

Pharmacologic Effect: Inhibits monoamine oxidase, thus increasing the concentration of endogenous epinephrine, norepinephrine, serotonin, dopamine in storage sites in CNS

Pharmacokinetics: PO: Metabolized by liver, excreted in kidneys, half-life not established

Side Effects: *CNS:* Dizziness, drowsiness, confusion, **headache,** anxiety, **tremors,** stimulation, weakness, *hyperreflexia,* mania, **insomnia, fatigue,** weight gain; *Peripheral:* Change in libido; **constipation, dry mouth,** nausea and vomiting, **anorexia,** diarrhea, rash, flushing, increased perspiration, jaundice, **orthostatic hypotension, hypertension, dysrhythmias,** hypertensive crisis, **blurred vision**

*Generally no longer available

Interactions

- Drug-drug: *Sympathomimetics (indirect or mixed acting):* Severe headache, hypertension, hyperpyrexia, and hypertensive crisis; sympathomimetic drugs include amphetamines, levodopa, tryptophan, methylphenidate, OTC compounds containing phenylpropanolamine, ephedrine, and pseudoephedrine, TCAs, other MAOIs, guanethidine, methyldopa, guanadrel, reserpine; *Anticholingeric drugs:* Additive effect; *Antihypertensives (diuretics, beta blockers, hydralazine, nitroglycerin, prazosin):* Hypotension
- Drug-food: *Tyramine-rich foods* (see text): Hypertensive crisis

Implications

Assess

- B/P (lying, standing), pulse; if systolic B/P drops 20 mm Hg, withhold drug, notify physician
- Blood studies: CBC, leukocyte count, cardiac enzyme levels (if patient is receiving long-term therapy)
- Hepatic studies: Hepatotoxicity may occur

Planning/Implementation

- Increased fluids, bulk in diet when constipation, urinary retention occur
- With food or milk for GI symptoms
- Gum, hard candies, or frequent sips of water for dry mouth
- Phentolamine for severe hypertension
- Storage in tight container in cool environment
- Assistance with ambulation during beginning of therapy because drowsiness or dizziness occurs
- Safety measures, including use of side rails
- Checking to see that PO medication is swallowed

Teaching

- That therapeutic effects may take 1-4 wk
- To avoid driving or other activities that require alertness
- To avoid ingesting alcohol, CNS depressants, or OTC medications for

cold, weight control, hay fever; to avoid cough syrups
- Not to discontinue medication quickly after long-term use
- To avoid high-tyramine foods, e.g., cheese (aged), caviar, dried fish, game meat, beer, wine, pickled products, liver, raisins, bananas, figs, avocados, meat tenderizers, chocolate, yogurt, increased caffeine, soy sauce
- Report headache, palpitations, neck stiffness

Evaluate
- Toxic effects: Increased headache, palpitations; discontinue drug immediately
- Mental status
- Urinary retention, constipation
- Withdrawal symptoms: Headache, nausea, vomiting, muscle pain, weakness

Treatment of Overdose: Lavage, activated charcoal, monitor electrolyte levels, VS, treat hypotension

Administration
Adult: PO 30 mg/day in divided doses, reduce to maintenance dose of 10-20 mg/day, if feasible
- Available forms include: Tabs 10 mg

Lamotrigine
LAMICTAL
(la-moé-tri-jeen) (Chapter 7)

Functional classification: Antiepileptic
Chemical classification: Phenyltriazine derivative
FDA pregnancy category: C

Indications: Adjunctive treatment for partial seizures; may have implications for more generalized seizures

Contraindications: Lactation
Cautious use: Impaired hepatic, renal, cardiac function

Pharmacologic Effects: Blocks sustained repetitive firing of neurons by prolonging the inactivation of sodium channels in animal models, probably resulting in decreased release of the excitatory neurotransmitters aspartate and glutamate

Pharmacokinetics: Lamotrigine is almost completely absorbed after oral ingestion, with or without food. Peak serum levels in 1.5 to 4 hr; half-life 25 hr, protein binding 55%

Side Effects: *CNS:* Dizziness (14%), diplopia (14%), somnolence (13%), headache (12%), ataxia (11%), asthenia (10%); *Peripheral:* Blurred vision, nausea, vomiting, rash (5% to 10%). Deaths have occurred r/t Stevens-Johnson syndrome. Disseminated intravascular coagulation has been reported

Interactions
- Carbamazepine, phenytoin, phenobarbital, primidone (all are enzyme-inducing agents): Decrease the half-life of lamotrigine to about 15 hr; carbamazepine serum levels are reported to increase, sometimes to toxic levels
- Valproic acid: Increases half-life of lamotrigine to about 60 hr; valproic acid concentrations decrease by about 25%

Implications
Assess
- History of hepatic, renal, or cardiac problems
- Lactation
- Baseline physical data, e.g. VS, B/P, skin, orientation

Planning/Implementation
- Monitor renal, hepatic, and cardiac functions
- Re-evaluate if abnormal test results are found
- Monitor drug dosage. Carefully assess when changing the dosage of another antiepileptic (because lamotrigine is an adjunctive agent)
- When discontinuing, taper drug over 2-wk period

Teaching
- Take drug as prescribed
- Do not stop drug abruptly because of possibility of withdrawal-precipitated seizures
- Avoid driving or working with hazardous machinery because of dizziness and somnolence
- Take drug with meals if GI upset occurs
- Self-assess skin changes: skin yellowing, fever, sore throat, mouth sores, unusual bleeding, skin rash, bruising, etc should all be reported. (See side effects section.)
- Wear MedicAlert bracelet so that others will have information about seizure disorder

L

Evaluate
- Seizure status
- Minimal effect of adverse reactions

Administration

Adults taking an enzyme-inducing antiepileptic (carbamazepine, phenytoin, phenobarbital, primidone): 50 mg once daily for 2 wk; then can increase to 50 mg twice a day for 2 more wk; then weekly changes of 100 mg/day up to a maintenance dosage of 300-500 mg/day in 2 doses. If valproic acid is being taken in addition to an enzyme-inducing drug, then the starting dose should be 25 mg qod for 2 wk followed by 25 mg/day for 2 wk. Then increase by 25-50 mg/day q 1-2 wk up to a maintenance dosage of 100-150 mg/day in 2 divided doses. If valproic acid is given alone, then the dosage of lamotrigine would be lower; *children and adolescents:* Not recommended for children <16 yr

Lithium Carbonate

CIBALITH-S, LITHANE, ESKALITH, LITHONATE, LITHOTABS, LITHOBID, LITHIUM CITRATE, LITHONATE-S
(lí-thee-um) (Chapter 5)

Functional classification: Antimanic
Chemical classification: Alkali metal ion salt
FDA pregnancy category: D

Indications: Manic-depressive illness (manic phase), prevention of bipolar manic depressive psychosis

Contraindications: Children <12 yr, hepatic or renal disease, brain trauma, lactation, schizophrenia, severe cardiac disease, severe dehydration, organic mental syndrome, sodium depletion

Cautious use: Concomitant neuroleptic therapy, elderly patients, hypothyroidism, seizure disorders, diabetes mellitus, systemic infection, urinary retention

Pharmacologic Effects: Alters sodium ion transport in nerve, muscle cells; affects norepinephrine reuptake and increases serotonin receptor sensitivity

Pharmacokinetics: PO: Onset rapid, peak 1-4 hr, half-life about 24 hr, depending on age; crosses blood-brain barrier, excreted in urine, crosses placenta, enters breast milk, well absorbed by oral method; sodium loading increases lithium excretion

Side Effects: *CNS:* Headache, drowsiness, dizziness, tremors, twitching, ataxia, seizure, slurred speech, restlessness, confusion, stupor, memory loss, clonic movements; *Peripheral:* Dry mouth, anorexia, nausea, vomiting, diarrhea, hypotension, leukocytosis, blurred vision, hypothyroidism, hyponatremia, muscle weakness

Interactions
- Haloperidol: Encephalopathy
- Neuromuscular blocking agents, phenothiazines: Increased effects of these drugs
- Sodium bicarbonate, acetazolamide, mannitol, aminophylline: Increased renal clearance
- Indomethacin, thiazide diuretics, NSAIDs: Increased toxic effects
- Theophylline, urinary alkalinizers: Decreased effects of lithium
- Carbamazepine: Neurotoxic effects
- Captopril, lisinopril (ACE inhibitors): Reported to produce a three- to fourfold increase in serum lithium levels (a potentially fatal combination)

Implications

Assess
- Initiate serum creatinine and thyroid function studies before starting lithium regimen
- Weigh daily, check for edema in legs, ankles, wrists; if present, report
- Sodium intake; decreased sodium intake with decreased fluid intake may lead to lithium retention; increased sodium and fluids may decrease lithium retention
- Skin turgor, at least daily
- Urine for albuminuria, glycosuria, uric acid during beginning of treatment, q 2 mo thereafter
- Neurologic status: Gait, motor reflexes, hand tremors

- Serum lithium levels weekly initially, then obtain lithium levels 8-12 hr after previous dose (therapeutic serum level 0.6-1.2 mEq/L)

Planning/Implementation

- With meals to avoid GI upset
- Adequate fluids (2-3 L/day) to prevent dehydration during initial treatment, 1-2 L/day during maintenance

Teaching

- Symptoms of minor toxic effects, i.e., vomiting, diarrhea, poor coordination, fine-motor tremors, weakness, lassitude; major toxic effects, i.e., coarse tremors, severe thirst, tinnitus, dilute urine
- Action, dosage, side effects; when to notify physician
- To monitor urine specific gravity
- That contraception is necessary because lithium may harm fetus
- Not to operate machinery until lithium serum levels are stable

Evaluate

- Reduction in manic symptoms
- Patient verbalizes understanding of side effects, symptoms of toxic effects, and need for compliance

Lab Test Interferences

- Increase: Potassium excretion, urine glucose, blood glucose, protein, BUN levels
- Decrease: VMA, T_3, T_4, PBI, I-131

Treatment of Overdose: Lavage, maintain airway, respiratory function; dialysis for severe intoxication

- Lithium levels <2 mEq/L: Diarrhea, vomiting, nausea, drowsiness, weakness
- Lithium levels 2 to 3 mEq/L: Giddiness, ataxia, blurred vision, tinnitus, slurred speech, blackouts, fasciculations, incontinence
- Lithium levels >3 mEq/L: Multiple organs and organ systems failure, seizures, vascular collapse, coma

Administration

Adult: PO 600 mg tid, maintenance 300 mg tid or qid; slow-rel tabs 450 mg bid, dose should be individualized to maintain blood levels at 0.5-1.5 mEq/L; maintenance serum concentrations are 0.6-1.2 mEq/L

- Available forms include: Caps 150, 300, 600 mg; tabs 300 mg; tabs slow-rel 300, 450 mg; syrup 8 mEq/5 mL (as citrate)

Lorazepam

ATIVAN

(lor-á-ze-pam) (Chapter 6)

Functional classification: Antianxiety
Chemical classification: Benzodiazepine
Controlled substance schedule IV
FDA pregnancy category: D

Indications: Anxiety

Contraindications: Hypersensitivity to benzodiazepines, narrow-angle glaucoma, psychosis, child <18 yr (inj), child 12 yr (oral)

Cautious use: Elderly or debilitated patients, hepatic or renal disease

Pharmacologic Effects: Apparently potentiates effects of GABA and other inhibitory transmitters by binding to specific benzodiazepine receptor sites; depresses subcortical levels of CNS, including limbic system and reticular formation

Pharmacokinetics: Speed of onset: Intermediate PO peak 1-6 hr, duration 3-6 hr, metabolized by liver, excreted by kidneys, crosses placenta, enters breast milk, half-life 15 hr

Side Effects: *CNS:* **Drowsiness, dizziness,** confusion, headache, anxiety, tremor, stimulation, fatigue, depression, insomnia; *Peripheral:* Photophobia caused by mydriasis, **blurred vision** caused by cycloplegia; sleeplike slowing of respirations with therapeutic doses, cough; **orthostatic hypotension, tachycardia,** hypotension; constipation, dry mouth

Interactions

- Alcohol and other CNS depressants: Increased risk of excessive CNS depression
- Cimetidine: Potentiation of CNS depression
- Digoxin: Increased risk of cardiac side effects from digoxin
- Levodopa: Decreased antiparkinson effect
- Phenytoin: Increased phenytoin serum levels

Implications

Assess

- Patient's level of anxiety and method of coping

L

- B/P, VS
- Establish baseline physical assessment data before medications are started

Planning/Implementation

- Monitor patient's response to medication
- Observe elderly, very young, and debilitated patients for paradoxic excitement
- Reduce dose of other depressant drugs
- Observe for signs of withdrawal when discontinuing antianxiety agent

Teaching

- To avoid operating dangerous machinery and performing other tasks requiring good reflexes
- To report ocular pain at once, as well as other visual disturbances
- Drug may be taken with food

Evaluate

- Whether patient achieves lower levels of anxiety without undue sedation
- Whether patient can follow prescribed regimen
- For physical dependence: withdrawal symptoms of headache, nausea, vomiting, muscle pain, weakness after long-term use

Lab Test Interferences

- Increase: AST, ALT, serum bilirubin level
- Decrease: RAIU
- False increase: 17-OHCS

Treatment of Overdose: Lavage, VS, supportive care; there have been few deaths, if any, from benzodiazepine overdose alone; deaths occur when benzodiazepines are mixed with other drugs

Administration

- Anxiety: *Adult:* PO 2-6 mg/day in divided doses, not to exceed 10 mg/day; take largest dose before bedtime; *geriatric:* Initially 1-2 mg/day in divided doses, adjust as needed or tolerated
- Insomnia: *Adult:* PO 2-4 mg hs
- IM: 0.05 mg/kg up to a maximum of 4 mg
- IV: Initially 2 mg or 0.044 mg/kg, whichever is smaller, not to exceed 2 mg/min
- Available forms include: Tabs 0.5, 1, 2 mg; IM/IV inj 2-4 mg/mL: must refrigerate

Loxapine Succinate/ Loxapine HCl

LOXAPAC,† LOXITANE, LOXITANE-C

(lox-á-peen) (Chapter 4)

Functional classifications: Antipsychotic, neuroleptic

Chemical classification: Dibenzoxazepine

FDA pregnancy category: C

Indications: Psychotic disorders

Contraindications: Hypersensitivity, blood dyscrasias, coma, child <16 yr, brain damage, bone marrow depression, alcohol and barbiturate withdrawal states

Cautious use: Lactation, seizure disorders, hypertension, hepatic disease, cardiac disease, glaucoma, urinary retention

Pharmacologic Effects: Antipsychotic drugs produce a neuroleptic effect characterized by sedation, emotional quieting, psychomotor slowing, and affective indifference; exact mode of action is not fully understood; antipsychotics primarily block dopamine D_2 receptors in the basal ganglia, hypothalamus, limbic system, brain stem and medulla; antipsychotics are also thought to depress certain components of the reticular activating system, that partially control body temperature, wakefulness, vasomotor tone, emesis, and hormonal balance; additionally, antipsychotics have significant anticholinergic and alpha-adrenergic blocking effects

Pharmacokinetics: PO: Onset 20-30 min, peak 2-4 hr, duration 12 hr; IM: Onset 15-30 min, peak 15-20 min, duration 12 hr; metabolized by liver, excreted in urine, crosses placenta, enters breast milk, initial half-life 5 hr, terminal half-life 19 hr

Side Effects: *CNS:* Parkinsonism, akathisias, dystonias, tardive dyskinesia, oculogyric crisis; *Peripheral:* Blurred vision (cycloplegia or paralysis of accommodation); ocular pain, photophobia, mydriasis, impaired vision; intolerance of extreme heat or cold, possible heat stroke or

†Available in Canada only.

fatal hyperthermia; nasal congestion, wheezing, dyspnea; **hypotension, especially orthostatic,** leading to dizziness, syncope; **tachycardia,** irregular pulse, arrhythmias; **dry mouth, constipation,** jaundice, abdominal pain; urinary retention, urinary hesitancy, galactorrhea, gynecomastia, impaired ejaculation, amenorrhea

Interactions

- Alcohol and other CNS depressants (barbiturates, antihistamines, antianxiety or antidepressant drugs): Increased CNS depression; increased risk of EPSEs
- Amphetamines: Possible decreased antipsychotic effect
- Antacids (magnesium and aluminum products): Possible decreased antipsychotic effect
- Anticholinergics (atropine, H_1-type antihistamines, antidepressants, etc): Increased risk of excessive atropine-like side effects or toxic effects
- Benztropine: Possible decreased antipsychotic effect, increased risk of severity of peripheral anticholinergic side effects
- Diazoxide: Possible severe hyperglycemia, prediabetic coma
- Guanethidine: Poor control of hypertension by guanethidine
- Hypoglycemia drugs (insulin, oral hypoglycemia agents): Poor diabetic control
- Lithium: Poor control of psychosis with combined therapy; can mask lithium toxic effects; neurotoxic effects with confusion, delirium, seizures, encephalopathy
- Meperidine, morphine: Increased risk of severe CNS depression, respiratory depression, hypotension
- Propranolol: Increased pharmacologic effects of either drug

Implications

Assess

- Establish baseline VS, laboratory values to assess side effects, allergic or hypersensitivity reactions
- Physiologic and psychologic status before therapy, to determine needs and evaluate progress
- For early stages of tardive dyskinesia by use of Abnormal Involuntary Movement Scale
- Identify concurrent symptoms that may be aggravated by antipsychotics, e.g., glaucoma, diabetes

Planning/Implementation

- Ensure that drug has been taken; check mouth for "cheeking"
- If giving liquid antipsychotics, use at least 60 mL of compatible beverage to mask taste; dilute and give immediately; take drug with food to minimize GI upset; give IM injections in lateral thigh
- Keep patient quiet after injection, to prevent falls associated with postural hypotension
- For dry mouth, give chewing gum, hard candies, lip balm
- Monitor urinary output; check for bladder distention in inactive patients, older men, and patients on high doses
- Assist with ambulation, if patient is having blurred vision; dim room lights for photosensitivity
- Ensure safety with hypotension; sit on side of bed before rising, head-low position for dizziness, avoid hot showers, wear elastic stockings
- Check B/P (supine, sitting, standing) and pulse before and after each dose when possible; observe for side effects
- Monitor body temperature for indications of neuroleptic malignant syndrome, e.g., muscle rigidity, fever, depressed neurologic status; ensure adequate hydration, nutrition, and ventilation
- Protect patient from exposure to extreme heat or cold
- Recognize impending hypersensitivity: pruritus or jaundice with hepatitis; flu or coldlike symptoms, evidence of bleeding with blood dyscrasia
- Observe for involuntary movements

Teaching

- About benefits and potential harm of antipsychotic drugs; weigh need to know against causing apprehension
- To comply with drug treatment
- To avoid activities requiring clear vision for a few weeks after treatment starts; to report eye pain immediately
- About the importance of exercise, fluids, and fiber in diet
- To watch for symptoms of heart failure, i.e., weight gain, dyspnea, distended neck veins, tachycardia

L

- Possible male sexual performance failure; suggest relaxed, stress-free environment
- To avoid conception; women should practice effective contraception
- To avoid exposure to sunlight; keep skin covered but with temperature-appropriate clothing
- That patient cannot become addicted to antipsychotic drugs

Evaluate

- Whether patient follows prescribed regimen, takes medications as ordered
- Avoids injury; reports dizziness or need for assistance
- Verbalizes reduced anxiety
- Experiences minimal or no adverse responses
- Uses appropriate interventions to minimize side effects
- Achieves improved mental status

Treatment of Overdose: Lavage, if orally ingested; provide an airway; do not induce vomiting

Administration

Adult >15 yr: PO 10 mg bid initially, may be rapidly increased depending on severity of condition, maintenance 20-60 mg/day, range 20-250mg/day; IM 12.5-50 mg q4-6h or more until desired response, then start PO form

- Mix concentrate in orange or grapefruit juice
- Available forms: Caps 5, 10, 25, 50 mg; conc 25 mg/mL; inj IM 50 mg/mL

Maprotiline HCl

LUDIOMIL

(ma-proé-ti-leen) (Chapter 5)

Functional classification: Antidepressant
Chemical classification: Tetracyclic
FDA pregnancy category: B

Indications: Depression, dysthymic disorder, bipolar–depressed, anxiety associated with depression

Contraindications: Hypersensitivity to TCAs, CV disease, convulsive disorders

Cautious use: Suicidal patients, severe depression, increased intraocular pressure, narrow-angle glaucoma, urinary retention, cardiac disease, hepatic disease, hypothyroidism, hyperthyroidism, ECT, elective surgery, elderly patients, lactation, child <18 yr, prostatic hypertrophy

Pharmacologic Effect: Blocks reuptake of norepinephrine, serotonin into nerve endings, increasing action of norepinephrine, serotonin in nerve cells; also r/t receptor sensitivity; therapeutic plasma levels 200-300 ng/mL

Pharmacokinetics: PO: Onset 15-30 min, peak 12 hr, duration up to 3 wk, steady state 6-10 days; metabolized by liver, excreted by kidneys and feces; crosses placenta, half-life 21-25 hr

Side Effects: *CNS:* **Sedation,** ataxia; confusion, delirium; *Peripheral:* **Blurred vision,** photophobia, increased intraocular pressure; decreased tearing, orthostatic hypotension; arrhythmias, tachycardia, palpitations, dry mouth, constipation, diarrhea, decreased sweating, **urinary retention, hesitancy**

Interactions

- Anticholinergic agents: Additive anticholinergic effects with atropine, antihistamines (H_1 blocker), antiparkinson drugs, antipsychotics, OTC cold and allergy drugs
- CNS depressants: Additive depressant effect
- Guanethidine, clonidine: Decreased antihypertensive effect
- MAOIs: Hypertensive crisis, atropine-like poisoning
- Oral contraceptives: Inhibit metabolism of TCAs
- Phenothiazines: May increase tricyclic serum level
- Quinidine: Additive effect, heart block possible
- Sympathomimetics: Potentiate sympathomimetic effects
- Thyroid preparations: Tachycardia, arrhythmias; may increase TCA effect

Implications

Assess

- Establish baseline data to aid recognition of adverse responses to medication, e.g., liver enzyme levels, VS, renal function, mental status, speech patterns, affect, weight
- For signs of noncompliance, e.g., poor therapeutic response
- Observe for major symptoms of depres-

sion, i.e., apathy, sadness, sleep disturbances, hopelessness, guilt, decreased libido, spontaneous crying
- Review history for contraindicated conditions, e.g., glaucoma, CV disease, GI conditions, urologic conditions, seizures, pregnancy

Planning/Implementation
- Monitor for "cheeking" or hoarding; check drug dosage carefully, because a small overdose may cause toxic effects
- Monitor for suicidal ideations; suicidal thought content may increase as antidepressants begin to "energize" patient
- Monitor VS; if hypotension, tachycardia, or arrhythmias occur, withhold TCAs
- Give most TCAs in a single dose hs
- Observe for early signs of toxic effects, e.g., drowsiness, tachycardia, mydriasis, hypotension, agitation, vomiting, confusion, fever, restlessness, sweating
- If CNS overstimulation occurs, e.g., hypomania, delirium, discontinue drug

Teaching
- Maprotiline may produce clinical effects faster than TCAs do, sometimes within 3-7 days; however, a lag time of 2-3 wk occurs in many patients
- To adhere to drug regimen
- To avoid OTC drugs, particularly those containing sympathomimetics or anticholinergics
- To avoid drugs listed in section on interactions
- About ways to deal with minor side effects, as follows: dry mouth, with hard candies, sips of water, mouth rinse; visual disturbances, with artificial tears, sunglasses, assistance with ambulation; constipation, with bulk-forming foods, increased fluids; urinary hesitancy, with adequate fluids, privacy; decreased perspiration, with appropriate clothing, avoidance of unnecessary exercise; orthostatic hypotension, with slow positional changes, avoidance of hot baths and showers; for drowsiness, take single dose hs with physician approval, avoid driving
- That abrupt discontinuance may result in cholinergic rebound, e.g., nausea, vomiting, insomnia, headache

Evaluate
- Desired therapeutic serum level
- Verbalize decrease in subjective symptoms
- Observe decrease in objective symptoms
- Minimal to no adverse drug effects
- Stable VS
- Less anxiety; sleep, talk, and feel better

Lab Test Interferences
- Increase: Serum bilirubin, blood glucose, alkaline phosphatase levels
- False increase: Urinary cathecholamines
- Decrease: VMA, 5-HIAA

Treatment of Overdose: ECG, monitoring, induce emesis, lavage, activated charcoal, rapid digitalization for CV failure, reduce tendency for convulsions, control hyperexia

Administration

Adult: PO 75 mg/day in moderate depression, may increase to 150 mg/day; not to exceed 225 mg in hospitalized patients; severely depressed patients who are hospitalized may be given 300 mg/day; *geriatrics:* 50-75 mg/day
- Available forms include: Tabs 25, 50, 75 mg

Mephenytoin*

MESANTOIN

(me-fen-i-toyn) (Chapter 7)

Functional classification: Antiepileptic

Chemical classification: Hydantoin derivative

FDA pregnancy category: C

Indications: Generalized tonic-clonic, psychomotor, focal seizures refractory to other agents

Contraindications: Hypersensitivity to hydantoins, sinus bradycardia, heart block, Adams-Stokes syndrome

Cautious use: Alcoholism, hepatic or renal disease, blood dyscrasias, CHF, elderly patients, respiratory depression, diabetes mellitus, lactation

Pharmacologic Effects: Inhibits spread of seizure activity in motor cortex

Pharmacokinetics: PO: Onset 30 min, duration 24-48 hr, metabolized by liver, excreted by kidneys, half-life unknown

*Infrequently used.

Side Effects: *CNS:* Drowsiness, dizziness, insomnia, paresthesias, depression, suicidal tendencies, aggression, headache; *Peripheral:* **Nausea, vomiting, constipation,** anorexia, weight loss, hepatitis, jaundice, nephritis, albuminuria, rash, agranulocytosis, leukopenia, aplastic anemia

Interactions

- Allopurinol, cimetidine, diazepam, disulfiram, alcohol (acute ingestion), phenacemide, succinimides, valproic acid: Increased effect of hydantoins
- Barbiturates, carbamazepine, alcohol (chronic use), theophylline, antacids, dietary calcium: Decreased effects of hydantoins
- Corticosteroids, dicumarol, digitoxin, doxycycline, haloperidol, methadone, oral contraceptives, dopamine, furosemide, levodopa: Decreased effects of these drugs

Implications

Assess

- Blood studies: CBC, platelet count q 2 wk until stabilized, then q mo for 12 mo, then q 3 mo; if neutrophils <1600 cells/mm^3, discontinue drug

Planning/Implementation

- Describe seizures accurately

Teaching

- All aspects of drug administration: route, action, dose
- To report side effects
- To avoid driving or operating dangerous equipment
- To practice good oral hygiene
- Not to discontinue abruptly
- To wear MedicAlert identification bracelet

Evaluate

- Mental status: Mood, sensorium, affect, memory (long-term, short-term)
- Respiratory depression
- Blood dyscrasias: Fever, sore throat, bruising, rash, jaundice
- Dilute with normal saline, never with water

Treatment of Overdose: Mean lethal dose in adults is thought to be 2-5 g; initial symptoms are nystagmus, ataxia; death is due to respiratory and circulatory depression; lavage, emesis, activated charcoal

Administration

Adult: PO 50-100 mg/day, may increase by 50-100 mg q 7 days, up to 200 mg tid (600 mg/day); *child:* Usually require 100-400 mg/day

- Available forms include: Tabs, 100 mg

Mephobarbital

MEBARAL

(me-foe-bar΄-bi-tal) (Chapter 7)

Functional classification: Antiepileptic (long-acting)
Chemical classification: Barbiturate
Controlled substance schedule IV
FDA pregnancy category: D

Indications: Generalized tonic-clonic, absence seizures

Contraindications: Hypersensitivity to barbiturates

Cautious use: Hepatic or renal disease, lactation, alcoholism, drug abuse, hyperthyroidism, myasthenia gravis, myxedema

Pharmacologic Effects: Depresses sensory cortex, motor activity

Pharmacokinetics: PO: Onset 30-60 min, duration 10-12 hr; metabolized by liver, excreted by kidneys, half-life 34 hr (mean)

Side Effects: *CNS:* **Somnolence, drowsiness,** lethargy, hangover headache, flushing, hallucinations, coma, **dizziness;** *Peripheral:* Nausea, vomiting, hypoventilation, bradycardia, hypotension, rash, urticaria, angioedema, local pain, swelling, necrosis, thrombophlebitis, blood dyscrasias

Interactions

- CNS depressants, other antiepileptics: Drugs that increase the effects of barbiturates (toxic effects)
- Acetaminophen, digitoxin, oral anticoagulants, oral contraceptives, TCAs, possibly phenytoin, griseofulvin, doxycycline: Drugs whose effects are decreased by barbiturates

Implications

Assess

- Blood studies, liver function tests during long-term therapy
- Check VS, neurologic values regularly

Planning/Implementation

- Describe seizure accurately
- Offer consistent emotional support
- Monitor for early signs of toxic effects (slurred speech, ataxia, respiratory and CNS depression)

Teaching

- To report any side effects or adverse reactions
- To avoid driving or operating dangerous equipment
- To change position slowly
- To take drugs as prescribed because mephobarbital is habit forming
- Not to discontinue drug abruptly
- To wear MedicAlert identification bracelet
- To consult physician before becoming pregnant

Evaluate

- Mental status
- Respiratory depression
- Blood dyscrasias: Fever, sore throat, bruising, rash, jaundice

Treatment of Overdose: 1 g can cause serious poisoning in an adult; 2-10 g can be fatal; toxic effects can be confused with drunkenness. Emesis, if feasible; gastric lavage, if conscious; 30 g activated charcoal, maintain airway, good nursing care to prevent pneumonia

Administration

- Epilepsy: *Adult:* PO 400-600 mg/day or in divided doses; *child* < *5 yr:* 16-32 mg tid or qid; *child* > *5 yr:* 32-64 mg tid or qid
- Available forms include: Tabs 32, 50, 100 mg

Methadone HCl

DOLOPHINE, METHADONE HCL

(meth́-a-done) (Chapter 10)

Functional classification: Narcotic analgesic

Chemical classifications: Opiate, synthetic diphenylheptane derivative

Controlled substance schedule II

FDA pregnancy category: C

Indications: Narcotic withdrawal, severe pain

Contraindications: Hypersensitivity, addiction (narcotic)

Cautious use: Addictive personality, lactation, increased intracranial pressure, asthma, hypotension, acute abdominal condition, respiratory depression, hepatic or renal disease, child <18 yr

Pharmacologic Effects: Acts on mu and kappa opiate receptors

Pharmacokinetics: PO: Onset 30-60 min, duration 4-6 hr; peak 2-6 hr, metabolized by liver, excreted by kidneys, crosses placenta, excreted in breast milk, half-life 15-30 hr

Side Effects: *CNS:* **Drowsiness, dizziness, confusion, headache, sedation, euphoria;** *Peripheral:* **Nausea, vomiting, anorexia, constipation, cramps,** increased urinary output, dysuria, rash, urticaria, bruising, flushing, diaphoresis, pruritus, **respiratory depression,** tinnitus, blurred vision, miosis, diplopia, palpitations, bradycardia, change in B/P

Interactions

- Alcohol, narcotics, sedative hypnotics, antipsychotics, skeletal muscle relaxants, rifampin, phenytoin: Increased CNS depression
- Droperidol: Hypotension
- Hydantoins: Increase effects of methadone
- MAOIs: Unpredictable, have caused fatalities when used with related drugs

Implications

Assess

- I&O ratio: Check for decreasing output; may indicate urinary retention

M

Planning/Implementation
- If nausea, vomiting occurs, give with antiemetic
- Rotate injection sites
- Assist with ambulation
- Safety measures: Side rails, night light, call bell within easy reach

Teaching
- To report any symptoms of CNS changes
- That dependency may result
- Withdrawal symptoms may occur, e.g., nausea, vomiting, cramps, fever, faintness, anorexia

Evaluate
- Therapeutic response
- CNS changes: Dizziness, drowsiness, hallucinations, euphoria, pupil reaction
- Respiratory dysfunction: Respiratory depression; if respirations are <12/min, notify physician
- Physical dependence

Lab Test Interferences: Increased amylase and lipase levels

Treatment of Overdose: Naloxone 0.2-0.8 mg IV, O_2, IV fluids, vasopressors

Administration
- Pain: *Adult:* PO/SC/IM 2.5-10 mg q3-4h prn
- Narcotic withdrawal: *Adult:* PO 15-20 mg/day individualized initially, then up to 40 or more mg/day as patient response indicates
- Available forms: Inj SC, IM 10 mg/mL; tabs 5, 10 mg; oral solution 5, 10 mg/5 mL, 10 mg/10 mL; dispersible tabs 40 mg, oral conc 10 mg/mL

Methamphetamine HCl

DESOXYN, DESOXYN GRADUMET

(meth-am-fet́-a-meen) (Chapters 12, 13, 15, 16)

Functional classification: Cerebral stimulant
Chemical classification: Amphetamine
Controlled substance schedule II
FDA pregnancy category: C

Indications: ADHD, exogenous obesity

Contraindications: Hypersensitivity to sympathomimetic amines, hyperthyroidism, hypertension, glaucoma, severe arteriosclerosis, parkinsonism, drug abuse, anxiety, MAOI use
Cautious use: Tourette's syndrome, lactation, child <3 yr

Pharmacologic Effect: Stimulates release of norepinephrine in cerebral cortex, brain stem, and reticular activating system and dopamine in the mesolimbic system; therapeutic plasma levels 5-10 μg/dL

Pharmacokinetics: PO: Duration 3-6 hr, metabolized by liver, excreted by kidneys, crosses blood-brain barrier, half-life 4-5 hr

Side Effects: *CNS:* **Hyperactivity, insomnia, restlessness, talkativeness,** dizziness, headache, chills, stimulation, dysphoria, irritability, aggressiveness; *Peripheral:* Nausea, vomiting, anorexia, dry mouth, diarrhea, constipation, weight loss, metallic taste, cramps; impotence, change in libido; **palpitations, tachycardia,** hypertension, hypotension

Interactions
- MAOIs or within 14 days of MAOIs: Hypertensive crisis
- Acetazolamide, antacids, sodium bicarbonate, ascorbic acid, ammonium chloride, phenothiazines, haloperidol: Increases half-life of amphetamine
- Barbiturates: Decreased effects of this drug
- Guanethidine, other antihypertensives: Decreased hypotensive effect

- Phenothiazines: Antagonize amphetamines

Implications
Assess
- VS, B/P because this drug may reverse antihypertensives; check patients with cardiac disease more often
- CBC, urinalysis; in diabetes, blood and urine glucose levels, insulin changes may need to be made, because eating may decrease
- **Height, growth rate in children (growth rate may be decreased)**

Planning/Implementation
- Give at least 6 hr before bedtime to avoid sleeplessness
- For obesity, only when patient is on weight-reduction program that includes dietary changes, exercise; tolerance develops, and weight loss will not occur without additional methods
- Gum, hard candies, frequent sips of water for dry mouth
- If drug is for obesity, 30-60 min before meals
- Dispense least amount feasible, to minimize risk of overdose

Teaching
- To decrease caffeine consumption (coffee, tea, cola, chocolate), which may increase irritability, stimulation
- Avoid OTC preparations unless approved by physician
- To taper off drug over several weeks, or depression, increased sleeping, lethargy may occur
- To avoid alcohol ingestion
- To avoid hazardous activities until condition is stabilized on medication
- To get needed rest; patients feel more tired at end of day
- Check to see that PO medication has been swallowed

Evaluate
- Mental status: Mood, sensorium, affect, stimulation, insomnia; aggressiveness may occur
- Physical dependency; should not be used for extended time; dose should be discontinued gradually
- **Withdrawal symptoms: Headache, nausea, vomiting, muscle pain, weakness**
- Drug tolerance develops after long-term use
- If tolerance develops, dosage should not be increased

Treatment of Overdose: Gastric evacuation if overdose occurred in preceding 24 hr; otherwise, acidify urine; administer fluids until urine flow is 3-6 mL/kg/hr; hemodialysis or peritoneal dialysis; antihypertensives for increased B/P; ammonium chloride for increased excretion; chlorpromazine for CNS stimulation

Administration
- ADHD: *Child >6 yr:* 2.5-5 mg qd or bid, increasing by 5 mg/wk; usual effective dose 20-25 mg/day
- Obesity: *Adult:* PO 5 mg 30 min ac or 10-15 mg long-acting qd in morning
- Available forms: Tabs 5 mg, long-acting tabs 5, 10, 15 mg

Methohexital

BREVITAL SODIUM, BRIETAL SODIUM†
(meth-oh-hex́-i-tal) (Chapter 11)

Functional classification: General anesthetic
Chemical classification: Barbiturate
Controlled substance schedule IV
FDA pregnancy category: D

Indications: General anesthesia for ECT

Contraindications: Hypersensitivity, status asthmaticus, porphyria

Pharmacologic Effect: Ultrashort-acting barbiturate depresses CNS to produce anesthesia

Pharmacokinetics: Highly lipophilic; onset rapid but of brief duration (5-7 min); produces anesthesia in 1 min; plasma half-life 3-8 hr

Side Effects: *CNS:* Delirium, headache, prolonged somnolence and recovery; *Peripheral:* Circulatory depression, arrhythmias, respiratory depression, apnea, laryngospasm, bronchospasm, nausea, vomiting

Interactions
- CNS depressants including alcohol: Additive effect

†Available in Canada only.

- Furosemide: Aggravates orthostatic hypotension

Implications
Assess
- VS q 3-5 min until recovered from ECT

Planning/Implementation
- Have emergency drugs and resuscitation equipment available

Evaluate
- Cardiac status
- Respirations
- Mental status

Treatment of Overdose: Usually occurs because of rapid injection, resulting in apnea and respiratory difficulties; discontinue drug, maintain airway, give oxygen prn; ventilatory assistance prn

Administration
Adult : IV 50-120 mg (5-12 mL of 1% solution); this amount provides anesthesia for 5-7 min
- Available forms include: Powder for IV inj; ampules 2.5, 5 g; vials 500 mg/50 mL, 2.5 g/250 mL, 5 g/500 mL

Methsuximide*

CELONTIN
(meth-sux́-i-mide) (Chapter 7)

Functional classification: Antiepileptic
Chemical classification: Succinimide
FDA pregnancy category: C

Indications: Second-choice drug for absence seizures

Contraindications: Hypersensitivity

Pharmacologic Effects: See ethosuximide

Pharmacokinetics: Onset in 15-30 min, peak level 1-4 hr, duration of effect 3-4 hr, excreted in urine, half-life 2.6-4 hr

Side Effects: *CNS:* Drowsiness, ataxia, and dizziness most common side effect; see ethosuximide for other CNS effects; *Peripheral:* See ethosuximide

Interactions: See ethosuximide

Implications: See ethosuximide

*Infrequently used.

Lab Test Interference: See ethosuximide

Treatment of Overdose: See ethosuximide

Administration
Adult and child: 300 mg/day at first, increase by 300 mg/day at weekly intervals as needed; do *not* exceed 1200 mg/day in divided doses
- Available forms: Caps half-strength 150 mg, caps 300 mg

Methylphenidate HCl

RITALIN, RITALIN SR
(meth-ill-feń-i-date) (Chapters 12, 13, 15, 16)

Functional classification: Cerebral stimulant
Chemical classification: Piperidine derivative
Controlled substance schedule II
FDA pregnancy category: C

Indications: ADHD, narcolepsy

Contraindications: Hypersensitivity to sympathomimetic amines, anxiety, Tourette's syndrome, history of seizures
Cautious use: Hypertension, severe depression, seizures, drug abuse, lactation

Pharmacologic Effect: Mild CNS stimulant, mechanism unknown

Pharmacokinetics: PO: Onset ½-1 hr, duration 4-6 hr, metabolized by liver, excreted by kidneys, half-life 1-3 hr

Side Effects: *CNS:* **Hyperactivity, insomnia, restlessness, talkativeness,** dizziness, headache, chills, stimulation, dysphoria, irritability, aggressiveness; *Peripheral:* Nausea, vomiting, anorexia, dry mouth, diarrhea, constipation, weight loss, metallic taste, cramps, impotence, change in libido, **palpitations, tachycardia,** hypertension, hypotension

Interactions
- MAOIs or within 14 days of MAOIs: Hypertensive crisis
- Acetazolamide, antacids, sodium bicar-

bonate, ascorbic acid, ammonium chloride, phenothiazines, haloperidol: Increases effects of amphetamine
- Barbiturates: Decreased effects of this drug
- Guanethidine, other antihypertensives: Decreased effects of this drug

Implications
Assess
- VS, B/P
- Appetite: May be decreased
- Height, growth rate in children may be decreased (see Chapters 15 and 16)

Planning/Implementation
- Give at least 6 hr before bedtime to avoid sleeplessness

Teaching
- To decrease caffeine consumption (coffee, tea, cola, chocolate), which may increase irritability, stimulation
- Avoid OTC preparations unless approved by physician
- To taper off drug over several weeks, or depression, increased sleeping, lethargy may occur
- To avoid alcohol ingestion
- To avoid hazardous activities until condition is stabilized on medication
- To get needed rest; patients feel more tired at end of day
- Check to see that PO medication has been swallowed

Evaluate
- Mental status: Mood, sensorium, affect, stimulation, insomnia; aggressiveness may occur
- Physical dependency; should not be used for extended time; drug should be discontinued gradually
- **Withdrawal symptoms: Headache, nausea, vomiting, muscle pain, weakness**
- Drug tolerance can develop
- If tolerance develops, dosage should not be increased

Treatment of Overdose: Supportive measures; protect against self-injury; evacuate gastric contents, if possible; maintain circulation; external cooling, if hyperpyrexia occurs

Administration
- ADHD: *Child >6 yr:* 5 mg before breakfast and lunch, increasing by 5-10 mg/wk, not to exceed 60 mg/day
- Narcolepsy: *Adult:* PO 10 mg bid-tid, 30-45 min before meals, may increase to 40-60 mg/day
- Available forms: Tabs 5, 10, 20 mg; tabs time-rel 20 mg

Molindone HCl
MOBAN
(moe-liń-done) (Chapter 4)

Functional classifications: Antipsychotic, neuroleptic
Chemical classification: Dihydroindolone
FDA pregnancy category: C

Indications: Psychotic disorders

Contraindications: Hypersensitivity, coma, child <12 yr, brain damage, bone marrow depression, alcohol and barbiturate withdrawal states
Cautious use: Lactation, hypertension, hepatic disease, cardiac disease

Pharmacologic Effects: Antipsychotic drugs produce a neuroleptic effect characterized by sedation, emotional quieting, psychomotor slowing, and affective indifference; exact mode of action is not fully understood; antipsychotics primarily block dopamine D_2 receptors in the basal ganglia, hypothalamus, limbic system, brain stem, and medulla; antipsychotics are also thought to depress certain components of the reticular activating system that partially control body temperature, wakefulness, vasomotor tone, emesis, and hormonal balance; additionally, antipsychotics have significant anticholinergic and alpha-adrenergic blocking effects

Pharmacokinetics: PO: Onset erratic, peak 1½ hr, duration 24-36 hr; metabolized by liver, excreted in urine and feces, may cross placenta, enters breast milk, half-life 10-20 hr

Side Effects: *CNS:* Parkinsonism, akathisias, dystonias, tardive dyskinesia, oculogyric crisis; *Peripheral:* Blurred vision (cycloplegia or paralysis of accommodation); ocular pain, photophobia, mydriasis, impaired vision; intolerance of extreme heat or cold, possible heat stroke or fatal hyperthermia; nasal congestion, wheezing, dyspnea; **hypotension, especially orthostatic,** leading to dizziness, syncope; **tachycardia,** irregular pulse,

M

arrhythmias; **dry mouth, constipation,** jaundice, abdominal pain; urinary retention, urinary hesitancy, galactorrhea, gynecomastia, menses in previously amenorrheic women

Interactions

- Alcohol and other CNS depressants (barbiturates, antihistamines, antianxiety or antidepressant drugs): Increased CNS depression; increased risk of EPSEs
- Amphetamines: Possible decreased antipsychotic effect
- Antacids (magnesium and aluminum products): Possible decreased antipsychotic effect
- Anticholinergics (atropine, H_1-type antihistamines, antidepressants, etc): Increased risk of excessive atropine-like side effects or toxic effects
- Benztropine: Possible decreased antipsychotic effect, increased risk of severity of peripheral anticholinergic side effects
- Diazoxide: Possible severe hyperglycemia, prediabetic coma
- Guanethidine: Poor control of hypertension by guanethidine
- Hypoglycemia drugs (insulin, oral hypoglycemia agents): Poor diabetic control
- Lithium: Poor control of psychosis with combined therapy; can mask lithium intoxication, neurotoxic effects with confusion, delirium, seizures, encephalopathy
- Meperidine, morphine: Increased risk of severe CNS depression, respiratory depression, hypotension
- Propranolol: Increased pharmacologic effects of either drug

Implications

Assess

- Establish baseline VS, laboratory values, to assess side effects, allergic or hypersensitivity reactions
- Physiologic and psychologic status before therapy, to determine needs and evaluate progress
- For early stages of tardive dyskinesia by use of Abnormal Involuntary Movement Scale
- Identify concurrent symptoms that may be aggravated by antipsychotics, e.g., glaucoma, diabetes

Planning/Implementation

- Ensure that drug has been taken; check mouth for "cheeking"
- If giving liquid antipsychotics, use at least 60 mL of compatible beverage to mask taste; dilute and give immediately; take drug with food to minimize GI upset
- Keep patient quiet after injection, to prevent falls associated with postural hypotension
- For dry mouth, give chewing gum, hard candies, lip balm; monitor urinary output; check for bladder distention in inactive patients, older men, and patients on high doses
- Assist with ambulation, if patient is experiencing blurred vision; dim room lights for photosensitivity
- Ensure safety with hypotension; sit on side of bed before rising, head-low position for dizziness, avoid hot showers, wear elastic stockings
- Check B/P (supine, sitting, standing) and pulse before and after each dose, when possible; observe for side effects
- Monitor body temperature for indications of neuroleptic malignant syndrome, e.g., muscle rigidity, fever, depressed neurologic status; ensure adequate hydration, nutrition, and ventilation
- Protect patient from exposure to extreme heat or cold
- Recognize impending hypersensitivity: pruritus or jaundice with hepatitis, flu or coldlike symptoms, evidence of bleeding with blood dyscrasia
- Observe for involuntary movements

Teaching

- About benefits and potential harm of antipsychotic drugs; weigh need to know against causing apprehension
- To comply with drug treatment
- To avoid activities requiring clear vision for a few weeks after treatment starts; to report eye pain immediately
- About the importance of exercise, fluids, and fiber in diet
- To watch for symptoms of heart failure: weight gain, dyspnea, distended neck veins, tachycardia
- To avoid conception; women should practice effective contraception
- To avoid exposure to sunlight; keep skin covered but with temperature-appropriate clothing

- That patient cannot become addicted to antipsychotic drugs

Evaluate

- Whether patient follows prescribed regimen, takes medications as ordered
- Avoids injury; reports dizziness or need for assistance
- Experiences minimal or no adverse responses
- Uses appropriate interventions to minimize side effects
- Achieves improved mental status

Lab Test Interferences: Alterations in blood glucose, BUN, and RBC levels are not clinically significant

Treatment of Overdose: If orally ingested, lavage, providing an airway; do not induce vomiting; symptomatic, supportive care

Administration

Adult >12 yr: PO 50-75 mg/day, increasing to 225 mg/day, if needed; maintenance dosage for mild condition is 5-15 mg tid-qid

- Concentrate mixed with orange or grapefruit juice
- Available forms include: Tabs 5, 10, 25, 50, 100 mg; conc 20 mg/mL

Naloxone HCl

NARCAN

(Nay-locks-own) (Chapter 10)

Functional classification: Narcotic antagonist

Chemical classification: Thebaine derivative

FDA pregnancy category: B

Indications: Narcotic-induced respiratory depression

Contraindications: Hypersensitivity

Cautious use: Children

Pharmacologic Effects: Competes with narcotics at opioid receptor sites

Pharmacokinetics: PO: Onset 2 min (IV), half-life 30-81 min; duration 1-4 hr; metabolized by liver, excreted by kidneys, crosses placenta

Side Effects: *CNS:* Stimulation, **drowsiness,** nervousness; *Peripheral:* Hypotension, hypertension, ventricular tachycardia, hyperpnea; withdrawal symptoms, e.g., nausea, vomiting, sweating, increased blood pressure, tremulousness

Interactions

- Potentially cardiotoxic drugs: Hypotension, hypertension, ventricular tachycardia
- Opioids: Loss of analgesia

Implications

Assess

- VS q 3-5 min

Planning/Implementation

- Remember that naloxone does not improve respiratory depression caused by nonnarcotic drugs
- Have resuscitative equipment nearby
- Give solutions prepared within 24 hr

Evaluate

- Signs of withdrawal in drug-dependent individuals
- Cardiac status: Tachycardia, hypertension
- Respiratory dysfunction: Respiratory depression, character, rate, and rhythm; if respirations are <10/min, respiratory stimulant should be administered

Lab Test Interferences: Urine VMA, 5-HIAA, urine glucose levels, pregnancy test

Administration

- Narcotic-induced respiratory depression: *Adult:* IV/SC/IM 0.4-0.8 mg; repeat q 2-3 min, if needed
- Postoperative respiratory depression: *Adult:* IV 0.1-0.2 mg q 2-3 min prn; *child:* IV/IM/SC 0.01 mg/kg q 2-3 min prn
- Available forms include: Inj IV, IM, SC 0.02, 0.4, 1 mg/mL

N

Naltrexone HCl

REVIA

(nal-trex́-one) (Chapter 10)

Functional classification: Narcotic antagonist

Chemical classification: Thebaine derivative

FDA pregnancy category: C

Indications: Treatment of alcohol dependence (reduces craving and increases abstinence); blockage of opioid analgesics, narcotic addiction; longer-acting than naloxone; prevention of readdiction

Contraindications: Patients receiving opioid analgesics; patients currently dependent on opioids; patients in acute opioid withdrawal; any individual who has failed the naloxone challenge test or who has a positive urine screen for opioids; any individual with a history of sensitivity to naltrexone; acute hepatitis or liver failure; child <18 yr

Cautious use: Anemia, hepatic or renal disease, Hodgkin's disease

Pharmacologic Effect: Thought to bind alcohol-released endogenous opioids; competes with narcotics at opioid receptor sites; blocks subjective effects of IV narcotics

Pharmacokinetics: PO: Onset 15-30 min, peak 1-2 hr, duration 4-6 hr; REC: Onset slow, duration 4-6 hr; metabolized by liver, excreted by kidneys, crosses placenta, excreted in breast milk, half-life 4 hr for naltrexone and 13 hr for active metabolite

Side Effects: *CNS:* Low energy (>10%), nervousness (4%) drowsiness, dizziness (10%), confusion, convulsion, headache (7%), flushing, hallucinations, coma; *Peripheral:* **Nausea, vomiting (>10%), diarrhea, constipation (<10%), decreased potency (<10%), rash (<10%), increased thirst (<10%),** anorexia, hepatitis; urticaria, bruising, tinnitus, hearing loss, rapid pulse, pulmonary edema, wheezing, hyperpnea, hypoglycemia, hyponatremia, hypokalemia

Interactions

- Potentially cardiotoxic drugs: Hypotension, hypertension, ventricular tachycardia
- Opioids: Loss of analgesia

Implications

Assess

- VS q 3-5 min

Planning/Implementation

- Remember that naltrexone may precipitate an abstinence syndrome

Teaching

- Naltrexone is part of the treatment plan
- Carry MedicAlert bracelet to alert health care provider
- That large doses of heroin might kill the patient

Evaluate

- Cardiac status: Tachycardia, hypertension
- Respiratory dysfunction: Respiratory depression, character, rate, and rhythm; if respirations are <10/min, respiratory stimulant should be administered

Lab Test Interferences: Liver test abnormalities

Treatment of Overdose: There is a lack of information concerning naltrexone overdose. Treat symptoms and possibly call poison control center for up-to-date information

Administration

- Alcohol treatment: *Adult:* PO: 50 mg once per day
- Narcotic dependence: *Adult:* Administer naloxone challenge first: (1) Do not give until patient opioid-free for 7 to 10 days (2) Give naloxone challenge test (see below)
- If opioid withdrawal signs are observed, do not treat with naltrexone

Naloxone Challenge Test:

IV challenge: Draw 2 ampules of naloxone, 2 mL into a syringe. Inject 0.5 mL. Leave needle in vein and observe for 30 seconds. If no signs of withdrawal occur, inject remaining 1.5 mL and observe for 20 minutes for signs and symptoms of withdrawal

SC challenge: Administer 2 mL (0.8 mg) SC, and observe the patient for signs and symptoms of withdrawal

Interpretation of challenge test: The elicitation of withdrawal signs and symptoms indicates a potential risk to the subject, and naltrexone should not be given

Withdrawal signs and symptoms: stuffiness or running nose, tearing, yawning, sweating, tremor, vomiting, piloerection, feeling of temperature change, joint, bone, muscle pain; abdominal cramps: skin crawling

- Slowly initiate treatment: Give 25 mg PO, may then give another 25 mg after 1 hr if there are no withdrawal symptoms; usual maintenance dose is 50 mg in 24-hr period. A more flexible dosing strategy may improve compliance, e.g., 100 mg qod or 150 mg every third day
- Available forms: Tabs 50 mg

Nefazodone HCl

SERZONE

ne-faź-oh-don) (Chapter 5)

Functional classification: Antidepressant (unique molecular configuration)

Chemical classification: Phenylpiperazine

FDA pregnancy category: C

Indications: Depression

Contraindications: Hypersensitivity to phenylpiperazine antidepressants

Cautious use: Patients susceptible to orthostatic hypotension; may activate mania

Pharmacologic Effects: Mechanism of action not known. Inhibits neuronal uptake of serotonin and norepinephrine. Inhibits cytochrome P-450 IIIA4 enzyme system

Pharmacokinetics: Nefazodone is rapidly and completely absorbed, but food will delay absorption and decrease bioavailability by 20%. It is extensively metabolized in the liver. Peak plasma levels occur in about an hour. Half-life 2-4 hours; protein binding 99%

Side Effects (at dose of 300 to 600 mg/day): *CNS:* Headache (36%), somnolence (25%), dizziness (17%), insomnia (11%), light-headedness (10%), confusion (7%); *Peripheral:* Dry mouth (25%), nausea (22%), constipation (14%), asthenia (11%)

Interactions

- Serious interactions may occur with monoamine oxidase inhibitors, terfenadine, and astemizole
- Triazolam, alprazolam: Increased serum levels of these benzodiazepines
- Drugs highly bound to plasma proteins: Because nefazodone is highly bound (99%), it could displace or be displaced, causing adverse effects
- Drugs that are metabolized by P-450 IIIA4: Increased levels of those drugs

Implications

Assess

- For history of pregnancy, cardiovascular illness, stroke, mania, hypomania, suicidal tendencies
- Establish baseline physical and psychologic status
- Signs of noncompliance, e.g., poor response to drug

Planning/Implementation

- Monitor for drug compliance
- Monitor for suicide as nefazodone may "energize" the patient to carry out plans to commit suicide
- Monitor B/P, particularly when patient complains of light-headedness

Teaching

- As with other antidepressants, several weeks may be needed for a full antidepressant response
- To adhere to drug regimen
- To avoid drugs listed in section on interactions
- About ways to deal with dry mouth, constipation, light-headedness, headache, insomnia

Evaluate

- Verbalize decrease in subjective symptoms
- Observe decrease in objective symptoms
- Minimal to no adverse effects
- Stable VS
- Less anxiety; able to sleep, eat, and talk better

Lab Test Interferences: Possible lowering of hematocrit through dilution

Treatment of Overdose: No serious overdoses of nefazodone have been reported

Administration

Adult: PO: 100 mg twice a day. Increase doses by 100-200 mg per day at 1-wk

intervals. Effective dose range is typically between 300 to 600 mg/day; *elderly:* PO 50 mg twice a day to start; *adolescents and children:* Not recommended for this age group
- Available forms: Tabs 100, 150, 200, 250 mg

Nortriptyline HCl

AVENTYL, PAMELOR
(nor-triṕ-ti-leen) (Chapter 5)

Functional classification: TCA
Chemical classification: Dibenzocycloheptene, secondary amine
FDA pregnancy category: C

Indications: Depression
Unlabeled use: Panic disorder

Contraindications: Hypersensitivity to TCAs, recovery phase of myocardial infarction
Cautious use: Convulsive disorders, prostatic hypertrophy, suicidal patients, severe depression, increased intraocular pressure, narrow-angle glaucoma, urinary retention, cardiac disease, hepatic disease, hyperthyroidism, ECT, elective surgery, children

Pharmacologic Effects: Blocks reuptake of norepinephrine, serotonin into nerve endings, increasing action of norepinephrine, serotonin in nerve cells; also r/t changes in receptor sensitivity; therapeutic plasma levels 50-150 ng/mL

Pharmacokinetics: PO: Steady state 4-19 days; metabolized by liver, excreted by kidneys, crosses placenta, excreted in breast milk, half-life 18-44 hr

Side Effects: *CNS:* **Sedation,** ataxia; confusion, delirium; *Peripheral:* **Blurred vision,** photophobia, increased intraocular pressure; decreased tearing, orthostatic hypotension, arrhythmias, tachycardia, palpitations, dry mouth, constipation, diarrhea, decreased sweating, **urinary retention, hesitancy**

Interactions
- Anticholinergic agents: Additive anticholinergic effects with atropine, antihistamines (H_1 blocker), antiparkinson drugs, antipsychotics, OTC cold and allergy drugs
- CNS depressants: Additive depressant effect
- Guanethidine, clonidine: Decreased antihypertensive effect
- MAOIs: Hypertensive crisis, atropine-like poisoning
- Oral contraceptives: Inhibits effects of TCAs
- Phenothiazines, methylphenidates: May increase tricyclic serum level
- Quinidine: Additive effect, heart block possible
- Sympathomimetics: Potentiate sympathomimetic effects
- Thyroid preparations: Tachycardia, arrhythmias; may increase TCA effect

Implications
Assess
- Establish baseline data, to aid recognition of adverse responses to medication, e.g., liver enzyme levels, VS, renal function, mental status, speech patterns, affect, weight
- For signs of noncompliance, e.g., poor therapeutic response
- Observe for major symptoms of depression, e.g., apathy, sadness, sleep disturbances, hopelessness, guilt, decreased libido, spontaneous crying
- Review history for contraindicated conditions, e.g., glaucoma, CV disease, GI conditions, urologic conditions, seizures, pregnancy

Planning/Implementation
- Monitor for "cheeking" or hoarding; check drug dosage carefully, because a small overdose may cause toxic effects
- Monitor for suicidal ideations; suicidal thought content may increase as antidepressants begin to "energize" patient
- Monitor VS; if hypotension, tachycardia, or arrhythmias occur, withhold TCAs
- Give most TCAs in a single dose hs
- Observe for early signs of toxic effects, e.g., drowsiness, tachycardia, mydriasis, hypotension, agitation, vomiting, confusion, fever, restlessness, sweating
- If CNS overstimulation occurs, e.g., hypomania, delirium, discontinue drug

Teaching
- That these drugs have a lag time of up to 1 month
- To adhere to drug regimen
- To avoid OTC drugs, particularly those containing sympathomimetics or anticholinergics

- To avoid drugs listed in section on interactions
- About ways to deal with minor side effects, as follows: dry mouth, with sugarless hard candies, sips of water, mouth rinses; visual disturbances, with artificial tears, sunglasses, assistance with ambulation; constipation, with bulk-forming foods, increased fluids; urinary hesitancy, with adequate fluids, privacy; decreased perspiration, with appropriate clothing, avoidance of unnecessary exercise; orthostatic hypotension, with slow positional changes, avoidance of hot baths and showers; for drowsiness, take single dose hs with physician approval, avoid driving
- That abrupt discontinuance may result in cholinergic rebound, e.g., nausea, vomiting, insomnia, headache

Evaluate

- Desired therapeutic serum level
- Verbalize decrease in subjective symptoms
- Observe decrease in objective symptoms
- Minimal to no adverse drug effects
- Stable VS
- Less anxiety; sleep, talk, and feel better

Lab Test Interferences

- Increase: Serum bilirubin, blood glucose, alkaline phosphatase levels
- False increase: Urinary catecholamines
- Decrease: VMA, 5-HIAA

Treatment of Overdose: ECG monitoring, induce emesis, lavage, activated charcoal, administer anticonvulsant, treat anticholinergic response, if needed

Administration

Adult: PO 25 mg bid or qid, may increase to 200 mg/day; may give daily dose hs; *adolescent and geriatric:* 30-50 mg/day in divided doses

- Available forms include: Caps 10, 25, 50, 75 mg; solution 10 mg/5 mL

Oxazepam

SERAX

(ox-á-ze-pam) (Chapter 6)

Functional classification: Antianxiety
Chemical classification: Benzodiazepine
Controlled substance schedule IV
FDA pregnancy category: D

Indications: Anxiety, alcohol withdrawal, anxiety and tension in elderly

Contraindications: Hypersensitivity to benzodiazepines, psychoses, narrow-angle glaucoma, psychosis, child <12 yr

Cautious use: Elderly or debilitated patients, hepatic or renal disease

Pharmacologic Effects: Apparently potentiates effects of GABA and other inhibitory transmitters by binding to specific benzodiazepine receptor sites; depresses subcortical levels of CNS, including limbic system and reticular formation

Pharmacokinetics: Speed of onset: Intermediate to slow PO: Peak 2-4 hr, metabolized by liver, excreted by kidneys, half-life 5-20 hr

Side Effects: *CNS:* **Drowsiness, dizziness,** confusion, headache, anxiety, tremor, stimulation, fatigue, depression, insomnia; *Peripheral:* Photophobia due to mydriasis, **blurred vision** due to cycloplegia; sleeplike slowing of respirations with therapeutic doses, cough; **orthostatic hypotension, tachycardia,** hypotension; constipation, dry mouth

Interactions

- Alcohol and other CNS depressants: Increased CNS depression
- Cimetidine: Potentiation of CNS depression
- Digoxin: Increased risk of cardiac side effects from digoxin
- Levodopa: Decreased antiparkinson effect
- Phenytoin: Increased phenytoin serum levels

Implications

Assess

- Patient's level of anxiety and method of coping
- B/P, VS

- Establish baseline physical assessment data before medications are started

Planning/Implementation

- Monitor patient's response to medication
- Observe elderly, very young, and debilitated patients for paradoxic excitement
- Reduce dose of other depressant drugs
- Observe for signs of withdrawal when discontinuing antianxiety drug

Teaching

- To avoid operating dangerous machinery and performing other tasks requiring good reflexes
- To report ocular pain at once, as well as other visual disturbances
- Drug may be taken with food

Evaluate

- Whether patient achieves lower levels of anxiety without undue sedation
- Whether patient can follow prescribed regimen
- For physical dependence: Withdrawal symptoms of headache, nausea, vomiting, muscle pain, weakness after long-term use

Lab Test Interferences

- Increase: AST/ALT, serum bilirubin level
- Decrease: RAIU
- False increase: 17-OHCS

Treatment of Overdose: Lavage, VS, supportive care; there have been few deaths, if any, resulting from benzodiazepine overdose alone; deaths occur when benzodiazepines are mixed with other drugs, especially alcohol

Administration

- Anxiety: *Adult:* PO 10-30 mg tid-qid; *geriatric:* 10 mg tid, up to 15 mg tid-qid (use cautiously)
- Alcohol withdrawal: *Adult:* PO 15-30 mg tid-qid
- Available forms include: Caps, 10, 15, 30 mg; tabs 15 mg

Paraldehyde

PARAL

(par-aĺ-de-hyde) (Chapter 7)

Functional classification: Anticonvulsant
Chemical classification: Cyclic ether
Controlled substance schedule IV
FDA pregnancy category: C

Indications: Refractory seizures, status epilepticus, alcohol withdrawal, tetanus, eclampsia, sedation

Contraindications: Hypersensitivity, gastroenteritis, asthma, hepatic disease, pulmonary disease
Cautious use: Labor, children

Pharmacologic Effects: CNS depressant; mechanism of action unknown

Pharmacokinetics: PO: Onset 10-15 min, peak 1 hr, duration 8-12 hr; REC: Onset slow, duration 4-6 hr; metabolized by liver, excreted by kidneys and lungs, crosses placenta, half-life 3-10 hr

Side Effects: *CNS:* **Stimulation, drowsiness,** dizziness, confusion, convulsions, headache, flushing, hallucinations, coma; *Peripheral:* **Foul breath,** irritation, nephrosis, **rash, erythema,** local pain, esophagitis, yellowing of eyes

Interactions

- Alcohol, CNS depressants, general anesthetics, disulfiram: Increased paraldehyde blood levels
- Sulfonamides: Increased crystallization in kidneys
- Disulfiram: Blocks metabolism of paraldehyde; avoid use

Implications

Assess

- VS q 30 min after parenteral route
- Hepatic studies: AST, ALT, bilirubin and creatinine levels

Planning/Implementation

- IM inj in deep, large muscle (Z-track) mass to prevent tissue sloughing; maximum, 5 mL at one site
- Give rectally, after diluting in cottonseed oil or olive oil, as retention enema or 200 mL NS for enema
- Give orally with juice or milk to cover taste and smell and decrease GI symptoms (orally)

- Ventilate room
- Use glass containers; not compatible with plastics
- Do not use if brownish or if vinegar odor is evident

Teaching
- That physical dependency may result when used for extended periods
- To avoid driving, other activities that require alertness
- Not to discontinue medication quickly after long-term use, taper over several weeks

Evaluate
- Mental status
- Respiratory dysfunction

Treatment of Overdose: Do not lavage; support respirations, treat acidosis

Administration
- Seizures: *Adult:* IM 5-10 mL; IV 0.2-0.4 mL/kg in NS inj; *child:* IM 0.15 mL/kg; REC 0.3 mL/kg q4-6h; IV 0.1-0.15 mL/kg mL NS inj
- For other uses see *PDR*
- Available forms include: Inj IM/IV, oral and rectal liquids 1 g/mL

Paramethadione*

PARADIONE
(par-a-meth-a-dyé-one)
(Chapter 7)

Functional classification: Antiepileptic
Chemical classification: Oxazolidinedione
FDA pregnancy category: D

Indications: Refractory absence seizures

Contraindications: Hypersensitivity, blood dyscrasias
Cautious use: Hepatic or renal disease

Pharmacologic Effects: Increases seizure threshold in cortex and basal ganglia

Pharmacokinetics: PO: Onset 15-30 min, peak 1-2 hr, duration 4-6 hr; metabolized by liver, excreted by kidneys, crosses placenta, excreted in breast milk, half-life 1-3½ hr

Side Effects: *CNS:* **Drowsiness,** dizziness, fatigue, paresthesia, irritability, headache; *Peripheral:* Vaginal bleeding, albuminuria, nephrosis, abdominal pain, weight loss, nausea, vomiting, bleeding gums, abnormal liver function test, **exfoliative dermatitis,** rash, alopecia, petechiae, erythema, photophobia, diplopia, epistaxis, retinal hemorrhage, hypertension, hypotension, thrombocytopenia, agranulocytosis, leukopenia, neutropenia, hemolytic anemia

*Infrequently used.

Interactions: None known

Implications

Assess
- Blood studies: Hematocrit, hemoglobin level, RBCs, serum folate level, vitamin D, if on long-term therapy
- Hepatic studies: ALT, AST, bilirubin and creatinine levels
- Skin: If rash occurs, withhold drug

Planning/Implementation
- Dilute oral solution with water
- Take orally with juice or milk to cover taste and smell and to decrease GI symptoms

Teaching
- To take with food, if GI upset
- To carry MedicAlert identification bracelet
- To notify physician, if visual disturbances, sore throat, etc, occur
- To avoid driving and other activities that require alertness
- Not to discontinue medication quickly after long-term use, because convulsions may result

Evaluate
- Mental status
- Renal and hematologic problems

Treatment of Overdose: Symptoms include nausea, drowsiness, dizziness, ataxia, visual disturbances; coma, if massive overdose; emesis, lavage, supportive care

Administration

Adult: PO 300 mg tid (900 mg/day), may increase by 300 mg/wk, not to exceed 600 mg qid (2400 mg/day); *child:* 300 to 900 mg/day in 3 or 4 equally divided doses; dilute with water because of high alcohol content
- Available forms include: Caps 150, 300 mg; sol 300 mg/mL (65% alcohol)

P

Paroxetine

PAXIL

(pah-rox́-a-teen) Chapter 5

Functional classification: Antidepressant
Chemical classification: Selective serotonin reuptake inhibitor
Pregnancy category: B

Indications: Depression

Contraindications: Use with MAO inhibitors; allow at least 2 wk after stopping paroxetine before starting an MAOI

Cautious use: history of seizures, history of mania or hypomania, renal or hepatic disorder; elderly, pregnancy, lactation, suicidal patients

Pharmacologic Effects: Inhibits CNS neuronal uptake of serotonin

Pharmacokinetics: Peak plasma level 5 hr; half-life 21 hr; protein binding 95%; steady state reached in about 10 days; elimination both renal (64%) and hepatic (36%)

Side Effects: *CNS:* Somnolence (23%), headache (17%), asthenia (15%), dizziness (13%), insomnia (13%); *Peripheral:* Nausea (26%), dry mouth (18%), constipation (14%), sweating (11%), diarrhea (11%), ejaculatory disturbance (13%), other male genital disorders (10%)

Interactions

- Cimetidine: Increases concentrations of paroxetine
- MAO inhibitors: A serious and sometimes fatal interaction. Serotonin syndrome may result and can be fatal. Wait 14 days after stopping paroxetine before initiating an MAOI. Wait at least 14 days after stopping MAOI before starting paroxetine
- Phenobarbital: Increases the half-life of paroxetine
- Phenytoin: Half-life of both drugs reduced
- L-tryptophan: May cause a serotonin syndrome
- Alcohol: Although impairment has not been observed, potential for CNS depression suggests caution
- Digoxin: Decreased therapeutic effect of digoxin
- Procyclidine, warfarin: Increased serum levels of these drugs

Implications

Assess

- B/P, VS
- Activation of mania
- Baseline physical data

Planning/Implementation

- Maintain safety
- Closely supervise patients with a high risk of suicide because there may be a relationship between suicide and alterations in serotonin levels

Teaching

- Take medication as prescribed even though feeling better before course of treatment is completed
- Caution about driving (although no impairment in driving ability has been recorded with use of paroxetine)
- To avoid alcohol (although no impairment resulting from this combination has been recorded)
- Caution about the use of OTC products
- Notify primary care provider if intending to become pregnant
- Notify primary care provider if rash develops

Evaluate

- Therapeutic effect: Depression
- Mental status

Lab Test Interferences: Unknown

Treatment of Overdose: No deaths have been reported with paroxetine alone or in combination with other drugs or alcohol. Signs and symptoms of overdose include: nausea, vomiting, drowsiness, sinus tachycardia, dilated pupils. There are no specific antidotes. Maintain airway, ensure adequate oxygenation, give activated charcoal or lavage; give emetic. Monitor VS. Dialysis and forced diuresis unlikely to help

Administration

Adult: PO: 20 mg/day as 1 dose given in the morning. Usual range is 20-60 mg/day. Dose changes should occur at a minimum of 1-wk intervals; *elderly, debilitated, or hepatic or renal impairment:* PO: 10 mg/day. Increase may be made if indicated. Maximum dosage 40 mg/day; *children and adolescents:* Not approved for children

Available forms: Tabs 20, 30 mg

Pemoline

CYLERT
(pem-oh-leen) (Chapters 13, 15, 16)

Functional classification: Cerebral stimulant
Chemical classification: Oxazolidinone derivative
Controlled substance schedule IV
FDA pregnancy category: B

Indications: ADHD

Contraindications: Hypersensitivity
Cautious use: Renal disease, child <6 yr

Pharmacologic Effects: Exact mechanism not known; may work through dopaminergic pathways

Pharmacokinetics: PO peak 2-4 hr, duration 8 hr, metabolized by liver, excreted by kidneys, half-life 12 hr

Side Effects: *CNS:* Hyperactivity, insomnia, restlessness, dizziness, depression, headache, stimulation, irritability, aggressiveness, hallucinations, seizures; *Peripheral:* Nausea, anorexia, diarrhea, abdominal pain, increased liver enzyme levels, hepatitis, growth suppression in children, rashes

Interactions: None known

Implications
Assess
- Hepatic function studies: ALT, AST, bilirubin and creatinine levels
- Growth rate because retardation may occur (see Chapters 15 and 16)

Planning/Implementation
- Give at least 6 hr before bedtime
- Gum, hard candies, frequent sips of water for dry mouth

Teaching
- To decrease caffeine consumption (coffee, tea, cola, chocolate) because caffeine may increase irritability
- To avoid OTC preparations unless approved by physician
- To taper off drug over several weeks
- To avoid alcohol ingestion
- To avoid hazardous activities until condition is stabilized on medication
- Therapeutic effect may take 3-4 wk

Evaluate
- Mental status

Treatment of Overdose: *Symptoms:* CNS overstimulation and excessive sympathomimetic effect; vomiting, agitation, tremors, twitching, convulsions; *Treatment:* Supportive measures, if not too severe; gastric contents may be evacuated; chlorpromazine may decrease CNS stimulation

Administration
Child >6 yr: 37.5 mg in morning, increasing by 18.75 mg/wk, not to exceed 112.5 mg/day; maintenance dose usually 37.25-75 mg/day
- Available forms include: Tabs 18.75, 37.5, 75 mg; chewable tabs 37.5 mg

Pentobarbital, Pentobarbital Sodium

NEMBUTAL SODIUM, NOVA-RECTAL,† PENTOGEN†
(pen-toe-bar-bi-tal) (Chapter 8)

Functional classifications: Sedative, hypnotic
Chemical classification: Barbiturate
Controlled substance schedule II
FDA pregnancy category: D

Indications: Insomnia, sedation, emergency control of seizures

Contraindications: Hypersensitivity, respiratory depression, barbiturate dependence, marked liver dysfunction, acute pain
Cautious use: Seizure disorders, elderly patients, lactation, children

Pharmacologic Effects: Short-acting barbiturate: depresses sensory cortex to produce drowsiness, sedation, and sleep

Pharmacokinetics: PO: Onset 10-15 min, duration 3-4 hr, half-life 15-50 hr

Side Effects: *CNS:* See secobarbital; *Peripheral:* See secobarbital

Interactions: See secobarbital

Implications: See secobarbital

†Available in Canada only.

Lab Test Interference: False increase: Sulfobromophthalein

Treatment of Overdose: Gastric lavage, activated charcoal, warm the patient; monitor VS, I&O; hemodialysis may be effective; roll patient from side to side q 30 min

Administration
- Insomnia: *Adult:* PO 100 mg hs
- Available forms: Caps 50, 100 mg; elix 18.2 mg/5 mL; rectal supp 30, 60, 120, 200 mg; IM inj, IV 50 mg/mL

Perphenazine

PHENAZINE, TRILAFON
(per-feń-a-zeen) (Chapter 4)

Functional classifications: Antipsychotic, neuroleptic
Chemical classifications: Phenothiazine, piperidine
FDA pregnancy category: C

Indications: Psychotic disorders, nausea, vomiting

Contraindications: Hypersensitivity, blood dyscrasias, coma, child <12 yr, brain damage, bone marrow depression, adynamic ileus
Cautious use: Lactation, seizure disorders, hypertension, hepatic disease, cardiac disease, glaucoma, renal impairment, ECT

Pharmacologic Effects: Antipsychotic drugs produce a neuroleptic effect characterized by sedation, emotional quieting, psychomotor slowing, and affective indifference; exact mode of action is not fully understood; antipsychotics primarily block dopamine D_2 receptors in the basal ganglia, hypothalamus, limbic system, brain stem, and medulla; antipsychotics are also thought to depress certain components of the reticular activating system that partially control body temperature, wakefulness, vasomotor tone, emesis, and hormonal balance; additionally, antipsychotics have significant anticholinergic and alpha-adrenergic blocking effects; antiemetic effect r/t inhibition of chemoreceptor trigger zone

Pharmacokinetics: PO onset erratic, peak 2-4 hr; IM onset 10 min, peak 1-2 hr, duration 6 hr, occassionally 12-24 hr; metabolized by liver, excreted in urine, crosses placenta, enters breast milk; therapeutic plasma levels 0.8-1.2 ng/mL

Side Effects: *CNS:* Parkinsonism, akathisias, dystonias, tardive dyskinesia, oculogyric crisis; *Peripheral:* Blurred vision (cycloplegia or paralysis of accommodation), ocular pain, photophobia, mydriasis, impaired vision; intolerance of extreme heat or cold, possible heat stroke or fatal hyperthermia; nasal congestion, wheezing, dyspnea; **hypotension, especially orthostatic,** leading to dizziness, syncope; **tachycardia,** irregular pulse, arrhythmias; **dry mouth, constipation,** jaundice, abdominal pain; urinary retention, urinary hesitancy, galactorrhea, gynecomastia, impaired ejaculation, amenorrhea

Interactions
- Alcohol and other CNS depressants (barbiturates, antihistamines, antianxiety or antidepressant drugs): Increased CNS depression, increased risk of EPSEs
- Amphetamines: Possible decreased antipsychotic effect
- Antacids (magnesium and aluminum products): Possible decreased antipsychotic effect
- Anticholinergics (atropine, H_1-type antihistamines, antidepressants, etc): Increased risk of excessive atropine-like side effects or toxic effects
- Benztropine: Possible decreased antipsychotic effect, increased risk of severity of peripheral anticholinergic side effects
- Diazoxide: Possible severe hyperglycemia, prediabetic coma
- Guanethidine: Poor control of hypertension by guanethidine
- Hypoglycemia drugs (insulin, oral hypoglycemia agents): Poor diabetic control
- Lithium: Poor control of psychosis with combined therapy; can mask lithium toxicity; neurotoxicity with confusion, delirium, seizures, encephalopathy
- Meperidine, morphine: Increased risk of severe CNS depression, respiratory depression, hypotension
- Propranolol: Increased pharmacologic effects of either drug

Implications

Assess

- Establish baseline VS, laboratory values, to assess side effects, allergic or hypersensitivity reactions
- Assess physiologic and psychologic status before therapy to determine needs and evaluate progress
- Assess for early stages of tardive dyskinesia by use of Abnormal Involuntary Movement Scale
- Identify concurrent symptoms that may be aggravated by antipsychotics, e.g., glaucoma, diabetes

Planning/Implementation

- Ensure that drug has been taken; check mouth for "cheeking"
- If giving liquid, use only water, fruit juices, and the like; do not use caffeinated drinks or tea; take drug with food to minimize GI upset; give IM injections in lateral thigh
- Keep patient quiet after injection, to prevent falls associated with postural hypotension
- For dry mouth, give chewing gum, hard candies, lip balm; monitor urinary output; check for bladder distention in inactive patients, older men, and patients on high doses
- Assist with ambulation, if patient is having blurred vision; dim room lights for photosensitivity
- Ensure safety with hypotension; sit on side of bed before rising, head-low position for dizziness, avoid hot showers, wear elastic stockings
- Check B/P (supine, sitting, standing) and pulse before and after each dose when possible; observe for side effects
- Monitor body temperature for indications of neuroleptic malignant syndrome, e.g., muscle rigidity, fever, depressed neurologic status; ensure adequate hydration, nutrition, and ventilation
- Protect patient from exposure to extreme heat or cold
- Recognize impending hypersensitivity: pruritus or jaundice with hepatitis; flu or coldlike symptoms, evidence of bleeding with blood dyscrasia
- Observe for involuntary movements

Teaching

- About benefits and potential harm of antipsychotic drugs; weigh need to know against causing apprehension
- To comply with drug treatment
- To avoid activities requiring clear vision for a few weeks after treatment starts; to report eye pain immediately
- About the importance of exercise, fluids, and fiber in diet
- To watch for symptoms of heart failure, e.g., weight gain, dyspnea, distended neck veins, tachycardia
- Possible male sexual performance failure; suggest relaxed, stress-free environment
- To avoid conception; women should practice effective contraception; phenothiazines may cause false positive result in pregnancy tests
- To avoid exposure to sunlight; keep skin covered but with temperature-appropriate clothing
- That patient cannot become addicted to antipsychotic drugs

Evaluate

- Whether patient follows prescribed regimen, takes medications as ordered
- Avoids injury
- Verbalizes reduced anxiety
- Experiences minimal or no adverse responses
- Uses appropriate interventions to minimize side effects
- Achieves improved mental status

Lab Test Interferences

- Increase: Liver function tests, cardiac enzyme levels, cholesterol, blood glucose, prolactin, bilirubin, cholinesterase, I-131 levels
- Decrease: Hormones (blood, urine)
- False positive: Pregnancy tests, PKU

Treatment of Overdose: Lavage, if orally ingested; provide an airway; do not induce vomiting, control EPSEs and hypotension

Administration

- Psychiatric indications: Psychiatric use in hospitalized patients: *Adults:* PO 8-16 bid-qid, gradually increased to desired dose, not to exceed 64 mg/day; IM 5 mg q6h, not to exceed 30 mg/day; *child >12 yr;* PO 8 mg in divided doses; *geriatric:* half to one third of adult dose
- Nonhospitalized patients: *Adult:* PO 4-8 mg tid; IM 5 mg q6h
- Do not mix concentrate with liquids containing caffeine, tannics, or pectinates

P

- Available forms include: Tabs 2, 4, 8, 16; conc 16 mg/5 mL; inj IM 5 mg/mL

Phenacemide*

PHENURONE
(fe-naś-e-mide) (Chapter 7)

Functional classification: Antiepileptic
Chemical classification: Acetylurea derivative
FDA pregnancy category: D

Indications: Refractory psychomotor seizures

Contraindications: Hypersensitivity, personality disorders
Cautious use: Hepatic or renal disease; use with other antiepileptics, blood dyscrasias, child <5 yr

Pharmacologic Effect: Increases seizure threshold

Pharmacokinetics: Metabolized by liver, excreted by kidneys, half-life not known

Side Effects: *CNS:* **Drowsiness** (4%), dizziness, insomnia, paresthesias, **psychiatric** (17%), depression, suicidal tendencies, aggression, headache; *Peripheral:* **Anorexia** (5%), weight loss, hepatitis, jaundice, nausea, nephritis, albuminuria, blood dyscrasias (primarily leukopenia) (2%), **rash** (5%), agranulocytosis, leukopenia, aplastic anemia

Interactions: Extreme caution if used with other antiepileptics, particularly ethotoin

Implications
Assess
- Blood, **liver function,** renal function studies
- Drug level: Drug is extremely toxic

Planning/Implementation
- Food decreases GI symptoms

Teaching
- All aspects of drug therapy: Action, dosage, side effects
- To notify physician when sore throat, fever, rash, fatigue, bleeding, bruising occur (blood dyscrasia)

Evaluate
- Mental status: Psychosis not uncommon
- Liver function, renal function
- Blood dyscrasias: Fever, sore throat, bruising, rash, jaundice

Treatment of Overdose: *Symptoms:* Excitement or mania, followed by drowsiness, ataxia, and coma; *Treatment:* Emesis, lavage, supportive care, careful evaluation of liver and kidney function

Administration
Adult: PO 250-500 mg tid, may increase by 500 mg/wk, not to exceed 5 g/day, usual maintenance dose 2-3 g/day; *child 5-10 yr:* half of adult dose at same intervals
- Available forms include: Tabs 500 mg

*Infrequently used.

Phenelzine Sulfate

NARDIL
(feń-el-zeen) (Chapter 5)

Functional classifications: Antidepressant, MAOI
Chemical classification: Hydrazine
FDA pregnancy category: C

Indications: Depression in treatment-resistant patients, patients with mixed anxiety-depression
Unlabeled uses: Bulimia, cocaine deterrent

Contraindications: Hypersensitivity to MAOIs, elderly patients (>60 yr), children <16 yr, hypertension, CHF, severe hepatic disease, pheochromocytoma, severe renal disease, severe cardiac disease
Cautious use: Suicidal patients, convulsive disorders, hyperactivity, diabetes mellitus, hypomania, agitation, hyperthyroidism

Pharmacologic Effect: Inhibits monoamine oxidase, thus increasing the concentration of endogenous epinephrine, norepinephrine, serotonin, dopamine in storage sites in CNS

Pharmacokinetics: Metabolized by liver, excreted by kidneys, half-life not established

Side Effects: *CNS:* **Dizziness,** drowsiness, confusion, **headache,** anxiety, **tremors,** stimulation, weakness, **hyper-**

reflexia, mania, **insomnia, fatigue,** weight gain; *Peripheral:* Change in libido; **constipation, dry mouth,** nausea and vomiting, **anorexia,** diarrhea, rash, flushing, increased perspiration, jaundice, **orthostatic hypotension, hypertension, arrhythmias,** hypertensive crisis, blurred vision

Interactions
- Drug-drug: *Sympathomimetics (indirect or mixed acting):* Severe headache, hypertension, hyperpyrexia, and hypertensive crisis; sympathomimetic drugs include amphetamines; levodopa; tryptophan; methylphenidate; OTC compounds containing phenylpropanolamine, ephedrine, and pseudoephedrine; TCAs, other MAOIs, guanethidine, methyldopa, guanadrel, reserpine; *Anticholingeric drugs:* Additive effect; *Antihypertensives (diuretics, beta blockers, hydralazine, nitroglycerin, prazosin):* Hypotension
- Drug-food: *Tyramine-rich foods* (see text): Hypertensive crisis

Implications
Assess
- B/P (lying, standing), pulse; if systolic B/P drops 20 mm Hg, withhold drug, notify physician
- Blood studies: CBC, leukocyte counts, cardiac enzyme levels (if patient is receiving long-term therapy)
- Hepatic studies: Hepatotoxic effects may occur

Planning/Implementation
- Increased fluids, bulk in diet, if constipation, urinary retention occur
- With food or milk for GI symptoms
- Sugarless gum, hard candies, or frequent sips of water for dry mouth
- Phentolamine for severe hypertension
- Storage in tight container in cool environment
- Assistance with ambulation during beginning of therapy because drowsiness or dizziness occurs
- Safety measures, including side rails
- Checking to see that PO medication is swallowed

Teaching
- That therapeutic effects may take 1-4 wk
- To avoid driving or other activities that require alertness
- To avoid ingesting alcohol and CNS depressants, or OTC medications for cold, weight loss, hay fever, cough
- Not to discontinue medication abruptly after long-term use
- To avoid high-tyramine foods, e.g., cheese (aged), caviar, dried fish, game meat, beer, wine, pickled products, liver, raisins, bananas, figs, avocados, meat tenderizers, chocolate, yogurt, increased caffeine, soy sauce
- Report headache, palpitations, neck stiffness

Evaluate
- Toxic effects: Increased headache, palpitations; discontinue drug immediately
- Mental status
- Urinary retention, constipation
- Withdrawal symptoms, e.g., headache, nausea, vomiting, muscle pain, weakness

Treatment of Overdose: Lavage, activated charcoal, monitor electrolyte levels, VS, treat hypotension

Administration
Adult: PO 15 mg tid, may increase to 60 mg/day, dose should be reduced to 15 mg/day, not to exceed 90 mg/day
- Available forms include: Tabs 15 mg

Phenobarbital, Phenobarbital Sodium

BARBITA, LUMINAL SODIUM, SOLFOTON
(fee-noe-baŕ̸-bi-tal) (Chapter 7)

Functional classification: Antiepileptic (long-acting)
Chemical classification: Barbiturate
Controlled substance schedule IV
FDA pregnancy category: D

Indications: Tonic-clonic, simple partial, complex partial, status epilepticus

Contraindications: Hypersensitivity to barbiturates, porphyria, hepatic disease, respiratory disease, nephritis, diabetes mellitus, elderly, lactation, barbiturate addiction

Cautious use: Anemia, cardiac disease, children, fever, hyperthyroidism

Pharmacologic Effects: Decreases impulse transmission, works at level of thalamus, increases seizure threshold at cerebral cortex level; therapeutic serum level 15-40 μg/mL

Pharmacokinetics: PO onset 20-60 min, peak 8-12 hr, duration 10-12 hr, metabolized by liver, excreted by kidneys, crosses placenta, excreted in breast milk, half-life 53-118 hr

Side Effects: *CNS:* **Somnolence, drowsiness,** lethargy, hangover headache, flushing, hallucinations, coma; *Peripheral:* **Nausea, vomiting,** hypoventilation, bradycardia, hypotension, rash, urticaria, angioedema, local pain, swelling, necrosis, thrombophlebitis, blood dyscrasias

Interactions
- CNS depressants, other antiepileptics: Drugs that increase the effects of barbiturates (toxic effects)
- Acetaminophen, digitoxin, oral anticoagulants, oral contraceptives, TCAs, possibly phenytoin: Drugs whose effects are decreased by barbiturates

Implications
Assess
- Blood studies, liver function tests during long-term therapy
- Check VS, neurologic values regularly

Planning/Implementation
- Describe seizure accurately
- Offer consistent emotional support
- Monitor for early signs of toxic effects (slurred speech, ataxia, respiratory and CNS depression)

Teaching
- To report any side effects or adverse reactions
- To avoid driving or operating dangerous equipment
- To change position slowly
- To take drugs as prescribed
- Not to discontinue drug abruptly
- To wear MedicAlert identification bracelet
- To consult physician before becoming pregnant

Evaluate
- Mental status
- Respiratory depression
- Blood dyscrasias: Fever, sore throat, bruising, rash, jaundice

Treatment of Overdose: 1 g can cause serious poisoning in an adult; 2-10 g can be fatal. Toxic effects can be confused with drunkenness. Emesis, gastric lavage, if conscious; 30 g activated charcoal, maintain airway, good nursing care to prevent pneumonia

Administration
- Seizures: *Adult:* PO 50-100 mg bid-tid or total dose hs; *child:* PO 3-5 mg/kg/day in 3 divided doses; may be given as single dose hs
- Status epilepticus: *Adult:* IV 200-300 mg, repeat in 6 hr if necessary, run no faster than 50 mg/min, may give up to 20 mg/kg; *child:* IV 15-20 mg/kg over 10-15 min, then 6 mg/kg q 20 min prn, maximum dose 40 mg/kg/24 hr, run no faster then 50 mg/min
- Available forms: Caps 16 mg; elix 15, 20 mg/5 mL; tabs 8, 16, 32, 65, 100 mg; inj 30, 60, 65, 130 mg/mL

Phensuximide*

MILONTIN
(fen-sux́-i-mide) (Chapter 7)

Functional classification: Antiepileptic
Chemical classification: Succinimide
FDA pregnancy category: D

Indications: Absence seizures (petit mal) refractory to other drugs

Contraindications: Hypersensitivity to succinimide derivatives
Cautious use: Lactation, hepatic or renal disease

Pharmacologic Effect: Inhibits spike and wave formation in absence seizures, depresses motor cortex

Pharmacokinetics: PO peak 1-4 hr, metabolized by liver, excreted by kidneys, half-life 4 hr

Side Effects: *CNS:* **Drowsiness, dizziness, fatigue, euphoria, lethargy;** anxiety, aggressiveness, irritability, depression, insomnia; *Peripheral:* **Nausea, vomiting,** heartburn, **anorexia, diarrhea,**

*Infrequently used.

abdominal pain, cramps, constipation, vaginal bleeding, hematuria, renal damage, urticaria, pruritic erythema, hirsutism, Stevens-Johnson syndrome, myopia, gum hypertrophy, tongue swelling, blurred vision, agranulocytosis, aplastic anemia, thrombocytopenia, leukocytosis, eosinophilia, pancytopenia (some blood dyscrasias have been fatal); urinary frequency

Interactions
- TCAs: Antagonist effect (imipramine, doxepin); also, lower seizure threshold
- Estrogens: Decreased effects of oral contraceptives
- CNS depressants: Increased CNS depression

Implications
Assess
- Renal studies: Urinalysis; BUN, urine creatinine levels
- Blood studies: CBC, hematocrit, hemoglobin level, reticulocyte counts
- Hepatic studies: AST, ALT, bilirubin and creatinine levels
- Drug levels during initial treatment

Planning/Implementation
- With food or milk, to decease GI symptoms
- Hard candies, frequent rinsing of mouth and gums, for dry mouth
- Assistance with ambulation during early part of treatment; dizziness occurs

Teaching
- To carry identification card or MedicAlert bracelet, stating drugs taken, condition, physician's name and phone number
- To avoid driving and other activities that require alertness
- To avoid ingestion of alcohol and CNS depressants, because increased sedation may occur
- Not to discontinue medication suddenly after long-term use

Evaluate
- Therapeutic response: Decreased seizure activity; document on patient's chart
- Mental status
- Allergic reaction: Red raised rash, exfoliative dermatitis; if these occur, drug should be discontinued; blood dyscrasias: fever, sore throat, bruising, rash, jaundice
- Toxic effects: Bone marrow depression, lupus have been reported

Administration
Adult and child: PO 500 mg-1 g bid or tid
- Available forms include: Caps 500 mg

Phenytoin, Phenytoin Sodium Extended, Phenytoin Sodium Prompt

DILANTIN, DILANTIN CAPSULES, DIPHENYLAN
(feń-i-toy-in) (Chapter 7)

Functional classification: Anticonvulsant
Chemical classification: Hydantoin
FDA pregnancy category: D

Indications: Drug of choice for tonic-clonic seizures; status epilepticus, psychomotor seizures; simple partial seizures

Contraindications: Hypersensitivity, psychiatric disease, sinus bradycardia (IV use), lactation
Cautious use: Allergies, hepatic or renal disease, hypotension, myocardial insufficiency

Pharmacologic Effect: Inhibits spread of seizure activity in motor cortex; therapeutic serum levels, 10-20 μg/mL

Pharmacokinetics: PO slowly absorbed, peak 4-12 hr (extended), 1½-3 hr (prompt); duration 5 hr; time to steady-state, 7-10 days; average half-life 22 hr, but dose dependent and has little clinical importance, metabolized by liver, excreted by kidneys

Side Effects: *CNS:* Nystagmus, ataxia, drowsiness, dizziness, insomnia, paresthesias, depression, suicidal tendencies, aggression, headache; *Peripheral:* **Nausea, vomiting, constipation,** anorexia, weight loss, hepatitis, jaundice, nephritis, albuminuria, rash, gingival hyperplasia, agranulocytosis, leukopenia, aplastic anemia

P

Interactions

- Allopurinol, cimetidine, diazepam, disulfiram, alcohol (acute ingestion) phenacemide, succinimides, valproic acid, others: Increased effect of hydantoins
- Barbiturates, carbamazepine, alcohol (chronic use) theophylline, antacids, dietary calcium: Decreased effects of hydantoins
- Corticosteroids, dicumarol, digitoxin, doxycycline, haloperidol, methadone, oral contraceptives, dopamine, furosemide, levodopa: Decreased effects of these drugs

Implications

Assess

- Blood studies: CBC, platelet count q mo until stabilized, discontinue drug, if marked depression of the blood cell count occurs

Planning/Implementation

- Observe for gingival hyperplasia
- Describe seizures accurately

Teaching

- All aspects of drug administration: Route, action, dose
- To report side effects
- To avoid driving or operating dangerous equipment
- To practice good oral hygiene
- Not to discontinue abruptly
- To wear MedicAlert identification bracelet

Evaluate

- Mental status
- Respiratory depression
- Blood dyscrasias: Fever, sore throat, bruising, rash, jaundice

Treatment of Overdose: Mean lethal dose in adults is thought to be 2-5 g; initial symptoms are nystagmus, ataxia; death is due to respiratory and circulatory depression; lavage, emesis, activated charcoal

Administration

- Seizures: *Adult:* IV loading dose 10-15 mg/kg, run at 50 mg/min; PO loading dose 1 g in 3 divided doses, then after 24 hr, 300 mg/day (extended) or divided tid (prompt); *child:* IV 15-20 mg/kg, 1-3mg/kg/min; PO 4-8 mg/kg/day in divided doses
- Use normal saline to avoid precipitation
- Available forms include: Suspension 30, 125 mg/5 mL; tabs, chewable 50 mg; inj 50 mg/mL; caps ext-rel 30, 100 mg; caps, prompt 30, 100 mg

Pimozide

ORAP

(pí-moe-zide) (Chapters 4, 15, 16)

Functional classifications: Antipsychotic, neuroleptic

Chemical classification: Diphenylbutylpiperidine

FDA pregnancy category: C

Indications: Tourette's syndrome

Contraindications: Hypersensitivity, CNS depression, coma, tics other than those of Tourette's syndrome, cardiac arrhythmias, long QT interval

Cautious use: Child <12 yr, lactation, seizure disorders, hypertension, hepatic or renal disease, cardiac disease, hypokalemia

Pharmacologic Effects: Blocks CNS dopamine D_2 receptors

Pharmacokinetics: PO peak 6-8 hr; metabolized by liver, excreted in urine, half-life 55 hr

Side Effects: *CNS:* Parkinsonism, akathisias, dystonias, tardive dyskinesia, oculogyric crisis; *Peripheral:* Blurred vision (cycloplegia or paralysis of accommodation), ocular pain, photophobia, mydriasis, impaired vision; intolerance of extreme heat or cold, possible heat stroke or fatal hyperthermia; nasal congestion, wheezing, dyspnea; **hypotension, especially orthostatic,** leading to dizziness, syncope; **tachycardia,** irregular pulse, arrhythmias; **dry mouth, constipation,** jaundice, abdominal pain; urinary frequency, galactorrhea, gynecomastia, impaired ejaculation, amenorrhea; prolonged QT interval, sudden death has occurred at doses >20 mg/day

Interactions

- Anticonvulsants: Decreased convulsive threshold
- Antiarrhythmics, phenothiazines: Increased QT interval

- Increased CNS depression: Alcohol and other CNS depressants
- Other antipsychotics: Increased EPSEs

Implications

Assess

- For prolonged QT interval
- Establish baseline VS, laboratory values, to assess side effects, allergic or hypersensitivity reactions
- Physiologic and psychologic status before therapy, to determine needs and evaluate progress
- For early stages of tardive dyskinesia by using Abnormal Involuntary Movement Scale
- Identify concurrent symptoms that may be aggravated by antipsychotics, e.g., glaucoma, diabetes

Planning/Implementation

- Ensure that drug has been taken; check mouth for "cheeking"
- Keep patient quiet after injection, to prevent falls associated with postural hypotension
- For dry mouth, give chewing gum, hard candies, lip balm, monitor urinary output; check for bladder distention in inactive patients, older men, and patients on high doses
- Assist with ambulation, if patient is having blurred vision; dim room lights for photosensitivity
- Ensure safety with hypotension; sit on side of bed before rising, head-low position for dizziness, avoid hot showers, wear elastic stockings
- Check B/P (supine, sitting, standing) and pulse before and after each dose when possible; observe for side effects
- Monitor body temperature for indications of neuroleptic malignant syndrome, e.g., muscle rigidity, fever, depressed neurologic status; ensure adequate hydration, nutrition, and ventilation
- Protect patient from exposure to extreme heat or cold
- Recognize impending hypersensitivity to pruritus or jaundice with hepatitis; flu or coldlike symptoms, evidence of bleeding with blood dyscrasia
- Observe for involuntary movements

Teaching

- To comply with drug treatment
- To avoid activities requiring clear vision for a few weeks after treatment starts; to report eye pain immediately
- About the importance of exercise, fluids, and fiber in diet
- To watch for symptoms of heart failure, e.g., weight gain, dyspnea, distended neck veins, tachycardia
- Possible male sexual performance failure; suggest relaxed, stress-free environment
- To avoid conception; women should practice effective contraception
- To avoid exposure to sunlight; keep skin covered but with temperature-appropriate clothing
- That they cannot become addicted to antipsychotic drugs

Evaluate

- Whether patient follows prescribed regimen, takes medications as ordered
- Avoids injury; reports dizziness or need for assistance
- Verbalizes reduced anxiety
- Experiences minimal or no adverse responses
- Uses appropriate interventions to minimize side effects
- Achieves improved mental status

Treatment of Overdose: Lavage, if orally ingested; provide an airway; monitor ECG; do not induce vomiting; *do not* use epinephrine for hypotension; observe patient for at least 4 days

Administration

Adult and child >12 yr: PO 1-2 mg qd in divided doses; increase dose qod, if needed; maintenance <0.2 mg/kg/day or 10 mg/day, whichever is less, not to exceed 0.2 mg/kg/day or 10 mg/day

- Available forms include: Tabs 2 mg

Prazepam

CENTRAX
(prá-ze-pam) (Chapter 6)

Functional classification: Antianxiety
Chemical classification: Benzodiazepine
Controlled substance schedule IV
FDA pregnancy category: D

Indications: Anxiety

Contraindications: Hypersensitivity, narrow-angle glaucoma, psychosis, children <18 yr

Pharmacologic Effects: Depresses CNS, including limbic and reticular areas, by potentiating GABA inhibitory neurotransmitters

Pharmacokinetics: Speed of onset: Slow PO peak levels 6 hr, half-life 30-100 hr, metabolized by liver, excreted in urine

Side Effects: *CNS:* Dizziness, drowsiness are main effects; see diazepam for other side effects; *Peripheral:* GI effects, i.e., dry mouth, nausea, vomiting; blurred vision, orthostatic hypotension; see diazepam for other side effects

Interactions
- Valproic acid: Increased effect of prazepam
- CNS depressants, alcohol, disulfiram: Increased CNS depression

Implications
Assess
- B/P

Planning/Implementation
- Give with food or milk to decrease GI upset
- Provide gum, hard candies for dry mouth
- Maintain safety

Teaching
- To avoid driving
- To avoid alcohol
- To check with clinician before taking OTC drugs

Evaluate
- Mental status
- Therapeutic response: Level of anxiety

Lab Test Interference
- Increase: AST, ALT, serum bilirubin level, LDH
- Decrease: RAIU
- False increase: 17-OHCS

Treatment of Overdose: Lavage, monitor VS, provide supportive care as indicated; there are no recorded deaths with benzodiazepines alone; death occurs when these drugs are mixed with other CNS depressants

Administration
Adult: PO 30 mg/day in divided doses, range is 20-60 mg/day; *geriatric:* 10-15 mg/day in divided doses, can be given as single dose hs
- Available forms: Caps 5, 10, 20 mg; tabs 10 mg

Primidone

MYSOLINE, SERTAN†
(prí-mi-done) (Chapter 7)

Functional classification: Antiepileptic
Chemical classification: Barbiturate derivative
FDA pregnancy category: D

Indications: Generalized tonic-clonic, complex partial seizures

Contraindications: Hypersensitivity, porphyria
Cautious use: Lactation

Pharmacologic Effects: Raises seizure threshold; metabolites (phenobaritol is one) have anticonvulsant properties; therapeutic serum level 5-12 μg/mL

Pharmacokinetics: PO peak 3 hr; excreted in breast milk; half-life 3-12 hr, but active metabolites are longer, i.e., phenylethylmalonamide (PEMA) (24-48 hr); phenobarbital (53-118 hr)

Side Effects: *CNS:* Ataxia, vertigo, fatigue, drowsiness, nystagmus; *Peripheral:* **Nausea, vomiting, anorexia; rash,** alopecia, lupuslike syndrome, diplopia, nystagmus, impotence, thrombocytopenia, leukopenia, megaloblastic anemia

Interactions
- Alcohol, heparin, carbamazepine, CNS depressants, isoniazid, phenytoin, phenobarbital: Increased levels of primidone

†Available in Canada only.

- Acetazolamide: Decreased effect of primidone

Implications
Assess
- Establish baseline data

Planning/Implementation
- Monitor for early signs of toxic effects

Teaching
- All aspects of drug administration: action, route, dose
- Not to withdraw drug quickly; withdrawal symptoms may occur
- Not to drive
- Notify physician if rash or symptoms of blood dyscrasia occur
- Wear MedicAlert identification bracelet

Evaluate
- Mental status
- Respiratory depression
- Blood dyscrasias: Fever, sore throat, bruising, rash, jaundice

Administration
Adult and child >8 yr: Day 1-3, 100-125 mg hs; day 4-6, 100-125 mg bid; day 7-9, 100-125 mg tid; day 10 and maintenance, 250 mg tid or qid; do not exceed 500 mg/day; *child <8 yr:* Day 1-3, 50 mg hs; day 4-6, 50 mg bid; day 7-9, 100 mg bid; day 10 and maintenance, 125-250 mg tid or 10-25 mg/kg/day
- Available forms include: Tabs 50, 250 mg; susp 250 mg/5 mL

Procyclidine
KEMADRIN
(proe-sýé-kli-deen)

Functional classification: Anticholinergic
Chemical classification: Tertiary amine
FDA pregnancy category: C

Indications: Parkinsonism, EPSEs

Contraindications: Hypersensitivity, narrow-angle glaucoma, duodenal obstruction, peptic ulcer, prostatic hypertrophy, myasthenia gravis, megacolon

Pharmacologic Effects: Blocks cholinergic receptors; may inhibit the reuptake and storage of dopamine

Pharmacokinetics: Peak 1.1-2 hr, half-life 11.5-12.6 hr; little pharmacokinetic information is known

Side Effects: *CNS:* Depression develops in 19% to 30% of patients; disorientation, confusion, memory loss, hallucinations, psychoses, agitation, delusions, nervousness; *Peripheral:* **Tachycardia,** palpitations, hypotension, **orthostatic hypotension, dry mouth,** nausea, vomiting, constipation, paralytic ileus, **blurred vision,** mydriasis, diplopia, urinary retention and hesitancy, elevated temperature

Interactions
- Amantadine: Increased anticholinergic effect
- Digoxin: Increased digoxin serum levels
- Haloperidol: Worsening of schizophrenia, decreased haloperidol serum levels
- Levodopa: Possible reduction of levodopa efficacy
- Phenothiazines: Increased anticholinergic effect, decreased antipsychotic effect

Implications
Assess
- VS, B/P
- For glaucoma
- Mental status

Planning/Implementation
- Provide instructions for anticholinergic responses, i.e., dry mouth, constipation, urinary hesitancy, decreased sweating

Teaching
- Give with meals
- May cause drowsiness, blurred vision, dizziness: emphasize safety
- Avoid alcohol and other CNS depressants
- For rapid or pounding heartbeat, notify physician
- Use caution in hot weather

Evaluate
- EPSE improvement
- For adverse effects
- Mental status: Confusion, delirium, memory

Treatment of Overdose: Emesis, lavage, activated charcoal, treat respiratory depression, hyperpyrexia

Administration
- EPSE: *Adult:* PO 2.5 mg tid, up to 10-20 mg/day
- Available form: Tabs 5mg

P

Promazine*

PROMANYL,† PROZINE, SPARINE
(proé-ma-zeen) (Chapter 4)

Functional classification: Antipsychotic
Chemical classification: Aliphatic phenothiazine
FDA pregnancy category: C

Indications: Psychosis; *infrequently used* as antipsychotic

Contraindications: Hypersensitivity, blood dyscrasias, coma, children <12 yr, bone marrow depression; see chlorpromazine

Pharmacologic Effects: Provides antipsychotic effect by antagonizing dopamine receptors; also antiadrenergic, anticholinergic, and antiemetic; see chlorpromazine for more extensive explanation

Pharmacokinetics: PO peak level 2-4 hr; IM onset 15 min, peak level 1 hr, duration 4-6 hr; metabolized by liver, excreted in urine, crosses placenta, enters breast milk

Side Effects: *CNS:* See chlorpromazine; *Peripheral:* See chlorpromazine

Interactions: See chlorpromazine

Implications: See chlorpromazine

Lab Test Interference: See chlorpromazine

Treatment of Overdose: Do *not* induce vomiting; lavage for oral dose; maintain airway and provide supportive care prn

Administration

- Psychosis: *Adult:* PO 10-200 mg q 4-6 hr; range 40-1200 mg/day; however, it is recommended dose not exceed 1000 mg/day; *severe agitation:* 50-150 mg IM; if not effective in 30 min, give additional doses up to total dose of 300 mg; *child* >12 yr: PO 10-25 mg q4-6 hr
- Available forms: Tabs 25, 50, 100 mg; inj IM, IV, 25, 50 mg/mL

*Infrequently used.
†Available in Canada only.

Propranolol HCl

INDERAL
(proe-prań-oh-lole) (Chapter 6)

Functional classifications: Antihypertensive, antianginal
Chemical classification: Beta-adrenergic blocker
FDA pregnancy category: C

Indications: Chronic stable angina pectoris, prophylaxis of angina pain; *unapproved use* for "stage fright" (use is controversial), anxiety, acute panic

Contraindications: Hypersensitivity to this drug, cardiac failure, cardiogenic shock, second- or third-degree heart block, asthma, sinus bradycardia

Cautious use: Diabetes mellitus, pheochromocytoma, hypotension, renal disease, lactation, CHF, hyperthyroidism, cardiopulmonary distress, peripheral vascular disease

Pharmacologic Effects: Nonselective beta blockers; reduces major symptoms of anxiety, e.g., tachycardia, palpitations, muscle tremors

Pharmacokinetics: PO onset 30 min, peak 1-1½ hr, duration 6 hr; IV onset 2 min, peak 15 min, duration 3-6 hr; half-life 3-5 hr, metabolized by liver, crosses placenta and blood-brain barrier, excreted in breast milk

Side Effects: *CNS:* Depression, hallucinations, dizziness, fatigue, lethargy, paresthesias; *Peripheral:* Dyspnea, respiratory dysfunction, bronchospasm; **bradycardia, hypotension,** CHF, palpitations, agranulocytosis, thrombocytopenia, nausea, vomiting, diarrhea, colitis, constipation, cramps, dry mouth, rash, pruritus, fever, sore throat, laryngospasm

Interactions

- Verapamil, disopyramide: Increased propranolol effect
- Reserpine: Increased effects
- Norepinephrine, isoproterenol, barbiturates, rifampin, dopamine: Reduced beta-blocking effects
- Cimetidine, morphine: Increased beta-blocking effect

- Quinidine, haloperidol: Increased hypotension

Implications
Assess
- B/P, pulse, respirations during beginning of therapy

Teaching
- That drug may be taken before stressful activity, e.g., exercise, sexual activity
- To avoid hazardous activities, if dizziness occurs
- Emphasize patient compliance with complete medical regimen
- To make position changes slowly, to prevent fainting

Evaluate
- Headache, light-headedness, decreased B/P; may indicate need for decreased dosage

Administration
Adult: Dose for stage fright is low, i.e., 10 mg before appearances
- Dysrythmia, hypertension, angina, myocardial infarction, pheochromocytoma, migraines: See *PDR*
- Available forms include: Caps ext-rel 60, 80, 120, 160 mg; tabs 10, 20, 40, 60, 80, 90 mg; inj 1 mg/mL, oral solution 4, 8, 80 mg/mL

Protriptyline HCl

VIVACTIL
(proe-triṕ-te-leen) (Chapter 5)

Functional classification: TCA
Chemical classification: Dibenzocycloheptene, secondary amine
FDA pregnancy category: C

Indications: Depression

Contraindications: Hypersensitivity to TCAs, recovery phase of myocardial infarction, convulsive disorders, prostatic hypertrophy
Cautious use: Suicidal patients, severe depression, increased intraocular pressure, narrow-angle glaucoma, urinary retention, cardiac disease, hyperthyroidism, ECT, elective surgery, children, MAOI therapy

Pharmacologic Effect: Blocks reuptake of norepinephrine, serotonin into nerve endings, therapeutic serum levels 100-200 ng/mL

Pharmacokinetics: PO onset 15-30 min, peak 24-30 hr, duration 4-6 hr; therapeutic effect 2-3 wk; metabolized by liver, excreted by kidneys, crosses placenta, half-life 67-89 hr

Side Effects: *CNS:* **Sedation,** ataxia; confusion, delirium; *Peripheral:* **Blurred vision,** photophobia, increased intraocular pressure; decreased tearing, orthostatic hypotension, arrhythmias, tachycardia, palpitations, dry mouth, constipation, diarrhea, decreased sweating, **urinary retention, hesitancy**

Interactions
- Anticholinergic agents: Additive anticholinergic effects with atropine, antihistamines (H_1 blocker), antiparkinson drugs, antipsychotics, OTC cold and allergy drugs
- CNS depressants: Additive depressant effect
- Guanethidine, clonidine: Decreased antihypertensive effect
- MAOIs: Hypertensive crisis, atropine-like poisoning
- Oral contraceptives: Inhibits metabolism of TCAs
- Phenothiazines: May increase TCA serum level
- Quinidine: Additive effect, heart block possible
- Sympathomimetics: Potentiates sympathomimetic effects
- Thyroid preparations: Tachycardia, arrhythmias; may increase TCA effect

Implications
Assess
- Establish baseline data, to aid recognition of adverse responses to medication, e.g., liver enzyme levels, VS, renal function, mental status, speech patterns, affect, weight
- For signs of noncompliance, e.g., poor therapeutic response
- Observe for major symptoms of depression, e.g., apathy, sadness, sleep disturbances, hopelessness, guilt, decreased libido, spontaneous crying
- Review history for contraindicated conditions, e.g., glaucoma, CV disease, GI conditions, urologic conditions, seizures, pregnancy

Planning/Implementation
- Monitor for "cheeking" or hoarding; check drug dosage carefully, because a small overdose may cause toxic effects
- Monitor for suicidal ideations; suicidal thought content may increase as antidepressants begin to "energize" patient
- Monitor VS; if hypotension, tachycardia, or arrhythmias occur, withhold TCAs
- Give most TCAs in a single dose hs
- Observe for early signs of toxic effects, e.g., drowsiness, tachycardia, mydriasis, hypotension, agitation, vomiting, confusion, fever, restlessness, sweating
- If CNS overstimulation occurs, e.g., hypomania, delirium, discontinue drug

Teaching
- That these drugs may have faster onset (1 wk) than other TCAs
- To adhere to drug regimen
- To avoid OTC drugs, particularly those containing sympathomimetics or anticholinergics
- To avoid drugs listed in section on interactions
- About ways to deal with minor side effects, as follows: dry mouth, with hard candies, sips of water, mouth rinses; visual disturbances, with artificial tears, sunglasses, assistance with ambulation; constipation, with bulk-forming foods, increased fluids; urinary hesitancy, with adequate fluids, privacy; decreased perspiration, with appropriate clothing, avoidance of unnecessary exercise; orthostatic hypotension, with slow positional changes, avoidance of hot baths and showers; for drowsiness, take single dose hs with physician approval, avoid driving
- That abrupt discontinuance may result in cholinergic rebound, e.g., nausea, vomiting, insomnia, headache

Evaluate
- Desired therapeutic serum level
- Verbalize decrease in subjective symptoms
- Observe decrease in objective symptoms
- Minimal to no adverse drug effects
- Stable VS
- Less anxiety; sleep, talk, and feel better

Lab Test Interferences
- Increase: Serum bilirubin, blood glucose, alkaline phosphatase levels
- False increase: Urinary catecholamines
- Decrease: VMA, 5-HIAA

Treatment of Overdose: ECG monitoring, induce emesis, lavage, activated charcoal, administer anticonvulsant, treat anticholinergic effects, if needed

Administration

Adult: PO 15-40 mg/day in divided doses, may increase to 60 mg/day; *adolescent and geriatric:* 5 mg tid, increase gradually if needed; CV monitoring is necessary for elderly patient receiving dosages > 20 mg/day
- Available forms include: Tabs 5, 10 mg

Risperidone

RISPERDAL

(ris-peeŕ-i-dohn) (Chapter 4)

Functional classification: Antipsychotic, neuroleptic, serotonin/dopamine antagonist

Chemical classification: Benzisoxazole

FDA pregnancy category: C

Indications: The management and manifestations of psychotic disorders

Contraindications: Hypersensitivity to risperidone

Cautious use: In the elderly, who are susceptible to orthostatic hypotension; patients with history of cardiovascular disease because risperidone is thought to lengthen the QT interval; history of seizures

Pharmacologic effects: Mechanism of action is unknown. Antipsychotic effect is thought to be related to risperidone's antagonism of both dopamine D-2 and serotonin 5HT-2 receptors. Theoretically, by blocking D-2 receptors in the mesolimbic area, positive symptoms respond, and by blocking 5HT-2 receptors in the cortex, negative symptoms respond

Pharmacokinetics: Risperidone is well absorbed. It is extensively metabolized in the liver to a major metabolite, 9-hydroxy-risperidone, which is equipotent. The half-life of both risperidone and its metabolite is about 24 hr. Protein binding is about 90% and 77%, respectively. Renal clearance is decreased, and the half-life is prolonged in elderly individuals

Side Effects: Risperidone does not antagonize muscarinic receptors so it causes few anticholinergic side effects. It also does not produce significant sedation (3%) (it has little affinity for histamine H_1 receptors); *CNS (at dose of <10 mg/day):* Orthostatic hypotension (blocks alpha-1 receptors); insomnia (26%), agitation (22%), headache (14%), anxiety (12%); EPSEs (17%) do occur but less so than with most antipsychotics; *Peripheral (at dose of <10 mg/day):* tachycardia (3%), rhinitis (10%), nausea (6%), constipation (7%); photosensitivity (1%); QT interval widening

Interactions
- Levodopa: Risperidone may antagonize the effect of levodopa
- Carbamazepine: Risperidone clearance increased so **decreased** serum levels
- Clozapine: chronic combined administration may decrease risperidone clearance and **increase** serum levels

Implications
Assess
- Establish baseline ECG, VS, laboratory values, and potential hypersensitivity to risperidone
- Physiologic and psychologic status before starting drug, to evaluate progress

Planning/Intervention
- Ensure drug is taken
- Be alert for hypotensive effect that could lead to falls
- If orthostatic hypotension occurs, have patient sit on side of bed before rising, place head in head-low position for dizziness, avoid hot showers, wear elastic stockings
- Check B/P, using orthostatic protocols
- Monitor temperature for potential NMS
- Observe for involuntary movements

Teaching
- Advise of risk of orthostatic hypotension, especially during period of initial dose titration
- Caution about operation of hazardous machinery
- Advise to notify health care provider if pregnant or intend to become pregnant; not to breast-feed while taking risperidone
- To notify care provider before taking OTC drugs (drug interaction?)
- Avoid exposure to ultraviolet light or sunlight (photosensitivity)

Evaluate
- Decrease in positive and/or negative symptoms
- Whether patient follows prescribed regimen, takes medications as ordered
- Avoids injury; reports dizziness
- Uses appropriate interventions to minimize side effects

Lab Test Interferences: None

Treatment of Overdose: No fatalities have been reported with risperidone overdose. In acute overdose establish and maintain airway and provide adequate oxygenation. Gastric lavage, activated charcoal, and laxatives are all reasonable approaches. Monitor ECG. There is no specific antidote to risperidone

Administration
- Psychosis: *Adult:* PO 1 mg twice daily on day 1; 2 mg twice daily on day 2; 3 mg twice daily on day 3 and thereafter. Further upward adjustments may be made at weekly intervals up to 16 mg/day. Typical daily dose is 4-6 mg/day; *elderly or debilitated patients:* Start with 0.5 mg twice a day. Increase by 0.5 mg twice daily. After reaching 1.5 mg twice daily, incremental changes should occur on weekly basis; *adolescents:* Not recommended for use with this age group
- When switching from another antipsychotic agent, minimize period of overlap
- Available forms: Tabs 1, 2, 3, 4 mg

R

Secobarbital, Secobarbital Sodium

SECONAL, SECOGEN SODIUM,† SECONAL SODIUM, SERAL†
(see-koe-bar̍-bi-tal) (Chapter 8)

Functional classifications: Sedative, hypnotic
Chemical classification: Barbitone
Controlled substance schedule II
FDA pregnancy category: D

Indications: Insomnia, status epilepticus, other uses

Contraindications: Hypersensitivity, respiratory depression, barbiturate dependency, liver impairment, blood dyscrasias

Pharmacologic Effects: Short-acting barbiturate, causing CNS depression in limbic and reticular areas

Pharmacokinetics: Onset 10-15 min, duration 3-4 hr, half-life 15-40 hr, metabolized by liver, excreted in urine; of barbiturates, secobarbital is the most lipophilic and has highest protein binding

Side Effects: *CNS:* Drowsiness, lethargy, hangover are primary CNS side effects; see phenobarbital for general barbiturate effects; *Peripheral:* Respiratory depression, laryngospasm, brochospasm, GI upset, blood dyscrasias; see phenobarbital

Interactions
- CNS depressants and alcohol: Additive CNS depression
- MAOIs: CNS depression
- Oral anticoagulants, corticosteroids: Decreased effects of these drugs
- Doxycycline: Decreased half-life

Implications
Assess
- B/P; blood studies, if indicated

Planning/Implementation
- IM in large muscles
- If given IV, have emergency equipment nearby
- Give ½ hr before bedtime
- Maintain safety

Teaching
- To avoid driving
- To avoid alcohol
- To avoid discontinuing drug abruptly (withdrawal)

Evaluate
- Therapeutic response, i.e., sleeping
- Mental status
- Dependence?
- Toxic effects

Lab Test Interference: False increase: Sulfobromophthalein

Treatment of Overdose: Gastric lavage, charcoal to absorb drug, monitor B/P, VS, I&O; warm patient; hemodialysis may be effective

Administration
- Insomnia: *Adult:* PO/IM 100-200 mg hs
- REC: 4-5 mg/kg
- Status epilepticus: *Adult and child:* IM/IV 5.5 mg/kg; repeat q3-4h; rate not to exceed 50 mg/15 sec
- Available forms: Caps 50, 100 mg; tabs 100 mg; inj IM, IV 50 mg/mL; rec inj 50 mg/mL

†Available in Canada only.

Selegiline HCl

ELDEPRYL
(sel-ee-gilĺ-ene) (Chapter 14)

Functional classification: Antiparkinson
Chemical classification: MAOI
FDA pregnancy category: C

Indications: Parkinsonism adjunct to carbidopa/levodopa

Contraindications: Hypersensitivity

Pharmacologic Effect: Inhibits monoamine oxidase type B, increasing dopamine

Pharmacokinetics: Rapidly absorbed, peak ½-2 hr; 3 active metabolites, including amphetamine (half-life 18 hr) and methamphetamine (half-life 20 hr); excreted in urine

Side Effects: *CNS:* Dizziness and lightheadedness (7%); parkinson-like symptoms; confusion (3%); hallucinations (3%); dyskinesias (2%); headache (2%), anxiety; *Peripheral:* **Nausea** (10%); abdominal pain (4%); dry mouth (3%); generalized aches, diarrhea, leg and back pain; urinary retention; weight loss

Interactions
- Meperidine: Fatalities have been reported with this combination

Implications
Assess
- B/P, respirations

Planning/Implementation
- Give with meals; limit protein taken with drug
- Keep doses <10 mg/day because monoamine oxidase inhibition may not be selective (may also inhibit monoamine oxidase type A, which could precipitate hypertensive crisis)

Teaching
- Patient may need to reduce levodopa
- Not to exceed 10 mg/day

Evaluate
- Therapeutic response: Decrease in symptoms of parkinsonism

Lab Test Interference
- False positive: Urine ketones, urine glucose
- False negative: Urine glucose
- False increase: Uric acid, urine protein
- Decrease: VMA

Treatment of Overdose: *Symptoms:* If selegiline nonselectively inhibits monoamine oxidase, look for symptoms similar to those found with MAOI overdose; see isocarboxazid

Administration
Adult: PO 5 mg at breakfast and at lunch (10 mg total); after 2-3 days, begin reducing carbidopa/levodopa by 10% to 30%
- Available forms: Tabs 5 mg

Sertraline

ZOLOFT
(seŕ-tra-leen) (Chapter 5)

Functional classification: Antidepressant
Chemical classification: Selective serotonin reuptake inhibitor (SSRI)
FDA pregnancy category: B

Indications: Depression

Contraindications: Hepatic dysfunction, renal impairment, lactation

Pharmacologic Effect: Inhibits CNS neuronal uptake of serotonin

Pharmacokinetics: Peak levels 4.5-8.4 hr; half-life 26-98 hr; sertraline undergoes extensive first-pass metabolism; excreted in urine; protein binding 98%

Side Effects: *CNS* (from premarketing trials): Headache (20%), dizziness (11%), tremor (10%), paresthesia (2%), insomnia (16%), somnolence (13%), agitation (5.6%); *Peripheral* (from premarketing trials): Dry mouth (16%), increased sweating (8%), palpitations (3.5%), rash (2%), diarrhea (17%), constipation (8%), dyspepsia (6%), vomiting (4%), gas (3%), anorexia (3%), abdominal pain (2.4%), sexual dysfunction (15.5%), abnormal vision (4%)

Interactions
- MAOIs: Fatal hypertensive crises (serotonin syndrome) have resulted from combining MAOIs and SSRIs
- Serotonergic drugs: The serotonin syndrome can result from combining SSRIs and serotonin-enhancing agents
- Drugs highly bound to plasma proteins: Displacement of sertraline or one of these drugs could result in adverse responses
- Alcohol: CNS depression
- Diazepam: Decreased clearance of diazepam

Implications
Assess
- B/P, VS
- Hepatic studies because of sertraline's extensive liver metabolism
- Weight loss
- Activation of mania

Planning/Implementation
- Maintain safety
- Closely supervise patients at high risk for suicide because some professionals believe that a relationship exists between suicide and alterations in serotonin levels
- Give with food to minimize first-pass metabolism

Teaching
- Caution about driving (although no impairment in driving ability has been recorded with use of sertraline)
- To avoid alcohol (although no impairment resulting from this combination has been recorded)
- Caution about use of OTC products

Evaluate
- Therapeutic effect: Depression
- Mental status

Lab Test Interference

Increase: AST, ALT; small increase in cholesterol, triglyceride, and serum uric acid levels

Treatment of Overdose: Deaths have occurred when SSRIs, including sertraline, have been combined with other serotonergic drugs. Some evidence indicates that treatment with methysergide, a serotonin antagonist, is effective. For overdose with sertraline alone, establish and maintain airway; administer oxygen prn; charcoal may inhibit absorption and may be more effective than induced vomiting

Administration

Adult: PO 50 mg initially, once daily (morning or evening); increases can be made weekly (because of long half-life); maximum dose, 200 mg/day
- Available forms: Tabs 50, 100 mg

Succinylcholine Chloride

ANECTINE, ANECTINE FLO-PACK, QUELICIN, SCALINE,† SUCOSTRIN†
(suk-sin-ill-koé-leen)
(Chapter 11)

Functional classification: Neuromuscular blocker (depolarizing, ultrashort)
FDA pregnancy category: C

Indications: Facilitates endotracheal intubation during ECT; reduces intensity of convulsions during ECT; other indications for use with general anesthesia are given in *PDR*

Contraindications: Hypersensitivity, malignant hyperthermia, **decreased plasma pseudocholinesterase,** elevated CPK

Cautious use: Cardiac disease, severe burns, fractures, lactation, children <2 yr, electrolyte imbalances, dehydration, neuromuscular disease, respiratory disease, collagen diseases, glaucoma, eye surgery, penetrating eye wounds, elderly or debilitated patients

Pharmacologic Effect: Inhibits transmission of nerve impulses by binding with cholinergic receptors at motor endplate; muscle depolarizes and can be seen as fasciculations head to foot; recovery follows a reverse process

Pharmacokinetics: IV onset 30-60 sec, peak 2-3 min, duration 4-6 min; IM onset 1-3 min; hydrolyzed by pseudocholinesterase to active and inactive metabolites

Side Effects: *Peripheral:* Bradycardia, tachycardia, increased and decreased B/P, sinus arrest, arrhythmias, **prolonged apnea,** bronchospasm, cyanosis, **respiratory depression,** increased secretions, increased intraocular pressure, weakness, muscle pain, **fasciculations,** prolonged relaxation, myoglobulinemia, rash, flushing, pruritus, urticaria, malignant hyperthermia

†Available in Canada only.

Interactions

- Phenelzine, promazine, oxytocin, beta blockers, procainamide, anticholinesterases; quinidine, local anesthetics, polymyxin antibiotics, lithium, thiazides, enflurane, isoflurane: Increased neuromuscular blockade
- Theophylline: Arrhythmias
- Diazepam: Reduction of neuromuscular block
- Narcotic analgesics: Bradycardia
- Do not mix with barbiturates in solution or syringe

Implications

Assess

- For electrolyte imbalances (K, Mg); may lead to increased action of this drug
- VS until fully recovered from ECT; rate, depth, pattern of respirations, strength of hand grip

Planning/Implementation

- Anticholinesterase to reverse neuromuscular blockade
- If communication is difficult during recovery from neuromuscular blockade, offer reassurance

Evaluate

- Therapeutic response: Paralysis
- Recovery
- Prolonged apnea, allergic reactions, i.e., rash, fever, respiratory distress, pruritus: Drug should be discontinued

Treatment of Overdose: Use peripheral nerve stimulator to determine whether in phase I or phase II block; if phase II, give anticholinesterase, monitor VS; may require mechanical ventilation

Administration

Adult: IV 25-75 mg (average dose 0.6 mg/kg), then 2.5 mg/min prn; IM 2.5 mg/kg, not to exceed 150 mg; *child:* IV 1-2 mg/kg, IM 3-4 mg/kg, not to exceed 150 mg IM

- Available forms include: Inj IM IV 20, 50, 100 mg/mL; powder for inj 100, 500 mg/vial, 1 g/vial

Temazepam

RESTORIL

(te-maź-e-pam) (Chapter 8)

Functional classifications: Sedative, hypnotic

Chemical classification: Benzodiazepine

Controlled substance schedule IV

FDA pregnancy category: X

Indications: Insomnia

Contraindications: Hypersensitivity to benzodiazepines, lactation

Cautious use: Sleep apnea, hepatic or renal disease, suicidal individuals, drug abuse, elderly patients, depression, child <18 yr

Pharmacologic Effect: Produces CNS depression

Pharmacokinetics: PO onset 2-3 hr, duration 6-8 hr, half-life 9.5-12.4 hr; metabolized by liver, excreted by kidneys, crosses placenta, excreted in breast milk

Side Effects: *CNS:* Euphoria, drowsiness, daytime sedation, dizziness, confusion, light-headedness, headache, depression, irritability; *Peripheral:* Nausea, vomiting, diarrhea, heartburn, abdominal pain, constipation, chest pain, palpitations

Interactions

- Cimetidine, disulfiram: Prolong half-life of benzodiazepines
- Alcohol, CNS depressants: CNS depression
- Antacids: Decrease effects of benzodiazepines
- Digoxin: Digoxin intoxication

Implications

Assess

- VS

Planning/Implementation

- For sleeplessness, ½-1 hr before bedtime
- If GI symptoms occur, may be taken with food
- Assistance with ambulation
- Side rails, night light, call bell within easy reach
- Checking to see that medication has been swallowed

Teaching

- To avoid driving or other activities requiring alertness until drug regimen is stabilized
- To avoid ingestion of alcohol or CNS depressants
- That it may take two nights for benefits to be noticed
- That hangover is common in elderly persons but less common than with barbiturates

Evaluate

- Therapeutic response: Ability to sleep at night, decreased amount of early-morning awakening when taking drug for insomnia
- Mental status
- Type of sleep problem, falling asleep, staying asleep

Lab Test Interferences

- Increase: ALT/AST, serum bilirubin level
- Decrease: RAIU
- False increase: Urinary 17-OHCS

Treatment of Overdose: Lavage, monitor electrolytes, VS, supportive care

Administration

Adult: PO 10-60 mg hs; *geriatric, debilitated:* 10-20 mg until individual response is determined

- Available forms include: Caps 15, 30 mg

Thioridazine HCl

MELLARIL, NOVORIDAZINE,† THIORIDAZINE

(thye-or-rid́-a-zeen) (Chapters 4, 17)

Functional classifications: Antipsychotic, neuroleptic

Chemical classifications: Phenothiazine, piperidine

FDA pregnancy category: C

Indications: Psychotic disorders, behavioral problems in children, anxiety, major depressive disorders

Contraindications: Hypersensitivity, blood dyscrasias, coma, child <2 yr, brain damage, bone marrow depression, parkinsonism

†Available in Canada only.

Cautious use: Lactation, seizure disorders, hypertension, hepatic disease, cardiac disease

Pharmacologic Effects: Antipsychotic drugs produce a neuroleptic effect characterized by sedation, emotional quieting, psychomotor slowing, and affective indifference; exact mode of action is not fully understood; antipsychotics primarily block dopamine D_2 receptors in the basal ganglia, hypothalamus, limbic system, brain stem, and medulla; antipsychotics are also thought to depress certain components of the reticular activating system that partially control body temperature, wakefulness, vasomotor tone, emesis, and hormonal balance; additionally, antipsychotics have significant anticholinergic and alpha-adrenergic blocking effects; least antiemetic of all phenothiazines

Pharmacokinetics: PO onset erratic, peak 2-4 hr; metabolized by liver, excreted in urine, crosses placenta, enters breast milk, half-life 26-36 hr

Side Effects: *CNS:* Parkinsonism, akathisias, dystonias, tardive dyskinesia, oculogyric crisis; *Peripheral:* Blurred vision (cycloplegia or paralysis of accommodation); ocular pain, photophobia, mydriasis, impaired vision; intolerance of extreme heat or cold, possible heat stroke or fatal hyperthermia; nasal congestion, wheezing, dyspnea; **hypotension, especially orthostatic,** leading to dizziness, syncope; **tachycardia,** irregular pulse, arrhythmias; **dry mouth, constipation,** jaundice, abdominal pain; urinary retention, urinary hesitancy, galactorrhea, gynecomastia, impaired ejaculation, amenorrhea

Interactions

- Alcohol and other CNS depressants (barbiturates, antihistamines, antianxiety or antidepressant drugs): Increased CNS depression, increased risk of EPSEs
- Amphetamines: Possible decreased antipsychotic effect
- Antacids (magnesium and aluminum products): Possible decreased antipsychotic effect
- Anticholinergics (atropine, H_1-type antihistamines, antidepressants, etc): Increased risk of excessive atropine-like side effects or toxic effects

- Benztropine: Possible decreased antipsychotic effect, increased risk of severity of peripheral anticholinergic side effects
- Diazoxide: Possible severe hyperglycemia, prediabetic coma
- Guanethidine: Poor control of hypertension by guanethidine
- Hypoglycemia drugs (insulin, oral hypoglycemia agents): Poor diabetic control
- Lithium: Poor control of psychosis with combined therapy; can mask lithium intoxication; neurotoxic effects with confusion, delirium, seizures, encephalopathy
- Meperidine, morphine: Increased risk of severe CNS depression, respiratory depression, hypotension
- Propranolol: Increased pharmacologic effects of either drug

Implications

Assess

- Establish baseline VS, laboratory values, to assess side effects, allergic or hypersensitivity reactions
- Physiologic and psychologic status before therapy, to determine needs and evaluate progress
- For early stages of tardive dyskinesia by use of Abnormal Involuntary Movement Scale
- Identify concurrent symptoms that may be aggravated by antipsychotics, e.g., glaucoma, diabetes

Planning/Implementation

- Ensure that drug has been taken; check mouth for "cheeking"
- If giving liquid antipsychotics, use at least 60 mL of distilled water or fruit juice to mask taste; dilute and give immediately; take drug with food to minimize GI upset
- Keep patient quiet after injection, to prevent falls associated with postural hypotension
- For dry mouth, give chewing gum, hard candies, lip balm; monitor urinary output; check for bladder distention in inactive patients, older men, and patients on high doses
- Assist with ambulation, if patient is having blurred vision; dim room lights for photosensitivity
- Ensure safety with hypotension; sit on side of bed before rising, head-low position for dizziness, avoid hot showers, wear elastic stockings
- Check B/P (supine, sitting, standing) and pulse before and after each dose when possible; observe for side effects
- Monitor body temperature for indications of neuroleptic malignant syndrome, e.g., muscle rigidity, fever, depressed neurologic status; ensure adequate hydration, nutrition, and ventilation
- Protect patient from exposure to extreme heat or cold
- Recognize impending hypersensitivity: pruritis or jaundice with hepatitis; flu or coldlike symptoms, evidence of bleeding with blood dyscrasia
- Observe for involuntary movements

Teaching

- About benefits and potential harm of antipsychotic drugs; weigh need to know against causing apprehension
- To comply with drug treatment
- To avoid activities requiring clear vision for a few weeks after treatment starts; to report eye pain immediately
- About the importance of exercise, fluids, and fiber in diet
- To watch for symptoms of heart failure, e.g., weight gain, dyspnea, distended neck veins, tachycardia
- Possible male sexual performance failure; suggest relaxed, stress-free environment
- To avoid conception; women should practice effective contraception; phenothiazines may cause false-positive result in pregnancy tests
- To avoid exposure to sunlight; keep skin covered but with temperature-appropriate clothing
- That patient cannot become addicted to antipsychotic drugs

Evaluate

- Whether patient follows prescribed regimen, takes medications as ordered
- Avoids injury; reports dizziness or need for assistance
- Verbalizes reduced anxiety
- Experiences minimal or no adverse responses
- Uses appropriate interventions to minimize side effects
- Achieves improved mental status

Lab Test Interferences

- Increase: Liver function tests, cardiac enzyme levels, cholesterol, blood

glucose, prolactin, bilirubin, PBI, cholinesterase, I-131 levels
- Decrease: Hormones (blood, urine)
- False positive: Pregnancy tests, PKU
- False negative: Urinary steroids

Treatment of Overdose: Lavage, provide an airway; do not induce vomiting; control EPSEs and hypotension

Administration
- Psychosis: *Adult:* PO 50-100 mg tid, *maximum dose* 800 mg/day; dosage is gradually increased to desired response, then reduced to minimum maintenance dose
- Depression, behavioral problems: *Adult:* PO 25 tid, range from 10 mg bid-qid to 50 mg tid-bid; *child 2-12 yr:* PO 0.5-3 mg/kg/day in divided doses
- Mix concentrate in distilled water or orange or grapefruit juice
- Available forms include: Tabs 10, 15, 25, 50, 100, 150, 200 mg; conc 30, 100 mg/mL; susp 25, 100 mg/5 mL

Thiothixene

NAVANE
(thye-oh-thix́-een) (Chapters 4, 15, 16)

Functional classifications: Antipsychotic, neuroleptic
Chemical classification: Thioxanthene
FDA pregnancy category: C

Indications: Psychotic disorders

Contraindications: Hypersensitivity, blood dyscrasias, child <12 yr, bone marrow depression
Cautious use: Lactation, seizure disorders, hypertension, hepatic disease

Pharmacologic Effects: Antipsychotic drugs produce a neuroleptic effect characterized by sedation, emotional quieting, psychomotor slowing, and affective indifference; exact mode of action is not fully understood; antipsychotics primarily block dopamine D_2 receptors in the basal ganglia, hypothalamus, limbic system, brain stem, and medulla; antipsychotics are also thought to depress certain components of the reticular activating system that partially control body temperature, wakefulness, vasomotor tone, emesis, and hormonal balance; additionally, antipsychotics have significant anticholinergic and alpha-adrenergic blocking effects

Pharmacokinetics: PO onset slow, peak 2-8 hr, duration up to 12 hr; IM onset 15-30 min, peak 1-6 hr, duration up to 12 hr; metabolized by liver, excreted in urine, crosses placenta, enters breast milk, half-life 34 hr

Side Effects: *CNS:* Parkinsonism, akathisias, dystonias, tardive dyskinesia, oculogyric crisis; *Peripheral:* Blurred vision (cycloplegia or paralysis of accommodation), ocular pain, photophobia, mydriasis, impaired vision; intolerance of extreme heat or cold, possible heat stroke or fatal hyperthermia; nasal congestion, wheezing, dyspnea; **hypotension, especially orthostatic,** leading to dizziness, syncope; **tachycardia,** irregular pulse, arrhythmias; **dry mouth, constipation,** jaundice, abdominal pain; urinary retention, urinary hesitancy, galactorrhea, gynecomastia, impaired ejaculation, amenorrhea

Interactions
- Alcohol and other CNS depressants (barbiturates, antihistamines, antianxiety or antidepressant drugs): Increased CNS depression, increased risk of EPSEs
- Amphetamines: Possible decreased antipsychotic effect
- Antacids (magnesium and aluminum products): Possible decreased antipsychotic effect
- Anticholinergics (atropine, H_1-type antihistamines, antidepressants, etc): Increased risk of excessive atropine-like side effects or toxic effects
- Benztropine: Possible decreased antipsychotic effect, increased risk of severity of peripheral anticholinergic side effects
- Diazoxide: Possible severe hyperglycemia, prediabetic coma
- Guanethidine: Poor control of hypertension by guanethidine
- Hypoglycemia drugs (insulin, oral hypoglycemia agents): Poor diabetic control
- Lithium: Poor control of psychosis with combined therapy; can mask lithium intoxication; neurotoxic effects with

confusion, delirium, seizures, encephalopathy
- Meperidine, morphine: Increased risk of severe CNS depression, respiratory depression, hypotension
- Propranolol: Increased pharmacologic effects of either drug

Implications

Assess

- Establish baseline VS, laboratory values, to assess side effects, allergic or hypersensitivity reactions
- Physiologic and psychologic status before therapy, to determine needs and evaluate progress
- For early stages of tardive dyskinesia by use of the Abnormal Involuntary Movement Scale
- Identify concurrent symptoms that may be aggravated by antipsychotics, e.g., glaucoma, diabetes

Planning/Implementation

- Ensure that drug has been taken; check mouth for "cheeking"
- If giving liquid antipsychotics, use at least 60 mL of compatible beverage to mask taste; dilute and give immediately; take drug with food to minimize GI upset; give IM injections in lateral thigh
- Keep patient quiet after injection, to prevent falls associated with postural hypotension
- For dry mouth, give chewing gum, hard candies, lip balm; monitor urinary output; check for bladder distention in inactive patients, older men, and patients on high doses
- Assist with ambulation, if patient is having blurred vision; dim room lights for photosensitivity
- Ensure safety with hypotension; sit on side of bed before rising, head-low position for dizziness, avoid hot showers, wear elastic stockings
- Check B/P (supine, sitting, standing) and pulse before and after each dose when possible; observe for side effects
- Monitor body temperature for indications of neuroleptic malignant syndrome, e.g., muscle rigidity, fever, depressed neurologic status; ensure adequate hydration, nutrition, and ventilation
- Protect patient from exposure to extreme heat or cold
- Recognize impending hypersensitivity: pruritus or jaundice with hepatitis; flu or coldlike symptoms, evidence of bleeding with blood dyscrasia
- Observe for involuntary movements

Teaching

- About benefits and potential harm of antipsychotic drugs; weigh need to know against causing apprehension
- To comply with drug treatment
- To avoid activities requiring clear vision for a few weeks after treatment starts; to report eye pain immediately
- About the importance of exercise, fluids, and fiber in diet
- To watch for symptoms of heart failure, e.g., weight gain, dyspnea, distended neck veins, tachycardia
- Possible male sexual performance failure; suggest relaxed, stress-free environment
- To avoid conception; women should practice effective contraception
- To avoid exposure to sunlight; keep skin covered but with temperature-appropriate clothing
- That patient cannot become addicted to antipsychotic drugs

Evaluate

- Whether patient follows prescribed regimen; takes medications as ordered
- Avoids injury; reports dizziness or need for assistance
- Verbalizes reduced anxiety
- Experiences minimal or no adverse responses
- Uses appropriate interventions to minimize side effects
- Achieves improved mental status

Lab Test Interferences

- Increase: Liver function tests, cardiac enzyme levels, cholesterol, blood glucose, prolactin, bilirubin, PBI, cholinesterase, I-131 levels
- Decrease: Uric acid

Treatment of Overdose: Lavage, if orally ingested; provide an airway; do not induce vomiting

Administration

Adult: PO 2-5 mg bid-qid, depending on severity of condition; dose is gradually increased to 20-30 mg, if needed; IM 4 mg bid-qid, maximum dose is 30 mg qd; administer PO dose as soon as possible

T

- Mix concentrate in orange or grapefruit juice
- Available forms include: Caps 1, 2, 5, 10, 20 mg; conc 5 mg/mL; inj IM 2 mg/mL; powder for inj 5 mg/mL

Tranylcypromine Sulfate

PARNATE
(tran-ill-siṕ-roe-meen)
(Chapter 5)

Functional classifications: Antidepressant, MAOI
Chemical classification: Nonhydrazine
FDA pregnancy category: C

Indications: Depression refractory to drug therapy

Contraindications: Hypersensitivity to MAOIs, elderly patients (>60 yr), children <16 yr, hypertension, CHF, severe hepatic disease, pheochromocytoma, severe renal disease, severe cardiac disease
Cautious use: Suicidal patients, convulsive disorders, schizophrenia, hyperactivity, diabetes mellitus, hypomania, agitation, hyperthyroidism

Pharmacologic Effect: Inhibits monoamine oxidase, thus increasing the concentration of endogenous epinephrine, norepinephrine, serotonin, dopamine in storage sites in CNS

Pharmacokinetics: Metabolized by liver, excreted by kidneys, excreted in breast milk, half-life not established

Side Effects: *CNS:* **Dizziness,** drowsiness, confusion, **headache,** anxiety, **tremors,** stimulation, weakness, **hyperreflexia,** mania, **insomnia, fatigue,** weight gain; *Peripheral:* Change in libido, **constipation, dry mouth,** nausea and vomiting, **anorexia,** diarrhea, rash, flushing, increased perspiration, jaundice, **orthostatic hypotension, hypertension, arrhythmias,** hypertensive crisis, blurred vision

Interactions
- Drug-drug: *Sympathomimetics (indirect or mixed acting):* Severe headache, hypertension, hyperpyrexia, and hypertensive crisis; sympathomimetic drugs include amphetamines, levodopa, tryptophan, methylphenidate, OTC compounds containing phenylpropanolamine, ephedrine, and pseudoephedrine; TCAs, other MAOIs, guanethidine, methyldopa, guanadrel, and reserpine; *Anticholinergic drugs:* Additive effect; *Antihypertensive drugs (diuretics, beta blockers, hydralazine, nitroglycerin, prazosin):* Hypotension
- Drug-food: *Tyramine-rich foods* (see text): Hypertensive crisis

Implications
Assess
- B/P (lying, standing), pulse; if systolic B/P drops 20 mm Hg, withhold drug, notify physician
- Blood studies: CBC, leukocyte count, cardiac enzyme levels (if patient is receiving long-term therapy)
- Hepatic studies: Hepatotoxicity may occur

Planning/Implementation
- Increased fluids, bulk in diet, if constipation or urinary retention occurs
- With food or milk for GI symptoms
- Gum, hard candies, or frequent sips of water for dry mouth
- Phentolamine for severe hypertension
- Storage in tight container in cool environment
- Assistance with ambulation during beginning of therapy because drowsiness or dizziness occurs
- Safety measures, including side rails
- Checking to see that PO medication is swallowed

Teaching
- That therapeutic effects may take 2 days to 3 weeks
- To avoid driving or performing other activities that require alertness
- To avoid alcohol ingestion, CNS depressants, or OTC medications for cold, weight, hay fever, cough
- Not to discontinue medication suddenly after long-term use
- To avoid high-tyramine foods, e.g., cheese (aged), caviar, dried fish, game meat, beer, wine, pickled products, liver, raisins, bananas, figs, avocados, meat tenderizers, chocolate, yogurt, increased caffeine, soy sauce
- Report headache, palpitations, neck stiffness

Evaluate
- Toxic effects: Increased headache, palpitations; discontinue drug immediately
- Mental status
- Urinary retention, constipation
- Withdrawal symptoms: Headache, nausea, vomiting, muscle pain, weakness

Treatment of Overdose: Lavage, activated charcoal, monitor electrolytes, VS, treat hypotension

Administration
Adult: 30 mg/day in divided doses; if no improvement after 2 weeks, increase by 10 mg/day in increments of 1-3 wk, maximum dose 60 mg/day
- Available forms include: Tabs 10 mg

Trazodone HCl
DESYREL
(traý-zoe-done) (Chapter 5)

Functional classification: Tricyclic-like antidepressant
Chemical classification: Triazolopyridine
FDA pregnancy category: C

Indications: Depression
Unlabeled uses: Cocaine withdrawal, aggressive behavior, panic disorder

Contraindications: Hypersensitivity to trazodone, child <18 yr
Cautious use: Suicidal patients, hypotension, priapism, narrow-angle glaucoma, urinary retention, cardiac disease, hepatic disease, hyperthyroidism, ECT, elective surgery

Pharmacologic Effects: Selectively inhibits serotonin uptake in brain; therapeutic plasma levels 800-1600 ng/mL

Pharmacokinetics: Metabolized by liver, excreted by kidneys and feces; peak 1 hr without food; half-life 4-9 hr (biphasic)

Side Effects: *CNS:* Anger, ataxia, confusion, delirium; *Peripheral:* **Blurred vision,** photophobia, increased intraocular pressure, decreased tearing, orthostatic hypotension, arrhythmias, tachycardia, palpitations, dry mouth, constipation, diarrhea, decreased sweating, **priapism**

Interactions
- CNS depressants: Additive depressant effect
- MAOIs: Hypertensive crisis, atropine-like poisoning
- Phenytoin: May increase phenytoin level

Implications
Assess
- Establish baseline data, to aid recognition of adverse responses to medication, e.g., liver enzyme levels, VS, renal function, mental status, speech patterns, affect, weight
- For signs of noncompliance, e.g., poor therapeutic response
- Observe for major symptoms of depression, e.g., apathy, sadness, sleep disturbances, hopelessness, guilt, decreased libido, spontaneous crying
- Review history for contraindicated conditions, e.g., glaucoma, CV disease, GI conditions, urologic conditions, seizures, pregnancy

Planning/Implementation
- Monitor for "cheeking" or hoarding; check drug dosage carefully, because a small overdose may cause toxic effects
- Monitor for suicidal ideations; suicidal thought content may increase as antidepressants begin to "energize" patient
- Monitor VS; if hypotension, tachycardia, or arrhythmias occur, withhold drug
- Observe for early signs of toxic effects, e.g., drowsiness, tachycardia, mydriasis, hypotension, agitation, vomiting, confusion, fever, restlessness, sweating
- If CNS overstimulation occurs, e.g., hypomania, delirium, discontinue drug

Teaching
- That this drug has a lag time of up to 2-4 wk
- To adhere to drug regimen
- To avoid alcohol and other depressants
- To avoid drugs listed in section on interactions
- About ways to deal with minor side effects, as follows: dry mouth, with hard candies, sips of water, mouth rinses; visual disturbances, with artificial tears, sunglasses, assistance with ambulation; constipation, with bulk-forming foods, increased fluids; urinary hesitancy, with adequate fluids, privacy; decreased perspiration, with appropriate clothing,

avoidance of unnecessary exercise; orthostatic hypotension, with slow positional changes, avoidance of hot baths and showers; for drowsiness, take single dose hs with physician approval, avoid driving
- To notify physician and discontinue use of the drug if prolonged, painful erection occurs
- To take with food

Evaluate
- Desired therapeutic serum level
- Verbalize decrease in subjective symptoms
- Observe decrease in objective symptoms
- Minimal to no adverse drug effects
- Stable VS
- Less anxiety; sleep, talk, and feel better

Lab Test Interferences
- Increases: Serum bilirubin, blood glucose, alkaline phosphatase levels
- Decreases: VMA, 5-HIAA

Treatment of Overdose: Deaths have occurred as a result of use of trazodone and another drug (i.e., alcohol); there is no antidote; supportive care of hypotension and excessive sedation, gastric lavage

Administration

Adult: PO 150 mg/day in divided doses, may be increased by 50 mg/day q 3-4 days, not to exceed 600 mg/day
- Available forms include: Tabs 50, 100, 150, 300 mg

Triazolam

HALCION

(trye-aý-zoe lam) (Chapter 8)

Functional classifications: Sedative, hypnotic

Chemical classification: Benzodiazepine

Controlled substance schedule IV

FDA pregnancy category: X

Indications: Insomnia

Contraindications: Pregnancy, hypersensitivity to benzodiazepines, lactation

Cautious use: Depression, hepatic or renal disease, elderly patients, drug abuse, narrow-angle glaucoma, child <18 yr

Pharmacologic Effect: Produces CNS depression

Pharmacokinetics: PO onset 1-2 hr, peak 0.5-2 hr, duration 6-8 hr, metabolized by liver, excreted by kidneys, crosses placenta, excreted in breast milk, half-life 1.5-5.5 hr

Side Effects: *CNS:* Anterograde amnesia, drowsiness, daytime sedation, dizziness, confusion, light-headedness, headache, irritability; *Peripheral:* Nausea, vomiting, diarrhea, heartburn, abdominal pain, constipation, chest pain, palpitations

Interactions
- Cimetidine, disulfiram: Prolong half-life of benzodiazepines
- Alcohol, CNS depressants: CNS depression
- Antacids: Decrease effects of benzodiazepines
- Digoxin: Digoxin intoxication
- Antifungals (ketoconazole, itraconazole): Triazolam can reach dangerous concentrations when mixed with these drugs

Implications

Assess
- VS

Planning/Implementation
- For sleeplessness, ½-1 hr before bedtime
- If GI symptoms occur, may be taken with food
- Assistance with ambulation
- Side rails, night light, call bell within easy reach
- Checking to see that medication has been swallowed

Teaching
- To avoid driving or other activities requiring alertness until drug is stabilized
- To avoid ingestion of alcohol or CNS depressants; serious CNS depression may result
- That it may take two nights to be able to sleep
- Triazolam should not be taken if a full night's rest cannot be obtained
- That hangover is common in elderly patients but less common than with barbiturates

Evaluate
- Therapeutic response: Ability to sleep at night, decreased amount of early-morning awakening, if taking drug for insomnia

- Mental status: Mood, sensorium, affect, memory (long-term, short-term)
- Blood dyscrasias: Fever, sore throat, bruising, rash, jaundice, epistaxis (rare)
- Type of sleep problem: Falling asleep, staying asleep

Lab Test Interferences
Increase: ALT, AST, serum bilirubin level
- Decrease: RAIU
- False increase: Urinary 17-OHCS

Treatment of Overdose: Lavage, monitor electrolytes, VS, supportive care

Administration
Adult: PO 0.125-0.5 mg hs; *elderly patient:* PO 0.125-0.25 mg hs
- Available forms: Tabs 0.125, 0.25 mg

Trifluoperazine HCl

NOVOFLURAZINE,† SOLAZINE,† STELAZINE, TERFLUZINE,† TRIFLURIN†
(trye-floo-oh-peŕ-a-zeen)
(Chapters 4, 9, 17)

Functional classifications: Antipsychotic, neuroleptic
Chemical classifications: Phenothiazine, piperazine
FDA pregnancy category: C

Indications: Psychosis, anxiety

Contraindications: Hypersensitivity, coma, child <6 yr

Pharmacologic Effects: Antipsychotic drugs produce a neuroleptic effect characterized by sedation, emotional quieting, psychomotor slowing, and affective indifference; exact mode of action is not fully understood; antipsychotics primarily block dopamine D_2 receptors in the basal ganglia, hypothalamus, limbic system, brain stem, and medulla; antipsychotics are also thought to depress certain components of the reticular activating system that partially control body temperature, wakefulness, vasomotor tone, emesis, and hormonal balance; additionally, antipsychotics have significant anticholinergic and alpha-adrenergic blocking effects

†Available in Canada only.

Pharmacokinetics: PO onset erratic, peak 2-4 hr, duration 4-6 hr; IM onset 15-30 min, peak 15-20 min, duration 4-6 hr; metabolized by liver, excreted in urine and feces, crosses placenta, enters breast milk

Side Effects: *CNS:* Parkinsonism, akathisias, dystonias, tardive dyskinesia, oculogyric crisis; *Peripheral:* Blurred vision (cycloplegia or paralysis of accommodation), ocular pain, photophobia, mydriasis, impaired vision; intolerance of extreme heat or cold, possible heat stroke or fatal hyperthermia; nasal congestion, wheezing, dyspnea; **hypotension, especially orthostatic,** leading to dizziness, syncope; **tachycardia,** irregular pulse, arrhythmias; **dry mouth, constipation,** jaundice, abdominal pain; urinary retention, urinary hesitancy, galactorrhea, gynecomastia, impaired ejaculation, amenorrhea

Interactions
- Alcohol and other CNS depressants (barbiturates, antihistamines, antianxiety or antidepressant drugs): Increased CNS depression, increased risk of EPSEs
- Amphetamines: Possible decreased antipsychotic effect
- Antacids (magnesium and aluminum products): Possible decreased antipsychotic effect
- Anticholinergics (atropine, H_1-type antihistamines, antidepressants, etc): Increased risk of excessive atropine-like side effects or toxic effects
- Benztropine: Possible decreased antipsychotic effect, increased risk of severity of peripheral anticholinergic side effects
- Diazoxide: Possible severe hyperglycemia, prediabetic coma
- Guanethidine: Poor control of hypertension by guanethidine
- Hypoglycemia drugs (insulin, oral hypoglycemia agents): Poor diabetic control
- Lithium: Poor control of psychosis with combined therapy; can mask lithium intoxication; neurotoxic effects with confusion, delirium, seizures, encephalopathy
- Meperidine, morphine: Increased risk of severe CNS depression, respiratory depression, hypotension

- Propranolol: Increased pharmacologic effects of either drug

Implications

Assess

- Establish baseline VS, laboratory values, to assess side effects, allergic or hypersensitivity reactions
- Physiologic and psychologic status before therapy, to determine needs and evaluate progress
- For early stages of tardive dyskinesia by use of Abnormal Involuntary Movement Scale
- Identify concurrent symptoms that may be aggravated by antipsychotics, e.g., glaucoma, diabetes

Planning/Implementation

- Ensure that drug has been taken; check mouth for "cheeking"
- If giving liquid antipsychotics, use at least 60 mL of compatible beverage to mask taste; dilute and give immediately; take drug with food to minimize GI upset; give IM injections in lateral thigh
- Keep patient quiet after injection, to prevent falls associated with postural hypotension
- For dry mouth, give chewing gum, hard candies, lip balm; monitor urinary output; check for bladder distention in inactive patients, older men, and patients on high doses
- Assist with ambulation, if patient is having blurred vision; dim room lights for photosensitivity
- Ensure safety with hypotension; sit on side of bed before rising, head-low position for dizziness, avoid hot showers, wear elastic stockings
- Check B/P (supine, sitting, standing) and pulse before and after each dose when possible; observe for side effects
- Monitor body temperature for indications of neuroleptic malignant syndrome, e.g., muscle rigidity, fever, depressed neurologic status; ensure adequate hydration, nutrition, and ventilation
- Protect patient from exposure to extreme heat or cold
- Recognize impending hypersensitivity to pruritus or jaundice with hepatitis; flu or coldlike symptoms, evidence of bleeding with blood dyscrasia
- Observe for involuntary movements

Teaching

- About benefits and potential harm of antipsychotic drugs; weigh need to know against causing apprehension
- To comply with drug treatment
- To avoid activities requiring clear vision for a few weeks after treatment starts; to report eye pain immediately
- About the importance of exercise, fluids, and fiber in diet
- To watch for symptoms of heart failure, e.g., weight gain, dyspnea, distended neck veins, tachycardia
- Possible male sexual performance failure; suggest relaxed, stress-free environment
- To avoid conception; women should practice effective contraception; phenothiazines may cause false positive results in pregnancy tests
- To avoid exposure to sunlight; keep skin covered but with temperature-appropriate clothing
- That patient cannot become addicted to antipsychotic drugs

Evaluate

- Whether patient follows prescribed regimen, takes medications as ordered
- Avoids injury; reports dizziness or need for assistance
- Verbalizes reduced anxiety
- Experiences minimal or no adverse responses
- Uses appropriate interventions to minimize side effects
- Achieves improved mental status

Lab Test Interferences

- Increase: Liver function tests, cardiac enzyme levels, cholesterol, blood glucose, prolactin, bilirubin, PBI, cholinesterase levels
- Decrease: Hormones (blood and urine)
- False positive: Pregnancy tests, PKU
- False negative: Urinary steroids, 17-OHCS

Treatment of Overdose: Lavage, if orally ingested; provide an airway; do not induce vomiting, control EPSEs and hypotension

Administration

- Psychosis: *Adult:* PO 2-5 mg bid, usual range 15-20 mg/day, may require 40 mg/day or more; IM 1-2 mg q4-6h; *child* >6 *yr:* PO 1 mg qd or bid, maximum up to 15 mg/day; IM not recom-

mended for children, but 1 mg may be given qd or bid
- Anxiety: *Adult:* PO 1-2 mg bid, not to exceed 6 mg/day; do not give for longer than 12 wk
- Available forms: Tabs 1, 2, 5, 10 mg; conc 10 mg/mL; inj IM 2 mg/mL

Triflupromazine*

VESPRIN
(trye-floo-proé-ma-zeen)
(Chapter 7)

Functional classification: Antipsychotic
Chemical classification: Aliphatic phenothiazine
FDA pregnancy category: C

Indications: Infrequently used for psychosis, schizophrenia

Contraindications: Hypersensitivity, children <2½ yr

Pharmacologic Effects: See chlorpromazine

Pharmacokinetics: PO peak levels 2-4 hr, duration 4-6 hr, IM onset 15-30 min, peak levels 15-20 min, duration 4-6 hr; metabolized by liver, excreted in urine and feces, crosses placenta, enters breast milk

Side Effects: *CNS:* EPSEs, drowsiness, seizures; *Peripheral:* Respiratory depression, laryngospasm, blood dyscrasias, dry mouth, GI disturbances, blurred vision, nausea and vomiting, orthostatic hypotension, tachycardia, hypertension

Interactions: See chlorpromazine

Lab Test Interference: See chlorpromazine

Treatment of Overdose: See chlorpromazine

Administration
- Psychosis: *Adult:* IM: 60 mg, up to 150 mg/day; *child >2½ yr:* IM 0.2-0.25 mg/kg, up to a maximum dose of 10 mg/day
- Available forms: Inj 10, 20 mg/mL

*Infrequently used.

Trihexyphenidyl

ARTANE
(tyre-hex-ee-feń-i-dill)

Functional classification: Anticholinergic, antiparkinson
Chemical classification: Tertiary amine
FDA pregnancy category: C

Indications: Parkinsonism, EPSEs

Contraindications: Hypersensitivity, narrow-angle glaucoma, duodenal obstruction, peptic ulcer, prostatic hypertrophy, myasthenia gravis, megacolon

Pharmacologic Effects: Blocks cholinergic receptors, may inhibit the reuptake and storage of dopamine

Pharmacokinetics: Peak 1-1.3 hr, half-life 5.6-10.2 hr; little pharmacokinetic information is known

Side Effects: *CNS:* Depression develops in 19% to 30% of patients; disorientation, confusion, memory loss, hallucinations, psychoses, agitation, delusions, nervousness; *Peripheral:* **Tachycardia,** palpitations, hypotension, **orthostatic hypotension, dry mouth,** nausea, vomiting, constipation, paralytic ileus, **blurred vision,** mydriasis, diplopia, urinary retention and hesitancy, elevated temperature

Interactions
- Amantadine: Increased anticholinergic effect
- Digoxin: Increased digoxin serum levels
- Haloperidol: Worsening of schizophrenia, decreased haloperidol serum levels
- Levodopa: Possible reduction of levodopa efficacy
- Phenothiazines: Increased anticholinergic effect, decreased antipsychotic effect

Implications
Assess
- VS, B/P
- For glaucoma
- Mental status

Planning/Implementation
- Provide instructions for anticholinergic responses, i.e., dry mouth, constipa-

tion, urinary hesitancy, decreased sweating

Teaching

- Give with meals
- May cause drowsiness, blurred vision, dizziness: Emphasize safety
- Avoid alcohol and other CNS depressants
- For rapid or pounding heartbeat, notify physician
- Use caution in hot weather

Evaluate

- EPSE improvement
- For adverse effects
- Mental status: Confusion, delirium memory

Treatment of Overdose: Emesis, lavage, activated charcoal, treat respiratory depression, hyperpyrexia

Administration

- Parkinsonism: *Adult:* PO initially, 1-2 mg first day, increase by 2-mg increments at 3- to 5-day intervals, up to a daily dose of 5-15 mg in 3 divided doses at mealtime
- EPSEs: To start, 1 mg with 1 mg every few hours until symptoms controlled; maintenance or prophylactic use, 5-15 mg/day

Trimethadione*

TRIDIONE

(trye-meth-a-dyé-one)

Functional classification: Antiepileptic
Chemical classification: Oxazolidinedione
FDA pregnancy category: D

Indications: Refractory absence seizures

Contraindications: Hypersensitivity, blood dyscrasias
Cautious use: Hepatic or renal disease

Pharmacologic Effects: Increases seizure threshold in cortex, basal ganglia; therapeutic serum level is 700 μg/mL

Pharmacokinetics: PO peak 30 min-2 hr; excreted in kidneys; half-life of 12-24 hr, with a half-life of 6-13 days for the active metabolite dimethadione

*Infrequently used.

Side Effects: *CNS:* **Drowsiness,** dizziness, fatigue, paresthesia, irritability, headache; *Peripheral:* Vaginal bleeding, albuminuria, nephrosis, abdominal pain, weight loss, nausea, vomiting, bleeding gums, abnormal liver function test, **exfoliative dermatitis,** rash, alopecia, petechiae, erythema, photophobia, diplopia, epistaxis, retinal hemorrhage, hypertension, hypotension, thrombocytopenia, agranulocytosis, leukopenia, neutropenia, hemolytic anemia

Interactions: None known

Implications

Assess

- Blood studies: Hematocrit, hemoglobin level, RBCs, serum folate and vitamin D values, if on long-term therapy regimen
- Hepatic studies: ALT, AST, bilirubin and creatinine levels
- Skin: If rash occurs, withhold drug

Planning/Implementation

- Dilute oral solution with water
- Oral with juice or milk to cover taste and smell, to decrease GI symptoms

Teaching

- To take with food, if GI upset occurs
- To carry MedicAlert identification bracelet
- To notify physician, if visual disturbances, sore throat, etc, occur
- To avoid driving and other activities that require alertness
- Not to discontinue medication abruptly after long-term use, because convulsions may result

Evaluate

- Mental status
- Renal and hematologic problems

Treatment of Overdose: Symptoms include nausea, drowsiness, dizziness, ataxia, visual disturbances; coma in cases of massive overdose; emesis, lavage, supportive care

Administration

Adult: PO 300 mg tid (900 mg/day), may increase by 300 mg/wk, not to exceed 600 mg qid (2400 mg/day); *child:* 300 to 900 mg/day in 3 or 4 equally divided doses

- Available forms include: Caps 300 mg, chew tabs 150 mg; oral sol 40 mg/mL

Trimipramine Maleate

SURMONTIL
(tri-miṕ-ra-meen) (Chapter 5)

Functional classification: TCA
Chemical classification: Tertiary amine
FDA pregnancy category: C

Indications: Depression

Contraindications: Hypersensitivity to TCAs, recovery phase of myocardial infarction, convulsive disorders, prostatic hypertrophy, children

Cautious use: Suicidal patients, severe depression, increased intraocular pressure, narrow-angle glaucoma, urinary retention, cardiac disease, hepatic disease, hyperthyroidism, ECT, elective surgery, MAOI therapy

Pharmacologic Effect: Inhibits serotonin and norepinephrine uptake; therapeutic plasma level 180 ng/mL

Pharmacokinetics: Metabolized by liver, excreted by kidneys, steady state 2-6 days; half-life 7-30 hr

Side Effects: *CNS:* **Sedation,** ataxia, confusion, delirium; *Peripheral:* **Blurred vision,** photophobia, increased intraocular pressure; decreased tearing, orthostatic hypotension, arrhythmias, tachycardia, palpitations, dry mouth, constipation, diarrhea, decreased sweating, **urinary retention, hesitancy**

Interactions

- Anticholinergic agents: Additive anticholinergic effects with atropine, antihistamines (H_1 blocker), antiparkinson drugs, antipsychotics, OTC cold and allergy drugs
- CNS depressants: Additive depressant effect
- Guanethidine, clonidine: Decreased antihypertensive effect
- MAOIs: Hypertensive crisis, atropine-like poisoning
- Oral contraceptives: Inhibit effects of TCAs
- Phenothiazines: May increase TCA serum level
- Quinidine: Additive effect, heart block possible
- Sympathomimetics: Potentiates sympathomimetic effects
- Thyroid preparations: Tachycardia, arrhythmias; may increase TCA effect

Implications

Assess

- Establish baseline data, to aid recognition of adverse responses to medication, e.g., liver enzyme levels, VS, renal function, mental status, speech patterns, affect, weight
- For signs of noncompliance, e.g., poor therapeutic response
- Observe for major symptoms of depression: apathy, sadness, sleep disturbances, hopelessness, guilt, decreased libido, spontaneous crying
- Review history for contraindicated conditions, e.g., glaucoma, CV disease, GI conditions, urologic conditions, seizures, pregnancy

Planning/Implementation

- Monitor for "cheeking" or hoarding; check drug dosage carefully, because a small overdose may cause toxic effects
- Monitor for suicidal ideations; suicidal thought content may increase as antidepressants begin to "energize" patient
- Monitor VS; if hypotension, tachycardia, or arrhythmias occur, withhold TCAs
- Give most TCAs in a single dose hs
- Observe for early signs of toxic effects, e.g., drowsiness, tachycardia, mydriasis, hypotension, agitation, vomiting, confusion, fever, restlessness, sweating
- If CNS overstimulation occurs, e.g., hypomania, delirium, discontinue drug

Teaching

- That these drugs have a lag time of up to 1 month
- To adhere to drug regimen
- To avoid OTC drugs, particularly those containing sympathomimetics or anticholinergics
- To avoid drugs listed in section on interactions
- About ways to deal with minor side effects, as follows: dry mouth, with hard candies, sips of water, mouth rinses; visual disturbances, with artificial tears, sunglasses, assistance with ambulation; constipation, with bulk-forming foods, increased fluids; urinary hesitancy, with adequate fluids, privacy; decreased perspiration, with appropriate clothing,

avoidance of unnecessary exercise; orthostatic hypotension, with slow positional changes, avoidance of hot baths and showers; for drowsiness, take single dose hs with physician approval, avoid driving
- That abrupt discontinuance may result in cholinergic rebound, e.g., nausea, vomiting, insomnia

Evaluate
- Desired therapeutic serum level
- Verbalize decrease in subjective symptoms
- Observe decrease in objective symptoms
- Minimal to no adverse drug effects
- Stable VS
- Less anxiety; sleep, talk, and feel better

Lab Test Interferences
- Increase: Serum bilirubin, blood glucose, alkaline phosphatase levels
- False increase: Urinary catecholamines
- Decrease: VMA, 5-HIAA

Treatment of Overdose: ECG monitoring, induce emesis, lavage, activated charcoal, administer anticonvulsant; treat anticholinergic effects, if needed

Administration

Adult: PO 75 mg/day in divided doses, may be increased to 300 mg/day; *adolescent and geriatric:* 50 mg/day to start, gradually increase to 100 mg/day
- Available forms: Caps 25, 50, 100 mg

Valproic Acid and Derivatives

DEPAKENE/DEPAKOTE
(val-proé-ic) (Chapter 7)

Functional classification: Anticonvulsant
Chemical classification: Carboxylic acid derivative
FDA pregnancy category: D

Indications: Drug of choice for tonic-clonic and absence seizures; psychomotor seizures

Contraindications: Hypersensitivity to valproic acid; hepatic disease or significant hepatic dysfunction; teratogenic birth defects have been reported with valproic acid

Cautious use: Children with metabolic disorders, lactation, children <2 yr

Pharmacologic Effects: Mechanism not known but may be related to increased brain levels of GABA; therapeutic serum levels are 50-100 μg/mL

Pharmacokinetics: PO rapidly absorbed, peak levels 1-4 hr, time to steady state 2-4 days, half-life 6-16 hr

Side Effects: Serious side effects are *not* common; *CNS:* Sedation but usually dissipates; *Peripheral:* **Nausea, vomiting, indigestion,** other GI symptoms; emotional upset; minor elevation in SGOT and LDH; severe hepatotoxicity may occur and has been linked to some fatalities; blood dyscrasias, **rash**

Interactions
- Alcohol and other CNS depressants: CNS depression
- Anticonvulsants: May increase serum levels of phenobarbital; clonazepam toxicity may be increased; phenytoin causes two opposite interactions: Increase in serum phenytoin and decrease in serum phenytoin levels
- Aspirin and warfarin: Prolonged bleeding time
- Chlorpromazine and aspirin: Increased valproic acid half-life
- Carbamazepine and phenytoin: Decreased valproic acid serum levels

Implications

Assess
- Blood studies, hepatic studies

Planning/Implementation
- Serious side effects are uncommon
- Do not dilute elixir with carbonated beverage

Teaching
- Take with food for GI upset
- Swallow tabs and caps whole, to avoid irritation
- Take hs to avoid drowsiness during day
- Notify that valproic acid alters blood and urine volume in diabetes
- Wear MedicAlert identification bracelet

Evaluate
- Efficacy of treatment

Treatment of Overdose: *Symptoms:* Coma and death have occurred; however, more typical symptoms of overdose include motor restlessness, visual hallucinations; supportive care, paying close attention to adequate urinary output. Because the fraction of the drug not bound to serum proteins is high in overdose, hemodialysis may be helpful. Naloxone has been reported to reverse the CNS depression associated with valproic acid overdose

Administration

- Seizure control: *Adult and child:* PO 15 mg/kg/day; increase at weekly intervals by 5-10 mg/kg/day until seizures are controlled or as side effects dictate; maximum dose 60 mg/kg/day; if total dose exceeds 250 mg/day, give in divided doses
- Bipolar disorder—manic phase: *Adult:* PO: Start with 750 mg/day in divided doses; increase daily dose by 250 mg every 2 to 3 days to achieve lowest therapeutic dose that produces the desired clinical effect or the desired serum concentrations. Maximum recommended dose 60 mg/kg/day; *children and adolescents:* Use of valproic acid in patients <18 yr has not been established
- Available forms: *Valproic acid:* Caps 250 mg; syr 250 mg/5 mL; *Valproate sodium-valproic acid:* Tabs 125, 250, 500 mg

Venlafaxine

EFFEXOR
(ven-lah-fackś-in)

Functional classification: Antidepressant
Chemical classification: Phenethylamine
FDA pregnancy category: C

Indications: Depression

Contraindications: Hypersensitivity to venlafaxine, pregnancy, lactation, use of MAOIs

Pharmacologic Effects: Inhibits norepinephrine and serotonin uptake

Pharmacokinetics: Venlafaxine is well absorbed (92%) and extensively metabolized. It undergoes significant first-pass metabolism but has a shorter half-life and lower protein binding than most antidepressants. Venlafaxine is metabolized to an active metabolite, O-desmethylvenlafaxine, that has similar biochemical properties. Venlafaxine's half-life is 5 hr; the active metabolite is 11 hr. Protein binding 27%; steady state achieved in 3-4 days; excreted in urine

Side effects: *CNS:* Headache (25%), somnolence (23%), dizziness (19%), insomnia (18%), nervousness (13%); *Peripheral:* Nausea (37%), dry mouth (22%), constipation (15%), asthenia (12%), sweating (12%), abnormal ejaculation/orgasm (12%), anorexia (11%), weight loss, hypertension (5%) at high doses (>200mg/day)

Interactions

- MAOIs: Risk of a serotonin syndrome, which can be fatal
- Cimetidine: Inhibits first-pass metabolism of venlafaxine
- Drugs that inhibit cytochrome P-450, IID6: Potential for interaction.

Implications

Assess

- Use of MAOIs
- B/P, VS, weight
- Baseline physical data
- Hepatic studies because of venlafaxine's extensive liver metabolism
- Activation of mania

Planning/Implementation

- Maintain safety
- Administer with food to decrease GI upset
- If discontinuing venlafaxine, do so gradually
- If switching to MAOI, wait 7 days after stopping venlafaxine; if switching from MAOI to venlafaxine, wait at least 14 days before starting venlafaxine

Teaching

- Take with food to avoid GI upset
- Inform about side effects that can occur and appropriate interventions to minimize them
- Avoid alcohol while on venlafaxine
- Report rash, hives, swelling, sore throat, etc, indicative of allergic reaction
- Report pregnancy, intent to become pregnant, or lactation
- Report use of OTCs
- Avoidance of operating hazardous machinery

Evaluate

- Depression
- Mental status
- Minimal side effects
- Weight loss

Lab Test Interference: Serum cholesterol increases (by 3 mg/dL)

Treatment of Overdose: Few overdoses have been reported, no fatalities have been reported, and symptoms, if any, are ill-defined. Treatment of overdose includes maintenance of an airway, oxygenation, monitoring of VS, and supportive care. Consider use of charcoal, emetic, or lavage. Dialysis or forced diuresis seems to hold little promise of benefit for the patient. No specific antidotes are known

Administration: *Adult:* PO: Starting dose is 75 mg/day in 2 or 3 divided doses taken with food. Dose may be increased to 150-225 mg/day in increments of 75 mg/day every 4 or more days. Severely depressed patients may respond to a higher dose up to 375-450 mg/day in 3 divided doses; *hepatic impairment:* Reduce adult dose by 50%; *geriatric:* No dose adjustment is required; *children and adolescents:* Not approved for use in children <18 yr

- Available forms; Tabs 25, 37.5, 50, 75, 100 mg

Zolpidem

AMBIEN
(zoĺ-pih-dem)

Functional classification: Sedative, hypnotic (nonbarbiturate)
Chemical classification: Imidazopyridine
Controlled substance schedule IV
FDA pregnancy category: B

Indications: Short-term treatment of insomnia

Contraindications: Hypersensitivity to zolpidem

Cautious use: Acute intermittent porphyria, impaired hepatic or renal function; susceptibility to respiratory problems; depression; history of drug dependence

Pharmacologic Effects: Modulation of GABA receptor chloride channels may be responsible for several therapeutic effects, including sedation

Pharmacokinetics: Onset 0.5-1 hr; rapid absorption from GI tract; half-life 2.6 hr; protein binding 92%; half-life and bioavailability increased in elderly and patients with hepatic function impairment; zolpidem is converted to inactive metabolites and excreted in urine

Side Effects: *CNS:* Headache (19%); drowsiness (8%); dizziness (5%); *Peripheral:* Myalgia (7%); nausea (6%); dyspepsia (5%)

Interactions

- Food: Peak concentrations are decreased, and time to concentration is prolonged

Implications

Assess

- Baseline physical data
- B/P, VS
- History of hypersensitivity
- History of hepatic or renal disorders

Planning/Implementation

- Carefully observe patients known to be suicidal
- Taper drug slowly if discontinuance is warranted
- Assistance with ambulation
- Side rails, night lite, call bell within reach

Teaching

- Avoid alcohol and other CNS depressants
- May cause drowsiness; use caution in operating hazardous machinery

Evaluate

- Therapeutic response: Ability to sleep at night, decreased amount of early-morning awakening
- Mental status
- Type of sleep problem: Falling asleep or staying asleep

Lab Test Interferences: None reported

Treatment of Overdose: With zolpidem alone, symptoms range from somnolence to light coma; recovery has been reported when 400 mg have been taken, which is 40 times the recommended dose; when mixed with CNS depressant agents, fatalities have occurred; supportive care is required, with immediate lavage; monitor hypotension and CNS depression; withhold sedating drugs, even if CNS excitement occurs; flumazenil may be useful; dialysis will probably not be very useful

Administration

Adult: PO: Usual dose is 5-10 mg immediately before bedtime. Maximum dose is 10 mg; *elderly or debilitated patients:* PO: Initially 5 mg immediately before bedtime; *children and adolescents:* Not approved for children <18 yr

- Available forms: Tabs 5, 10 mg

Z

APPENDIX

Controlled Substance Chart

Drugs	United States	Canada
Heroin, LSD, peyote, marijuana, mescaline	Schedule I	Schedule H
Opiates such as morphine and meperidine, amphetamines, cocaine, short-acting barbiturates (amobarbital, secobarbital), hydromorphone	Schedule II	Schedule G
Glutethimide, paregoric, cerebral stimulants used to treat obesity (benzphetamine, phendimetrazine)	Schedule III	Schedule F
Chloral hydrate, benzodiazepines, cerebral stimulants used to treat obesity (mazindol, fenfluramine), meprobamate, mephobarbital, pemoline, phenobarbital	Schedule IV	Schedule F
Antidiarrheals with opium, antitussives	Schedule V	

FDA Pregnancy Categories

A No risk demonstrated to the fetus in any trimester

B No adverse effects in animals, no human studies available, or if adverse effects in animals, none demonstrated in human studies

C Only given after risks to the fetus are considered; animal studies have shown adverse reactions, no human studies available, or no animal studies and inadequate human studies

D Definite fetal risks, may be given in some situations because of mother's condition

X Absolute fetal abnormalities; risk outweighs potential benefit

Abbreviations

ac	Before meals	**mL**	Milliliter
ADHD	Attention deficit hyperactivity disorder	**μg**	Microgram
		mo	Month
ALT	Alanine aminotransferase, serum	**Na**	Sodium
		ng	Nanogram
AST	Aspartate aminotransferase, serum	**NMS**	Neuroleptic malignant syndrome
bid	Twice a day	**NPO**	Nothing by mouth
B/P	Blood pressure	**OTC**	Over-the-counter
BUN	Blood urea nitrogen	**PBI**	Protein-bound iodine
cap	Capsules	**PDR**	*Physicians' Desk Reference*
CBC	Complete blood cell count	**PKU**	Phenylketonuia
		PO	By mouth
CHF	Congestive heart failure	**PTSD**	Posttraumatic stress disorder
CNS	Central nervous system		
conc	Concentrate	**prn**	As needed
CPK	Creatinine phosphokinase	**q**	Every
CV	Cardiovascular	**qd**	Every day
ECG	Electrocardiogram	**qh**	Every hour
EEG	Electroencephalogram	**qid**	Four times a day
ECT	Electroconvulsive therapy	**qod**	Every other day
elix	Elixir	**q2h**	Every 2 hours, and so forth
EPSEs	Extrapyramidal side effects		
		RAIU	Radioactive iodine uptake
ext rel	Extended release	**RBC**	Red blood cell count
5HT	5-hydroxytryptamine (serotonin receptor)	**REC**	Rectal
		r/t	Related to
g	Gram	**SC**	Subcutaneous
GABA	Gamma-aminobutyric acid	**17-OHCS**	17-hydroxycorticosteroids
		SGOT	Serum glutamic-oxaloacetic transaminase
gr	Grain		
GI	Gastrointestinal	**SMA-12**	Sequential multiple-analysis-12
GU	Genitourinary		
5-HIAA	5-Hydroxyindoleacetic acid	**SRI**	Serotonin reuptake inhibitor
hr	Hour	**SSRI**	Selective serotonin reuptake inhibitor
hs	At bedtime		
I-131	Thyroid uptake	**supp**	Suppository
IM	Intramuscular	**susp**	Suspension
inj	Injection	**Syr**	Syrup
I&O	Intake and Output	**tabs**	Tablets
IV	Intravenous	**TCA**	Tricyclic antidepressant
kg	kilogram	**tid**	Three times a day
L	Liter	**time-rel**	Timed-release
LDH	Lactic dehydrogenase	**UA**	Urinalysis
MAOIs	Monoamine oxidase inhibitors	**VMA**	Vanillylmandelic acid
		VS	Vital signs
mEq	Milliequivalent	**WBC**	White blood cell count
mg	Milligram		

Food and Drug Administration (FDA) Drug Approval Process

FACTS ABOUT THE DRUG APPROVAL PROCESS

- Time from experimental drug development to druggist's shelf: 15 years
- For each 5000 experimental compounds entered into preclinical testing, only 5 are tested on humans (clinical trials), and of those only 1 is eventually approved for human use (FDA approved)
- Average cost of taking drug from laboratory to druggist's shelf: $359 million

STAGES IN THE APPROVAL PROCESS (LENGTH OF TIME IN YEARS)

1. **Preclinical** (6.5 years): evaluating for safety and biologic activity on nonhuman subjects
2. **Clinical trials**
   A. **Phase I** (1 year): 20 to 80 healthy human volunteers used to determine safety
   B. **Phase II** (2 years): 100 to 300 patient volunteers used to evaluate effectiveness and side effects
   C. **Phase III** (3 years): 1000 to 3000 patient volunteers used to verify effectiveness and monitor long-term adverse reactions
3. **FDA Review/Approval Process:** (2.5 years)
4. **Phase IV:** Postapproval evaluation

Modified from Beary JF: The drug development and approval process, *New Medicine in Development for Mental Illnesses* Pharmaceutical Research and Manufacturers of America, 4:7, 1996.

General Index

A

C

E

F

G

I

J

K

L

N

GENERAL INDEX

O

GENERAL INDEX

Q

R

S

U

V

W

Y

Z

GENERAL INDEX

Disorders Index

A

N

O

P

Drug Index

A

C

E

F

M

Q

R

S

T

344RUS
02/19/98 39255
INFORMATION CONSERVATION, INC.